Fundamentals of Biomedical Science

Haematology

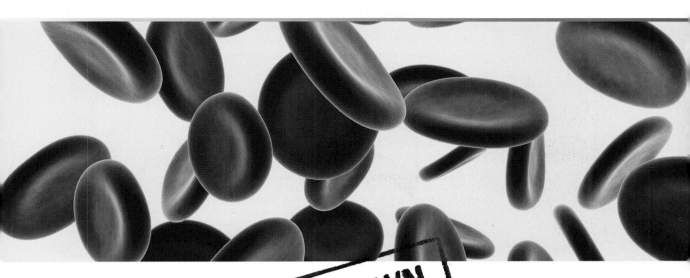

Dr. Gary W. Moore
BSc DBMS CSci FIBMS CBiol MSB CertMHS
Consultant Biomedical Scientist
Centre for Haemostasis and Thrombosis
St Thomas' Hospital, London

Gavin Knight
BSc. (Hons.) MSc. CSci. FIBMS FHEA
Senior Lecturer in Haematology
School of Pharmacy and Biomedical Science
University of Portsmouth

Dr. Andrew D. Blann
PhD FRCPath FIBMS CSci.
Consultant Clinical Scientist and Senior Lecturer in Medicine
University of Birmingham Centre for Cardiovascular Sciences
Department of Medicine, City Hospital, Birmingham

OXFORD
UNIVERSITY PRESS

OXFORD

UNIVERSITY PRESS

Great Clarendon Street, Oxford OX2 6DP

Oxford University Press is a department of the University of Oxford.
It furthers the University's objective of excellence in research, scholarship,
and education by publishing worldwide in

Oxford New York

Auckland Cape Town Dar es Salaam Hong Kong Karachi
Kuala Lumpur Madrid Melbourne Mexico City Nairobi
New Delhi Shanghai Taipei Toronto

With offices in

Argentina Austria Brazil Chile Czech Republic France Greece
Guatemala Hungary Italy Japan Poland Portugal Singapore
South Korea Switzerland Thailand Turkey Ukraine Vietnam

Oxford is a registered trade mark of Oxford University Press
in the UK and in certain other countries

Published in the United States
by Oxford University Press Inc., New York

British Library Cataloguing in Publication Data

Data available

Library of Congress Cataloging in Publication Data

Data available

Typeset by MPS Limited, A Macmillan Company
Printed in Italy
on acid-free paper by
LEGO SpA – Lavis TN

ISBN 978-0-19-956883-3

3 5 7 9 10 8 6 4 2

Contents

An introduction to the Fundamentals of Biomedical Science series

Biomedical Scientists form the foundation of modern healthcare, from cancer screening to diagnosing HIV, from blood transfusion for surgery to food poisoning and infection control. Without Biomedical Scientists, the diagnosis of disease, the evaluation of the effectiveness of treatment, and research into the causes and cures of disease would not be possible.

However, the path to becoming a Biomedical Scientist is a challenging one: trainees must not only assimilate knowledge from a range of disciplines, but must understand—and demonstrate—how to apply this knowledge in a practical, hands-on environment.

The *Fundamentals of Biomedical Science* series is written to reflect the challenges of biomedical science education and training today. It blends essential basic science with insights into laboratory practice to show how an understanding of the biology of disease is coupled to the analytical approaches that lead to diagnosis.

The series provides coverage of the full range of disciplines to which a Biomedical Scientist may be exposed – from microbiology to cytopathology to transfusion science. Alongside volumes exploring specific biomedical themes and related laboratory diagnosis, an overarching Biomedical Science Practice volume provides a grounding in the general professional and experimental skills with which every Biomedical Scientist should be equipped.

Produced in collaboration with the Institute of Biomedical Science, the series

- Understands the complex roles of Biomedical Scientists in the modern practice of medicine.

- Understands the development needs of employers and the Profession.

- Places the theoretical aspects of biomedical science in their practical context.

Learning from this series

The *Fundamentals of Biomedical Science* series draws on a range of learning features to help readers master both biomedical science theory, and biomedical science practice.

Case studies illustrate how the biomedical science theory and practice presented throughout the series relates to situations and experiences that are likely to be encountered routinely in the biomedical science laboratory. Answers to questions posed in some Case Studies are available in the book's Online Resource Centre.

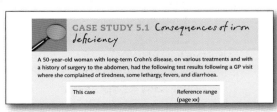

CASE STUDY 5.1 Consequences of iron deficiency

A 50-year-old woman with long-term Crohn's disease, on various treatments and with a history of surgery to the abdomen, had the following test results following a GP visit where she complained of tiredness, some lethargy, fevers, and diarrhoea.

	This case	Reference range (page xx)

BOX 6.1 Warm and cold

Most of our body operates at 37 °C, and many antibodies bind to their target optimally at this temperature. However, at a different (lower) temperature, binding may not occur. By contrast, some antibodies may not bind at normal body temperature, but may readily react at a cooler temperature such as 30 °C, at room temperature (18–25 °C), or in the cold (4 °C). This is important clinically because the skin is clearly cooler than the liver, so antibodies may react in the peripheral tissues and circulation but not elsewhere. It

Additional information to augment the main text appears in **boxes**

 METHOD Staining for iron

The key stain for iron is Perls' stain, developed by the German pathologist, Max Perls. Samples of bone marrow or peripheral blood spread out on glass slides are air-dried and then fixed with methanol for 10–20 min. When dry, they are exposed to acidified potassium ferrocyanide for a further 10 min, washed with tap water and then distilled water, and then exposed for around 10–15 s to a second stain such as aqueous neutral red or eosin as a counter-

A modification of the technique can be u thology laboratory to stain body tissues ferritin nor apoferritin take up Perls' stai undergoes degradation to generate ha can be detected in tissue macrophages cells) and spleen.

When the body is overloaded with iron, i in other tissues, including cardiac tissue. Si

Method boxes walk through the key protocols that the reader is likely to encounter in the laboratory on a regular basis.

can make the detection of parasites difficult. Where uncertainty exists, the entire thin film should be examined with a × 100 objective, which will take in the region of 30 minutes per operator.

Key Points

Cells containing parasites are inevitably heavier than non-parasitized cells so it is worth looking at the tails and edges of a thin film where larger and heavier cells can predominate.

Key points reinforce the key concepts that the reader should master from having read the material presented, while **Summary** points act as an end-of-chapter checklists for readers to verify that they have remembered correctly the principal themes and ideas presented within each chapter.

can be sudden. The acute phase can be accompanied by diarrhoea, joint bleeding gums which are followed by progressive muscle wastage, fever, tosplenomegaly. Some patients have lymphadenopathy. Death is often parasite itself but **opportunistic infections** such as pneumonia, tubercu because of a weakened immune system. In immunocompromised patient human immunodeficiency virus (HIV) infection, visceral leishmaniasis be tunistic infection.

Development of a normochromic, normocytic anaemia is common, with as low as 70 g/L. Splenomegaly can give rise to anaemia, leucopenia, and and liver dysfunction can affect blood coagulation due to the reduced pro tion factors.

opportunistic infection
An infection caused by organisms that do not normally cause disease in the presence of a competent immune system.

Key terms provide on-the-page explanations of terms with which the reader may not be familiar; in addition, each title in the series features a **glossary**, in which the key terms featured in that title are collated.

and may or may not lead to low folate, but almost always leads to hyperhomocysteinaemia. Hereditary folate malabsorption has been described but is extremely rare.

SELF-CHECK 5.9

What are primary causes of vitamin B$_{12}$ deficiency?

Treatment of vitamin and folate deficiency

The cause of the deficiency should always be defined and remedied for its complete resolution. However, in the short term, the standard treatment is replacement therapy. For vitamin

Self-check questions throughout each chapter provide the reader with a ready means of checking that they have understood the material they have just encountered; answers to self-check questions are presented in the book's Online Resource Centre.

l lymphocyte morphology, monocytosis, eosinopenia, or a reactive he recovery phase.

enia is common in malaria infection, resulting from a combination of creased pooling / clearance in the spleen, and reduced platelet lifespan nses. The platelet count can drop to around 100 × 10⁹/L and sometimes evere disease. In addition, blood coagulation can be activated in malaria y with P. falciparum, as a result of the following:

is the cytokine storm produced in response to the infection which can tting mechanisms.

e red cell membrane so that coagulation-promoting phospholipids are

Cross reference
You can find explanations of white cell abnormalities in Chapter 8.

You were introduced to blood coagulation in Chapter 2 and will meet more details about its activation in Chapter 13.

Cross references help the reader to see biomedical science as a unified discipline, making connections between topics presented within each volume, and across all volumes in the series.

Online learning materials

The *Fundamentals of Biomedical Science* series doesn't end with the printed books. Each title in the series is supported by an Online Resource Centre, which features additional materials for students, trainees, and lecturers.

online resource centre

www.oxfordtextbooks.co.uk/orc/fbs

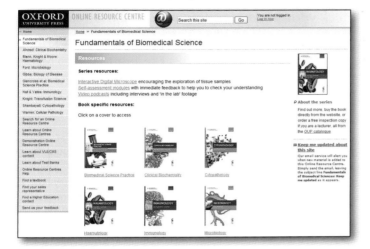

Guides to key experimental skills and methods

Multimedia walk-throughs of key experimental skills—including both animations and video—to help you master the essential skills that are the foundation of Biomedical Science practice.

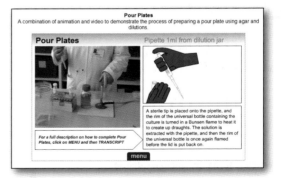

Biomedical science in practice

Interviews with practising Biomedical Scientists working in a range of disciplines, to give you valuable insights into the reality of work in a Biomedical Science laboratory.

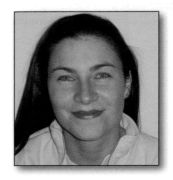

Jane Worthington, Specialist Biomedical Scientist in Microbiology at St Peters Hospital, Chertsey.

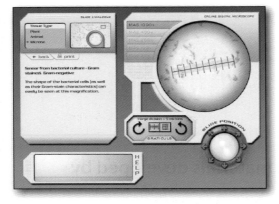

Digital Microscope

A library of microscopic images for you to investigate using this powerful online microscope, to help you gain a deeper appreciation of cell and tissue morphology.

The Digital Microscope is used under licence from the Open University.

'Check your understanding' learning modules

A mix of interactive tasks and questions, which address a variety of topics explored throughout the series. Complete these modules to help you check that you have fully mastered all the key concepts and key ideas that are central to becoming a proficient Biomedical Scientist.

We extend our grateful thanks to colleagues in the School of Health Science at London Metropolitan University for their invaluable help in developing these online learning materials.

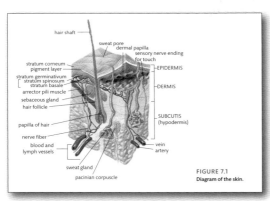

FIGURE 7.1
Diagram of the skin.

Lecturer support materials

The Online Resource Centre for each title in the series also features figures from the book in electronic format, for registered adopters to download for use in lecture presentations, and other educational resources.

To register as an adopter visit **www.oxfordtextbooks.co.uk/orc/moore** and follow the on-screen instructions.

Any comments?

We welcome comments and feedback about any aspect of this series.
Just visit **www.oxfortextbooks.co.uk/orc/feedback/** and share your views.

Contributors

Mr David A. Gurney MSc, CSci, FIBMS
Senior Biomedical Scientist/Platelet Specialist, Centre for Haemostasis & Thrombosis, GSTS Pathology, Guy's & St Thomas' NHS Foundation Trust, London, UK

Ms Alexis Henley MBA, MSc, CSci, FIBMS
Divisional Manager Blood Sciences, Bart's and The London NHS Trust London, UK

Ms Pam Holtom
Senior Biomedical Scientist, Heartlands Hospital, Birmingham, UK

Dr Ian Jennings PhD, CSci, FIBMS
Scientific Programme Manager, UKNEQAS (Blood Coagulation), Sheffield, UK

Dr Sukhjinder Marwah PhD, CSci, FIBMS
Clinical Scientist, Department of Haematology and Blood Transfusion, City Hospital, Birmingham, UK

Dr Jane Needham PhD, CSci, FIBMS
Principal Biomedical Scientist, Haemophilia, Haemostasis & Thrombosis Centre, Basingstoke & North Hampshire NHS Foundation Trust, UK

Online materials developed by

Sheelagh Heugh, Principal Lecturer in Biomedical Science, Faculty of Human Sciences, London Metropolitan University

Dr Ken Hudson, Lecturer in Biomedical Science, Faculty of Human Sciences, London Metropolitan University

William Armour, Lecturer in Biomedical Science, Faculty of Human Sciences, London Metropolitan University

Table 1: Reference Ranges

Red Cells	Reference range
Haemoglobin (Hb)	
Male	13.3–16.7 g/dL, 133–167 g/L
Female	11.8–14.8 g/dL, 118–148 g/L
Red blood cell count (RBCC)	
Male	$4.3–5.7 \times 10^{12}$/L
Female	$3.9–5.0 \times 10^{12}$/L
Haematocrit (Hct)	
Male	0.35–0.53 L/L
Female	0.33–0.47 L/L
Reticulocytes	$25–125 \times 10^{9}$/L
	(0.5–3.5% of total red cell count)
Red cell distribution width (RDW)	
As coefficient of variation	10.3–15.3 %
As standard deviation	34.5–50.5 fL
Red cell indices	
Mean cell volume (MCV)	77–98 fL
Mean cell haemoglobin (MCH)	26–33 pg
Mean cell haemoglobin concentration (MCHC)	33–37 pg/dL, 330–370 pg/L
Erythrocyte sedimentation rate (ESR)	<10 mm/hour
Micronutrients and Plasma Proteins	
Iron	10–37 µmol/L
Total iron binding capacity	
Men	54–72 µmol/L
Women	55–81 µmol/L
Transferrin	2–4 g/L
Transferrin saturation	
Men	18–40%
Women	13–37 %
Ferritin	
Male	25–380 µg/L
Post menopausal female	28–365 µg/L
Pre-menopausal female	7.5–224 µg/L
Vitamin B_{12}	160–925 ng/L
	120–680 pmol/L
Vitamin B_6*	5–30 µg/L
	23–129 nmol/L
	3.0–15.0 µg/L
Folate	4–30 nmol/L
Serum	160–640 µg/L
Red blood cell	360–1460 nmol/L
	0.08–0.28 µmol/L
Methylmalonic acid	1.5–1.72 mPa/s at 25°C
Plasma viscosity	1.16–1.33 mPa/s at 37°C

(Continued)

Table (*Continued*)

White Blood Cells

White cell count (WCC)	$4.0–10.0 \times 10^9/L$
The differential:	Absolute
Neutrophils	$2.0–7.0 \times 10^9/L$
Lymphocytes	$1.0–3.0 \times 10^9/L$
Monocytes	$0.2–1.0 \times 10^9/L$
Eosinophils	$0.02–0.5 \times 10^9/L$
Basophils	$0.02–0.1 \times 10^9/L$
Blasts/atypical cells	$\sim0.01 \times 10^9/L$

Haemostasis

Platelets	$143–400 \times 10^9/L$
Fibrinogen	1.5–4 g/L
Prothrombin time (PT)	11–14 seconds
Partial thromboplastin time (PTT)	24–34 seconds
International normalized ratio (INR)	2–3 or 3–4
D-dimers	<500 units/mL (strongly dependent on method)

* Vitamin B_6 has several isoforms; pyridoxal 5′-phosphate is most commonly reported.

Notes

1. These reference ranges are pooled from recent authoritative textbook and guidelines. The figures vary with time, with location, and according to the method of analysis, and must reflect the nature of the population that the Hospital serves. Accordingly, the Practitioner **MUST** work to their local reference range.

2. The Authors also stress that units for the indices are also subject to change. The unit for haemoglobin is in transition from g/dL to g/L. This means that a result of 13.5 may well become 135.

Abbreviations

A23187	calcium ionophore
Ab	antibody
ABC	activated B-cell-like
ABL	Abelson
α_2AP	alpha 2-antiplasmin
α_2M	alpha 2-macroglobulin
ACA	anticardiolipin antibodies
aCML	atypical chronic myeloid leukaemia
ADAMTS-13	a zinc- and calcium-dependent disintegrin and metalloprotease with thrombospondin type 1 motifs, member 13
ADCC	antibody directed cellular cytotoxicity
ADP	adenosine diphosphate
AF	atrial fibrillation
Ag	antigen
AHG	antihuman globulin
AIDS	acquired immunodeficiency syndrome
AIHA	autoimmune haemolytic anaemia
AITL	angioimmunoblastic T-cell lymphoma
ALA	aminolevulinic acid
ALCL	anaplastic large cell lymphoma
ALK	anaplastic lymphoma kinase
ALK-1	activin receptor-like kinase 1
ALL	acute lymphoblastic leukaemia
AMKL	acute megakaryoblastic leukaemia
AML	acute myeloid leukaemia
AML–MRC	acute myeloid leukaemia with myelodysplasia-related changes
ANAE	alpha-naphthyl acetate esterase
APA	antiphospholipid antibodies
APC	activated protein C
APC	antigen presenting cell
APCR	activated protein C resistance
API2	apoptosis inhibitor 2
APL	acute promyelocytic leukaemia
APS	antiphospholipid syndrome

APTT	activated partial thromboplastin time
ARF	alternate reading frame
ARU	aspirin reaction units
ASLA	activated seven lupus anticoagulant assay
AT	antithrombin
ATL	adult T-cell leukaemia
ATM	ataxia telangiectasia mutated
ATP	adenosine triphosphate
ATPase	adenosine triphosphatase
ATRA	all-*trans* retinoic acid
AVWD	acquired von Willebrand's disease
B-CLL	B-cell chronic lymphocytic leukaemia
BCR	B-cell receptor
β_2GPI	beta 2-glycoprotein I
β_2GPI Ab	beta 2-glycoprotein I antibodies
BCR	breakpoint cluster region
BCSH	British Committee for Standards in Haematology
bFGF	basic fibroblast growth factor
BL	Burkitt lymphoma
BM	bone marrow
BNF	British National Formulary
BNLI	British National Lymphoma Investigation
BPI	bacterial permeability inducing factor
B-PLL	B-cell prolymphocytic leukaemia
BSH	British Society for Haematology
BSS	Bernard–Soulier syndrome
BU	Bethesda unit
C4bBP	C4b-binding protein
CAE	chloroacetate esterase
c-ALL	common-acute lymphoblastic leukaemia
CBF	core binding factor
Cbl	cobalamin
CCR	chemokine receptor
CD	cluster of differentiation

CDA	congenital dyserythropoietic anaemia
CDK	cyclin-dependent kinase
CDR	complementarity determining region
CEBPA	CCAAT enhancer binding protein α gene
CEL	chronic eosinophilic leukaemia
CFU	colony-forming unit
CFU-Baso	CFU for basophils
CFU-E	CFU for erythrocytes
CFU-EMk	CFU for erythrocytes and megakaryocytes
CFU-Eo	CFU for eosinophils
CFU-GEMM	CFU for granulocytes, erythrocytes, monocytes, and megakaryocytes
CFU-GMo	CFU for granulocytes and monocytes
CFU-L	CFU for lymphocytes
CFU-M	CFU for monocytes
CFU-Mk	CFU for megakaryocytes
CFU-N	CFU for neutrophils
CGH	comparative genomic hybridization
CGL	chronic granulocytic leukaemia
C_H	constant domain of an antibody heavy chain
CHL	classical Hodgkin lymphoma
Cip/Kip	CDK inhibitory proteins
CKI	cyclin kinase inhibitor
C_L	constant domain of an antibody light chain
CLL	chronic lymphocytic leukaemia
CLP	common lymphocyte progenitors
CMAF	cellular musculoaponeurotic fibrosarcoma
CML	chronic myeloid leukaemia
CMML	chronic myelomonocytic leukaemia
CMPD	chronic myeloproliferative disease
CMPD-u	chronic myeloproliferative disease—unclassified
CMV	cytomegalovirus
CNL	chronic neutrophilic leukaemia
CNS	central nervous system
CNS DLBCL	central nervous system diffuse large B-cell lymphoma
CoA	coenzyme A
COPD	congestive obstructive pulmonary disease
COSHH	Control of Substances Hazardous to Health
COX	cyclooxygenase
CPA UK	Clinical Pathology Accreditation (UK) Ltd
CPD	continuing professional development

CRAB	hyper**c**al**c**aemia, **r**enal insufficiency, **a**naemia, **b**one lesions
CRP	C-reactive protein
CSF	colony-stimulating factor
CSR	class-switching recombination
CYP	cytochrome P
2,3-DPG	2,3-diphosphoglycerate
Da	dalton
DAB	3,3′-diaminobenzidine
DAF	decay accelerating factor
DAPTT	dilute activated partial thromboplastin time
DARC	Duffy antigen receptor for chemokines
DAT	direct antiglobulin test
DBA	Diamond–Blackfan anaemia
DBL-EBP	Duffy binding-like erythrocyte-binding protein
DDT	dichlorodiphenyltrichloroethane
del	deletion
DIC	disseminated intravascular coagulation
DLBCL	diffuse large B-cell lymphoma
DMT-1	divalent metal transporter-1
DNA	deoxyribonucleic acid
DNMT	DNA methyltransferases
DPT	dilute prothrombin time
DRVVT	dilute Russell's viper venom time
DS	Down syndrome
DS-AMKL	Down syndrome-associated acute megakaryoblastic leukaemia
DSCR	Down syndrome critical region
dsDNA	double-stranded DNA
DSPA	Desmodus salivary plasminogen activator
DTI	direct thrombin inhibitor
DTS	dense tubular system
DVT	deep vein thrombosis
EBER	Epstein–Barr virus-encoded RNA
EBV	Epstein–Barr virus
EBNA	Epstein-Barr virus nuclear antigen
ECP	eosinophil cationic protein
EDN/EPX	eosinophil-derived neurotoxin/eosinophil protein X
EDTA	ethylene diamine tetra-acetic acid

EGIL	European Group for the Immunological Classification of Leukaemias
ELF-EMF	extremely low-frequency electromagnetic field
ELIFA	enzyme-linked immunofiltration assay
ELISA	enzyme linked immunosorbent assay
EPCR	endothelial protein C receptor
Epo	erythropoietin
EpoR	erythropoietin receptor
EQA	external quality assessment
ESR	erythrocyte sedimentation rate
ET	ecarin time
ET	essential thrombocythaemia
ETO	eight-twenty-one
EVI1	ecotropic viral integration site-1
FA	Fanconi anaemia
FAB	French–American–British
FBC	full blood count
Fc	crystallizable fraction (of an immunoglobulin)
FCγR	gamma receptor for the IgG fragment crystallizable region
FDC	follicular dendritic cell
FDP	fibrin(ogen) degradation products
FGF	fibroblast growth factor
FGFR	fibroblast growth factor receptor
FII	factor II or prothrombin
FIIa	activated factor II or thrombin
FISH	Fluorescence *in situ* hybridization
FITC	fluorescein isothiocyanate
FIX	factor IX
FIXa	activated factor IX
fL	femtolitre (10^{-15} litre)
FLIFA	fluorescence-linked immunofiltration assay
FLT3	fms-related tyrosine kinase 3
FPA	fibrinopeptide A
FPB	fibrinopeptide B
FRET	fluorescence resonance energy transfer
FSC	forward scatter
FV	factor V
FVa	activated factor V

FVII	factor VII
FVIIa	activated factor FVII
FVIII	factor VIII
FVIIIa	activated factor VIII
FVL	factor V Leiden
FX	factor X
FXa	activated factor X
FXI	factor XI
FXIa	activated factor XI
FXIII	factor XIII
FXIIIa	activated factor XIII
G0-phase	quiescent phase (of the cell cycle)
G1-phase	Gap 1 phase
G2-phase	Gap 2 phase
G6PD	glucose-6-phosphate dehydrogenase
GCB	germinal centre-like B-cell-like
G-CSF	granulocyte colony-stimulating factor
GLA	gamma-carboxyglutamic acid
Glut	glutamine
GM-CSF	granulocyte macrophage colony-stimulating factor
GMNPT	geometric mean normal prothrombin time
GP	general practitioner
GP	glycoprotein
GPC	glycophorin C
GPI	glycosyl phosphatidylinositol
GPIa	glycoprotein Ia
GPIb	glycoprotein Ib
GPIb– IX-V	glycoprotein Ib– IX– V complex
GPIIbIIIa	glycoprotein IIb–IIIa complex
GPLU	(Ig)G (anti)phospholipid unit
GPVI	glycoprotein VI
GS	glutathione
GSH	reduced glutathione
GT	Glanzmann's thrombasthenia
H	histone
H&E	Haematoxylin and Eosin
Haly-PA	Haly plasminogen activator
HAT	histone acetyltransferase

Hb	haemoglobin
HbF	fetal haemoglobin
HBS	heparin binding site (of antithrombin)
HbS	sickle haemoglobin
HC II	heparin cofactor II
HCL	hairy cell leukaemia
Hct	haematocrit
HDAC	histone deacetylase
HES	hypereosinophilic syndrome
HH	hereditary haemochromatosis
HHT	hereditary haemorrhagic telangiectasia
HHV8	human herpesvirus 8
HIT	heparin-induced thrombocytopenia
HIV	human immunodeficiency virus
HL	Hodgkin lymphoma
HLA	human leucocyte antigen
HMW	high molecular weight
HMWK	high molecular weight kininogen
HPC	Health Professions Council
hpf	high-power field
HPLC	high-performance/pressure liquid chromatography
HRG	histidine-rich glycoprotein
HRP-1	histidine-rich protein 1 (likewise HRP-2, and HRP-3)
HRS	Hodgkin–Reed–Sternberg
HS	hereditary spherocytosis
HTLV-1	human-lymphotrophic virus-1
HUS	haemolytic uraemic syndrome
IAP	inhibitor of apoptosis
IAT	indirect antiglobulin test
IBMS	Institute of Biomedical Science
ICAM	intercellular adhesion molecule
ICSH	International Committee for Standards in Haematology
IEF	isoelectric focusing
IF	intrinsic factor
IFN	interferon
Ig	immunoglobulin
IGH	immunoglobulin heavy chain gene
IGVH	immunoglobulin variable heavy chain gene
IL	interleukin
IM	infectious mononucleosis
IMF	idiopathic myelofibrosis
INK	inhibitors of CDK4
INR	International Normalized Ratio
inv	inversion
IPSID	immunoproliferative small intestine disease
IPSS	International Prognostic Scoring System
IQC	internal quality control
IRMA	immunoradiometric assay
IRP	International reference preparation
IRS	indoor residual spraying
ISCN	International System for Human Cytogenetic Nomenclature
ISI	International Sensitivity Index
ITD	internal tandem duplication
ITN	insecticide-treated net
ITP	idiopathic thrombocytopenic purpura
IU	International unit
JAK	Janus activated kinase
Jak2	Janus kinase 2
JBL	journal-based learning
JMML	juvenile myelomonocytic leukaemia
KAHRP	knob-associated histidine-rich protein
KCT	kaolin clotting time
LA	lupus anticoagulant
LBL	lymphoblastic lymphoma
LDCHL	lymphocyte-depleted classical Hodgkin lymphoma
LDH	lactate dehydrogenase
LDT	lymphocyte doubling time
LGL	large granular lymphocytes
LIA	latex immunoassay
LLIN	long-lasting insecticidal nets
LMAN-1	lectin mannose binding protein 1
LMP	latent membrane protein 1
LMWH	low molecular weight heparin
LPL	lymphoplasmacytic lymphoma
LPS	lipopolysaccharide
LRM	leucine-rich motif
LV-PA	Lachesis venom plasminogen activator
MAb	monoclonal antibody

MAHA	microangiopathic haemolytic anaemia	NADP	nicotinamide adenine dinucleotide phosphate
MALT	mucosa-associated lymphoid tissue	NADPH	nicotinamide adenine dinucleotide phosphate hydrogen
MBD	methyl-binding domain	NEQAS	National External Quality Assessment Scheme
MBP	major basic protein		
MCCHL	mixed cellularity classical Hodgkin lymphoma	NFκB	nuclear factor kappa B
MCFD2	multiple coagulation factor deficiency 2	NHL	non-Hodgkin lymphoma
MCH	mean cell haemoglobin	NHS	National Health Service
MCHC	mean cell haemoglobin concentration	NK	natural killer (cell)
		NPM	nucleophosmin
MCL	mantle cell lymphoma	NSAID	non-steroidal anti-inflammatory drug
MCR	Manchester comparative reagent	NSCHL	nodular sclerosis classical Hodgkin lymphoma
M-CSF	macrophage colony-stimulating factor	NTBI	non-transferrin bound iron
MCV	mean cell volume	NuMA	nuclear matrix associated
MDS	myelodysplastic syndrome	NUP214	nucleoporin 214 kDa
MDS-U	myelodysplastic syndrome unclassified	NuRD	nucleosome remodelling (and histone) deacetylation (complex)
MESA	mature erythrocyte surface antigen		
MF	mycosis fungoides	OAF	osteoclast activating factors
MF	myelofibrosis	OD	optical density
MGUS	monoclonal gammapathy of undetermined significance	OPG	osteoprotegerin
		Pa	pascal
MHC	Major Histocompatibility Complex	PA	pernicious anaemia
MI	myocardial infarction	PAF	platelet activating factor
MIB-1	molecular immunology Bortsel-1	PAI-1	plasminogen activator inhibitor type 1
MIP-1α	macrophage inflammatory protein-1α	PAI-2	plasminogen activator inhibitor type 2
MiRNA	microRNA	PAI-3	plasminogen activator inhibitor type 3
MKL1	megakaryoblastic leukaemia-1	PAR-1	protease-activated receptor-1
MLL	mixed lineage leukaemia	PAS	Periodic acid–Schiff
MM	multiple myeloma	PAU	platelet-aggregation units
MMA	methyl-malonic acid	PB	Paul Bunnell
MMSET	multiple myeloma SET domain	PBX1	pre-B cell leukaemia homeobox 1
M-phase	mitosis phase	PC	protein C
MPLU	(Ig)M (anti)phospholipid unit	PCH	paroxysmal cold haemoglobinuria
MPO	myeloperoxidase	PCI	protein C inhibitor
M-protein	monoclonal protein	PCL	plasma cell leukaemia
MRC	myelodysplasia-related changes	PCR	polymerase chain reaction
mRNA	messenger RNA	pDC	plasmacytic dendritic cells
MTHFR	methylene tetrahydrofolate reductase	PDGFR	platelet-derived growth factor receptor
MZL	marginal zone lymphoma	PE	pulmonary embolism
NAD	nicotinamide adenine dinucleotide	PEG	polyethylene glycol
NADH	nicotinamide dinucleotide hydrogen	PF4	platelet factor 4

PfEMP 1	*Plasmodium falciparum* erythrocyte membrane protein 1		RANKL	receptor activator of nuclear factor κB ligand
PfEMP 2	*P. falciparum* erythrocyte membrane protein 2		*RARA*	retinoic acid receptor alpha gene
PfEMP 3	*P. falciparum* erythrocyte membrane protein 3		RARE	retinoic acid response element
PfLDH	*P. falciparum* lactate dehydrogenase		RARS	refractory anaemia with ringed sideroblasts
pg	picogram (10^{-12} gram)		RASA	ring-infected erythrocyte membrane surface antigen
PGF	platelet growth factor		RBC	red blood cell
Ph[1]	Philadelphia chromosome		RBCC	red blood cell count
PiCT	prothrombinase-induced clotting time		RBM15	RNA binding motif protein 15
PIVKA	Proteins Induced by Vitamin K absence/antagonism		RCC	refractory cytopenia of childhood
PK	prekallikrein		RCM	red cell mass
PK	pyruvate kinase		RCMD	refractory cytopenia with multilineage dysplasia
PKDL	post kala-azar dermal leishmaniasis		RDW	red cell distribution width
pLDH	*Plasmodium* lactate dehydrogenase		RE	restriction enzyme
PLZF	promyelocytic leukaemia zinc finger		REAL	Revised European and American classification of Lymphoid (neoplasms/malignancies)
PMBL	primary mediastinal large B-cell lymphoma		Rh	rhesus
PML	promyelocytic leukaemia gene		RhAG	rhesus-associated glycoprotein
PN-2	protease nexin-2		RIA	radio-immunoassay
PNH	paroxysmal nocturnal haemoglobinuria		RIPA	ristocetin-induced platelet aggregation
PNP	platelet neutralization procedure		RN	refractory neutropenia
POCT	point-of-care test		RNA	ribonucleic acid
PPP	platelet-poor plasma		RPN1	ribophorin 1
pRB	retinoblastoma protein		RS	reactive site
PRCA	pure red cell aplasia		RT	refractory thrombocytopenia
PRP	platelet-rich plasma		RT	reptilase time
PRU	$P2Y_{12}$ reaction units		RUNX	runt-related transcription factor
PS	protein S		s	second
PT	prothrombin time		SAK	staphylokinase
PV	parasitophorous vacuole		SAO	South-east Asian ovalocytosis
PV	polycythaemia vera		SBB	Sudan black B
PVM	parasitophorous vacuole membrane		SCF	stem cell factor
PZ	protein Z		SCOCS	surface connected open canalicular system
QBC	quantitative buffy coat		SCT	silica clotting time
RA	refractory anaemia		SDS-PAGE	sodium dodecyl sulphate polyacrylamide gel electrophoresis
RA	rheumatoid arthritis		Serpin	serine protease inhibitor
RAEB	refractory anaemia with excess blasts		SHM	somatic hypermutation
RAEB-t	refractory anaemia with excess blasts in transformation		SK	streptokinase
RANK	receptor activator of nuclear factor κB		SLE	systemic lupus erythematosus
			SLL	small lymphocytic lymphoma

smIg	surface membrane immunoglobulin
SMMHC	smooth muscle myosin heavy chain
SMZL	splenic marginal zone lymphoma
SOP	standard operating procedure
S-phase	synthesis phase
SSC	side scatter
STAT	signal transducer and activator of transcription
sTfR	soluble transferrin receptor
t	translocation
TAFI	thrombin activatable fibrinolysis inhibitor
TAM	transient abnormal myelopoiesis
t-AML	therapy-related acute myeloid leukaemia
T_c	cytotoxic T-cell
TC	transcobalamin
TCR	T-cell receptor
TEG	thromboelastography
TEL	translocation ETS leukaemia
TF	tissue factor
TFPI	tissue factor pathway inhibitor
TfR	transferrin receptor
TGF	transforming growth factor
TGFβ1	tumour growth factor β1
T_H	helper T cell
T-LGL	T-cell large granular lymphocytic leukaemia
TM	thrombomodulin
TMD	transient myeloproliferative disease
t-MDS	therapy-related myelodysplastic syndrome
t-MDS/ MPN	therapy-related myelodysplastic/ myeloproliferative neoplasm
TNF	tumour necrosis factor
TNFα	tumour necrosis factor-α
TopoII	topoisomerase II
t-PA	tissue plasminogen activator
T-PLL	T-prolymphocytic leukaemia
TPM3	tropomyosin 3
Tpo	thrombopoietin
TRAP	thrombin receptor agonist peptide
TSG	tumour suppressor gene
TSV-PA	*Trimeresurus stejnegeri* viper plasminogen activator

TSVT	Taipan snake venom time
TT	thrombin time
TTP	thrombotic thrombocytopenic purpura
TXA_2	thromboxane A_2
u	unit
U&E	urea and electrolytes
U46619	9,11-dideoxy-9α,11α-methanoepoxy PGF$_{2\alpha}$
UFH	unfractionated heparin
UK NEQAS	United Kingdom National External Quality Assurance Scheme
UKAS	United Kingdom Accreditation Service
u-PA	urinary plasminogen activator (or urokinase)
u-PAR	urinary plasminogen activator receptor
V/Q	ventilation/perfusion
VCA	viral capsid antigen
V_H	variable domain of an antibody heavy chain
VKORC1	vitamin K epoxide reductase complex subunit 1
V_L	variable domain of an antibody light chain
VSG	variant surface glycoproteins
VTE	venous thromboembolism
VW Ag II	von Willebrand antigen II
VWD	von Willebrand's disease
VWF	von Willebrand factor
VWF:Ag	von Willebrand factor: antigen
VWF:CB	von Willebrand factor: collagen binding (activity)
VWF:FVIIIB	von Willebrand factor: factor VIII binding
VWF:RCo	von Willebrand factor: ristocetin co-factor (activity)
WAS	Wiskott–Aldrich syndrome
WASp	Wiskott–Aldrich syndrome protein
WBC	white blood cell
WBCC	white blood cell count
WCC	white cell count
WHO	World Health Organization
WM	Waldenström macroglobulinaemia
ZAP-70	zeta-associated protein 70
ZPI	protein Z-dependent protease inhibitor

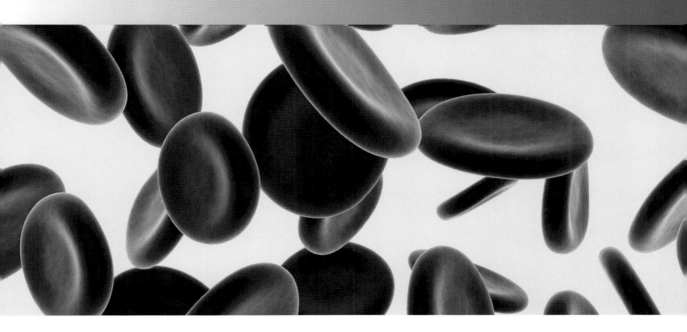

PART 1

Haematology and Haemopoiesis

1

Introduction to haematology

Alexis Henley, Gary W. Moore, and Andrew D. Blann

This chapter introduces haematology, not only as the science of the study of blood itself but also about how the subject relates to other disciplines in pathology. You will also get a feel for haematology in the wider aspects of healthcare, and how you will need to relate to professional bodies.

Learning objectives

After studying this chapter, you should confidently be able to:

- Explain key aspects of the science of haematology.
- Appreciate the role of the biomedical scientist in the haematology laboratory.
- Describe the role of haematology in the provision of healthcare.
- Outline the overlap of haematology and other pathology disciplines.
- Comment on the role of professional and regulatory bodies.

1.1 What is haematology?

Put simply, haematology is the study of blood. The haematology laboratory in a healthcare setting is concerned with the diagnosis and monitoring of diseases of the blood and blood-forming organs. Blood cells are manufactured in **bone marrow** and released into the **peripheral blood** once they are mature. Blood is a dynamic and crucial fluid providing molecular and cellular transport and many regulatory functions. Blood interfaces with all organs and tissues in the body, carrying essential substances such as oxygen and nutrients to the cells, and waste products away from cells to the excretory organs. As such it has a very important role in ensuring adequate whole-body physiology and **homeostasis**. It follows that adverse changes to the blood will have numerous consequences, many of which can be serious and life-threatening.

Conversely, adverse changes to organs and tissues may translate into changes in the make up of the blood that are secondary to the primary disease. It is in this latter capacity that blood can be used in the clinical laboratory for the detection and monitoring of various diseases and their treatments.

bone marrow
Soft tissue located inside hollow bones responsible for the production and maturation of blood cells.

peripheral blood
The blood that is contained within the circulatory system.

homeostasis
The maintenance of stable physiological systems.

Blood is composed of approximately 45% blood cells, which are classified into three main types:

- **Red blood cells** (RBC) that carry oxygen to the tissues.
- **White blood cells** (WBC) that function primarily as defence against infection.
- **Platelets** that prevent blood loss at sites of injury by combining with specialized proteins to form a clot.

The remaining 55% is **plasma**, which is an aqueous solution that acts as the transport medium for blood cells, dissolved nutrients, and plasma proteins, including those involved in **blood coagulation**.

Biomedical scientists working in the haematology laboratory perform an array of diverse blood tests that are concerned with the investigation of the number, structure, and function of the cellular elements of blood and the investigation and control of bleeding and clotting disorders.

Blood tests are performed either on whole blood, plasma or **serum** depending on the investigation required. Blood is collected by **venepuncture** into specially designed bottles. Blood tests that require whole blood or plasma are collected into blood tubes containing **anticoagulants** to prevent the blood clotting before it is analysed; tests on serum are collected into plain tubes.

SELF-CHECK 1.1

Name the three different types of blood cell.

1.2 **A classification of haematology**

Haematology tends to be considered under the three main areas of red blood cells, white blood cells and **haemostasis** which are then further subclassified.

Red blood cells

Haematologists are interested in the number and function of red blood cells, their size, and the amount and quality of the **haemoglobin** that they carry. The most common condition concerning red bloods cell is **anaemia**. The main physiological consequence of anaemia is reduced oxygen-carrying capacity of the blood, which leads to clinical symptoms of lethargy, weakness, dizziness, and feeling faint. If the anaemia worsens, patients can experience shortness of breath, palpitations, headaches, and sore mouth and gums. The different types of anaemia result from a variety of underlying medical disorders.

Common causes of anaemia are:

- Iron deficiency, which results in a defect in production of the haem (iron containing) component of haemoglobin due to the lack of ferrous iron.
- Vitamin B_{12} and/or folate deficiency, which affect the production of DNA.
- Other diseases such as malignancy, renal disease, liver disease, lead poisoning, and infection.
- Hereditary conditions, such as **sickle cell disease** and **thalassaemia** where there is a defect in haemoglobin production.
- Acute and chronic blood loss.

Cross references

Red blood cells and their associated disease states are described in further detail in Chapters 4–6.

White blood cells and associated disease states are described in further detail in Chapters 8–12.

Platelets and their associated disease states are described in further detail in Chapters 13–15.

blood coagulation
The process where specialized proteins interact to form a clot (in conjunction with platelets).

serum
The fluid that remains after the blood has been allowed to clot.

venepuncture
The process of obtaining intravenous access to obtain a sample of blood via a needle.

anticoagulant
A physiological or pharmacological mechanism that retards clotting processes.

haemostasis
The interplay of cellular and molecular processes that generate blood clots at sites of injury, regulate clot formation, and degrade clots.

haemoglobin
Metalloprotein inside red blood cells that is responsible for oxygen transport.

sickle cell disease
An inherited disorder of haemoglobin of varying severity. The name arises from the deformed shape the red blood cells take when the abnormal haemoglobin inside them polymerizes at low oxygen concentrations.

thalassaemia
A spectrum of inherited disorders of haemoglobin where there is an imbalance in globin chain production.

White blood cells

Leucocytes (white blood cells), of which there are five recognizable types, are part of the immune system. They help protect the body against **infections** caused by microbes such as viruses and bacteria. The most common serious disease of white blood cells is **leukaemia**, a type of **neoplasia**.

The haematology laboratory investigates the number of each type of white blood cell in the peripheral blood and whether they are mature or immature cells.

- Raised numbers of normally functioning white cells can be seen in bacterial, viral, and fungal infections where extra cells become available to deal with the microorganisms.
- Raised numbers of immature white cells are commonly found in many leukaemias. These represent the uncontrolled proliferation of malignant **clones** in the bone marrow or lymphoid tissue entering the peripheral blood.
- Low numbers of white blood cells can be caused by some medications and cytotoxic chemotherapy. Reduced numbers of white cells can be seen in diseases such as **aplastic anaemia**. The consequence of depleted numbers of white blood cells is the body's inability to fight infection effectively.

Haemostasis

Haemostasis comprises an integrated group of balanced cellular and molecular processes designed to minimize the loss of blood upon damage to blood vessels, i.e. **haemorrhage**, a condition which can be life-threatening. However, excessive and/or inappropriate activity of the coagulation system, generally resulting in **thrombosis**, can also be dangerous. Unimpaired platelet function and certain coagulation proteins are crucial to effective haemostasis.

Haematologists are also involved in the diagnosis and management of patients whose blood has a predisposition to clot and of those people who have an underlying bleeding disorder, e.g. **haemophilia**.

The haemostasis laboratory plays a key role in monitoring patients who are receiving medication for thrombosis. Anticoagulant medication inhibits the ability of the blood to clot, but too much can cause the patient to haemorrhage, therefore regular monitoring is required.

In addition to the categories of diseases discussed above haematologists are also involved in the diagnosis of some parasitic blood infections, such as **malaria**.

SELF-CHECK 1.2

What are the three main areas of haematology?

Cross references

Anaemia—this major spectrum of diseases of red blood cells is described in Chapters 5 and 6.

Leukaemia and related disorders are described in further detail in Chapters 8–12.

infection

The presence of sufficiently high numbers of a microorganism that invoke clinical symptoms and provoke a defensive response.

leukaemia

A haemoproliferative disorder characterized by increased numbers of blood cells in the bone marrow and peripheral blood.

neoplasia

An abnormal proliferation of cells that can be benign or progress to malignancy. (The word comes from the Greek *neo* = new, *plasia* = formation.)

clone

A cell, group of cells, or organism descended from and genetically identical to a single common ancestor.

aplastic anaemia

A serious disease where the bone marrow does not produce enough blood cells.

haemorrhage

Excessive bleeding caused by a breakdown in haemostasis.

thrombosis

The process of the (generally inappropriate) formation of blood clots.

haemophilia

Hereditary bleeding disorder caused by a deficiency in clotting factors.

malaria

An infectious disease found in tropical and subtropical regions. It is caused by protozoan parasites of *Plasmodium* species that are carried by mosquitoes.

Cross reference

Haemorrhage, thrombosis, and haemostasis are fully explained in Chapters 13–16.

BOX 1.1 *What will this book achieve?*

All the diseases you have just been introduced to, and their detection in the laboratory by biomedical scientists, will be discussed in more detail in the chapters that follow:

- Chapter 2 will introduce basic blood tests.
- Chapter 3 will describe how the blood cells develop.
- Chapters 4–6 will consider the red blood cell in health and disease.
- Chapter 7 will introduce you to blood-borne parasites.
- Chapters 8–12 will discuss white blood cells in health and disease.
- Chapters 13–16 will focus on haemostasis and the consequences of its failure.

1.3 The role of the biomedical scientist in the haematology laboratory

Biomedical scientists carry out a wide range of laboratory tests to produce and interpret results that assist clinicians in their diagnosis and treatment of disease. The biomedical scientist specializing in haematology plays an essential role in supporting many hospital departments, such as accident and emergency, intensive care, operating theatres, special care baby units, and **oncology**. Without the contribution of the biomedical scientist these departments could not function as effectively.

The biomedical scientist working in the haematology laboratory is particularly important in supporting the clinical haematologist in the specialist areas of **haemato-oncology**, haemostasis, and **haemoglobinopathies**. Indeed as your career progresses you may decide to specialize in one of these subdisciplines.

Many of the analytical techniques employed in haematology are also common to other pathology disciplines, e.g. immunoassay, molecular techniques (such as polymerase chain reaction), and microscopy, which will equip you with transferable scientific skills, whilst other scientific methods are specific to haematology.

oncology

The area of medicine that deals with the development, diagnosis, treatment, and prevention of tumours.

haemato-oncology

Cancers of the blood.

haemoglobinopathy

Disease (such as thalassaemia and sickle cell disease) resulting from mutations in the globin genes and so abnormal haemoglobin synthesis.

Common haematology techniques

Whilst haematology laboratories employ a wide range of analyses and analytical techniques there are some that are performed in large numbers on a daily basis throughout the UK. Many are basic screening tests that form a diagnostic springboard for the initiation of follow-up investigations to identify and characterize specific disease states.

Full blood count

The **full blood count** (FBC) is the single most commonly performed routine haematolgical blood test. It provides information on the numbers and size of red blood cells, white blood cells and platelets. It also measures the concentration of haemoglobin in the blood. The FBC is performed on highly specialized automated analysers. This is a first-line test that is important in providing information on the type of follow-up investigation that may be required.

BOX 1.2 *A rewarding career*

One fascinating aspect of practice as a biomedical scientist in haematology is that the nature of many haematological diseases is evident when marrying FBC data with blood film appearances and other results. You literally see the disease for yourself when examining a blood film. Indeed, it is not unknown for biomedical scientists to discover serious disorders such as leukaemia and malaria before they are clinically evident to medical staff and that can be immensely rewarding.

Blood films

Microscopy has an important role in the haematology laboratory as it enables the size, maturity, shape, and content of blood cells to be assessed. A drop of blood is smeared onto a glass slide, dried, and stained. Different cells take up different stains so that they can be identified under a microscope. **Blood films** are used to investigate the various causes of anaemia, white cell disorders, and parasitic infections of the blood. Haematological disease, and many disorders generating secondary haematological changes, give rise to a vast array of abnormal **morphological** findings that can be apparent on a stained blood film. Building up the knowledge and skills to be able to identify the myriad morphological changes that can be encountered in haematological practice will be one of the biggest and most fascinating challenges of your career. Bone marrow is also examined in a similar way to whole blood.

Erythrocyte sedimentation rate

An **erythrocyte sedimentation rate** (ESR) is performed to empirically assess the inflammatory response to tissue injury and response to treatment and has clinical value in monitoring diseases like **rheumatoid arthritis**. However, an abnormal ESR may also be present in non-inflammatory disease such as cancer and anaemia. The ESR is a physical property not of blood cells, nor of the plasma proteins, but of whole blood, and measures the **rheological** properties of the blood. The ESR is a test that can be performed either manually or on a specific autoanalyser. A test allied to the ESR is **plasma viscosity**, which assesses how thick or how thin the plasma component of the blood has become.

Coagulation screen

This group of tests measures the time it takes for blood plasma to clot in response to specific stimuli, and identifies which particular areas of the biochemistry of blood coagulation may be abnormal. These are front-line tests routinely employed in hospitals to monitor patients who are bleeding or undergoing an operation. A test called the **International Normalized Ratio** (INR) is used to monitor patients who are on the therapeutic anticoagulant drug **warfarin**. **Coagulation screens** can be performed manually, but are now more commonly performed on automated coagulation analysers.

Haematinic assays

This type of assay directly measures the concentration of iron, **ferritin**, vitamin B_{12}, or folate to indicate nutritional and other causes of anaemia. Due to the type of random access analyser that performs the analyses **haematinic** assays are often performed in the biochemistry laboratory.

Cross reference
Details of the full blood count are provided in Chapter 2, and also throughout the book.

morphological
The external appearances (of cells).

rheumatoid arthritis
An inflammatory disease that mainly affects the joints.

rheology/rheological
The study of the physical nature of blood or plasma principle measurement are ESR and viscosity.

International Normalized Ratio
A system established by the WHO to standardize prothrombin time (PT) reporting system for patients receiving oral anticoagulants.

warfarin
A common oral anticoagulant drug used to prevent the recurrence of thrombosis.

ferritin
The main storage protein for iron.

Immunophenotyping

This is a highly specialized technique that allows the measurement of multiple physical characteristics of a single cell. Pretreated cell preparations are analysed in an instrument called a **flow cytometer**. This technique is essential in the differential diagnosis of leukaemia.

Haemoglobin-variant detection

Separation methods such as **electrophoresis** and **high-pressure liquid chromatography** (HPLC) are used to identify variants of haemoglobin. These techniques are important in the diagnosis of haemoglobinopathies such as sickle cell anaemia and thalassaemia.

Molecular techniques

Analysis of DNA is an important tool for the investigation of many inherited haematological disorders such as haemophilia and haemoglobinopathies. Molecular analysis is also important in the management of leukaemia because specific molecular defects can indicate the severity of disease and the intensity of the treatment required.

All these techniques, plus many others, are described in detail in later chapters within this book.

Point-of-care testing

Traditionally, blood tests are performed in a centralized laboratory by specifically educated, trained, and registered practitioners, who are usually biomedical scientists. Technological advances have led to the development of portable analytical devices with limited or single test repertoires that allow basic pathology tests to be performed away from the centralized laboratory, either at the bedside or in the outpatient clinic. This has had two major effects on professional practice:

1. Biomedical scientists can, on occasions, practise away from the central laboratory and enjoy a degree of patient contact.

2. Other healthcare staff, and even patients, can access and operate the devices.

Point-of-care testing is more commonly available for analytes associated with the biochemistry laboratory, one major exception being the INR for warfarin monitoring.

1.4 Additional roles of biomedical scientists

As well as analytical investigations, biomedical scientists have responsibility for a number of other important areas that maintain effective laboratory practice.

Quality management

A key role of all biomedical scientists is to ensure that the quality of the results produced by each technique and operator is maintained, which is achieved in a variety of ways.

---

flow cytometer
Cells treated with fluorescent dyes move in a liquid stream past a laser beam. Analysis is based on the size, granularity, and fluorescence of the individual cell.

electrophoresis
Migration of dispersed particles (perhaps molecules) relative to a fluid under the influence of an electric field.

high-pressure [/performance] liquid chromatography
Column chromatography technique used to separate, identify, and quantify compounds.

The laboratory will participate in **external quality assessment** (EQA) programmes for all the tests they perform. Examples of such a scheme are those run by the National External Quality Assessment Scheme (NEQAS) in the UK. Additionally **internal quality controls** (IQC) are performed to monitor the performance of an assay in real time.

Quality is also maintained by assessing the competency of laboratory staff, at initial training and at regular intervals, and by the laboratory operating a quality management system which encompasses document control and a rolling audit programme. Much of the document control centres around **standard operating procedures** (SOP), which as the name suggests, are documents that explicitly state how every aspect of a given procedure must be performed. This is a way of ensuring, as far as is possible, that every test is performed the same way—irrespective of the operator—in order to achieve consistent high-quality results. The SOPs are regularly reviewed and updated where necessary.

Pathology laboratories have their own quality assessment body, **Clinical Pathology Accreditation (UK) Ltd** (CPA UK). Each medical laboratory is expected to meet a number of defined standards and are assessed at least every four years against these standards. It is a requirement of CPA UK that all laboratories have a quality manager who ensures compliance to accreditation standards.

Cross reference

There is a chapter in the *Biomedical Science Practice* volume in this series that covers quality assurance in more detail.

BOX 1.3 *Quality definitions*

It is important to recognize the difference between EQA and IQC because they assess the quality of results in different contexts.

External Quality Assessment (EQA)

A central agency supplies all registered laboratories with blood samples for analysis by locally employed techniques for each test performed. Local results are compared to those from laboratories throughout the UK to identify consensus or performance anomalies. It must be noted that EQA is only a retrospective evaluation of performance.

Internal Quality Control (IQC)

Samples of known values that are analysed simultaneously with patient samples to monitor the performance of an assay.

BOX 1.4 *Clinical Pathology Accreditation (UK) Ltd*

CPA is under the umbrella of the United Kingdom Accreditation Service (UKAS). All pathology laboratories must be registered with the CPA. The standards cover quality, health and safety, personnel, and analytical processes.

Health and safety

The clinical laboratory can be a dangerous place. The nature of the work means that potentially biohazardous blood specimens are handled and that the analytical work involves the use of chemicals many of which may be harmful if not controlled. Although their use has declined substantially over the last decade, some laboratories still use radioactive isotopes in investigations.

As with all workplace environments, laboratories are subject to legislative health and safety requirements, e.g. Control of Substances Hazardous to Health (COSHH). **Risk assessments** need to be performed for each procedure in the laboratory's repertoire. Laboratory personnel must be exposed to minimal risk which is achieved in a variety of ways, including the use of personal protective equipment such as laboratory coats, gloves, and safety goggles. Automated procedures have reduced the necessity of the individual coming into direct contact with blood and reagents. In hospital laboratories a biomedical scientist is often designated as the health and safety officer.

Risk assessment

The determination and documentation of the quantitative or qualitative value of risk related to a specific situation/procedure and a recognized hazard.

Cross reference

Health and safety is covered in more detail within the *Biomedical Science Practice* volume in this series.

Training and education

Many hospital laboratories have approved training status. Training is overseen by a biomedical scientist who is designated as the training officer and is often the link between the laboratory and the university. Laboratories may have BSc students on work placement or have staff attending university to obtain higher degrees. Healthcare scientists must prove that they are competent to perform each individual procedure/assay, and competency assessment records are kept for each employee.

Ongoing professional development is a requirement of all qualified biomedical scientists. Each laboratory needs to demonstrate how it assists personnel to develop. This may be by organizing journal clubs or ongoing lecture/tutorial programmes.

As additional educational resources, many departments arrange in-house lectures/courses delivered by internal and external speakers. Early in your career you will likely be a delegate, but later you could be asked to contribute presentations of your own. Further into your career, when you have amassed sufficient knowledge and experience, you may be invited to be a visiting lecturer at a university to educate the next generation of biomedical scientists.

SELF-CHECK 1.3

What are the major roles of the biomedical scientist in the haematology laboratory?

1.5 The role of haematology in the provision of healthcare

The UK spends 4% of its annual healthcare budget on pathology. Haematology laboratories are performing an increasing number and broader range of tests than ever before for the healthcare community.

As healthcare professionals we aim to provide a framework for the identification and treatment of human disease. Broadly speaking, this can be envisaged as comprising two stages: initially when the individual self-refers to their general practitioner (GP), which is termed the **primary care** setting. However, any particular case may require additional investigations or treatments not generally available to the GP, so that the patient is referred to and then cared for by a hospital, which is **secondary care**. Some haematology tests have a role in primary care, where the GP may call on the pathology laboratories for help in diagnosis and (if needed) to monitor the effects of treatment. However, the haematology laboratory is important in virtually all aspects of secondary care.

Exceptionally difficult or complex cases may demand additional tests that could be beyond the scope of a routine laboratory. If so, then referral to a specialist centre at a different hospital may be required—this is described as **tertiary care**. Such specialist centres are often linked to a university, i.e. will be part of a university teaching hospital.

There are many ways to classify human disease. As an example to give you a flavour of the contribution of haematology diagnostics to overall healthcare, one model is to consider three broad areas of pathology—cancer, connective tissue disease (such as rheumatoid arthritis, osteoarthritis, and their allied conditions), and cardiovascular disease (to include its risk factors such as diabetes and hyperlipidaemia). Together, these constitute 70–80% of the healthcare burden of the developed world. The remaining conditions include, for example, infectious diseases and psychiatric illness.

For many patients, one of the first presentations to their GP will be for a group of symptoms that could indicate anaemia. As you will see in Chapters 4–6, this may be due to problems with the red blood cells but may also be due to disease of the blood vessels, heart disease, and/or lung disease. This group of symptoms may be caused by cardiovascular disease, by a connective tissue disease, or by cancer—the symptoms of anaemia (whether actual anaemia or not) are common in all three conditions. However, patients with cancer or connective tissue disease will have a separate group of signs and symptoms, as well as abnormal blood results.

The winter months bring their excess burden of colds and influenza, especially to the elderly, and so with it sequelae such as secondary bacterial throat infections and chest infections. A common prescription to deal with these infections is broad-spectrum antibiotics. These infections can have several effects on the blood—notably an increase in the white blood cell count and changes to the ESR. However, the necessity for a prolonged prescription of antibiotics over several months may suggest something more serious, especially if accompanied by symptoms of anaemia, such as leukaemia where the malignant cells are made at the expense of normal cells. The late stages of this serious disease include an increased risk of bruising and bleeding, signs that can be investigated by the haematologist.

In cardiovascular disease the terminal event in almost all deaths is the cessation of the heart beat. In turn, the most common reason for this is the presence of clots within the coronary arteries that prevent blood flow to the **myocardium**. Once deprived of this blood, with its life-giving oxygen and glucose, the muscle cells of the heart will fail and die, leading to the often terminal heart attack. It follows that the causative process is the development of clot (thrombus), which may erupt from areas of damage (lesions) within the coronary artery itself, or by thrombus formation elsewhere in the body which travel to the heart and there become lodged. The final details of these processes (**atherosclerosis** and **atherogenesis**) are considered in the *Biology of Disease* textbook in this series. Thus, one role of the haematology laboratory in the care of the patient with cardiovascular disease is to provide knowledge of the coagulation system. However, patients with cancer are also at risk of thrombosis, and, conversely, a small proportion of people who find themselves with an unexplained clot in the legs or the lungs will go on to develop cancer.

Cross reference

The disease processes that lead to cancer, cardiovascular disease, and rheumatoid disease are further explained in the *Biology of Disease* textbook in this series.

myocardium
Heart muscle.

atherosclerosis
A major disease of blood vessels that is the underlying pathology in cardiovascular disease.

atherogenesis
The process of the development of atherosclerosis, often involving blood vessel damage, thrombosis, and hypercholesterolaemia.

SELF-CHECK 1.4

What percentage of the annual healthcare budget is spent on pathology?

Thus the haematology laboratory can help with the diagnosis and management of all three of the major human disease groups.

1.6 The overlap with other pathology disciplines

Although most biomedical scientists will specialize within a particular pathology discipline, it is important to remember that each area contributes information towards a complete understanding of disease.

Blood transfusion

blood transfusion
The science of ensuring the safe transfer of blood and other substances from one person to another.

The position of the **blood transfusion** laboratory is clear, as in the vast majority of pathology departments the haematology and blood transfusion laboratory are scientifically and organizationally linked. Most biomedical scientists specializing in haematology will also have trained in blood transfusion. However, the many differences between these two arms of biomedical science is emphasized by the requirement to deal with each part in a separate textbook of this series.

Cross reference
Blood transfusion is the subject of a separate textbook in this series, namely *Transfusion and Transplantation Science.*

The blood transfusion laboratory is concerned with the preparation of blood and blood products for transfusion, which includes compatibility testing between donor and recipient blood. The findings of anaemia, thrombocytopenia, or abnormal blood coagulation in the haematology laboratory can lead to requests for the blood transfusion laboratory to prepare red cells, platelets, or plasma for infusion into the patient.

Immunology

Immunology involves the study of the immune system and its disorders. Deficiencies of the immune system are investigated together with their association to infection, tumour growth, autoimmunity (e.g. rheumatoid arthritis), and allergies. The immunology laboratory is also involved in tissue-matching for organ transplants, and plays an important role in monitoring and treating patients with the acquired immune deficiency syndrome (AIDS).

immunophenotyping
A technique that labels cells with antibodies to identify the presence or absence of cell markers to characterize cell lineage.

There is a clear link between the immunology and haematology disciplines. Immunology is concerned with white cell function and antibody production and haematology looks at white cell numbers, morphology, and some aspects of function. There is an inevitable crossover; for instance, leukaemias are recognized initially from the FBC, blood film, and bone marrow results and then characterized using **immunophenotyping**, all of which are performed by biomedical scientists in the haematology laboratory.

Clinical biochemistry

The biochemistry laboratory is concerned with the study of changes in the chemical composition of blood and other body fluids to assist in the diagnosis and monitoring of disease, e.g. blood sugar in diabetes and liver function tests in liver disease. The laboratory is also involved in toxicology investigation, prenatal screening for Down's syndrome, and neural tube defects.

There is overlap with haematology as conditions such as liver disease may also exhibit abnormal blood cells and deranged blood clotting. Renal function is investigated in the biochemistry laboratory but the resultant anaemia is diagnosed and monitored in a haematology laboratory. The anaemia occurs due to reduction of a hormone produced in the kidneys that stimulates red cell production.

Bacteriology

Bacteriology, which is a branch of the microbiology laboratories, is involved in the identification of microorganisms that cause infections such as food poisoning, meningitis, and septicaemia. Microorganisms are cultured and subjected to tests to establish their identity. Subsequent tests identify which antibiotics will be effective in treating the specific organisms that have been isolated. Infection is also of interest to the haematologist as an infection can result in a high white blood cell count; in cases of severe septicaemia very abnormal clotting is seen accompanied by depleted platelet numbers, which have severe consequences for the patient. White cells can adopt abnormal morphology in response to infection.

The bacteriology laboratory is increasingly involved in the monitoring of hospital acquired infections and also investigates for gut parasites. Malaria is a parasitic infection with a life-cycle phase that occurs partly in the bloodstream and thus it is detected in the haematology laboratory, as are other blood-borne parasites.

Cross reference
You will meet blood-borne parasites and their laboratory detection in Chapter 7.

Virology

The virology laboratory diagnoses infectious diseases such as hepatitis, rubella, chlamydia, human immunodeficiency virus (HIV), and influenza. The hepatitis virus causes liver disease which will lead to both abnormal biochemistry and haematology results. The treatment for conditions such as infection with HIV can lead to a low white blood cell count, therefore the haematology laboratory will be co-involved in the monitoring of the patient's treatment. Some viral infections, such as infectious mononucleosis (glandular fever), present with characteristic morphological changes in white cells that are detected microscopically in the haematology laboratory. The haematology laboratory will also test for antibodies in patient plasma which indicate infectious mononucleosis.

Histopathology

The histopathology laboratory processes biopsy, surgical resections, and post-mortem tissue samples. The most closely related area to haematology is examining trephines from bone marrow and biopsies from lymphoma patients.

Cross reference
Infectious mononucleosis and its investigation are discussed in detail in Chapter 8.

Cytology

In cytology, cell samples are examined for the presence of cancerous and precancerous cells, including cervical screening.

Cytogenetics

Cytogeneticists study chromosomes, which is key to understanding genetic disease. Cytogenetics plays an important role in the clinical management of leukaemia and lymphomas, and clinicians need to marry the results from both laboratories when diagnosing subtypes of haematological malignancies and making treatment decisions.

Cross reference
Cytogenetic analysis will be discussed in much greater detail in Chapters 9–12.

Stem cell laboratory

Stem cell laboratories prepare harvested stem cells for transfusion into patients. Stem cells are important for the treatment of some patients with leukaemia. Cytogenetics and stem cell laboratories are only found in teaching hospitals.

SELF-CHECK 1.5

Which discipline is most closely related to haematology?

1.7 **The role of the professional body**

A **professional body** is a learned organization that represents a particular profession by maintaining control or oversight of the legitimate practice of that profession. It seeks to further the profession, the interests of individuals engaged in that profession, and to safeguard the public interest.

The major professional body for biomedical scientists employed in UK pathology laboratories is the **Institute of Biomedical Science**. However, the diversity in the biomedical sciences and the requirement to specialize often demands additional professional bodies. As far as haematology is concerned, this is the **British Society for Haematology**, which predominantly represents medical practitioners but also other healthcare staff whose practice involves/ encompasses haematology.

The Institute of Biomedical Science

The Institute of Biomedical Science (IBMS) is the professional body for biomedical scientists in the United Kingdom. The institute was founded in 1912 and aims to promote biomedical science and its practitioners. There are approximately 16,000 members. The main roles of the IBMS include setting standards of practice to protect patients, assessing competence for biomedical scientists to practise, accrediting university degrees, providing postgraduate professional qualifications, and organizing a **continuing professional development** (CPD) scheme. Additionally the Institute plays a key role in assessing qualifications for registration with the Health Professions Council (HPC).

The IBMS holds a biannual conference and publishes monthly *The Biomedical Scientist* which contains science articles, news, and job adverts. The Institute's scientific publication is the *British Journal of Biomedical Science* containing peer-reviewed scientific papers. It is not mandatory for biomedical scientists to be members of the IBMS, but there are many benefits, including the authority to adopt designatory initials that indicate the class of membership, such as MIBMS (member) or FIBMS (fellow).

The IBMS website gives full details. http://www.ibms.org

The British Society for Haematology

The British Society for Haematology (BSH) is the main haematology society in the UK; its main objective is to advance the study and practice of haematology. The BSH provides education, information, and networking to haematologists. The Society holds an annual scientific meeting and publishes the peer-reviewed journal *British Journal of Haematology*.

BOX 1.5 *Continuing professional development*

The material learnt during your undergraduate degree that qualifies you to enter the profession will not provide you with all the knowledge you need for your entire career. Medicine, biomedical science, and technology progress at a rapid pace and it is a requirement that health professionals constantly strive to maintain and update their knowledge and professional practice. The IBMS has a mature scheme that allocates credits for a range of professional and educational activities. If a practitioner accrues sufficient credits within a specified time period they are awarded a CPD Diploma.

CPD activities must be varied in nature to update different areas of practice. Suitable CPD activities include attending conferences and lectures, learning new laboratory procedures/techniques, reading up-to-date research articles, attending journal clubs, giving lectures/tutorials, publishing scientific papers, and writing reflective statements on workplace learning. The IBMS publishes monthly journal-based learning (JBL) exercises where practitioners read a relevant article and then answer questions that have been set by IBMS examiners. Essay titles are also set twice a year for practitioners to explore a relevant subject in depth by structured reading, and the essays are marked by IBMS examiners. Pass marks in JBL and structured reading attract additional CPD points.

A major role of the BSH is to publish guidelines from the British Committee for Standards in Haematology.

For full information about the BSH see http://www.b-s-h.org.uk

Health Professions Council

It is mandatory that all healthcare scientists practising in the NHS in the UK are registered with the Health Professions Council (HPC). The HPC is the regulator and exists to protect the public. Practitioners have to reach specific standards of education and professional competence to gain entry onto the register and attain the status of a registered healthcare professional. All healthcare professionals are required to continue to keep their knowledge and skills up to date while they are registered and practising in their profession. At re-registration a percentage of individuals are selected at random for audit, whereby they are expected to provide a summary of practice for the previous two years, evidence of varied CPD activities, and a statement with evidence that demonstrates how they have met the standards.

The HPC website gives full details: http://www.hpc-uk.org

Chartered Scientist (CSci)

CSci represents a single chartered mark for all scientists, recognising high levels of professionalism and competence in science. Being chartered is the mark of professional recognition, and being a Chartered Scientist allows all scientists working at the full professional level to be recognised on an equal footing. It gives an assurance of current competence through mandatory revalidation, and encapsulates the interdisciplinary nature of science in the 21st century. By benchmarking professional scientists at the same high level, CSci aims to re-engage public trust and confidence in science and scientists.

All those working in the practice, application, advancement or teaching of science can become CSci with the appropriate combination of qualifications and experience. Chartered Scientists work in an ever-growing diversity of settings, from food science to nuclear physics, and mathematical modelling to chemical engineering.

In order to be awarded CSci status, applicants must demonstrate various competencies including the ability to deal with complex issues and communicate their conclusions to a range of audiences. They must show originality in problem solving and substantial autonomy in planning and implementing tasks. Through a commitment to continuing professional development, Chartered Scientists will continue to advance their knowledge, understanding and competence throughout their career.

Practitioners seeking CSci status are advised to contact the IBMS.

SELF-CHECK 1.6

What are the major roles of the professional body?

SELF-CHECK 1.7

Why is CPD important to effective professional practice as a biomedical scientist?

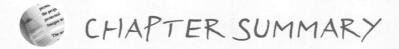 CHAPTER SUMMARY

- Haematology is the study of diseases of the blood and blood-forming organs.

- The biomedical scientist in haematology performs analyses that assist clinicians in the differential diagnosis of disease.

- Haematology inevitably overlaps with other physiologies and disciplines within pathology.

- The roles of the various professional bodies include setting professional, scientific, educational, and quality control standards.

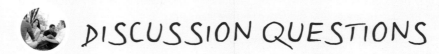 DISCUSSION QUESTIONS

1.1 Why is haematology considered a discrete discipline when the white cell elements could be part of the immunology discipline and most other elements contained within biochemistry?

1.2 What effect would the loss of a haematology service have on healthcare delivery in a hospital?

Answers to self-check questions, case study questions, and discussion questions are provided in the book's Online Resource Centre, visit www.oxfordtextbooks.co.uk/orc/moore

2

Major haematology parameters and basic techniques

Andrew D. Blann and Gary W. Moore

In this chapter we will introduce you to the principal haematology parameters (such as the full blood count) and many of the basic techniques that are used to define particular indices, such as haemoglobin.

Learning objectives

After studying this chapter, you should confidently be able to:

- Appreciate the importance of different anticoagulants and glass/plastic tubes for the different blood tests requested.
- Describe major haematology techniques: spectrometry, microscopy, light scatter, impedance technology and calibration.
- Be aware of the major components of the full blood count, which are the red blood cell indices, the white blood cell indices, and platelets.
- Describe the differences in the values of the Erythocyte Sedimentation Rate (ESR) and plasma viscosity.
- Understand coagulation screening.
- Grasp the important aspects of the micronutrients iron, vitamin B_{12}, and folate, as well as plasma proteins such as transferrin and ferritin.

2.1 Obtaining a blood sample

Venepuncture is the process of obtaining a sample of blood, generally from a vein (usually the median cubital vein) on the inside of the elbow joint (hence venous blood). The skin at this location is very soft, and veins are close to the surface of the skin (that is, they are superficial) (Figure 2.1). Until recently, most blood samples were obtained using a needle that had to be fitted onto a syringe. However, this method has been superseded in many hospitals by the

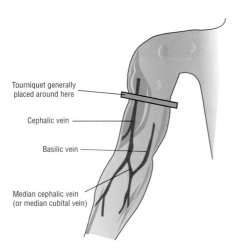

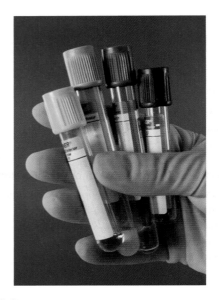

FIGURE 2.1

Anatomy of the arm showing superficial veins suitable for venepuncture.

FIGURE 2.2

Vacutainers commonly used in haematology. They have different coloured tops that indicate a particular anticoagulant (or lack thereof) and a label for patient details. © Claire Paxton & Jacqui Farrow/Science Photo Library.

use of **vacutainers**, glass tubes with an inbuilt vacuum, which draws blood directly from the vein without the use of a syringe (Figure 2.2). Venepuncture itself is a learned skill that requires completion of a training course. These are generally organized by the training section of the hospital. However, small quantities of blood can be obtained from soft tissues of the thumb, the ear lobe, or the heel. This is done by making a small incision in the soft tissue with a sharp needle called a lancet and then allowing the blood to drip directly into a blood collection tube—this method is particularly useful if a full blood sample is not required, or if a sample is required from a child or an infant from whom venepuncture may be difficult.

All blood cells arise from the bone marrow, the anatomical site where blood cells are generated. In many conditions, examination of the bone marrow can be very informative. However, obtaining a sample of the bone marrow can be difficult. Two approaches are common. The first is to drive a heavy-duty needle into a particular bone (such as the breast-bone or the hip), and then suck out some of the bone marrow. This procedure is referred to as a **bone marrow aspiration**. The second is to obtain a larger sample of bone that will include bone tissue as well as bone marrow. This is called a **trephine procedure**, and requires an even more substantial needle and should only be used to biopsy tissue from the hip.

2.2 **Anticoagulants**

Once removed from the body, blood will rapidly (in perhaps 2–5 minutes) form a semi-solid mass of cells (the clot) and a fluid. Separation of the clot from the fluid in a **centrifuge** provides a clear, often yellowish liquid called serum. The serum is required for the estimation of **micronutrients**, such as iron and vitamin B_{12}, proteins, and for other tests. A large number of blood cells and coagulation proteins (such as **fibrinogen**) will make up the clot, so it cannot be used for most tests of red blood cells, white blood cells, platelets and the proteins involved

Cross reference

The bone marrow and the process of bone marrow aspiration are discussed in more detail in Chapters 3 and 10.

micronutrients

Minerals and vitamins absorbed from the diet and required in trace amounts for the correct function of a cell or biochemical process.

fibrinogen

Fibrin precursor and ligand that facilitates platelet–platelet aggregation and forms a mesh that is the basis of the thrombus.

in coagulation. So in order to be able to analyse these cells and proteins, we must ensure the blood does not clot, and do so with anticoagulants. In many cases, vacutainers, are supplied with an anticoagulant already present. Other vacutainers can be obtained with no anticoagulant and will therefore ultimately provide serum.

Different blood tests require different anticoagulants:

- **A full blood count** (FBC), which provides information about the numbers of red blood cells, white blood cells, and platelets performed on blood that is anticoagulated with a sodium or potassium salt of ethylene diamine tetra-acetic acid (**EDTA**). This blood sample can also be used for more specialized tests, such as for analysing the integrity of the membrane of the red blood cell and for producing a blood film.

- **Coagulation** tests are invariably performed on plasma obtained from whole blood that has been anticoagulated with **sodium citrate** (of course, if blood was allowed to clot the coagulation proteins would have been used in the clotting process). The plasma itself is obtained after the vacutainer, or other tube containing the blood, has been centrifuged. The blood cells, lying below the plasma, are generally discarded. However, at least one common coagulation test (the International Normalized Ratio, INR) *can* be performed on whole blood.

- The erythrocyte sedimentation rate (ESR), which gives a global score of a physical property of the blood, can be assessed on blood that is held within its own dedicated glass tube: blood clotting in this tube is also prevented by sodium citrate. However, some haematology analysers are designed to be able to provide an ESR result on the same sample of blood as is used for the FBC.

Key Points

EDTA functions as an anticoagulant by irreversibly chelating the calcium ions that are essential in the blood clotting processes you will meet in Chapter 13. Chelating agents such as EDTA form soluble complex molecules upon binding to certain metal ions which inactivate the metal ions. The word 'chelate' is derived from the Greek for the claw of a lobster because there are two calliper-like groups in the molecule that function as associating units and fasten to the central atom to produce heterocyclic rings.

Tri-sodium citrate functions as an anticoagulant by forming a loose and reversible ionic complex with calcium ions. This makes it ideal for coagulation tests because many of them involve the addition of reagents containing calcium ions to initiate clotting *in vitro*. Additionally, platelets retain functional ability in citrate-anticoagulated blood but not in EDTA, so platelet function testing is performed on citrated samples.

Like the ESR, the plasma viscosity test provides information on another global property of the plasma; specifically, it describes the 'thickness' or 'thinness' of plasma. Rarely, blood may be anticoagulated with **heparin**—for example, when we wish to perform cytogenetic analysis on a sample or immunopherotype the white cells. This natural anticoagulant can also be used as a therapy to reduce the risk of thrombosis, as may occur after surgery for hip replacement, for example. The process of minimizing the risk of thrombosis in a clinical setting (called **therapeutic anticoagulation**) demands an entire section of its own (Chapter 16).

One problem with some anticoagulants is that they interfere with the blood itself. The best known artefacts of anticoagulants include a swelling of red blood cells and platelets by EDTA. It follows that the FBC needs to be analysed within a few hours if we are to be sure that the indices of red blood cell and platelet volume remain accurate.

Cross references

Red blood cells, and diseases associated with them, are described in considerable detail in Chapters 4–6, blood-borne parasites in chapter 7.

White blood cells are discussed in more detail in Chapters 8–12.

We discuss platelets further in Chapters 13–16.

Details of the anticoagulant action of heparin are given in Chapter 16.

sodium citrate
An anticoagulant chemical added to blood to allow the measurement of coagulation proteins, prothrombin time and the activated partial thromboplastin time.

heparin
A natural anticoagulant often added to blood to allow additional analyses of white blood cells.

therapeutic anticoagulation
The use of anticoagulants as a treatment for the increased risk of thrombosis.

SELF-CHECK 2.1

What are the major differences between serum and plasma?

SELF-CHECK 2.2

What are the two major laboratory anticoagulants, and which of these is required for each of the major blood tests?

SELF-CHECK 2.3

Which micronutrients are essential for the production of healthy blood cells?

2.3 Major techniques

Once a blood sample has been obtained, it must be analysed. Almost all routine haematology results are obtained from tests performed on highly sophisticated machines, or from viewing blood films that have been stained with special dyes (which allows them to be seen with a microscope). Without doubt the routine haematology laboratory (and, indeed, the biochemistry laboratory) is dominated by one or more autoanalysers that will provide the FBC, and others that provide coagulation test results. Although there are technical variations, these autoanalysers all use a small number of basic techniques. These are generally spectrometry, impedance, cytochemistry, and flow cytometry. Plasma proteins are often quantified by an immunoassay.

Key Points

Relating a particular result (such as a high white blood cell count) to a particular clinical condition (such as septicaemia) is often one of the more rewarding aspects of haematology. However, time and time again an experienced practitioner will be called on to provide details of the basic science underlying an unusual test or to explain an atypical observation.

Spectrometry

Cross reference

Different types of haemoglobin are described in Chapter 4.

This technique is used to provide the haemoglobin result. A small sample of blood is mixed with a non-ionic detergent that destroys the membrane of the red blood cell so that a red/pink 'soup' is created, of which the dominant component is haemoglobin. However, there are several different subtypes of haemoglobin, so an additional chemical (such as a mixture of potassium, ferricyanide, and cyanide ions, known as Drabkin's solution) is required to convert them to a single species, the concentration of which is measured by a spectrometer. This technique converts most types of haemoglobin to cyanmethaemoglobin and is recommended by the World Health Organization (WHO) for measuring haemoglobin concentrations. The machine assesses the extent to which the passage of a beam of light is reduced by the density of the solution. Thus the density of the red/pink colour is proportional to the haemoglobin present in the original blood sample.

Impedance

This process relies on the ability of an ionic fluid (an electrolyte) to assist the passage of electricity from one electrode to another. However, this passage of electricity can be interrupted by particles. In haematology autoanalysers, this principle is exploited in a chamber with a small pore that allows blood cells to pass through. Each time a blood cell passes through this pore, the passage of electricity is impeded by an amount proportional to the size of that cell. Hence the higher the number of cells present, the greater is the frequency of disturbances in the flow of electricity. Sophisticated software can convert the number of disturbances not only to the number of cells but also the size of the cell that is responsible for impeding the current. This method is capable of providing a red blood cell count, white cell count, platelet count, and the mean cell volume (MCV).

Cytochemistry

Cytochemistry utilises the presence of certain enzymes (such as peroxidase) and other molecules (such as fats and iron) within some normal white blood cells, and also in abnormal cells such as in certain types of leukaemia to identify cells of a particular lineage. This technique can be used by an autoanalyser, but it can also be used on a film of blood dried onto a glass slide.

Cross reference
Cytochemistry is also important in investigating leukaemia, as you will see in Chapter 10.

Flow cytometry

This process is allied to both microscopy and chemistry. It relies on the scattering of a fine beam of light, perhaps provided by a laser. The degree to which this beam of light is scattered is proportional to the size of the cell, and the frequency of the interruptions of the beam of light gives the number of cells. In some analysers, chemicals are used to strip the cytoplasm from the cell so that only the nucleus is analysed. This technique can be extended, with the use of antibodies conjugated to fluorochromes, so that different subtypes of cells (mostly white cells) can be quantified. Such an instrument is called a fluorescence activated cell scanner (FACS).

Cross reference
Use of flow cytometry in leukaemia classification is outlined in Chapters 10–12.

Microscopy

Literally, 'small viewing', this essential technique provides a view of the morphology of red cells, white cells, and platelets. Whilst the value of autoanalysers is established, they cannot provide for all eventualities, and in many cases the skill of an experienced scientist provides considerably greater surety. Cells can be viewed using standard stains, mostly of the nucleus and cytoplasm. However, the microscope can also tell of intracellular parasites such as malaria, and, with the help of a special stain, of the amount of iron within a cell.

Cross reference
Chapter 7 shows several blood-borne parasites.

Immunoassays

Whilst they are not part generally of routine screening, immunoassays are commonly used as follow-up tests to measure the plasma concentrations of various proteins, including those involved in coagulation and others to do with iron and vitamins. Immunoassays use antibodies that recognize a specific protein, or a specific section of a protein, to capture the molecule, which can then be subjected to a variety of detection methods. Immunoassay methods in common use include:

- **Enzyme-linked immunosorbent assays (ELISA)**
- Latex immunoassays (LIA)
- Immunonephelometry

Enzyme-linked immunosorbent assay (ELISA)
An important technique in many disciplines of biomedical science, generally for detecting molecules within fluids.

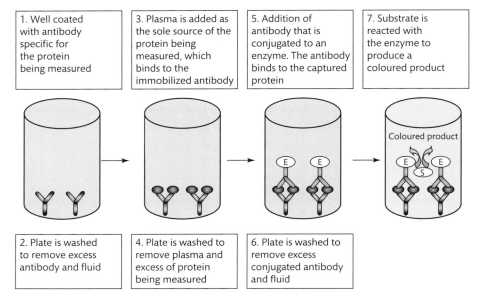

1. Well coated with antibody specific for the protein being measured

3. Plasma is added as the sole source of the protein being measured, which binds to the immobilized antibody

5. Addition of antibody that is conjugated to an enzyme. The antibody binds to the captured protein

7. Substrate is reacted with the enzyme to produce a coloured product

Coloured product

2. Plate is washed to remove excess antibody and fluid

4. Plate is washed to remove plasma and excess of protein being measured

6. Plate is washed to remove excess conjugated antibody and fluid

FIGURE 2.3

Principle of ELISA technique. This is referred to as a sandwich ELISA because the protein is indeed sandwiched between the capture and tag antibodies.

You can see in Figure 2.3 that the ELISA technique uses an antibody immobilized in a well to capture the protein being measured. To facilitate the testing of multiple samples, plastic or polystyrene plates containing 96 wells are used. The plates are referred to as the solid-phase of the assay. Patient plasmas, often in diluted form, are then added to the wells so that the protein being measured will bind to the immobilized antibody in direct proportion to its concentration. A second antibody specific to the protein being measured is then added. This antibody has an enzyme (such as horseradish peroxidase) attached to it and is often referred to as the 'tag' or 'secondary antibody'. The enzyme is then supplied with a substrate which produces a coloured product when cleaved by the enzyme, the intensity of which is measured by spectrometry. The colour intensity is directly proportional to the amount of enzyme available as a result of binding to the captured protein. Therefore, the more protein that binds to the capture antibody, the greater the measured colour intensity at the detection stage of the assay. A patient deficient in the protein will generate a lower colour intensity. The results are read off a standard curve that is assayed in the same plate.

METHOD *Standard curves*

Standard curves are used in the measurement of concentrations of substances such as proteins or DNA. An assay is first performed with various known concentrations of the substance being measured; these measurements are referred to as the standards. Each concentration will generate a different end-point reading. Examples of end-points are optical density, luminescence, fluorescence, radioactivity, or clotting times.

You can see in Figure 2.4 that the standard curve is prepared by plotting concentration on the x-axis and endpoint value on the y-axis. A line or curve is fitted through the points for the standards. Note in Figure 2.4 that the standard curve is in fact a straight line. This is the most accurate and so scientifically the most acceptable part of the standard curve. Above and below this straight line section the relationship between the concentration and the end-point value is difficult to interpret and so is of less rigorous scientific value.

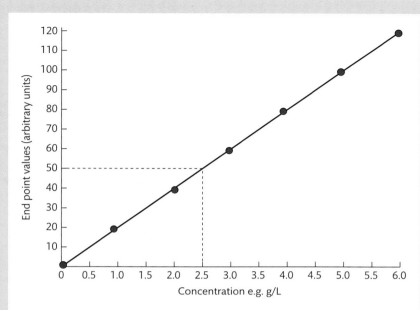

FIGURE 2.4

Standard curve. The result for each standard is plotted against concentration and a line drawn to connect the points. The diagram shows a patient sample with an endpoint result of 50 being read off the standard curve to generate a result of 2.5 g/L.

Once the standard curve is prepared the assay can be performed both on control samples and on patient samples containing unknown concentrations of the analyte. For each patient sample endpoint result, the graph is read horizontally across from its value on the y-axis until it intersects with the standard curve. This value is then read off the x-axis by reading down vertically. The concentration of the analyte in the patient sample is the value on the x-axis. Most analysers will automatically prepare the standard curves and read the values of controls and patient samples.

In LIA techniques the capture antibody is immobilized on microscopic latex beads. You can see in Figure 2.5 that adding a plasma sample to a solution of these beads causes agglutination of the beads in direct proportion to the amount of protein present. The degree of agglutination is measured by light scatter.

The technique of light scatter is also the basis of **nephelometry**, which measures the intensity of light scatter that occurs when light is transmitted through a reaction mixture containing particulate matter. Nephelometry is performed in a nephelometer. Antibodies to the antigen of choice (such as the marker of inflammation, **C-reactive protein**; CRP) are mixed in an optimum concentration of each so that exceptionally small aggregates are formed. Light (such as may be provided by a laser) will be scattered in proportion to the concentration of the aggregates, and from this the concentration of the molecule being measured can be determined. Because this process uses antibodies it is more correctly referred to as immunonephelometry. A closely related technique is **turbidimetry**, which measures the loss of intensity of light transmitted through a reaction mixture containing particulate matter, whereby the unscattered light is measured. Turbidimetry is performed using a turbidimeter.

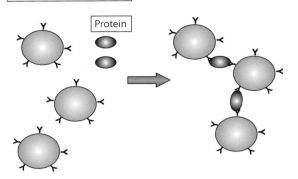

Latex particles coated with antibody to the protein being measured

Agglutination measured turbidimetrically

Protein

FIGURE 2.5
Latex particles act as the solid phase to anchor the capture antibody. The protein being measured in the patient's plasma acts as a bridge between coated latex particles, leading to a degree of agglutination in direct proportion to the amount of measured protein in the plasma. The amount of agglutination is measured by turbidimetry.

Immunoassays rarely used nowadays include radioimmunoassay (RIA), immunoradiometric assay (IRMA), and immunodiffusion. Because of the inherent danger of radioisotopes, the former are being replaced by ELISA. Immunodiffusion suffers from a lack of sensitivity. However, in exceptional circumstances, these methods may be called upon.

BOX 2.1 What's the difference between a standard and an internal control?

A standard is a preparation with a known, exact concentration (or other value such as INR) for use in the generation of standard curves. A control preparation has no fixed value, but has a range of expected values. Such internal controls are analysed at regular intervals for tests that are performed throughout the day and night, such as FBC or **prothrombin time** (PT), or each time a batch of samples is performed for tests that may be analysed just once a day, a few times a week, or less frequently. We recognize that operator, reagent, and analyser variability mean that you won't get exactly the same result each time a sample is analysed. As long as the difference in results is within acceptable limits of analytical variability and will not alter clinical decision-making, then a result, or batch of results, can be reported. Controls are used to check that a procedure is generating results within an acceptable range.

prothrombin time
One of the major coagulation tests: used to assess key aspects of the coagulation pathway.

Cross references
Further details of quality control procedures are given in the *Biomedical Science Practice* text in this series.

Further details on spectrometry, automation, immunoassay, and microscopy are present in the *Biomedical Science Practice* text in this series.

Key Points

Immunoassays merely capture the protein and measure its concentration but not its function. In the context of immunoassays, the protein being measured is referred to as the antigen.

SELF-CHECK 2.4

What are the commonalities and differences between ELISA and LIA techniques?

2.4 **The blood film**

The blood film provides the opportunity to view the components of blood under a microscope. A drop of blood, generally from the same tube that provides the full blood count, is smeared onto a glass slide and allowed to dry in air at room temperature and fixed in methanol. It is then covered with stains such as those originally developed by **Romanowsky** but subsequently refined by workers such as Jenner, Giemsa, and Leishman. After a set time, the stains are washed off with buffered saline and the slide is once more allowed to air-dry. Figure 2.6 shows a blood film, where a drop of blood has been spread out from left (where it is thickest) to the right (where the film is thin).

The slide is now ready to be viewed by light microscopy. But first we need to establish the correct degree of magnification. Multiplying the eyepiece magnification (often ×10) by the magnification of the objective lens (for example ×40) provides the total magnification (in this example ×400). Please refer to Figure 8.22 for the basic structure of a modern microscope. If this is too low (such as ×100) we will be unable to establish fine details of the cells, but a very high magnification (such as ×1000) permits many fine details to be seen, but generally only one or two cells at a time—this is too slow for a busy laboratory. Therefore the midpoint, perhaps a magnification of ×400, is preferred as the fine details of many cells can be viewed at the same time.

The second thing we must do is to find the correct place on the film to examine the sample so we can adequately assess the blood cells. The best place for these observations is where the cells are close together—not too far away from each other where the film is too thin, nor where the film is too thick so that individual cells cannot accurately be defined. This is illustrated by Figure 2.7, which shows three parts of the same slide and the differences in the density of the blood cells. In Figure 2.7(a) the cells are far apart, but in Figure 2.7(c) they are too close together and clearly overlap. Choose an area such as in Figure 2.7(b).

Having established the power of magnification and where on the slide to look, we can begin our examination of blood cells. Figure 2.8 shows a typical blood film. The principal feature is a white blood cell (top left), characterized by a three-lobed nucleus that had taken up stains so that it now appears dark purple/black. A second feature is the large number of roughly round cells that are all a single colour – these are red blood cells. A close viewing of these cells reveals some degree of variety in both the size of the cells and the density of the grey colouring. The importance of this variation in size and degree of coloration has significance, as we will see in Chapters 4–6. The third feature is the presence of small purple bodies—these are platelets.

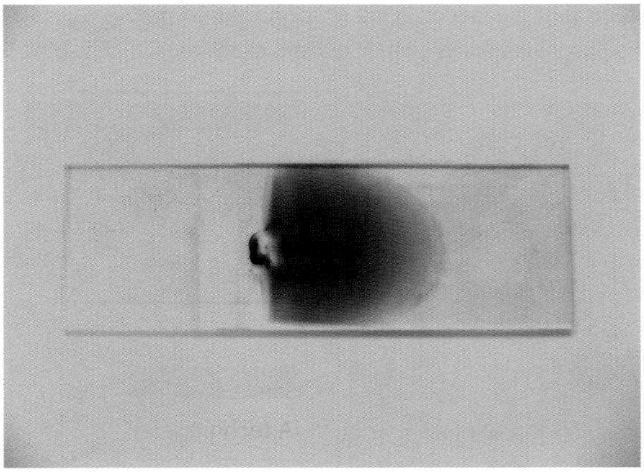

Romanowsky

A type of stain specially developed to enable the examination of different blood cells. Romanowsky stains contain polychromed methylene blue and eosin.

Cross reference

Microscopy is discussed in greater detail in Chapter 8. See the chapter on microscopy in the *Biomedical Science Practice* text in this series for more information about magnification.

FIGURE 2.6
The appearance of a blood film. As the blood is drawn out from left to right, cells become more spread out and so fine details of individual cells can be noted. © Institute of Biomedical Science (IBMS) and Sysmex Haematology Morphology Training CD-ROM, 2009.

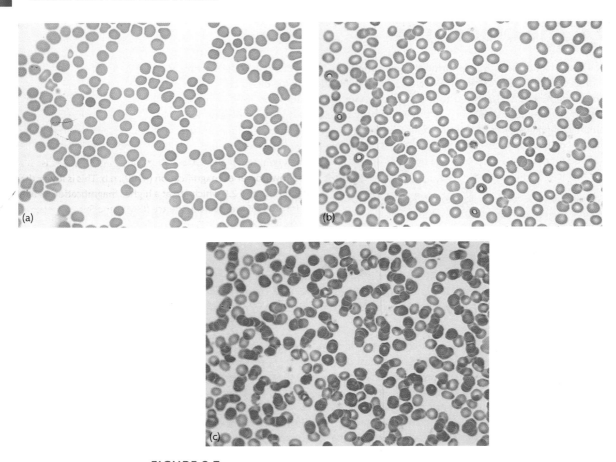

FIGURE 2.7

Peripheral blood film examination. Blood smears are stained with a Romanowsky stain. When viewing morphology, choose an area of the film where red cells are close together, i.e. (b). Incorrect places are where the cell layer is too thin and cells become flattened (a), and where the film is too thick and the cells overlap (c). Note that there are no white blood cells present. (Magnification ×400.) © Institute of Biomedical Science (IBMS) and Sysmex Haematology Morphology Training CD-ROM, 2009.

With the advent of automated autoanalysers that can provide an excellent breakdown of the different types of blood cells, the blood film has become less important and now is not routinely examined. However, there is still a place for the microscopic examination of a blood

FIGURE 2.8

A typical blood film at a high power of magnification, showing red cells, a white cell, and platelets. Different blood cells can be identified by the different patterns of dye uptake. This figure shows a single white blood cell – a neutrophil (with its purple and irregular nucleus of three lobes), many slightly smaller red blood cells, and a smaller number of platelets (small purple dots). (Magnification ×800.)

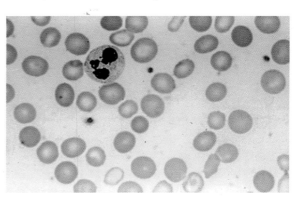

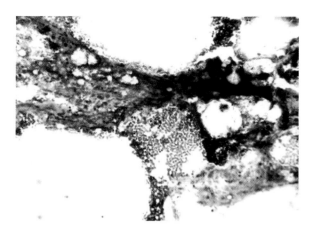

FIGURE 2.9

The appearance of a bone marrow aspiration on a glass slide at a low power of magnification (×100). n.b. This is lower than figures 2.7 and 2.8 which are at a higher magnification ×400–800. © Institute of Biomedical Science (IBMS) and Sysmex Haematology Morphology Training CD-ROM, 2009.

film; such examination may be necessary to confirm the autoanalyser's profile or to perform other assessments of the blood, such as for malarial parasites, the presence of bodies inside the red blood cell, for unusual white blood cells, or to look for evidence of partially destroyed or damaged red blood cells.

The same principle is also used to prepare bone marrow. The bone marrow aspirate is also spread out on a glass slide, dried, and stained. However, because the bone marrow sample is considerably thicker, it has a different appearance to peripheral blood, as is illustrated in Figure 2.9, and a bone marrow sample is harder to smear thinly than a blood sample. The principal difference is that a bone marrow sample contains numerous non-haematological cells (such as fat cells and endothelial cells) as well as non-cellular material (such as reticulin and collagen fibres).

2.5 The full blood count

The full blood count is the most requested and most important blood test in haematology. It provides a package of information on red blood cells, white blood cells, and platelets.

Red blood cells

Red blood cells, with a diameter of approximately 7 μm when mature, are unusual among cells of the body as they lack a nucleus. Consequently, they are easy to identify in a blood film (Figures 2.7 and 2.8). The full analysis of red blood cells includes several tests.

Haemoglobin (Hb) is undoubtedly the index most frequently referred to in biomedical haematology. It is an iron-containing protein that absorbs oxygen from areas of high-oxygen content (that is, at the lungs), and then releases it in areas where oxygen levels are low (i.e. in the tissues). The reference range for haemoglobin varies between the sexes. Pre-menopausal women lose blood with each menstrual period, but in post-menopausal women levels are still lower than age-matched men as the latter produce testosterone which stimulates red cell production. Men who have lost their testes to disease or through trauma generally have a haemoglobin level comparable to that of post-menopausal women.

The level of haemoglobin in a sample of venous blood is reported by the laboratory in grams per litre (g/L), so that an adult result of 138 g/L would be within the reference range. This notation has recently changed, under the advice of the International Council on Standardization in Haematology. Previous units were g/dL, so that the same result would have been

Cross reference

Reference ranges are included in Table 1 of this book and are further discussed in Section 2.9 of this Chapter.

13.8 g/dL, Thus in practice it is simply a question of moving the decimal point one place. Some laboratories continue to report haemoglobin levels in g/dL.

Haemoglobin is normally carried in the blood inside red blood cells, which are also called **erythrocytes** (*erythro* = red, *-cyte* = cell). There are approximately 640 million molecules of haemoglobin in each red cell. The number of red blood cells in a sample of blood is reported as the **red blood cell count**. Because these cells lack a nucleus and they are biconcaved discs, they have flexibility to penetrate the smallest capillaries. They are the most abundant cell in the blood, and numbers can also vary in health between the sexes, and also in various diseases. The function of the red cells is to carry oxygenated haemoglobin (often described as oxyhaemoglobin) from the lungs to the tissues (where oxygen is given up), and then the deoxygenated haemoglobin returns back from the tissue to the lungs via the venous circulation. Thus a crucial component of this cell is the ability of oxygen to pass freely into the cell at the lungs and out of the cell at the tissues, and this in turn demands a highly specialized cell membrane. The lack of a nucleus means that mature red blood cells cannot repair or divide, so the lifespan of the red blood cell is relatively short at 120 days compared to most nucleated cells.

The process of red blood cell production starts in the bone marrow, where cells pass through various stages of development, becoming increasingly mature. The **reticulocyte** is the final stage of the development of the red blood cell before full maturation. Indeed, reticulocytes may be seen as being the 'teenagers' of the life cycle of the red blood cells. Present in normal blood in very low numbers (perhaps one for each 100 mature red cells), increased numbers are maybe the product of a pathological process or could be the body's response to pregnancy, iron, B_{12} or folate therapy, or to blood loss. However, reticulocytes are not always part of the full blood count and so, if required, need to be specially requested.

Cross reference

The process of the development of red blood cells is described in Chapter 3.

The **haematocrit** (Hct) expresses as a decimal (e.g. 0.42/L) or as a percentage (e.g. 42%) that proportion of whole blood that is taken up by all the blood cells. Since there are approximately 1000 more red blood cells per unit volume than either white blood cells or the comparatively tiny platelets, then red cells make up the major proportion of blood and so the haematocrit. Consequently, at the practical level, the haematocrit provides an idea of the proportion of the mass of the red blood cells that make up the whole blood pool.

The red blood cell indices comprise three measures of different aspects of the red blood cell, its size, and the amount of haemoglobin it contains. These indices are:

- The **mean cell volume** (MCV, typically about 92 femtolitres (fL); 1 fL = 10^{-15} L) is the volume of the average (mean) red blood cell. Note the stress is on 'average', as each index is the mean of thousands of individual cells. As it is measured directly in the blood, it takes no account of the number of red bloods cells or the haemoglobin result.

- **Mean cell haemoglobin** (MCH, typically about 29.5 picograms (pg); 1 pg = 10^{-12} g), as the name implies, reports the average amount (mass) of haemoglobin in the average cell. It does not take into account the volume of the cell.

- **Mean cell haemoglobin concentration** (MCHC, typically about 330 g/L) is the average concentration of haemoglobin inside the average cell.

Most laboratory autoanalysers measure haemoglobin, the red cell count and mean cell volume (MCV) directly from the blood. Three other indices (Hct, MCH, and MCHC) are calculated from these three root measurements:

- The Hct is obtained by multiplying together the red blood cell count (RBCC) and the MCV, then dividing the result by 1000, so that:

$$Hct = (MCV \times RBCC)/1000$$

For example, if the MCV is 85 fL and the RBCC is 4.2×10^{12}/L, then the Hct = 0.357/L. In practice this could be rounded up to 0.36. However, this result may also be expressed as whole numbers as a percentage, which would be 36% (see Figure 2.16).

- The MCH is obtained by dividing the haemoglobin result by the red blood cell count, so that:

$$MCH = Hb/RBCC$$

For example, if the Hb is 138 g/L and the RBCC is 4.2×10^{12}/L, then the MCH = 32.8 pg. In practice this could be rounded up to 33 pg.

- The MCHC is obtained by dividing the haemoglobin result by the product of the MCV and the red blood cell count, and then multiplying by 100. But note that the red blood cell count and the MCV also make up the Hct. So that:

$$MCHC = \{Hb/(MCV \times RBCC)\} \times 100$$

For example, if the Hb is 138 g/L, the MCV is 85 fL, and the RBCC is 4.2×10^{12}/L, then the MCHC is 386 g/L.

Thus because these three latter red cell values (Hct, MCH, MCHC) are mathematically derived from the three root measurements (Hb, MCV, RBCC), it is entirely possible for either one or more of the Hct, the MCH, or the MCHC to be outside the reference range whilst the other indices are apparently normal. Indeed, in the third example above, the Hb, MCV, and RBCC are all within the reference range, but their mathematical product, MCHC, is outside the reference range. Thus one must consider all six red cell indices (and possibly some other blood tests) together to obtain a full picture.

Similarly, consider a haematocrit such as 0.42/L. Because the Hct is the product of two other indices (the MCV and the RBCC), then the same Hct would be present in one sample whose RBCC is 6×10^{12}/L and whose MCV is 70 fL and in a different sample where the RBCC is 7×10^{12}/L but whose MCV is 60 fL. This is because $(6 \times 70)/100$ is the same as $(7 \times 60)/100$, that is 0.42. As we will see in Chapters 5 and 6, this may have consequences for the way in which we interpret these results.

Each blood sample has an MCV that is the average size of all red cells in that sample. However, this average masks the possibility of considerable variation in the range of possible sizes within that same sample. The variation in the sizes of the red cell population can be assessed by the **red cell distribution width (RDW)**. This is derived by the Haematology Autoanalyser from all the measured red cell volumes which contribute to the MVC. Suppose our MCV is 90 fL. This average number may be derived from a population whose actual cells vary from 80 fL to 100 fl, or in a different sample whose cells vary from 85 fL to 95fL. The greater the RDW, then the greater the variation in the sizes of the red blood cells. A common reason for an increased RDW is the presence of reticulocytes. This index may be also useful in establishing a diagnosis, and we will return to it in Chapter 6.

SELF-CHECK 2.5

List the red cell indices?

Key Points

A greater overall burden of human disease can be accounted for by abnormalities in red blood cell functioning than in the pathology of white blood cells or platelets.

White blood cells

White blood cells (WBCs), or **leucocytes** ((*leuco-* = white, *-cyte* = cell) are collectively responsible for defending us from attack by microorganisms such as viruses, bacteria and parasites, when raised levels of white blood cells can be expected. The process by which certain white blood cells ingest and destroy pathogens is called **phagocytosis**, and the cells that perform this function are phagocytes. Increased numbers of white blood cells (i.e. a **leucocytosis**) may also be present in a number of conditions such as rheumatoid arthritis, cancer, after surgery, and, as we shall see in detail, in leukaemia. Haematologists currently recognize five different types of white blood cells that can be found in the (normal) blood—the **neutrophil**, **lymphocyte**, **monocyte**, **eosinophil**, and **basophil**. Each type of leucocyte can be defined on morphological grounds, but also by their function (Table 2.1).

These five types of cell are present in different proportions. The **white blood cell differential** reports the proportion of these cells in a sample. A typical distribution may be neutrophils 70%, lymphocytes 20%, monocytes 7%, eosinophils 2%, and basophils <1% (see the Reference range: Appendix 1; and Table 2.2). However, in pathology, these proportions will be altered. The differential may also be reported as the absolute number of each type of cell. So if the WBCC is 7.5×10^9/L, then the number of lymphocytes will be 1.5×10^9/L if the differential, as above, is 20%. However, in a reaction to a virus, the lymphocyte count may rise fourfold, to, for example, 6.0×10^9/L. If the relative quantities of all the other leucocytes remain the same, then the total WBCC will have increased to 12.0×10^9/L, which is outside the reference range, and the proportion of lymphocytes will have increased to 50%, also above the reference range.

phagocytosis

The process of the ingestion and destruction of foreign and unwanted material, such as bacteria and effete red blood cells. Phagocytosis is performed by phagocytes—principally neutrophils and monocyte/macrophages.

leucocytosis

An increase in the total white blood cell count above the top of the reference range.

Cross reference

Leukaemia is described in detail in Chapters 9–12.

TABLE 2.1 Functional characteristics of white blood cells.

Neutrophils	• Phagocytosis of bacteria and yeast • Participation in inflammation • Scavenging and removal of debris
Lymphocytes	• Generation of antibodies (B lymphocytes) • Cooperation in antibody production (T lymphocytes) • Destruction of cells infected with viruses (T lymphocytes)
Monocytes	• Phagocytosis of bacteria and yeast • Participation in inflammation • Scavenging and removal of debris • Cooperation with lymphocytes in generating antibodies (as macrophage antigen-presenting cells) • Release of cytokines (such as interleukins) • Participation in haemostasis (expression of tissue factor)
Eosinophils	• Protection against parasitic infection (such as helminths) • Participation in allergic responses • Release of histamine
Basophils	• Participation in hypersensitivity reactions • Release of histamine and heparin

Additional details of the functions of leucocytes are presented in Chapter 8.

TABLE 2.2 The WBC differential.

	Absolute ($\times 10^9$/L)	Percentage (%)
Neutrophils	2–7	40–75
Lymphocytes	1–3	20–45
Monocytes	0.2–1.0	2–10
Eosinophils	0.02–0.5	1–6
Basophils	0.02–0.1	<1
Blasts/atypical cells	~0.01	<1

White blood cells can be classified by the size and shape of the nucleus, and by the presence or absence of granules in the cytoplasm. Those cells with an irregular nucleus (which can vary in shape from cell to cell) are named **polymorphonuclear leucocytes**, often abbreviated to '**polymorphs**'. Polymorphs include neutrophils, eosinophils, and basophils. These cells are defined by the presence and properties of granules in their cytoplasm, so can be called **granulocytes**. Many of these granules contain enzymes and chemicals that are used in the process of phagocytosis. Alternatively, the white blood cell may have a round and regular shaped nucleus and are generally free of granules – these cells are called **mononuclear leucocytes**. Table 2.3 summarizes these differences.

Neutrophils are the most common leucocytes, and also the most common polymorphonuclear leucocyte. They are called neutrophils because they take up dyes at a neutral pH. A further characterization is of having a nucleus with many possible different and irregular shapes, or lobes, usually three or four in each cell. Neutrophils are also characterized by the presence of cytoplasmic granules (i.e. they are also granulocytes). The white blood cell in Figure 2.8 is a neutrophil (note the three purple/black lobes of the nucleus). Figure 2.10 also shows a neutrophil, which also has three lobes.

TABLE 2.3 Key morphological features of white blood cells.

Mononuclear leucocytes	Lymphocytes: small, the nucleus occupies perhaps 95% of the cell.
	Monocytes: large, the nucleus occupies perhaps 70–80% of the cell, Rarely there may be granules in the cytoplasm.
Polymorphonuclear leucocytes, or granulocytes	Neutrophils: the nucleus generally has 3–5 lobes. Intracytoplasmic constituents are generally at a neutral pH, resulting in purple granules.
	Eosinophils: the nucleus generally has 2 large lobes. Intracytoplasmic constituents react with the acidic component of dyes (such as eosin), resulting in red–brown granules.
	Basophils: the nucleus generally has 2 lobes. Intracellular constituents have an affinity for the basic component of dyes, resulting in dense purple/black granules that often obscure the nucleus.

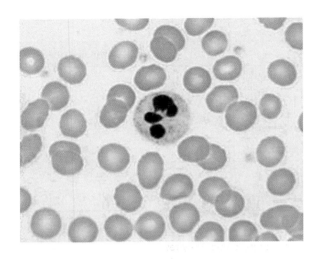

FIGURE 2.10

The neutrophil. These cells are both polymorphonuclear and granulocytic. The nucleus stains dark purple but granules take up the pH neutral part of the stain and are pinkish in colour. The nuclei generally have 3–5 lobes—this one has four lobes. Note that the cell is markedly larger than nearby red blood cells. (magnification ×800.) © Institute of Biomedical Science (IBMS) and Sysmex Haematology Morphology Training CD-ROM, 2004.

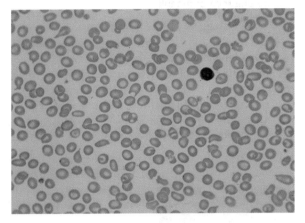

FIGURE 2.11

The lymphocyte. Lymphocytes are *mononuclear* cells—that is to say, their nucleus is often very round and regular, and generally occupies over 95% of the cell. Lymphocytes are only slightly larger than red cells. (Magnification ×400.) © Institute of Biomedical Science (IBMS) and Sysmex Haematology Morphology Training CD-ROM, 2004.

The second most frequent group of leucocytes are the lymphocytes. These differ principally from neutrophils by the structure of their nucleus, which is round and regular (hence: mono-nuclear, and thus mononuclear leucocyte) compared to the neutrophil's numerous irregular shapes. Lymphocytes are also smaller than neutrophils, often only slightly larger than red cells, and do not have granules. But a major feature is that almost all of the cell is nucleus—the cyto-plasm may take up as little as 2–5% of the cell (Figure 2.11).

Monocytes often resemble lymphocytes. They have an irregular, isolated nucleus, and can also be described as a mononuclear leucocyte (Figure 2.12). However, monocytes are the largest of the normal peripheral blood white cells, and the nucleus of most monocytes does not take up as much of the cell, maybe up to 80%, whereas the lymphocyte nucleus frequently occupies over 95% of the cells. It is often suggested that many monocytes are only temporarily in the blood (circulating for perhaps 20–40 hours), and are in fact on their way to the tissues (such as the skin, liver, spleen, and lung) where they are described as macrophages, with a lifespan often measurable in months.

Eosinophils are so-called because of their reddish colour, due to the chemical make-up of their granules, which take up eosin-like stains. The nucleus is composed of just two parts, linked together by a small thread. Basophils are the least frequent of the normal leucocytes, contain numerous granules that take up different dyes (that is, are basophilic), and so appear

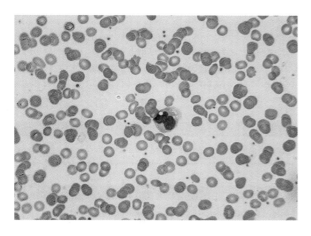

FIGURE 2.12

The monocyte. Monocytes are large mononuclear cells. Their nuclei are often kidney-shaped and the cytoplasm is said to have a ground-glass appearance. They may also have vacuoles in the cytoplasm, as shown in this example. Monocytes are the largest blood cell, considerably larger than red cells. (Magnification ×400.) © Institute of Biomedical Science (IBMS) and Sysmex Haematology Morphology Training CD-ROM, 2004.

black or dark blue. They resemble eosinophils in size but the nucleus shape is often obscured by the presence of granules. Eosinophils and basophils also have an irregular nucleus and have granules, so that others may consider these cells also to be polymorphs and granulocytes (Figures 2.13 and 2.14, respectively).

There will generally be great agreement amongst haematologists about the definitions of the five major subtypes of white blood cells. However, the occasional cell appears in the blood

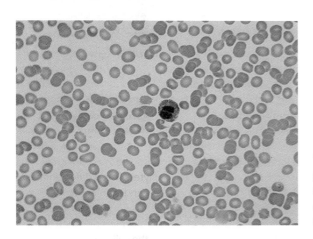

FIGURE 2.13

The eosinophil. These cells are also granulocytes. The granules stain with the acidic (eosin) part of the stain and are orangey-red. The nucleus has two lobes. (Magnification ×400.)

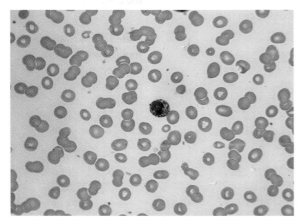

FIGURE 2.14

The basophil. Basophils are also granulocytes. The granules stain purple/black with the basic part of the stain, and are so numerous that they usually obscure the nucleus. (Magnification ×400.)

blast (or atypical cells)
A stage of differentiation of a blood cell as it passes from the stem cell stage to the mature cell stage that should only be found within the bone marrow in low numbers.

that defies this simple classification. Such cells, often with unusual characteristics, may be described as **blasts**, unclassifiable cells, or atypical cells. However, in certain diseases, as will be outlined below, increased numbers of blasts carry pathological implications, some of which are profound. An example of this occurs in several types of acute leukaemia, where the abnormal cells have such a strange morphology that they are described as blasts, and can be of the lymphoid or nyeloid family. This is developed in Chapters 9–12.

SELF-CHECK 2.6

What are the differences between the two major groups of white blood cells?

SELF-CHECK 2.7

What are the morphological characteristics of the two most frequent white blood cells?

Platelets

thrombus
Technical name for a clot, formed by aggregating platelets within a fibrin mesh. Red blood cells may also be present in a thrombus, especially if formed in a vein.

Platelets are small fragments of the cytoplasm of a larger cell found only in the bone marrow, the **megakaryocyte**. Platelets form a clot, or **thrombus**, when aggregated together with the help of the blood protein **fibrin** and so reduce blood loss. However, platelets are not simply inert participants in stemming blood flow but are in fact extremely dynamic, and have numerous granules containing molecules that promote haemostasis. Platelets circulate in the blood for 7–10 days, and are then destroyed in the spleen and the liver.

Cross reference
Platelets and coagulation are explained in full detail in Chapters 13 and 14.

A low platelet count (possibly caused by drugs, such as quinine, sulphonamides, and other antibiotics; poor production of platelets, as may be present in disease of the bone marrow; or their excessive consumption) is called **thrombocytopenia**. This condition can lead to an increased risk of bruising and bleeding, and will be considered in greater detail in Chapter 14. The converse, a raised count, is **thrombocytosis**, and is often present in many physiological and pathological situations. These include infections, after surgery, some autoimmune diseases (such as inflammatory bowel disease and rheumatoid arthritis), and after short but intense bouts of physical activity platelet counts also rise in patients with iron deficiency anaemia. A high platelet count may lead to thrombosis.

Platelets appear in a blood film as light-purple or grey bodies that are very much smaller than red blood cells. They are anucleate (that is, they do not have a nucleus) and contain granules. Indeed, to the untrained eye they could be mistaken for debris (Figures 2.8 and 2.10–2.15).

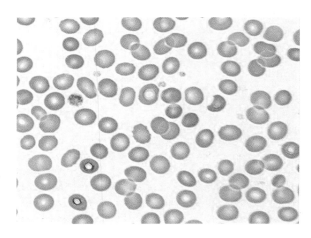

FIGURE 2.15
The platelet. These appear as small pale-blue/purple staining cells that are considerably smaller than red blood cells. However, one platelet, near the left margin, is large. (Magnification ×600.) © Institute of Biomedical Science (IBMS) and Sysmex Haematology Morphology Training CD-ROM, 2004.

What are the key aspects of the platelet?

Key Points

The full blood count is undoubtedly the most important set of results that the haematology laboratory can offer our colleagues on the ward, in the operating theatre, and in the clinic. No competent biomedical scientist can practise without a sound knowledge of how it is obtained and the implications of major abnormalities.

2.6 Rheology

Rheology provides information on the physical properties of the blood, and is therefore unlike other tests in that there is no measurement of a defined molecule or cell. The two most common tests are erythrocyte sedimentation rate (ESR) and plasma viscosity testing. However, it is also possible that some services offer whole blood viscosity.

rheology/rheological
The study of the physical nature of blood or plasma—principal measurements are ESR and viscosity.

The ESR is a global score of physical aspects of the whole blood. The result is obtained by allowing a thin column of anticoagulated blood in a vertically aligned tube to settle down under the influence of gravity. As it does so, the blood cells will separate from the plasma, so that after an hour, a band of clear plasma will sit on top of the column of blood cells. The fall in the level of the blood cells is then recorded at a rate of millimetres per hour (mm/h). It is therefore unique in requiring no sophisticated machine and few technical skills. Reference ranges for the ESR should take into account patient age. As patients age, their ESR rises. An ESR can be abnormal in a large number of conditions. These include inflammation, infection, the acute phase response, after surgery, anaemia, leukaemia, and almost all forms of cancer. Indeed, it follows that an abnormal ESR is present in most patients in hospital.

Key Points

In reality the units for ESR should be reported as millimetres in the *first* hour because the rate of sedimentation falls as time progresses—there is only so far the cells can fall before they form a compact layer at the bottom of the tube. Despite this, most laboratories use mm/h purely for convenience.

Plasma viscosity provides an idea of how thick or thin the plasma has become—whether or not it is thinner, and more like water (tending towards a low result of less than 1.5 mPa/s), or thicker and more like treacle (tending towards a high result, over 1.72 mPa/s). Viscosity records a global property of the plasma, not individual molecules. Indeed, the molecules that make up the major component of plasma viscosity include the clotting proteins fibrinogen and **von Willebrand factor** (VWF), and also albumin and immunoglobulins. There is also a relationship between plasma viscosity and total plasma protein concentration, and often with the haematocrit and the amount of water in the blood. The viscosity of the blood as a whole (i.e. whole blood viscosity, that is therefore influenced by blood cells) can also be assessed but is less informative (and is requested far less frequently) than plasma viscosity. Indeed, abnormalities in the red blood cell are commonly found in several diseases, leading to difficulty in interpretation.

von Willebrand factor
A large protein that enables platelets to bind to exposed subendothelium and also stabilizes coagulation Factor VIII.

TABLE 2.4 **Types of disorder associated with the different areas of haemostasis.**

Area of haemostasis	Causes of bleeding disorders	Causes of thrombotic disorders
Vascular integrity	Inability to support a clot as it forms due to structural defects of blood vessels	Secondary vessel structural changes such as those seen in cholesterol deposition
Primary haemostasis	Reduced concentration or impaired function of VWF. Reduced numbers or impaired function of platelets	High levels of VWF. Elevated platelet numbers or platelets with enhanced function
Secondary haemostasis	Reduced concentration or impaired function of one or more of the coagulation enzymes or co-factors	Elevated levels of one or more of the coagulation enzymes or co-factors
Inhibitors	Enhanced inhibitor function (extremely rare)	Reduced concentration or impaired function of an inhibitor or co-factor
Fibrinolysis	Increased activation of fibrinolysis	Reduced concentration or impaired function of plasminogen. Reduced regulation

FIGURE 2.16
FBC/ESR result. The right-hand column is the abbreviation of the particular test. To the left are the result, the unit, and the reference range (in brackets).

Sandwell and West Birmingham Hospitals NHS Trust.   Haematology, City Hospital

| Surname | SMITH | Address | | Unit No: | RXK3269324 | OPD - CITY |

Forename ROB
D.O.B. 12.07.53   Consultant/GP Prof.D.G.Beevers
Sex Male
NHS No: Lab No. C, 09.4250530.Q

Ethnic group: White–Any other   Clinical Details:

HB	13.9	g/dL	(12.5–18.0)		ESR	10	mm/h	(1–14)
MCV	87.4	fL	(79.0–99.0)
WBC	6.0	10*9/L	(4.0–11.0)
PLT	267	10*9/L	(150–450)
RBC	4.59	10*12/L	(3.50–6.50)
HCT	40.1	L/L	(38.0–54.0)
MCH	30.3	pg	(27.0–34.5)
MCHC	34.7	g/dL	(31.6–36.5)
NEUT	3.81	10*9/L	(1.70–7.50)
LYMPH	1.60	10*9/L	(1.00–4.50)
MONO	0.56	10*9/L	(0.20–0.80)
EOS	0.05	10*9/L	(0.00–0.50)
BASO	0.01	10*9/L	(0.00–0.10)

Tests: ESR, FBC   Date collected **06.02.09**
Report Run: 359   Specimen: Blood   Check Clinician   Date received **06.02.09 19:05**
                                                        Date reported **06.02.09**

Perhaps the single most important haematological disease where plasma viscosity is grossly abnormal is the white blood cell malignancy **myeloma**, which is characterized by anaemia and, generally, a high ESR and increased plasma viscosity. Viscosity is high because the abnormal lymphocytes are often generating excessive amounts of protein.

Plasma viscosity and ESR are often closely related as they are both influenced by plasma proteins. However, there is debate regarding the clinical value of both tests being offered by the same laboratory, and most offer only one of the two. Indeed, a more precise marker of inflammation is the plasma protein CRP, so much so that some laboratories offer CRP as an alternative to an ESR.

The FBC and ESR are generally printed out together in a standard form that can be inserted in the folder of patient's clinical details. Figure 2.16 shows a routine report of an FBC and an ESR from a middle-aged male.

SELF-CHECK 2.9

What are the two major tests of rheology?

2.7 Haemostasis

Haemostasis is the balanced orchestration of interactions between blood vessels, blood cells, plasma proteins, and some small molecules that maintain blood in a fluid state and also limit and arrest bleeding upon damage to the blood vessel. There are five main components of the system:

1. *Vascular integrity*—intact blood vessels promote mechanisms that maintain circulating blood in a fluid state. When the vessel is damaged, exposed subendothelial structures in the vessel wall (such as collagen) promote blood clotting processes.

2. *Primary haemostasis*—VWF binds to structures exposed by vessel damage and then captures platelets at the site of injury. The captured platelets become activated and recruit more platelets allowing them to aggregate to each other and form the initial physical barrier for preventing blood loss and the entry of microorganisms into the wound.

3. *Secondary haemostasis*—a clot made entirely of platelets is not robust enough to withstand the blood pressure in many blood vessels and thus needs a strengthening mechanism. This comes in the form of a series of interlinked enzyme reactions culminating in the generation of the enzyme **thrombin** from its precursor prothrombin. This crucial enzyme then converts fibrinogen, a soluble plasma protein, into an insoluble polymerized form called fibrin. The fibrin forms a mesh around the platelet clot to impart greater structural integrity. This complex series of enzyme reactions is termed **blood coagulation**. The enzymes are referred to as **coagulation factors** and circulate in the plasma as inactive precursors, the majority of which are converted to their active forms by other activated coagulation factors.

4. *Inhibitors*—although thrombin is a crucial component of coagulation, it is also a potentially lethal enzyme. Consequently, a group of plasma and membrane-bound proteins exist to regulate and eventually shut down the blood coagulation reactions. Other coagulation factors also have their own inhibitors.

5. *Fibrinolysis*—blood clots need to be removed once bleeding has stopped and the wound has healed. Platelets are cellular in origin and have autolytic mechanisms. The fibrin clot is digested by the enzyme plasmin which is generated and controlled in a similar fashion to thrombin by a separate group of activators and inhibitors.

The main events of haemostasis are summarized in Figure 2.17, and the fine detail of the coagulation process is explained in Chapter 13.

Abnormalities in the different areas of haemostasis can lead to disorders that predispose the patient to either **haemorrhagic** or **thrombotic** disease. Table 2.4 outlines the types of disorders that can be associated with abnormalities in each area. Although bleeding or thrombotic disorders are associated with each area, the most common bleeding disorders occur in the areas of primary and secondary haemostasis, whilst the most common thrombotic disorders are a result of abnormalities in the inhibitory mechanisms of blood coagulation.

haemorrhagic disease
Disorders that lead to excessive bleeding.

thrombotic disease
Disorders that lead to thrombosis, which is a partial or complete obstruction of a blood vessel by a blood clot.

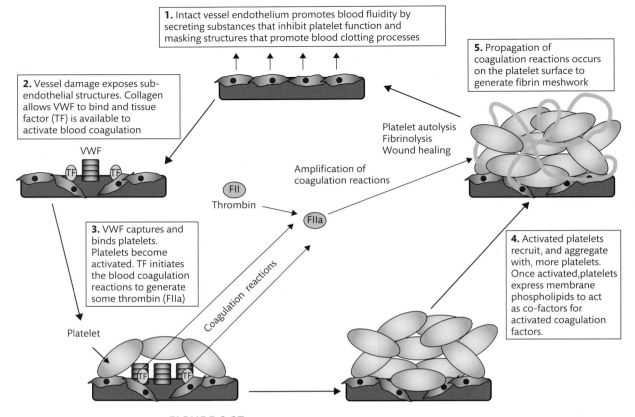

1. Intact vessel endothelium promotes blood fluidity by secreting substances that inhibit platelet function and masking structures that promote blood clotting processes

5. Propagation of coagulation reactions occurs on the platelet surface to generate fibrin meshwork

2. Vessel damage exposes sub-endothelial structures. Collagen allows VWF to bind and tissue factor (TF) is available to activate blood coagulation

VWF

Platelet autolysis
Fibrinolysis
Wound healing

Amplification of coagulation reactions

FII
Thrombin

FIIa

3. VWF captures and binds platelets. Platelets become activated. TF initiates the blood coagulation reactions to generate some thrombin (FIIa)

Coagulation reactions

4. Activated platelets recruit, and aggregate with, more platelets. Once activated, platelets express membrane phospholipids to act as co-factors for activated coagulation factors.

Platelet

TF   TF

FIGURE 2.17

Main events of haemostasis. 1. Intact blood vessel endothelium is active in dampening down clotting processes. 2. Structures exposed upon damage to the endothelium promote primary and secondary haemostasis. 3. VWF binds to collagen and then tethers platelets whilst tissue factor initiates the first series of coagulation reactions. 4. Platelets activated at tethering recruit more platelets to the clot and express surface phospholipid. 5. The small amount of thrombin generated at initiation of coagulation promotes further coagulation reactions on the surface of platelets leading to fibrin formation that strengthens the platelet clot. Upon wound healing, the clot is destroyed (fibrinolysis).

The haemostasis laboratory of a haematology department plays a critical role in the detection and characterization of haemostatic disease in a variety of patients and clinical circumstances, such as:

- Patients with bleeding symptoms
- Patients with thromboses
- Patients with other disorders that have secondary effects on haemostasis
- Preoperative checks for patients who may have haemostatic disorders that only manifest upon significant challenge
- Monitoring treatment of bleeding disorders
- Monitoring treatment with therapeutic anticoagulants

Complex specialized laboratory tests are required to characterize the nature of functional platelet abnormalities or to identify specific deficiencies of blood coagulation or inhibitory proteins. It is not possible to perform every test on every patient. Consequently, biomedical scientists perform screening tests that assess overall coagulation function, which, if abnormal, can be further investigated with appropriate specialized tests.

Cross reference

You will meet the design and use of specialized diagnostic haemostasis tests in Chapters 14 and 15.

SELF-CHECK 2.10

What are the five areas of haemostasis and their main roles?

Key Points

Deficiencies can result from:

- Absence of a particular protein
- Reduced concentration of a normally functioning molecule
- Normal concentration of an abnormally functioning molecule
- Reduced concentration of an abnormally functioning molecule

Screening tests

The nature of disorders of blood vessels means that abnormalities affecting haemostasis cannot be subjected to laboratory-based investigations in the routine diagnostic setting. However, you will meet the skin bleeding time in Chapter 14 where a small incision is made in the patient's arm and the time taken for bleeding to stop is recorded. Abnormalities of blood vessels, VWF, and platelets can lead to an abnormally long bleeding time. You will also meet analysers in Chapter 14 that assess global VWF and platelet function. They are mainly used for patients whose clinical symptoms suggest a disorder of primary haemostasis.

By far and away the most commonly performed haemostasis screening tests are those for coagulation screening and platelet counts, the latter having been covered earlier in this chapter. Coagulation screening tests artificially segregate groups of coagulation factors into three discrete compartments so that patterns of abnormal results, if present, can indicate which subsequent tests should be chosen to identify single or multiple factor deficiencies. The three discrete compartments are:

- The extrinsic pathway
- The intrinsic pathway
- The common pathway

Look at Figure 14.1 on page 484 and you will see that the end product of both the extrinsic and intrinsic pathways is activated factor X (FXa) which is the enzyme that begins the common pathway, culminating in fibrin generation. Each screening test is designed to activate the coagulation reactions at a different starting point, but they all have the same endpoint of fibrin generation. The coagulation screening tests in regular use are:

- Prothrombin time
- Activated partial thromboplastin time
- Thrombin time
- Quantitative measurement of fibrinogen activity

Prothrombin time (PT)

The prothrombin time uses a reagent called thromboplastin that activates coagulation at the start of the extrinsic pathway, which subsequently activates the common pathway. The time taken from the addition of thromboplastin to the patient's plasma to the generation of a fibrin clot is the PT itself, which is recorded in seconds. The coagulation factors of the intrinsic pathway take no part as there is nothing in the reagent to activate them.

Activated partial thromboplastin time (APTT)

The patient's plasma is incubated with the APTT reagent which specifically activates the intrinsic pathway, but only up to the point where calcium ions are required. After the incubation period, which is typically three or five minutes, calcium ions are added, allowing the intrinsic pathway to progress to activation of the common pathway and subsequent clot formation. The time taken to clot from the addition of the calcium ions is the APTT itself and is also recorded in seconds.

Thrombin time (TT)

The thrombin time merely involves adding thrombin to the patient's plasma to bypass all the other coagulation factors and just convert their fibrinogen to fibrin. It is mainly used as a quick method to check the patient's fibrinogen level and is also recorded in seconds.

Fibrinogen

Cross reference

You can find further detail about coagulation screening tests in Chapter 14 on bleeding disorders.

Presence of an adequate level of fibrinogen is crucial if the preceding coagulation factor reactions are to have their desired effect. Measuring fibrinogen activity is performed using a modified version of the TT where the patient's plasma is diluted and then clotted with a calibrated thrombin reagent. Now that automated analysers are available to perform this test many laboratories no longer perform TTs.

Analytical platforms

Although the endpoint for all coagulation screening tests is a fibrin clot there are in fact three main analytical methods for detecting clot formation.

Tilt-tube technique—the biomedical scientist manually pipettes reagents and plasma into test tubes in a 37 °C water bath and estimates clotting times using a stopwatch. Upon addition of the final reagent, the test tube is removed from the water bath, held horizontally and returned 2–3 times/second (to maintain temperature) until the reaction mixture is seen to have clotted.

Mechanical clot detection—reagents and plasma (or whole blood) are manually pipetted into a rotating cuvette, which contains a small metal ball sitting within a magnetic field. The cuvette is contained within a coagulometer that reads the endpoint when formation of the fibrin clot removes the metal ball from the magnetic field. Automated versions are available that use robotics to deliver reagents and plasma and to time the clot formation.

Photo-optical clot detection—robotics are used to deliver reagents and plasma and endpoints are timed automatically. Reaction cuvettes are placed in the light path of a fixed beam and the increase in turbidity upon fibrin formation alters the light-scatter, which is detected photo-optically by either turbidimetry or nephelometry. The analyser plots the change in light transmittance or scatter over time for each test as a coagulation curve, an example of which you can see in Figure 2.18.

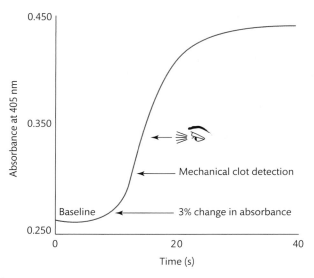

FIGURE 2.18

Coagulation curve for a normal prothrombin time. At the addition of the thromboplastin reagent the analyser plots a baseline of light transmittance or scatter which remains constant until fibrin clot formation begins. Polymerization of fibrin increases the turbidity of the reaction mixture leading to reduced transmission of light through the cuvette and an increase in light scatter. The analyser can be pre-set to detect a clot at a defined percentage of change in transmittance or increased scattered light intensity as low as a 3% difference from the baseline. You can see from the graph that mechanical clot detection is less sensitive to the early stages of fibrin formation, yet its design means that clots are detected at the point of coagulation of the entire reaction mixture. Photo-optical systems are often pre-set closer to this level. Tilt-tube techniques that rely on the skill and visual acuity of the operator are inevitably less sensitive.

What do the results tell us?

If a patient has reduced function of one or more coagulation factors it will cause a 'bottleneck' in the coagulation reactions. Consequently, one or more of the screening tests will take longer to clot than normal when compared to a reference range for each test. There is no definitive reference range for each test because reagents vary between manufacturers and an individual reagent may perform differently on alternative analytical platforms. Some laboratories report PT, APTT, and TT results as ratios by dividing the clotting time of the patient's plasma with that of a normal-pool control plasma. Representative reference ranges are given in Table 2.5.

TABLE 2.5 Representative coagulation reference ranges.

Screening test	Reference range (s)	Reference range (ratio)
Prothrombin time	11–14	0.90–1.10
APTT	24–34	0.85–1.15
Thrombin time	12–15	0.80–1.20

Fibrinogen is reported as a concentration, a typical reference range being 1.5–4.0 g/L.

Most hereditary coagulation factor deficiencies affect just one factor, the most common being haemophilia A which is a deficiency of factor VIII. Look again at Figure 14.1 on page 484 and you will see that an isolated deficiency in the extrinsic pathway will prolong only the PT, one in the intrinsic pathway will prolong only the APTT, and a common pathway deficiency will prolong both PT and APTT. A fibrinogen deficiency will be evident from its direct measurement and will prolong PT, APTT, and TT. Assessing the screening test results allows biomedical scientists and medical staff to make informed decisions about which specific coagulation factors should be measured with more complex tests to identify the deficiency.

Key Points

Remember that PT, APTT, and TT are artificial ways of causing plasma to clot *in vitro* and the clotting times we generate in the laboratory do not necessarily equate to *in vivo* clotting times where coagulation interacts with other physiological processes.

Some primary disorders lead to a secondary reduction in production or an increased consumption of coagulation factors and generate abnormal clotting screen results. For instance, most coagulation factors are synthesized in the liver, so if the patient's primary condition is a diseased liver a secondary effect can be reduced levels of coagulation factors. Similarly, some of the clotting factors require **vitamin K** for their effective production. If the patient does not have enough vitamin K in their diet or a diseased gut impairs its absorption, the vitamin K-dependent factors will not be produced in sufficient amounts. Coagulation can be overactivated in some patients with sepsis, malignancy, or even following surgery, leading to a secondary disorder called **disseminated intravascular coagulation** (DIC) where coagulation factors (and platelets and inhibitors) are used up faster than they can be replaced.

Inflammation and pregnancy can increase levels of factor VIII and fibrinogen such that they accelerate *in vitro* coagulation reactions and cause the APTT to fall below the reference range. In some instances, this can mask another abnormality.

Use of screening tests to monitor anticoagulant therapy

Many patients who have had a thrombosis or are at risk of developing a thrombosis are treated with **anticoagulant** drugs that reduce the ability of their coagulation mechanisms to form a clot. The anticoagulant effects of two of the most commonly used drugs, warfarin and **unfractionated heparin** (UFH), can be assessed using standard coagulation screening tests.

unfractionated heparin
An injectable anticoagulant whose effect is monitored by the APTT.

UFH works by binding to one of the circulating inhibitors of coagulation, **antithrombin**, and amplifying its anticoagulant effect. Antithrombin in its natural state does not interfere with coagulation screening tests but can markedly prolong the APTT and TT in a patient receiving UFH. The TT is oversensitive to UFH so patients are monitored by APTT, the aim being to keep their APTT ratio between 1.5 and 2.5. There is no equivalent to **International Sensitivity Index** (ISI) for APTT reagents. In many cases, UFH has been superseded by an improved formulation, **low molecular weight heparin** (LMWH). The advantage of this preparation over UFH is that it generally does not need to be monitored. However, if its activity is needed, this can be determined by the anti-factor Xa assay.

low molecular weight heparin (LMWH)
An injectable anticoagulant used principally to treat or reduce the risk of venous thromboembolism.

Warfarin achieves therapeutic anticoagulation by interfering with the synthesis of the vitamin K-dependent factors—which are factors II, VII, IX and X. Patients continue to synthesize these factors but their biological activity is diminished. Warfarin is monitored using the PT because most of the factors that contribute to the clotting time are vitamin K-dependent. Patients are tested at regular intervals to ensure that their dose of warfarin is not too high or too low. If too high, they are at risk of developing dangerous bleeding symptoms because they may not clot at all even when they need to. If the dose is too low, there will be insufficient protection against developing a thrombosis.

For patients on warfarin, their PT is converted to a parameter called the International Normalized Ratio (INR). The INR is derived from the ratio between the time blood or plasma takes to clot normally compared to the time it takes to clot due to warfarin. So if a normal PT is 12 seconds, and on warfarin the PT is 24 seconds, then the ratio is 2.0. In view of reagent and analytical platform variability, this ratio is then calculated to the power of a previously calibrated mathematical expression of the sensitivity of the reagent to the effects of warfarin, the ISI. In our example, if the ISI was 1.0, the ratio would remain as 2.0. If the ISI was 1.3, the resultant INR would be 2.46.

The INR/ISI system ensures that patients get equivalent results irrespective of the reagents and analytical platform used to generate the PT to prevent unnecessary and potentially dangerous dose alterations. Someone at a relatively low risk of thrombosis receives warfarin doses to maintain their INR between 2.0 and 3.0. However, those at high risk of thrombosis would be prescribed enough warfarin to maintain an INR between 3.0 and 4.0. Approximately 1% of the UK population are receiving warfarin at any one time, and so PT/INR testing forms a large part of the workload in a routine haemostasis laboratory. Fortunately, new anticoagulants in development may well replace warfarin in many situations and for many patients. Some of these new drugs interfere with thrombin, others inhibit factor Xa.

SELF-CHECK 2.11

Name the main coagulation screening tests and the areas of coagulation they assess.

SELF-CHECK 2.12

Which two therapeutic anticoagulants can be monitored with which routine coagulation screening tests?

Cross reference

You will learn more detail about therapeutic anticoagulation and the role of the laboratory in its monitoring in Chapter 16.

Table 2.4 gave a summary of the key laboratory aspects of haemostasis.

2.8 Haematinics

Haematinics considers what may be described as a vital supporting cast to the main players of red blood cells, white blood cells, and platelets. The major micronutrients (iron, vitamin B_{12}, vitamin B_6, and folate) must be provided in the diet. Other micronutrients, essential to other aspects of physiology (but less important in haematology) include iodine and copper. The liver and other organs and cells synthesize key plasma proteins crucial to micronutrient metabolism.

Micronutrients

Deficiencies in any one of four micronutrients many result in impaired production of red blood cells by the bone marrow and therefore anaemia.

The oxygen-carrying molecule haemoglobin is a mixture of proteins (globin) and non-proteins (haem). At the centre of the haem molecule is an atom of iron, and this is where the oxygen binds. This iron must be provided in the diet, but we also need healthy intestines to absorb it from our food, and it must be carried from the intestines to the bone marrow. Thus lack of iron, either in the diet or because of failure to absorb iron across the intestinal wall, can lead to a particular type of anaemia, called iron deficiency anaemia, where the red blood cells are smaller then usual.

Possibly more complex are the biochemical steps in the synthesis of DNA that rely on vitamins B_6 and B_{12}, and folate. The vitamins are required by metabolic enzymes. Folate is converted by the enzyme folic acid reductase to dihydrofolic acid, itself a root molecule for the production of a thymidine, ultimately a constituent of DNA. Failure of the bone marrow to be provided with enough of these micronutrients, either by a poor diet or by inadequate absorption across the gut wall, will lead to a particular type of anaemia, called megaloblastic anaemia, where the red blood cells become larger than usual. This complex process will be explained in Chapter 4, and the diseases that follow when the process is faulty will be described in Chapters 5 and 6.

Insufficient vitamin B_{12} or folate will, unlike insufficient iron, also lead to certain changes in white blood cells, and also other cells such as those of the nervous system. One of the principal white blood cell changes is that the nucleus of the neutrophil condenses into a larger number of lobes than usual (often five or more, compared with the normal three or four lobes). This is called hypersegmentation—and the cell that exhibits this is called a **hypersegmented neutrophil**. Most autoanalysers are unable to detect this change, but it can be seen on a blood film; yet another example where the skill of the Scientist comes into its own!

Cross references

Chapters 5 and 6 describe the many different types of anaemia.

Further details of the involvement of iron, folate, and vitamins B_6 and B_{12} in the synthesis of haemoglobin are presented in Chapter 4.

Key Points

The importance of trace amounts of micronutrients can be demonstrated by the marked abnormalities that accompany the deficiencies of iron and the B vitamins.

Plasma proteins

Once iron has been absorbed from the diet by the gastrointestinal tract and passes into the blood, it must be collected and moved to the bone marrow by a specialized blood protein, **transferrin**. Without this protein, free iron in the plasma may be excreted by the kidney, so that a lack of transferrin (possibly because of liver disease) may also lead to a deficiency of iron and, hence, anaemia. Iron is a valuable resource, and the body has developed a number of strategies to ensure it has enough stored up to guard against times of possible shortage. **Ferritin** is a specialized plasma protein that can collect and store many atoms of iron in organs such as the liver, spleen and bone marrow. There are also several other plasma proteins of interest to haematologists, such as the one which carries vitamin B_{12} from the intestines (where it is absorbed) to the cells where it is needed. This particular protein is called **transcobalamin**, and is found in three forms: transcobalamin I, and transcobalamin II.

The laboratory and haematinics

The study and measurement of haematinics is an area where haematology and biochemistry have shared interests. From the purely practical viewpoint, the measurement of 'haematology'

TABLE 2.6 **Key haematinics.**

Micronutrients	• Iron: low levels are present in some forms of anaemia. However, high levels may be dangerous and can lead to organ failure • Vitamin B_{12}, Vitamin B_6, and folate: low levels are present in some forms of anaemia.
Plasma proteins	• Ferritin: a molecule that stores iron. • Transferrin: a molecule that carries iron from the intestines to the bone marrow

plasma proteins and vitamins demands complex analysers and techniques, some of which are common to other proteins that many may see as being part of the 'biochemistry' profile. Consequently, the exact laboratory where these analyses take place varies from hospital to hospital because of the nature of the particular analyser. Furthermore, analysis of some vitamins is so complex that many smaller labs will find it more convenient to send their samples to a reference laboratory, which may be staffed by haematologists or biochemists.

Table 2.6 summarizes haematinics.

SELF-CHECK 2.13

What are the key haematinics?

2.9 **The reference range**

The purpose of the haematology laboratory is to facilitate the diagnosis and then confirm the effect (or lack of effect) of treatment. A key component of this is the need to know what we hope a blood result should be. This is the set of results we refer to, and hence the term, 'reference range'. We prefer this name to alternatives such as 'normal range' or 'range'.

The expression 'normal range' is inadequate simply because a result that is normal (that is, is present in a lot of individuals) in a population does not mean it is desirable. A good example of this is a low haemoglobin level that may be endemic in some parts of the world, possibly because of malnutrition, genetics, and parasites—none of which we would consider healthy. In addition, merely because someone appears healthy (that is, is asymptomatic), it does not automatically follow that their blood result is satisfactory, and vice versa. Similarly, 'target range' is not fully appropriate as it implies a level of a result that we are trying to achieve; this may never be possible in some individuals, resulting in disappointment and a sense of failure. However, there are cases where a target is a useful objective.

It is also worthwhile discussing where 'normal values' come from. Who is normal? Many of us have unsuspected asymptomatic diseases that may well impact on haematology. In the past, results from blood donors were considered to be representative of being 'normal', but we now recognize the shortcoming in this definition as blood donors are in fact highly motivated and health-aware individuals who are therefore, on the whole, 'healthier' than the general population. This is a classic example of selection bias.

It is important to note that reference ranges vary both from hospital to hospital and over time. The former is because different autoanalysers may well give a slightly different result on the same sample of blood. Furthermore, the reference range should serve the local population that the hospital serves, and local populations can vary a great deal. As we improve our knowledge of biomedical science it becomes clear that some reference ranges need to be changed. In the 1975 edition of a major practical textbook, the middle of the 'normal' range for MCV in the adult was given as 85 fL. In the 2001 edition, in the 'reference range and normal values' table, the mean MCV is given as 92 fL. In 1975 the reference range for neutrophils was 2.0–7.5 $\times$ 10^9/L, but in the 2001 edition the range is 2.0–7.0 $\times$ 10^9/L. It follows that in 1975 a result of 7.25 was considered to be within the 'normal' range, whereas 26 years later the same result is outside this range, and so may be described as a mild neutrophil leucocytosis. Whether or not this is actionable is another question.

A note on units. Not only do the units of blood tests vary around the world (such as total cholesterol being reported in mmol/L in the UK, as mg/L in the USA) but also in time. Historically, haemoglobin has been described as a percentage, but at present the many UK laboratories report haemoglobin in units of g/dL (as per Figure 2.16, that is 13.9 g/dL). However, the unit (dL, decilitre) is not fully part of the international system, which reports in terms of the litre (L). Hence the haemoglobin unit is transforming into g/L, so that the result of 13.9 g/dL simply becomes 139 g/L. In the present volume, the authors have decided to refer to levels of haemoglobin with units of g/L because it is now the internationally recommended format.

Interpretation

All routine haematology (and biochemistry) results sent out from the laboratory are accompanied by a reference range, which are a set of numbers enclosed by brackets (see Figure 2.16). In addition, the laboratory will often draw the reader's attention to those results that are considered to be out of range and therefore worthy of attention. There may be an asterisk or other flag along these results. Indeed, for this reason the reference range may also be considered a 'concern range'. This is because a result fractionally outside the reference range does not always carry a serious health hazard. However, the further a particular result is outside the reference range then the more seriously we must address the result as it may well be the consequence of actual disease, and so should be actioned.

The reference ranges for this volume are presented as Table 1 on page xvii.

SELF-CHECK 2.14

In your practice, why should you not use the reference values given in a textbook?

Key Points

Position statement

The Authors present a set of reference ranges that they consider appropriate. It does not follow that your particular laboratory is wrong merely because it has a different set of ranges. Each practitioner must work to their own local reference range, not to those presented in this volume. They are provided here for perspective and to allow for comparison in the various case studies and examples we will be presenting.

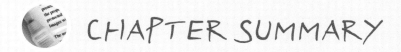

CHAPTER SUMMARY

- Anticoagulants are used to prevent blood from clotting. These include EDTA, tri-sodium citrate, and lithium heparin.

- Modern laboratories rely on an autoanalyser to provide the FBC, but the blood film is also an essential tool, especially to examine cell morphology.

- The full blood count comprises haemoglobin, the red blood cell count, haematocrit, three red cell indices (MCV, MCH, MCHC), the white blood cell count and differential, and the platelet count.

- Erythrocyte sedimentation rate and plasma viscosity provide information on physical characteristics of the blood (rheology).

- Haemostasis is the balanced orchestration of vascular integrity, primary and secondary haemostasis, regulatory mechanisms, and fibrinolysis. They maintain blood fluidity and limit and arrest bleeding upon vessel damage.

- Disorders of the different areas of haemostasis can lead to bleeding or thrombotic disorders.

- Blood coagulation disorders are first detected in the laboratory with the coagulation screening tests prothrombin time, activated partial thromboplastin time, thrombin time, and fibrinogen estimation. Particular result patterns inform subsequent diagnostic pathways.

- Crucial micronutrients include iron, vitamin B_{12}, and folate. Key plasma proteins include transferrin and ferritin. Together these are often described as haematinics.

- The reference range, generally composed of indices of thousands of presumed healthy individuals, provides an indication of the level of concern about a particular result.

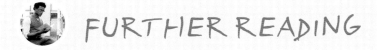

FURTHER READING

- Blann AD. *Routine Blood Results Explained*, 2nd edn. M&K Update, Keswick, 2007.

- Dale DC, Boxer L, Liles WC. The phagocytes: neutrophils and monocytes. *Blood* 2008:**112**;935–45.

- Hoffbrand AV, Pettit JE, Moss PAH. *Essential Haematology*, 4th edn. Blackwell, Oxford, 2001.

- Kern WF. *PDQ Haematology*. BC Decker, Hamilton, Ontario, 2002.

- Lewis SM, Bain BJ, Bates I (ed.). *Dacie and Lewis: Practical Haematology*, 9th edn. Churchill Livingstone, London, 2001.

Answers to self-check questions, case study questions, and discussion questions are provided in the book's Online Resource Centre, visit www.oxfordtextbooks.co.uk/orc/moore

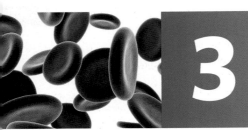

3

Haemopoiesis and the bone marrow

Andrew Blann

This chapter will outline the origin and development of blood cells, a process called **haemopoiesis**. Haemopoiesis describes the process of the maturation of blood cells—red blood cells, white blood cells, and platelets—as they progress from being precursor stem cells in the bone marrow to fully functioning mature cells found in the blood. Much of this knowledge has been obtained from the analysis of bone marrow itself.

Learning objectives

After studying this chapter you should confidently be able to:

- Explain the importance of effective haemopoiesis
- List the major components of bone marrow
- Describe the mechanisms of haemopoiesis and the importance of growth factors
- Explain the value of the analysis of bone marrow
- Comment on the uses of major cytochemical and flow cytometry methods in haematology

3.1 Overview of the cellular constituents of the blood

cytokines
Small hormone-like intercellular mediators with a diverse range of functions including the stimulation of the immune system in response to an encounter with a pathogen.

growth factors
Cytokines produced by one type of cell that initiate or promote the growth or differentiation of another cell.

Effective **haemopoiesis**, the process of the development of blood cells, is crucial to the health of the individual: it generates mature, functional blood cells that transport oxygen, defend us from infection, and participate in haemostasis. In adult life, haemopoiesis predominantly occurs in the **bone marrow**, the soft tissue within the centre of bones where blood cells develop. However, in exceptional circumstances (such as in certain pathological conditions) it may also happen in other tissues, including the liver, lymph nodes, and spleen. The situation is different in the foetus and the neonate, however, where it is normal for haemopoiesis to occur in the bone marrow, lymph nodes, liver, and spleen, as well as in the yolk sac of the embryo.

In a healthy individual, some $5-10 \times 10^{11}$ blood cells are produced by the bone marrow each day by a process that is highly balanced and regulated by **cytokines**, **growth factors**, and environmental factors, including the amount of oxygen in the body. Ideally, the number of cells produced each day exactly matches the number of cells that have come to the end of their life cycle thus maintaining a steady state. Irregularities in the production of blood cells can lead to disease. A thorough understanding of the structure and function of the bone marrow and haemopoiesis is necessary in order to grasp the concepts of these diseases, which include aplastic anaemia (where there is a reduction in cell production) and the **haemoproliferative disorders**, some of which are life-threatening. The most common haemoproliferative disorder is **leukaemia**, where often, an excess of blood cells is produced.

As indicated in the opening chapter, blood cells are relatively easy to classify into one of three types: red cells, white cells, and platelets. The mature cells that are present in the blood all have their origins in the bone marrow, which is the location of the **stem cells** that ultimately give rise to the mature cells found in blood. Red cells and white cells mature under the influence of **lineage-specific growth factors**, which act on only one set of cells and on no other (for example, on cells of the red cell series, but not on cells of the granulocyte series). In doing so, they pass through reasonably well-defined stages of maturity, beginning with blast stages, such as the **myeloblast** stage. Mature platelets are fragments of the cytoplasm of their own dedicated precursor, the megakaryocyte.

SELF-CHECK 3.1

Why do we need a good knowledge of haemopoiesis?

3.2 Ontogeny of haemopoiesis

Ontogeny effectively means 'where it takes place'. Haemopoiesis begins in the yolk sac of the embryo, but, after about a month, the liver and spleen slowly take over to become the dominant sites of blood cell production. Between the second and seventh months of gestation, the liver becomes the major site of haemopoiesis. The bone marrow begins to take over during the fifth to ninth months of gestation so that, at birth, it is normally the only place where haemopoiesis occurs. Infant haemopoiesis can occur in all bones. As the child develops, however, this falls back into the axial skeleton and proximal ends of the long bones, primarily the femur. In the adult, the major sites of haemopoiesis are the sternum and iliac crests; other sites include the skull, vertebrae and ribs (Figure 3.1). The importance of these locations will be clear in the study of haemoproliferative disorders, as will be explained in Chapter 5.

Haemopoiesis occurring within the bone marrow is termed **intramedullary**. By contrast, neonate and adult production at other sites (for example, in the liver, lymph node and spleen) is called **extramedullary haemopoiesis** ('outside the bone marrow'). In the adult, extramedullary haemopoiesis is present only in pathological conditions—for example, when the bone marrow becomes infiltrated with fibrous tissue (**myelofibrosis**), when there is chronic bleeding, in haemoglobinopathy, or when there is severe **haemolytic anaemia**. In these cases, the extension of haemopoiesis to sites beyond the bone marrow (the liver and spleen) is simply the body's response to a severe lack of functioning red blood cells and platelets.

SELF-CHECK 3.2

Where does haemopoiesis take place at different times in the development of the individual?

---

haemoproliferative disorder

A condition characterized by inappropriately increased numbers of circulating blood cells and their precursors.

myeloblast

A blast cell of the myeloid lineage.

Cross references

We discuss aplastic anaemia in more detail in Chapter 5.

Additional details of the importance of bone marrow and its analysis are presented in Chapter 10.

We present full details of leukaemia in Chapters 11 and 12.

Cross references

Myelofibrosis can also be a cause of anaemia, as discussed in Chapters 5 and 11.

Haemoglobinopathy, and its consequences, and different types of haemolytic anaemia will be discussed in Chapter 6.

haemolytic anaemia

The consequences of the premature destruction of red blood cells in the circulation and/or the spleen.

3.3 **Bone marrow architecture and cellularity**

The major structural function of bone is to provide support and pivot points for muscles, ligaments, and tendons; protection for delicate tissues (such as the brain and spinal cord); and physical support for body organs (liver, spleen, etc.). While many of these physical demands are met by virtue of the strength of bone as a hard and supportive connective tissue, many bones are 'hollow' and are extremely dynamic organs. Spaces within bone that are not there for structural reasons are host to haemopoietic tissues and the blood vessels and other supportive cells that serve them. Fat cells are very common, and a ratio of fat cells to haemopoietic cells of 1:1 is often found (although this varies with age). The complex microenvironment that ultimately gives rise to the blood cells can be seen as having three components:

- The haemopoietic tissues, sometimes described as cords, which consist of the stem cells and their progeny, the immature but developing blood cells such as myeloblasts and erythroblasts. More details of these are presented in the sections that follow.
- Sinuses—the vascular spaces or pools of blood that are lined with **endothelial cells** to regulate the release of mature and immature cells into the blood.
- Non-haemopoietic cells that support the bone marrow and often produce growth factors. These include:
  - stromal cells (such as **fibroblasts**) that produce the scaffolding (such as collagen) that supports other cells
  - **macrophages** that produce growth factors, promote red blood cell production (erythropoiesis), store iron, and perform routine debris removal
  - adipocytes that store energy in the form of fat

A close physical association of various cells is necessary to ensure the correct development of particular mature blood cells via cell–cell contact, with secretion and binding of growth factors.

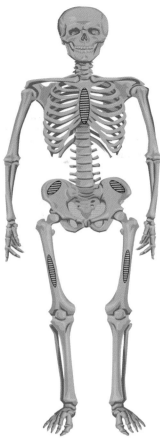

⊘ = major sites of physiological haemopoiesis (sternum, femurs, pelvis)

FIGURE 3.1

The skeleton showing major sites of haemopoiesis. The major sites of haemopoiesis in the adult are the sternum, femur and pelvis. Access to the latter is via the iliac crest. Minor sites include the ribs.

endothelial cell

A specialized cell that forms the internal lining of the blood vessels and sinuses.

Cross reference

Additional details of the importance of bone marrow and its analysis are presented in Chapters 9 and 10.

SELF-CHECK 3.3

What are the major types of cell within the bone marrow and what are their particular roles?

Key Points

Good production of blood cells requires not only the progenitor stem cells, but also a healthy bone marrow microenvironment that is composed of several different types of supporting cells. However, in certain circumstances, production of blood cells can occur outside the bone marrow in organs such as the liver and spleen.

3.4 **Models of differentiation, stem cells, and growth factors**

Blood cells pass through a series of well-defined stages of development and maturation, possibly in different compartments of the bone marrow. Haemopoiesis begins with a common primitive **pluripotent stem cell** (often also called the haemopoietic stem cell) that has the capacity to independently replicate, proliferate and differentiate into the various **lineage-specific stem cells** that will ultimately give rise to mature blood cells. These relationships are described in Figure 3.2. Pluripotent stem cells have a frequency of perhaps 1 per 1000–2000 marrow cells, and are impossible to recognize using normal morphological criteria (resembling, as they do, **lymphocytes**); most are in the resting stage of the cell cycle—stage G_0. However, stem cells (such as the myeloblast) can be recognized by the presence of a certain molecule (**CD34**) on their surface (although CD34 is also present on many non-stem cells). Nevertheless, an important practical aspect of the CD34 molecule is that it can be used to harvest stem cells from the peripheral blood as required for bone marrow transplantation.

lymphocyte

A small white blood cell with immunological properties, such as antibody production or the destruction of cells infected with viruses.

SELF-CHECK 3.4

What is the difference between a pluripotent stem cell and a unipotent stem cell?

Cross reference

The cell cycle is described in greater detail in Chapter 9.

Colony-forming units

Much of the current theory of the differentiation and development of blood cells is extrapolated from animal models and from tissue culture work in the laboratory where stem cells, also known as **colony-forming units** (CFUs), can be grown from samples of actual bone marrow cells. The CFU has and continues to be essential in our understanding of the different stages and pathways through which cells develop. These CFUs are presumed to be analogous to stem cells within the bone marrow.

Several different models of haemopoiesis exist. One of the current models is illustrated in Figure 3.2. This model first recognizes the haemangioblast, a stem cell from which develop endothelial cells and all blood cells. The stem cell that gives rise only to blood cells is called the pluripotent stem cell, which in turn gives rise to two stem-cell CFUs, each dedicated to particular cell lineages. One of these CFUs, often referred to as the common myeloid precursor, will ultimately give rise to **granulocytes**, **erythrocytes**, **monocytes**, and **megakaryocytes**, and so is abbreviated to CFU-GEMM. A second CFU, often described as the common lymphoid precursor, is dedicated to the production of **lymphocytes** alone, and as such is abbreviated to CFU-L.

The CFU-GEMM then gives rise to two additional stem cells, one progenitor specific for both the erythrocyte and the megakaryocyte (CFU-EMk), and another progenitor for granulocytes and monocytes (the CFU-GMo). The CFU-EMk then gives rise to lineage-specific erythroid (CFU-E) and megakaryocyte (CFU-Mk) stem cells, which ultimately produce the precursors and blasts specific for each mature cell, respectively, the red blood cell and the platelet.

The CFU-GMo gives rise to four lineage-specific CFUs, three dedicated to each of the granulocyte lineages (hence CFU-Eo for **eosinophils**, CFU-N for **neutrophils**, and CFU-Baso for **basophils**) and a CFU specific for **monocytes**—the CFU-Mo. The development pathway for lymphocytes is similar. The CFU-L arising from the haemopoietic stem cell gives rise directly to three lymphoid cells—the B lymphocyte, the natural killer (NK) cell, and the T lymphocyte. However, T lymphocytes must pass through the thymus to become fully functional. In parallel, B lymphocytes may also need to mature outside the bone marrow, but this has not been fully established.

This complex development of blood cells is driven and controlled by local growth factors and hormones, many of which are cytokines. These cytokines are produced by haemopoietic and non-haemopoietic cells both within the bone marrow and in other organs. Some growth factors act specifically on a single lineage of CFUs; others act broadly on CFUs for different classes of blood cell.

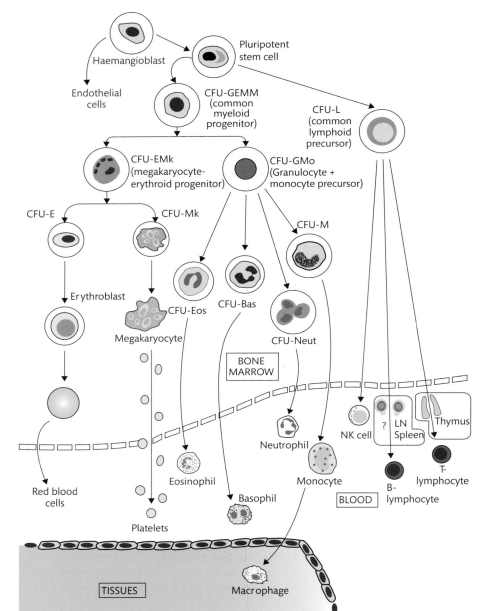

FIGURE 3.2

Cell lineages, haemopoiesis, and cell distribution. The different cell lineages give rise to immature and mature cells within the bone marrow. Mature cells pass from the bone marrow to the blood, and some then pass into the tissues. CFU = colony forming unit, GEMM = granulocyte, erythrocyte, monocyte, megakaryocyte. E = erythroid, Eos = eosinophil, Bas(o) = basophil, Neut = neutrophil, M = monocyte, NK = natural killer, LN = lymph node.

The blast cell

Whilst the CFU may be seen as a theoretical stage in haemopoiesis, and certainly can be defined in the research laboratory, a blast is a stage in development that can be identified in the bone marrow, and, in certain diseases, in the peripheral blood. In the adult, blast cells are almost exclusively found in the bone marrow because they are part of the normal and healthy process of haemopoiesis. In physiology, there are a number of different types of blast cells, and each has an additional qualifying name, which identifies the particular lineage of the mature

BOX 3.1 *Recognition of cells*

The primary tool in the identification of different classes of blood cells is the light microscope. Armed with standard stains (for example, **Romanowsky**) and specialized techniques (such as immunocytochemistry), various precursor and mature blood cells of the different cell lineages can be identified in samples of bone marrow that have been aspirated from a bone such as the sternum.

The ability to accurately recognize particular types of cell is a skill developed over years of patient observation. However, the development of new techniques, such as for intracellular granules, and for cell-surface molecules of the CD (cluster of differentiation) series, have greatly improved the reliability of cell identification.

The ability of the flow cytometer to accurately identify subpopulations of cells, such as those co-expressing a number of different CD molecules, has revolutionized cell analysis. A good example of this is the ability to detect cells that occur a low frequency (such as residual leukaemic cells), whose detection would not be possible by conventional light microscopy. These issues are expanded upon in Chapter 10.

Romanowsky

A type of stain specially developed to enable the examination and differentiation between different blood cells.

Cross references

We discuss granulocytes, eosinophils, basophils, neutrophils, monocytes, and lymphocytes in Chapters 2 and 8.

Lymphocytes are discussed in more detail in the *Immunology* volume in this series.

We discuss blasts and leukaemia in more detail in Chapters 8–12.

cell to which it belongs and the type of mature cell it will become upon release into the blood. For example:

- Myeloblast—a blast of the myeloid pathway
- Lymphoblast—blast of the lymphocyte pathway
- Erythroblast—blast of the erythrocyte (red blood cell) pathway

However, haemoproliferative diseases such as leukaemia and myeloma are characterized by abnormalities in haemopoiesis. An important aspect of leukaemia is the expansion of blasts (such as myeloblasts) from the bone marrow and the inappropriate appearance of increased numbers of these primitive cells in the peripheral circulation.

SELF-CHECK 3.5

What are the differences between CFUs, stem cells, and blast cells?

The role of growth factors

The bone marrow microenvironment is crucial for successful haemopoiesis: cells must be able to communicate directly with each other. However, there are also a host of crucial hormone-like molecules that can indirectly pass messages between cells. These cytokine growth factors—both proteins and glycoproteins—are essential for the developmental control of cells from stage to stage. They are released by one type of cell (such as a macrophage or a stromal cell) to act on different stem cells and blast cells to promote the process of cell development. For example, stem-cell factor SCF (also known by some as interleukin (IL) -11) is a ligand for the c-kit receptor, which in turn moves the cell along the cell-cycling pathway. These growth factors are listed in Table 3.1, and the role of growth factors in cell development is illustrated in Figure 3.3.

TABLE 3.1 Haemopoietic growth factors.

Interleukins (ILs)	• IL-1 stimulates production of GM-CSF, G-CSF, M-CSF, and IL-6 from a variety of cells within the bone marrow, including stromal cells. • IL-3, IL-4, and IL-6 act on early multipotential cells. • IL-5 is eosinophil CSF.
Colony stimulating factors (CSFs)	• Granulocyte CSF (G-CSF) stimulates the differentiation of granulocyte precursors (such as the myeloblast) and also the activity of mature granulocytes. • Granulocyte–macrophage CSF (GM-CSF) stimulates the differentiation and maturation of granulocytes and macrophages, and also the function of these cells once mature.
Other factors	• Stem cell factor acts on pluripotent stem cells, causing them to differentiate further, and also has effects on the later maturation of several cell lineages. • Erythropoietin is released mostly from the kidney and travels in the blood to the bone marrow where it acts on erythroid precursors to stimulate red blood cell production. • Thrombopoietin, produced principally by the liver, stimulates megakaryocyte maturation and thus platelet production. • Tumour necrosis factor (TNF) has actions similar to IL-1.

IL – interleukin; CSF – colony stimulating factor; TNF – tumour necrosis factor.

Molecules released by leucocytes that act on other leucocytes and non-leucocytes are **interleukins**, and some of these molecules may also have some non-growth factor activity, such as assisting in antibody production. However, in the present setting, the regulation of haemopoiesis is dominated by a series of **colony-stimulating factors** (CSFs, such as SCF mentioned in the previous paragraph) that act on various precursors, either generally or specifically. Growth factors may act on a single cell lineage at a single stage of its development, or on a series of cells at different stages of development. Further, growth factors may be autocrine (acting on cells of the same lineage), or paracrine (acting on cells of a different lineage). Thus various supporting cells within the bone marrow, such as fibroblasts, macrophages, endothelial cells, etc., and stem cells themselves, may both release and be acted on by various growth factors.

An important concept in cell biology is that of programmed cell death, or **apoptosis**. The basis of this process is that cells require the continual receipt of growth factor signals, effectively to keep them alive. Failure to receive these signals (or 'survival factors'), which include **erythropoietin**, triggers physiological changes within the cell. In the case of erythropoietin, the target cell would be a **normoblast**, and a lack of growth factor sets in motion a train of biochemical events that leads to the activity of certain enzymes (such as those of the caspase family), which in turn lead to the death of the cell. Consequently, apoptosis is sometimes considered to be 'cell suicide'. For many cells in the bone marrow, and elsewhere, growth factors are the crucial signal needed for the cell to remain viable.

Advances in biotechnology now allow the large-scale production of many of these growth factors, which have consequently become available as therapeutics for a variety of conditions. For example, patients with renal failure may become anaemic because their kidney fails to produce the erythropoietin required to stimulate the production of red blood cells. This growth factor can now be exogenously supplied as a therapeutic agent in particular cases of

erythropoietin

A growth factor, generally derived from the kidney, that promotes the development of red blood cells.

Cross reference

The full implications of apoptosis upon haematological cancer are described in Chapter 9.

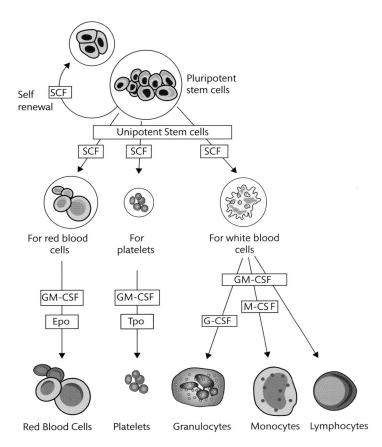

FIGURE 3.3

Simplified role of growth factors in haemopoiesis. Relationships between stem cells and their progeny, and their generation of mature blood cells. Note that GM-CSF can non-specifically stimulate the differentiation of all blood cells, whilst certain growth factors act specifically only on one particular lineage. SCF = stem cell factor, GM-CSF = granulocyte–monocyte colony stimulating factor, Epo = erythropoietin, Tpo = thrombopoietin, G-CSF = granulocyte colony-stimulating factor, M-CSF = monocyte colony-stimulating factor.

anaemia, and can facilitate a rise in the red cell count, which can rectify the anaemia. Similarly, **thrombopoietin** can be used to stimulate platelet production, and GM-CSF is used to stimulate neutrophil production. However, the most potent use of growth factors is in stimulating stem cell expansion *in vitro* and their subsequent use *in vivo* to aid bone marrow transplantation. Another use of these growth factors is to stimulate cell production in a bone marrow that has been suppressed by cancer chemotherapy or radiotherapy.

A further example of the promiscuous and complex nature of the growth factors is illustrated by the fact that G-CSF, GM-CSF, IL-6, M-CSF, and SCF all act on granulocyte colony formation. Furthermore, IL-6 also acts on non-haemopoietic cells such as hepatocytes, neuronal precursor cells, mesangial cells, and osteoclasts.

SELF-CHECK 3.6

What are the molecular signals that promote haemopoiesis?

3.5 Specific lineage haemopoiesis

Each mature blood cell is the end product of the well-regulated differentiation of stem cells and blast cells of a specific lineage, although, as we have noted in Figures 3.2 and 3.3, the initial stages are common to all cell types. Let us now go on to consider the development of the specific cell lines in more detail.

Erythrocyte production (**erythropoiesis**)

The earliest stem cell in the red cell pathway is the common myeloid precursor (the CFU-GEMM), although this cell can also give rise to other stem cells that are independent of red cells, such as granulocytes and monocytes (Figure 3.2). The CFU-GEMM gives rise to the megakaryocyte/erythroid precursor (CFU-EMk) which, in turn, produces the earliest recognizable red-cell lineage-specific stem cell, the CFU-E. From the CFU-E arises the earliest morphologically recognizable erythrocyte precursor, the proerythroblast. Further steps are marked by a steady reduction in the size of the particular blast cell through the normoblast (or **erythroblast**) stage, then the nucleated red blood cell. The cell then loses its nucleus entirely to become a **reticulocyte**. This juvenile red blood cell contains remnants of ribosomal ribonucleic acid which, when reacting with certain basic dyes such as new methylene blue, produces a blue or purple precipitate visible by light microscopy. Reticulocytes can also be numerated by flow cytometry, as fluorescent dyes such as auramine O and thiazole orange specifically bind to ribonucleic acid. The final step is the transformation of the reticulocyte into the mature red blood cell, a process that takes 3–4 days.

Thus the key steps in the development of the red blood cell from the blast cell to the fully functioning erythrocyte involve a slow and steady reduction in size, with loss of the nucleus. This process occurs in parallel with the development of **haemoglobin**, the oxygen-carrying protein within red blood cells, which becomes more and more prominent as the red cell approaches adult life as a mature cell. Several crucial steps in erythropoiesis depend on a red cell specific growth factor, erythropoietin. Additional details regarding erythropoiesis will be presented in Chapter 4.

Granulocyte production (**granulopoiesis**)

As we have discussed in Chapter 2, the granulocytes consist of three distinct cells—the neutrophil, the eosinophil, and the basophil, and each have different sets of **granules** in their cytoplasm. The precise make up of granules is important to the correct function of each of the three types of granulocytes, such as in the destruction of bacteria. Small numbers of granules may also be present in other white blood cells, such as monocytes and occasionally lymphocytes.

The development of granulocytes can be traced from the haemopoietic stem cell to the common myeloid progenitor (the CFU-GEMM). The CFU-GEMM then gives rise to four CFUs: one for basophils (i.e. CFU-Baso), a second for neutrophils (the CFU-Neut), a third for eosinophils (the CFU-Eos), and a fourth for monocytes (CFU-M) (Figure 3.2). From each of the three granulocyte CFUs (CFU-Neut, CFU-Eos, CFU-Baso) arise neutrophils, eosinophils, and basophils that are found in the blood.

The earliest identifiable neutrophil precursor cell to arise from the CFU-G that can be recognized by conventional light microscopy is the **myeloblast** (10–20 μm in diameter), which subsequently develops into the promyelocyte. As the latter differentiates into the

---

normoblast, or erythroblast

Blast of the erythrocyte (red blood cell) pathway.

reticulocyte

The final stage of the development of red blood cell before it reaches maturity.

Cross reference

Erythropoiesis is discussed further in Chapter 4.

granulopoiesis

The development of granulocytes.

granules

Small bodies within the cytoplasm of granulocytes that contain bioactive molecules such as enzymes.

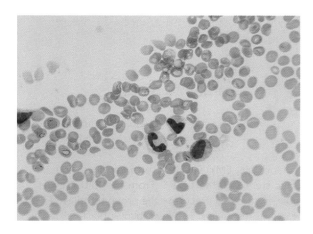

FIGURE 3.4

Metamyelocytes. These are the final 'immature' stage in the development of the neutrophil. The nucleus of the cell on the left has the typical 'stab' or 'band' morphology, the nucleus on the right has a 'kidney bean' shape. (Magnification ×400.)

myelocyte and then the **metamyelocyte** (with its kidney-bean shaped nucleus, often described as a stab cell), granules appear in larger numbers and become more prominent and dense. Figure 3.4 shows three metamyelocytes. The final step is the shrinking and lobulation of the nucleus, which marks the mature neutrophils. Figures 2.8 and 2.10 in Chapter 2 are examples of mature neutrophils. The entire process of granulopoiesis is shown in Figure 3.5.

The lineage-specific precursors of mature neutrophils, eosinophils, and basophils can be recognized at the myelocyte stage by the pattern and staining properties of their granules. These granules contain enzymes such as myeloperoxidase and collagenase, and other molecules such as heparin, lactoferrin, and histamine.

The final stages of cell development are the condensation of the nucleus into the distinct lobule pattern (generally 3–5 small lobes for the neutrophils, and 2 lobes for the eosinophil and basophil) and the presence of specific granules.

In the eosinophil, the granules stain deep-red with Romanowsky stains; by contrast, the granules of basophils are coloured black. Just as the dominant granulocyte in the blood is the neutrophil, the dominant metamyelocyte in the bone marrow is of the neutrophil lineage.

metamyelocyte

The final stage of the development of a granulocyte before it becomes a mature polymorphonuclear leucocyte.

Cross references

The full importance of granules will be developed in Chapter 8.

The three types of granulocytes (neutrophils, eosinophils, and basophils) are shown as Figures 2.10, 2.13, and 2.14 in Chapter 2.

BOX 3.2 Sex and the neutrophil

The sex of an individual is defined as the presence of two X chromosomes for females, and an X and a Y chromosome for males. An interesting characteristic of neutrophils is that, during the process of nuclear condensation, one of the two X chromosomes in females becomes fully condensed, so that it appears as a small 'dumb-bell' structure. This inactivated X chromosome, or Barr body, was so named following the work of Barr and Bertram in 1949. So although absence of a neutrophil Barr body does not prove male sex, its presence implies female sex. Now see if you can detect a Barr body in Figure 2.8. The neutrophil in Figure 2.10 does not have a Barr body.

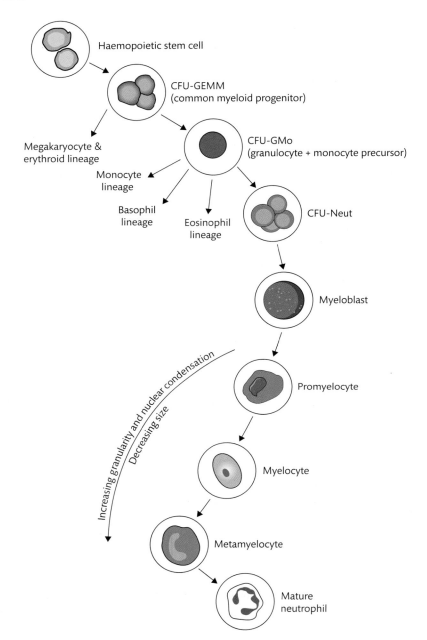

FIGURE 3.5

Neutrophil development. Stages in the development on the neutrophil within the bone marrow. Early stages involve the derivation of the lineage specific colony forming unit (CFU) for neutrophils from the multipotent stem cells (CFU-GEMM and the CFU-GMo). Later stages see the development of cells which, as they pass through the blast stage with developing maturity, form a multilobed nucleus and generate intracellular granules, many of which contain bacteriocidal enzymes.

However, it should theoretically be possible to identify both eosinophil metamyelocytes and basophil metamyelocytes in a sample of bone marrow.

SELF-CHECK 3.7

How can you distinguish between the three different types of granulocyte?

BOX 3.3 *Granules*

The three granulocytes are so named because of the presence of intracellular granules. The precise make-up of these enzymes is specific for each granulocyte.

Neutrophil granules include enzymes such as alkaline phosphatase, elastase, gelatinase, myeloperoxidase, lysozyme, and cathepsins. These granules also include the coagulation protein plasminogen.

Eosinophil granules include the enzyme peroxidase and a molecule called MBP, which has a relative molecular mass of 10 kDa. MBP can also cause the release of histamine from basophils

Basophil granules include histamine, heparin, hyaluronidase, and serotonin. These molecules may also be chemotactic for neutrophils and eosinophils.

Some of these granules, especially in the neutrophil, are important in the digestion of pathogens by the process of phagocytosis.

Cross reference
White blood cell granular contents are reviewed in depth in Chapter 8.

Platelet production (thrombopoiesis)

thrombopoiesis
The development of platelets (also known as thrombocytes).

The platelet's lineage-specific progenitor cell, the CFU-Mk, arises from the joint erythroid/megakaryocyte progenitor, the CFU-EMk, a cell which resembles a small lymphocyte. From the CFU-Mk, which expresses the CD34 membrane antigen, arises the **megakaryoblast**, and then the mature megakaryocyte, which is found in normal bone marrow at a frequency of about one in 2000 nucleated cells. Notably, some megakaryocytes leave the bone marrow and migrate to the lungs, which may provide an additional site for platelet production.

The megakaryocyte is so named not only because it is very large—the meaning of 'mega'—but because of its unique characteristic of carrying more than the usual numbers of chromosomes. All somatic cells of the body have 46 chromosomes, and are described as diploid (denoted 2N). By contrast, the non-somatic cells, the gametes (sperm and ova), have 23 chromosomes, and are described as being haploid (denoted N). However, megakaryocytes often have not merely 46 chromosomes (that is, are 2N), but possibly several multiples of this, such as 3N (with 69 chromosomes) or even higher. Indeed, the ploidy number for over half of the megakaryocyte population is 16N. This property of multiple sets of chromosomes is known as **polyploidy**. As a consequence, the megakaryocyte is very large and has a large and irregular nucleus, often with numerous lobes. This large number of chromosomes is achieved through the process of **endomitotic replication**, essentially mitosis without cytokinesis.

Cross reference
Chromosomal complement and ploids are further discussed in Chapter 9.

Developing megakaryocytes can also be identified by presence of major membrane glycoproteins on the surface of the cell, many of which are also present on mature platelets (Table 3.2). Megakaryocytes of 2–4N ploidy produce platelet peroxidase and von Willebrand factor but have no **alpha granules**, the intracellular organelles within mature platelets that contain molecules active in coagulation (Table 3.2).

Not surprisingly, the size of the megakaryocyte reflects the degree of ploidy—2N cells may have a diameter of 20 μm, whilst 64N cells may be as large as 56 μm. This is in contrast to the 'average' nucleated bone marrow cell which is likely to have a diameter of 14 μm and the red blood cell of 7–8 μm.

TABLE 3.2 Identification of megakaryocytes and platelets.

Membrane glycoproteins	Contents of the cytoplasm
CD41a (the gpIIb/IIIa complex, also known as $\alpha_{IIb}\beta_3$)	Alpha granules, dense granules, lysosomal vesicles
CD69P (P-selectin), CD41b (gpIIb), CD61 (gpIIIa)	von Willebrand factor, platelet factor 4, β-thromboglobulin
CD42a (gpIX), CD42b (gpIb), CD51 (αV)	Fibrinogen, coagulation factors V and VIII

N.B. there are different subpopulations of alpha granules: for example, some are rich in von Willebrand factor and poor in fibrinogen, whilst other granules have the opposite composition, being rich in fibrinogen but poor in von Willebrand factor.

thrombopoietin
A growth factor that stimulates megakaryocyte maturation and platelet production.

thrombocytopenia
Low numbers of platelets in the blood, often cited as less than 100 000 per mL.

The key growth factor for thrombopoiesis that mirrors the role of erythropoietin in erythropoiesis is **thrombopoietin**. This growth factor is produced by the liver and other organs (such as the kidney and bone marrow stromal cells) and is encoded for by a gene called *Tpo* on chromosome 3, which produces a protein of relative molecular mass 80–100 kDa. The growth factor itself 'switches on' its target cells—the megakaryocyte and its precursors such as the CFU-Mk—by interacting with a specific receptor coded for by a gene called *c-Mpl*. Thrombopoietin is required by the megakaryocyte to enable cell growth and the production of platelets, but it also acts on platelets themselves to stimulate their participation in coagulation. Indeed, the absence of either *c-Mpl* or *Tpo* results in very low numbers of platelets in the blood (**thrombocytopenia**) in mice, but also to reduced numbers of megakaryocytes and their precursors in the bone marrow. A similar abnormality in *c-Mpl*, which leads to the defective expression or function of the thrombopoietin receptor in our species, also leads to the very rare condition called congenital amegakaryocytic thrombocytopenia.

Thrombopoietin may also act on erythroid precursors, possibly because it shares a high degree of its amino acid sequence (structural homology) with erythropoietin. Plasma levels of thrombopoietin are in the order of 100 pg/L, but this can increase several fold in thrombocytopenia and aplastic anaemia, and in acute inflammation.

Platelets, which are generated at a rate of 10^{11} every day, are simply fragments of the cytoplasm of the megakaryocyte. How do these fragments arise? Pseudopodial projections of the cytoplasm called proplatelets break off and pass into the circulation. This process eventually consumes all of the cytoplasmic constituents of the megakaryocyte—the cytosol, granules, mitochondria, and other organelles, as well as coagulation molecules, etc. (Table 3.2). Hence after the production of perhaps 1500–4000 platelets nothing is left of the remainder of the megakaryocyte except its nucleus. The remnant of the megakaryocyte is eliminated by phagocytosis mediated by bone marrow macrophages, although apoptosis may also be involved.

During the final stage of proplatelet development, the intracellular contents of what will be the mature platelet are delivered by microtubules. The precise signal for shedding proplatelets from the megakaryocyte is unknown, but does not involve thrombopoietin.

The 'juvenile' platelet, like the 'juvenile' red blood cell (that is, the reticulocyte), has a slightly larger diameter and volume (2.0–4.0 μm and 8–11 fL, respectively) than the final mature platelet (diameter 1.5–3.5 μm, volume 6–9 fL). A further feature of juvenile platelets is that they also have intracellular inclusions such as messenger RNA, which can be specifically stained, allowing the 'reticulated platelet' to be detected.

Mature platelets can also bind thrombopoietin as they bear the thrombopoietin receptor, although their ability to detect this does not have a place in the routine laboratory. However, the binding of thrombopoietin enhances the secretion of alpha granules, and also promotes aggregation by agonists such as ADP, collagen, and thrombin.

Cross reference

The structure and function of platelets is described in Chapter 2, whilst the role of the platelet in coagulation is described in Chapter 13.

SELF-CHECK 3.8

What are the similarities between the juvenile form of red blood cells and platelets and their respective mature cells?

Monocyte production

Monocytes share a common stem cell with granulocytes (the CFU-GMo), but production of the mature cell passes to a more focused and dedicated lineage-specific precursor, the CFU-M, which produces only monocytes. At least two species of immature monocytes can be found in the bone marrow—the **monoblast**, which gives rise to the **promonocyte**. The mature monocyte develops from the promonocyte and passes from the bone marrow into the blood. After a period in the circulation (which can vary between hours and days), monocytes migrate into the tissues (such as the skin, the lung, the liver, the lymph nodes, and the spleen).

Once monocytes have arrived in the tissues, they differentiate into macrophages. Some then acquire additional properties, and transform further still into highly specialized cells, such as the Langerhans' cell (specific for the spleen), the Kupffer cell (specific for the liver), and antigen-presenting cells (most often found in lymph nodes, occasionally in the skin, and in association with lymphocytes). Granules are often to be found in the cytoplasm of both monocytes and macrophages. This is entirely possible because the monocyte shares a common stem cell with the granulocyte—the CFU-GMo (Figure 3.2).

Lymphocyte production

Cross reference

Additional details of monocytes and lymphocytes are presented in Chapter 8.

The common lymphoid progenitor stem cell (the CFU-L) arises directly from the pluripotent haemopoietic stem cell, and its development is independent of the other blood cells. CFU-L then gives rise to immature **lymphoblasts**, which then differentiate into the mature lymphocytes. Two *major* types of lymphocyte are recognized: B cell and T cells. The former synthesize antibodies and the latter cooperate in antibody production, but also recognize and destroy cells that are infected with viruses. A third lymphocyte, the NK (natural killer) cell is also recognized.

In mammals, the thymus is essential for the development of T lymphocytes, so much so that infants with the congenital disorder DiGeorge syndrome lack a thymus and also T lymphocytes. This is important because it leads to a condition known as **immunodeficiency**, whereby white blood cells fail to provide an adequate immunological response to a microbial pathogen such as a virus or bacterium. The same maturation process for B lymphocytes in birds requires the presence of the Bursa of Fabricius. This organ does not seem to have a mammalian equivalent, and it is assumed that immature B cells gain additional differentiating signals in the bone marrow, liver, lymph nodes, and possibly elsewhere. As is the case for the B lymphocyte, the site of maturation (if it exists) of the NK cell has also not been determined.

SELF-CHECK 3.9

Where do the different types of lymphocytes complete their maturation?

> *Key Points*
>
> The development of the different blood cells is complex, but certain patterns are present. All mature blood cells are the product of a slow and steady process of maturation that passes through progenitor stages and which relies on the presence of growth factors.

3.6 Bone marrow sampling and analysis

Knowledge of the interrelationships between different cells of the bone marrow is important in numerous diseases, such as aplastic and sideroblastic anaemia, and in myeloma, myelofibrosis, and leukaemia.

In the healthy adult, the number of white blood cell (that is, myeloid) precursors exceeds the number of red blood cell (that is, erythroid) precursors by a ratio of about 3–4 : 1. However, this myeloid/erythroid (M/E) ratio can vary with different diseases, as summarized in Table 3.3. For example, in leukaemia, the marrow will be dominated by leucocyte precursors such as myelocytes and metamyelocytes, so that the M/E ratio will be closer to 2. By the same principle, a bone marrow aspirate can also be used to examine the ratio between different types of white blood precursors. For example, the ratio of granulocyte precursors to lymphocyte precursors may vary between 1:1 and 17:1, especially in neoplastic diseases and in viral infections (when we expect more lymphocyte precursors) or bacterial infections (when we expect more neutrophil precursors).

In an anaemia related to lack of vitamin B_{12} we expect the presence of **megaloblasts**. Infiltration by metastatic tumours from a distant primary site such as lung, prostate, or breast

megaloblasts
Literally 'large blast cells' present in the bone marrow as a result of lack of vitamin B_{12}.

TABLE 3.3 **The myeloid/erythroid ratio. This ratio provides information on the relative numbers of white blood cells and their precursors compared to red blood cell precursors. In Health: At birth 2 : 1; 0–1 years raised, e.g. 7 : 1; 1–20 years generally 3 : 1; Adult between 3 : 1 and 4 : 1.**

M/E ratio increased	• Myeloid leukaemia • Most infections • Leukaemoid reactions • Depression of erythropoiesis (as in pure red cell aplasia) • Late myeloma
M/E ratio normal	• Myelosclerosis • Early myeloma • Aplastic anaemia (both myeloid and erythroid compartments are concurrently reduced)

M/E ratio reduced	• Myelopoiesis suppressed (perhaps by chemotherapy or viral infections
	• Erythropoiesis enhanced, as may be found:
	  − following severe blood loss
	  − in iron deficient anaemia
	  − in polycythaemia vera

carcinoma can be studied using a bone marrow aspirate. In both these cases the M/E ratio will generally be unaltered.

Thus the contents of the bone marrow provide an important opportunity to confirm or deny a diagnosis made on peripheral blood. In addition, sampling the bone marrow at different stages of a particular disease, such as after a round of chemotherapy, can tell us of the success (or not) of that procedure.

In practice, the only method of assessing haemopoiesis is to examine the contents of the bone marrow. A sample of bone marrow is obtained via the process of **bone marrow aspiration**. This can be achieved in one of two ways. The first is essentially an extension of the method for obtaining a peripheral blood sample from a vein on the inside of the elbow (venepuncture). In this case, however, a heavy-gauge needle is driven part of the way into the bone, such as the sternum or the iliac crest, to aspirate some marrow. The second method is to deliberately harvest bone tissue itself in the form of a **trephine** biopsy, which also provides a view of the internal architecture of the bone marrow. This process demands a considerably more robust needle. Both the aspirate and hephic require anaesthetic.

Once aspirated, bone marrow can be smeared onto a glass slide and stained in the same way as a sample of peripheral blood, for example by a Romanowsky stain. Once stained, bone marrow examination can provide useful information as to the relative proportions of the different types of cells in different stages of maturation (that is, the M/E ratio). Particular white blood cell precursors may be recognized by certain characteristics, such as the presence of prominent nucleoli in a myeloblast. Further, infiltrating cells, perhaps cancer, and even infections (by bacteria or fungi) can also be detected. Figure 3.6 shows a low-power magnification of a bone marrow aspiration. Compare the greatly increased density of the bone marrow aspiration with Figure 3.7, a low-power figure of peripheral blood, in which only two white blood cells are present.

Cross references

Additional details of the importance of bone marrow and its analysis are presented in Chapter 10.

Additional details of the consequences of a vitamin B_{12} deficiency are to be found in Chapter 5.

Aplastic anaemia, myeloma, myelofibrosis and leukaemia are described fully in Chapters 5 and 9–12.

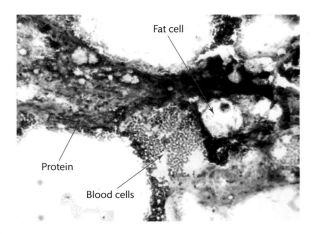

FIGURE 3.6

Bone marrow. This low-power photomicrograph shows a sample of bone marrow aspirate that has been spread on to a glass slide, dried in air, fixed and then stained with different dyes that are taken up by different cells and tissues. The figure is dominated by a central streak of blue and purple, with several unstained areas. These approximately circular patterns are fat cells that fail to take up any of the dyes. The blue dye has stained acellular protein material such as collagen, which provides physical support to the bone marrow. The other major colouration (purple) results from the uptake of other dyes by developing blood cells. Their approximate circular pattern is clearly visible, but the low-power magnification does not permit other analyses. (Magnification ×100.) © Institute of Biomedical Science (IBMS) and Sysmex Haematology Morphology training CDROM, 2009.

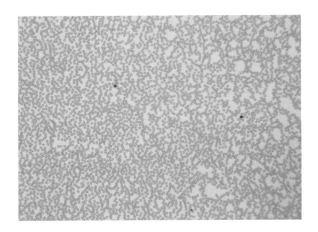

FIGURE 3.7

Peripheral blood. This shows a peripheral blood film at the same low-power magnification as the bone marrow aspiration in Figure 3.6. The two purple cells are possibly a neutrophil on the left and a monocyte on the right. (Magnification ×100.)

Cross references

The importance of bone marrow examination in diseases such as leukaemia will be developed in Chapter 10.

Aspects of the examination of tissues (cellular pathology, or histopathology) are described in the *Histopathology* volume in this series.

As a trephine biopsy provides actual bone, this tissue must be processed as if it was a piece of normal tissue, and will require decalcification before histological examination.

Much of our knowledge of growth factors such as erythropoietin has been obtained from tissue culture experiments. Bone marrow harvested from volunteers can be grown and characterized in tissue culture, and so can be used as a model for the effect of various CSFs on stem cells. For example, incubation of bone marrow with a certain highly purified cocktail of growth factors may well result in the growth or maturation of granulocytes, but not of monocytes. However, in this highly artificial *in-vitro* system, we cannot be sure if the events we witness are truly representative of the situation within our own bone marrow *in vivo* in either health or in disease. Nonetheless, the clinical provision of exogenous CSFs such as thrombopoietin as a specialized therapy to those with a failing bone marrow (as in cases of chemotherapy or following bone marrow transplantation) is of undoubted benefit.

SELF-CHECK 3.10

What are the principal reasons for examining the bone marrow?

SELF-CHECK 3.11

What are the main differences between bone marrow aspiration and the trephine sample?

Key Points

Analysis of the bone marrow is a complex process requiring expert interpretation, and as such provides essential information about the functioning of this organ.

Special investigations

There are two different types of special investigations that can provide crucial information regarding the pathology of different cells in the peripheral blood and also in the bone marrow. The first, **cytochemistry**, exploits the way that the components of the cytoplasm, and particularly granules, react with certain chemicals in a system akin to conventional haematological staining (such as with the Romanowsky stains). The second, **flow cytometry**, assesses cell populations according to the presence of different molecules on the surface of the cell, although it can be modified to look at molecules within the cytoplasm. This technique uses monoclonal antibodies to defined cell-surface glycoproteins such as CD34, a marker of stem cells.

Cytochemistry is a technique used to probe peripheral blood and bone marrow cells for the presence of different cytoplasmic enzymes and other chemicals, and has been developed and refined over decades. Cells are spread onto a glass slide, dried, and then subjected to various dyes, chemicals, and buffers. Cytochemistry can be used to study both red blood cells and white blood cells, although the focus is on the latter. Without doubt, the greatest use of these special stains is in the investigation of malignancies such as different leukaemias, which we will explore more fully in Chapter 10. The most common staining techniques include:

- Myeloperoxidase, an enzyme that is present most strongly in granulocytes and their pre-cursors, but may also be present in red cells and their precursors.
- Sudan black, which stains a component of the granules of granulocytes and monocytes, and so often provides the same information as does myeloperoxidase.
- Neutrophil alkaline phosphatase, an enzyme found predominantly in mature neutrophils.
- Acid phosphatase, an enzyme found in granulocytes, but which is generally used to define certain lymphocytic leukaemias in peripheral blood. However, in the bone marrow, mac-rophages and megakaryocytes are strongly positive. The use of acid phosphatase is one of the few methods that can be used to detect platelets.
- Periodic acid–Schiff (PAS), a stain used to stain glycogen and related polysaccharides. Although granulocyte precursors stain weakly, if at all, mature neutrophils show intense staining.
- The esterases, a family of enzymes that are generally used to investigate different leukaemias.

Abnormalities in red cell biology can be investigated using **Perls' stain**, which is also known as Prussian blue. This stain detects the presence of iron-containing molecules inside the cell and so, if found in a red cell, defines a **siderocyte**. The same stain when applied to a bone marrow aspirate can identify iron within red blood cell precursors such as **sideroblasts**—these are erythroblasts with inappropriate deposits of iron, and are associated with a particular type of anaemia. This stain is therefore important in identifying different types of anaemia, as will be discussed in more detail in Chapters 5 and 6.

SELF-CHECK 3.12

What are the most common cytochemical tests?

Flow cytometry, by contrast, is a much more recently developed technique. It relies on a complex analytical machine (the flow cytometer) and sophisticated reagents (monoclonal antibodies conjugated to a fluorochrome). Together, scientists use this machine and reagents to define different populations of cells in the peripheral blood and in the bone marrow. Different cells can be identified according to the presence of certain molecules on their surface, and hence cell populations can be quantified. As well as detecting cell-surface molecules, flow cytometry can also investigate molecules in the cytoplasm.

---

cytochemistry
A technique that uses chemical stains which react with cytoplasmic components and so define different cells in the blood and bone marrow.

flow cytometry
A technique that identifies blood and bone marrow cells according to the presence of different molecules on the cell surface or in the cytoplasm.

Cross references
Flow cytometry and cytochemistry are discussed further in Chapter 10.

Sideroblasts and siderocytes, and their places in anaemia, are presented in Chapter 5.

siderocyte
A red blood cell containing granules of non-haem iron complexed to other molecules.

sideroblasts
An erythroblast—therefore generally found in the bone marrow—containing granules of non-haem iron complexed to other molecules.

TABLE 3.4 CD molecules and the cell types on which they are found.

CD molecules	Cell type
CD2, CD3, and CD7	T lymphocytes
CD10, CD19, CD20, and CD22	B lymphocytes
CD13, CD33, and CD117	Myeloid cells
CD14	Monocytes
CD34	Haemopoietic precursors (stem cells)
CD45	All white blood cells

This list is certainly not intended to be specific nor exhaustive. CD = cluster of differentiation.

Like cytochemistry, flow cytometry is used most frequently by biomedical scientists to investigate different leukaemias. Most cell-surface molecules (and some intracellular molecules) are classified according to an internationally agreed system—the 'cluster of differentiation', abbreviated to CD. The most well-known molecules of this system, and the cells on which they are present, are shown in Table 3.4.

In practice, many laboratories will focus on a panel of only a few selected monoclonal antibodies that can be used to screen for the most common pathological conditions. However, care is required as the expression of a particular CD molecule may well be altered in diseases such as leukaemia. For example, the supposedly specific T-lymphocyte marker CD7 may be found on some granulocyte precursors in an acute myeloid leukaemia.

Cross reference

The importance of CD molecules for the investigation of leukaemia and other haematological neoplasia is presented in Chapters 10–12.

SELF-CHECK 3.13

Discuss the value of the common cell-surface markers used in flow cytometry.

Key Points

Special investigation such as flow cytometry and cytochemistry are useful tools for identifying different types of cells in both the bone marrow and in the peripheral blood.

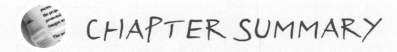

CHAPTER SUMMARY

- The production of blood cells occurs in a process called haemopoiesis.

- In the healthy adult, haemopoiesis occurs only in the bone marrow: in the neonate it may also occur in the liver and spleen.

- Haemopoietic tissue consists of stem cells and supportive tissue such as fibroblasts, macrophages, and endothelial cells.

- Haemopoiesis is driven by growth factors such as erythropoietin, interleukins, and thrombopoietin.

- Each major group of blood cell has its own specific haemopoietic pathway: erythropoiesis for red blood cells; thrombopoiesis for platelets; and granulopoiesis for granulocytes. Lymphocytes and monocytes also have their own specific pathways.

- Bone marrow aspiration is required to confirm diseases (such as myeloma) suspected of having an origin in this tissue, and to monitor the effect of treatment. In this respect the M/E ratio is useful.

- Special analyses include cytochemistry and flow cytometry. These are most often used to investigate different types of leukaemia.

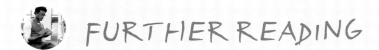 FURTHER READING

- **Ballmaier M, Germeshausen M.** Advances in the understanding of congenital amegakaryocytic thrombocytopenia. *British Journal of Haematology* 2009:**146**;3–16.

- **Deutsch VR, Tomer A.** Megakaryocyte development and platelet production. *British Journal of Haematology* 2006:**134**;453–66.

- **Italiano JR, Battinelli EM.** Selective sorting of alpha-granule proteins. *Journal of Thrombosis and Haemostasis* 2009:**7**(Suppl. 1):173–6.

- **Kaushansky K.** Historical review: megakaryocytopoiesis and thrombopoiesis. *Blood* 2008:**111**;981–6.

- **Metcalf D.** Haemopoietic cytokines. *Blood* 2008:**111**;485–91.

- **Orkin SH, Zon LI.** Haematopoiesis: An evolving paradigm for stem cell biology. *Cell* 2008:**132**;631–44.

- **Ottersbach K, Smith A, Wood A, Gottgens B.** Ontogeny of haematopoiesis: recent advances and open questions, *British Journal of Haematology* 2010:**148**;343–55.

Answers to self-check questions, case study questions, and discussion questions are provided in the book's Online Resource Centre, visit www.oxfordtextbooks.co.uk/orc/moore

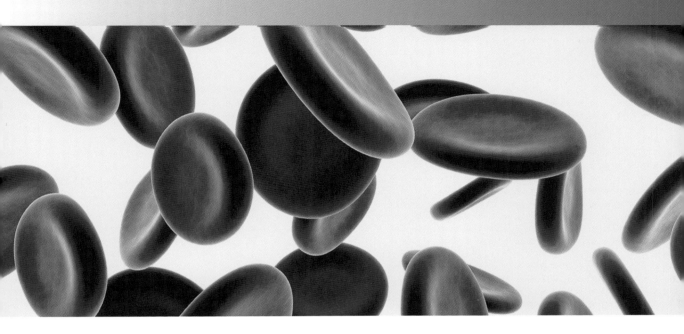

PART 2

Peripheral Blood Cells
in Health and Disease

4

The physiology of the red blood cell

Andrew Blann and Pam Holtom

Chapters 1 and 2 introduced some basic aspects of the red blood cell (also called an erythrocyte) and mentioned how it provides a number of major components of the full blood count (FBC), namely: the haemoglobin (Hb), the number of red blood cells (i.e. the red blood cell count, RBCC), the haematocrit (Hct), and the red cell indices. The latter include the mean cell volume (MCV), the mean cell haemoglobin (MCH), and the mean cell haemoglobin concentration (MCHC). Chapter 3 briefly described the development of the red blood cell. In the present chapter we go further to describe the structure and function of the red blood cell, and how it is adapted for its purpose of carrying oxygen. We will also consider the morphology of the cell, and interrelationships between size, shape, and colour. Once we have studied how the red cell operates in health (that is, the normal physiology of the cell), only then can we go on to study it in disease (that is, pathology). The principal disease associated with the red blood cell is anaemia, the diagnosis of which is impossible without knowledge of the haemoglobin concentration. We will address these complex conditions in Chapters 5 and 6.

Learning objectives

After studying this chapter you should confidently be able to:

- Explain how the red blood cell is adapted for its purpose.
- List the different types of haemoglobin and understand the relationship between their structure and function.
- Describe the structure of the red blood cell membrane.
- Discuss the importance of the red blood cell enzymes and metabolic intermediates.
- Identify major variations in the morphology of the red blood cell.

The red blood cell is one of the body's most highly specialized cells and this is manifested in numerous ways; for example its membrane is modified for the free and easy passage of oxygen both in and out of the cell. An additional consequence of specialization is that it has a relatively 'uncluttered' cytoplasm, with only those organelles and molecules directly required for its unique function, the carriage of oxygen by haemoglobin. The degree of specialization is so extreme that

TABLE 4.1 Relationship between structure and function of the red blood cell.

Feature	Advantage	Disadvantage
Uncomplicated cell membrane	Simple passage of oxygen	Fragile, so relatively susceptible to damage
Lack of a nucleus, enzymes	Flexibility to penetrate fine capillaries	Unable to synthesize essential protective and maintain membrane integrity
Membrane lacks HLA molecules	Relatively easy to transplant (that is, as a blood transfusion)	None (?)
All features	Highly specialized	Short lifespan (~120 days)

it has dispensed with the need for a nucleus. However, this modification comes at a price: the red blood cell is unable to regenerate itself or produce proteins as efficiently as nucleated cells. A consequence of this is a relatively short lifespan—often cited at 120 days for a healthy cell. These specialized features are summarized in Table 4.1. But before examining these specializations in detail, we will review how the red blood cell develops—the process of erythropoiesis.

4.1 The development of the red blood cell: erythropoiesis

As introduced in Chapter 3, almost all the development of the red blood cell occurs within the bone marrow. This process, called erythropoiesis, involves a series of steps that begin with multipotent stem cells (for instance, the CFU-GEMM), and moves via intermediate stages (such as the lineage-specific, colony-forming unit; CFU-E) to the **proerythroblast** (Figure 4.1). The largest of the red cell blasts (14–19 μm in diameter), the proerythroblast steadily shrinks through progressive cell divisions as it passes into the erythroblast (or normoblast) stage (10–15 μm diameter), where haemoglobin synthesis begins. The stage after the erythroblast/normoblast sees the emergence of the **nucleated red blood cell**, with a diameter of 9–12 μm. These stages are shown in Figures 4.1(a)-(d).

nucleated red blood cell
A stage in the development of the red blood cell when it still retains a nucleus and before it becomes a reticulocyte.

Several of these stages occur, in association with specialized bone marrow macrophages, in niches for erythropoiesis called **erythroblastic islands** (Figure 4.2). In the past it was believed that bone marrow macrophages were present simply to scavenge and phagocytose extruded nuclei. However, it is now becoming clear that the key role of the macrophage is to provide the cytokines and other signals that are crucial to the promotion of erythropoiesis. The close physical proximity of the macrophage, and its characteristic cytoplasmic protrusions, promote the maturation and proliferation of proerythroblasts and erythroblasts into more mature cells such as nucleated red blood cells, reticulocytes, and ultimately the red blood cell itself. This close proximity is promoted by the interaction of adhesion molecules on both cell types.

As erythroid maturation proceeds, the erythroblastic island migrates to regions of the bone marrow (the sinusoids) which are close to blood vessels, probably to facilitate the migration of reticulocytes and erythrocytes into the circulation. Erythroblastic islands are not bone marrow-specific: they have been noted in the embryonic yolk sac, fetal liver, and in the spleen. Despite this, it is still unclear whether or not the nurturing macrophages directly provide iron to the erythroblasts, or if the iron is collected by the erythroblast from the general plasmatic environment of the bone marrow.

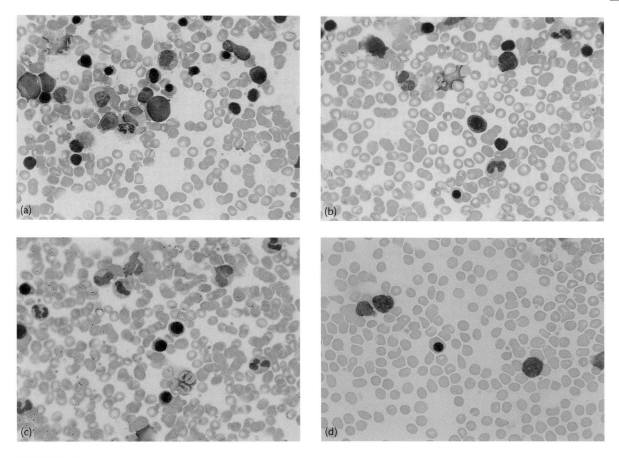

FIGURE 4.1

Erythroid precursors. As erythroid precursors develop in the bone marrow and transform into mature red blood cells they become progressively smaller and the cytoplasm loses its blue colour. The large cell in the centre of (a) is a proerythroblast, figures (b–d) show erythroblasts in the early, intermediate and large stages of differentiation respectively. (Magnification ×400.)

Erythropoietin

Much of the process of cell development described above is driven by growth factors such as stem cell factor and erythropoietin. The latter is an essential erythroid-specific factor for developing proerythroblasts and erythroblasts, which is also thought to influence CFU-E progenitor cell survival. Erythropoietin, with a relative molecular mass of 30–4 kDa (Daltons), interacts with its target cells via a specific structure embedded in the cell membrane—the erythropoietin receptor (EpoR). Upon binding of erythropoietin to its receptor, an intracellular signalling protein tyrosine kinase enzyme (**JAK2**) is activated. This sets in train a series of events that lead to the transcription of a number of genes, whose downstream effect is to promote cell proliferation and differentiation. We will revisit JAK2 in Chapters 6 and 11 as it is implicated in a certain red blood cell disease (**polycythaemia**) where the red blood cell count is raised, often markedly.

Erythropoietin is synthesized mainly by the peritubular interstitial cells of the kidney, often in response to low levels of oxygen (a condition known as hypoxia). Consequently, individuals with renal disease frequently have im-paired erythrocyte production, leading to low numbers

JAK2

An enzyme activated by the binding of erythropoietin to its receptor that ultimately results in cell proliferation and differentiation.

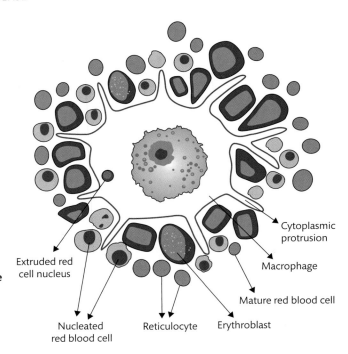

FIGURE 4.2

Eythroblastic islands. Erythropoiesis occurs in a defined microenvironment within the bone marrow—the erythroblastic island. Each centres on a macrophage which is surrounded by a ring, or crown, of developing erythroid cells. Cytoplasmic protrusions of the macrophage increase the effective cell membrane surface to allow more erythroid cells to be in contact with the macrophage. Within the macrophage, nuclei extruded from nucleated red blood cells are present, and are likely to be recycled.

of circulating red blood cells. However, erythropoietin is not the only growth factor to influence red blood cell production. The male sex hormone testosterone also acts as a red blood cell growth factor; this partially explains why men have more red blood cells and haemoglobin, and a higher haematocrit, than do women.

Fully functioning erythropoiesis also requires a host of minerals and vitamins, such as iron, cobalt, vitamin C, copper, vitamin E, vitamins B_6 and B_{12}, thiamine, and riboflavin, in addition to the thyroid hormone thyroxine. Anaemia may result from a deficiency of any of these micronutrients and hormones, as will be explored in Chapters 5 and 6.

The reticulocyte

The next step in the maturation of the red cell involves the loss of its nucleus, marking its transformation into the reticulocyte (diameter 7–10 μm and a volume of perhaps 150 fL). The loss of the nucleus is termed 'nuclear extrusion'. Much of the protein and nucleic acids within the nucleus are then recycled during the formation of new blasts and stem cells. The extruded nuclei express phosphatidyl serine on their surface, as do apoptotic cells, which may provide the signal to phagocytic macrophages.

The final step in erythropoiesis is the maturation of the reticulocyte into the mature erythrocyte, which then passes into the blood. However, some reticulocytes pass directly into the circulation for an additional 1 or 2 days, following which they differentiate into mature red blood cells with a diameter 7–8 μm and a volume generally between 80 and 100 fL (Figure 4.3). The reticulocyte can be differentiated from the mature erythrocyte not only by its slightly larger size, but also because it contains remnants of messenger RNA for haemoglobin, detectable by supra vital special stains such as brilliant cresyl blue. However, although reticulocytes generally cannot be specifically identified by conventional Romanowsky staining, a proportion do stain a slightly bluer colour than mature red blood cells. This bluish tinge is referred to as **polychromasia**.

polychromasia

A finding on the blood film that translates as 'many colours'. In practice, there will be red blood cells of a normal colour, but others (reticulocytes) with a blue tinge.

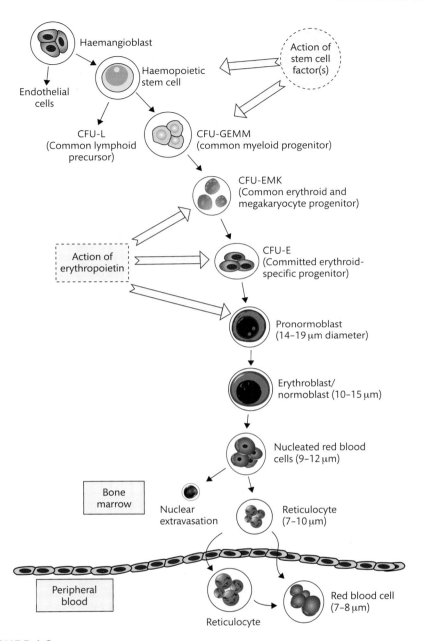

FIGURE 4.3

Erythropoiesis. Stages in the development of the mature red blood cell (erythrocyte) in the bone marrow and peripheral blood. A pathway of stem or precursor cells can be identified, commencing with the haemangioblast, and passing to various colony forming units (CFU) and ultimately to the mature cell. The 'early' stems such as the CFU-GEMM are stimulated primarily by stem cell growth factors, whereas 'late' stem cells such as the CFU-E are stimulated by erythropoietin. As this pathway proceeds, cells become smaller and as they do haemoglobin synthesis becomes more prominent. A crucial stage is the extravasation of the nucleus from the nucleated red blood cell as it becomes a reticulocyte. Some reticulocytes remain in the bone marrow where they mature into erythrocytes, although other reticulocytes pass from the bone marrow into the peripheral circulation where their own final maturation takes place.

As this final step in red cell maturation can take place in the peripheral blood as well as in the bone marrow, small numbers of reticulocytes (perhaps 0.5–1.5% of the entire red cell population) may be present in healthy blood. However, larger numbers of reticulocytes, perhaps greater than 2.5%, imply an abnormality, such as in certain types of anaemia, as will be described in Chapters 5 and 6. Similarly, nucleated red blood cells are seen so rarely in healthy adult blood that their presence is inevitably the result of a pathological process, although nucleated red blood cells may rarely be seen in healthy neonatal blood.

The regulation of erythropoiesis

The process of erythropoiesis is generally very tightly regulated to ensure the generation of approximately 5×10^{10} erythrocytes each day, enough to replace those cells destroyed by a particular disease process or simply by the cell's old age. However, this number may change: many diseases of the bone marrow, such as leukaemia, lead to a reduced production of red blood cells, and, consequently, anaemia. Increased numbers of red blood cells can also be produced by the bone marrow. When an increased red cell count is the response of the bone marrow to excessive red blood cell destruction, the increased count is said to be **erythrocytosis**. On the other hand, an increased red cell count due to a proliferative disease of the red cells is called polycythaemia. Unlike erythrocytosis, which is essentially the over-response of the bone marrow to external processes, polycythaemia is characterized by serious abnormalities in the stem cells within the bone marrow. It can also develop into diseases of white blood cells and platelets. Additional details of both these conditions will be presented in Chapter 6.

Cross reference

We discuss leukaemia in more detail in Chapters 10–12, and discuss erythrocytosis and polycythaemia in Chapters 6 and 11.

SELF-CHECK 4.1

How does the red cell differ from almost all other cells of the body, and how does this relate to function?

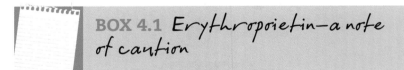

BOX 4.1 Erythropoietin—a note of caution

Until recently, erythropoietin was often considered a novel treatment for many different types of anaemia. However, this has been challenged as the indiscriminate use of erythropoietin may not be advisable, especially in patients with cancer and/or chronic kidney disease. One of the characteristics of cancer is that it is often associated with anaemia, so that it has been believed (quite reasonably) that such patients would benefit from treatment with erythropoietin. However, an additional characteristic of tumours is their reliance on, and extra sensitivity to, certain growth factors. It is now clear that certain cancers can respond to erythropoietin, which seems likely to explain (against expectation) an adverse effect of this growth factor on cancer survival rates, due mainly to tumour progression. Similarly, the presumption that the anaemia often associated with chronic kidney disease can be beneficially treated with (recombinant) erythropoietin has been challenged by a study which reported an increased risk of death in those using this hormone. Another study showed that, although erythropoietin did indeed increase levels of haemoglobin, and several indices of quality of life, there were safety issues connected with its use.

What are the principal differences between the reticulocyte and the mature red blood cell?

Key Points

Erythropoiesis is the process of the development of the red blood cell. Beginning in the bone marrow, immature stages include the erythroblast, the nucleated red blood cell, and the reticulocyte. The key growth factor is erythropoietin. Under-production of red cells leads to anaemia, while over-production leads to erythrocytosis and polycythaemia.

4.2 The red blood cell membrane

A complex cell membrane is required for a whole host of physiological functions, as may be carried out by such cells as the fibroblasts, lymphocytes, and smooth muscle cells. However, the red blood cell is so highly specialized for oxygen transport that it need not undertake many of the tasks of other cells. Principal among these specializations is the lack of a nucleus or other organelles such as mitochondria. So, relieved of the burden of the nucleus, the red cell has a physical flexibility or deformability that allows it to pass along the smallest capillaries and so deliver oxygen to the tissues. By contrast, a nucleus would severely restrict this freedom of movement. Indeed, the flexibility of the red blood cell is so highly developed that it can deform to an extent that its length increases by 250%, whereas an increase in surface area of only 3–4% is likely to lead to cell lysis. Furthermore, a normal 8-µm red blood cell can deform to pass through a 3-µm blood vessel lumen.

However, this high degree of specialization also brings disadvantages, such as a susceptibility to pathological factors and the extremes of physiology that would not normally be a problem for the membrane of a nucleated cell.

The red cell membrane has three components:

- A double layer consisting of equivalent amounts of phospholipids and cholesterol.
- Various proteins and glycoproteins embedded within the double phospholipid layer, but which may also have sections inside and/or on the exterior surface of the cell. The molecules which interface with the plasma are collectively called the glycocalyx.
- An internal cytoskeletal scaffold or skeleton that gives the red blood cell its characteristic round but flattened shape—a biconcave disc.

Perhaps 50% of the red cell membrane is protein, the remainder being fat (40%) and carbohydrates (10%); the general composition of the red cell membrane is illustrated in Figure 4.4(a). The lipoprotein bilayer is not symmetrical. Instead, the external layer is rich in phosphatidylcholine and sphingomyelin, whilst the internal layer is dominated by phosphatidylserine and phosphatidylethanolamine. Cholesterol is believed to be equally distributed. However, the phospholipids can move between the inner and outer membrane layers under the direction of different enzymes such as 'flippases', floppases', and 'scramblases'. The different proportions of lipids are important because macrophages, primarily in the spleen, are programmed to recognize and destroy (by the process of phagocytosis) those cells that have a high proportion of phosphatidylserine. The fluidity of the lipid component of the membrane is crucial in facilitating the lateral movements of floating 'rafts' made up of complexes of glycoproteins.

Within the lipid bilayer are embedded more than 50 glycoproteins at a frequency which varies from only a few hundred to over a million copies per cell. These have functions that include ion and gas transport and adhesion, whilst others are enzymes (Table 4.2). Principal among these

TABLE 4.2 Glycoprotein components of the red blood cell membrane.

Proteins with transport function	• Band 3 (CD233, the major anion transporter and central to gas exchange by exchanging the bicarbonate ion for the chloride ion, linked to blood group Diego. Also links the membrane to the cytoskeleton) • Aquaporin 1 (transporter of water, oxygen and carbon dioxide, linked to blood group Colton) • Aquaporin 3 (transporter of water and glycerol, linked to blood group Gill) • Glut -1 (glucose and L-dehydroascorbic acid transport) • Kidd antigen (urea transport) • RhAg (CD241, essential for the expression of rhesus (Rh) molecules, but is also a gas transporter, probably carbon dioxide and/or ammonia/the ammonium ion) • Rh complex (RhD [= CD240D], RhCcEe [= CD240 CE], possibly involved in ammonia/ammonium ion, and/or oxygen/carbon dioxide transport) • $Na^+/K^+/2Cl^-$ co-transporter • Na^+/K^+ co-transporter • Na^+/Cl^- co-transporter • K^+/Cl^- co-transporter
Enzymes	• Na^+/K^+ ATPase • Ca^{++} ATPase • Carbonic anhydrase (binds to a domain on Band 3) • Kell glycoprotein (CD238, a peptidase that cleaves big endothelin-1) • Acetylcholinesterase (associated with Yt blood group)* • 5'-nucleotidase* • Alkaline phosphatase* • Caeruloplasmin (involved in iron and copper transport and oxidation*
Proteins with adhesive, receptor or structural functions	• Intercellular adhesion molecule-4 (CD242, an integrin-binding protein, associated with blood group LW) • Lutheran glycoprotein (Lu, CD329, laminin-binding protein) • CD47 (part of the Band3/Rh complex, interacts with macrophages) • Duffy antigen receptor for chemokines (DARC)(CD234) • Complement component 3b/4b receptor (CD35) • CD151 (might associate with integrins and laminins) • Glycophorins A, B, C and D (CD235A, CD235B, CD236C and CD236D respectively, link the membrane to the internal cytoskeleton and may contribute to the glycocalyx. • Glycosyl phosphatidylinositol (an anchoring molecule) • CD59 (membrane inhibitor of reactive lysis – a complement regulatory protein)* • CD55 (decay accelerating factor – a complement regulatory protein)*

This table is not intended to be exhaustive. Note also that several of these molecules have CD designations between 233 and 242 (the 'red cell' area). Furthermore, many molecules may also be present on other cells such as those of the kidney (Band 3), white blood cells and platelets (glycosyl phosphatidylinositol) and the endothelium (DARC).

*These molecules are anchored to the membrane by glycosyl phosphatidylinositol. Many of these membrane molecules come together to form multi-molecular complexes (Figures 4.4a and b).

transmembrane glycoproteins are **Band 3**, **glycophorin A (GPA)**, **glycophorin C (GPC)**, and **Rh-associated glycoprotein ((RhAG)**, the function of many of which have been discovered (Table 4.2, which also lists other membrane components). The unusual names of these proteins (such as band 3) reflect the method of their discovery by techniques such as electrophoresis. GPA has a crucial presence on the outside of the cell as it is a structure from which the blood group structures A and B are presented. These A and B structures form the basis of the ABO blood group system and are important in blood transfusion.

The cell surface and cross-membrane molecules associate into two different groupings which interact with the major structural molecules inside the cell (**alpha- and beta-spectrins**) with, respectively, the Band 3/Rh macrocomplex and the 4.1R complex (Figures 4.4(b), (c)).

The interrelationships between the molecules of the cell membrane are crucial in giving the cell its flexibility and its unique double concave shape. Indeed, the normal biconcave discoid shape maintained by the spectin skeleton gives the cell a surface area 40% greater than a sphere of similar overall volume. Defects in these structural glycoproteins, some of which are genetic, give rise to changes in the shape and flexibility of the red blood cell. For example, lack of the glycophorins means that the cell cannot express other molecules, such as those of the ABO blood group system, on the outside of the cell membrane.

Many of these changes to the membrane of the red blood cell can lead to a particular pathological condition such as anaemia. We will revisit the consequences of defects in these membrane components in Chapter 6, one of which is due to problems with glycosyl phosphatidylinositol (GPI). An important 'housekeeping' function of the body is its ability to recognize and destroy abnormal cells using a complex series of plasma proteins called **complement**; red cells with these defects are detected and eliminated, potentially resulting in anaemia.

Notably, an additional feature of the membrane of the red blood cell is that it lacks **human leukocyte antigen (HLA)** molecules. These are highly specialized molecules, which are important in our defence against viruses—which is a good thing. However, their existence also frustrates our attempts to ensure viable organ transplantation, such as of the kidney. By contrast, red blood cells are far easier to transplant (for example, as a blood transfusion) than a solid organ such as the heart because of the absence of these HLA molecules.

A further consequence of the high degree of specialization of the red cell membrane is that it is far more fragile than the membranes of nucleated cells. One manifestation of this is a susceptibility to extremes of certain physiological conditions, such as pH and temperature, which are not a problem for nucleated cells. In the laboratory, the fragility of red blood cells can be assessed by their responses to different concentrations of sodium chloride in the osmotic fragility test.

A final important function of the red cell membrane is participation in the processes of maintaining the MCV at around 90 fL. The homeostasis of MCV depends upon the amount of water within the cell, which in turn involves the laws of osmosis. In order to maintain an MCHC of perhaps 330 g/L and retain flexibility, the red cell is dependent on the volume of water in the cell, and thus also on the balance between sodium (low levels relative to those of the plasma), potassium (high levels relative to those of the plasma), and calcium cations (which are normally undetectable in the cell). These must also be balanced by the sum of intracellular anions, principally chloride and bicarbonate.

The cell achieves a balance between these ions with a number of regulatory co-transporter molecules (also described as pumps, many of which require ATP), which collectively regulate the passage of water and these ions in and out of the cell (Table 4.2). However, if there is a shortage of ATP then the pumps may be unable to maintain the ionic homeostasis of the cell, leading to changes in cell shape and volume. For example, the consequences of an increase in the intracellular calcium for the cell are a loss of potassium and water leading to shape change, dehydration, less

Band 3, glycophorin A, glycophorin C, Rh-associated glycoprotein
Components of the membrane of the red cell that provide recognition, transport, and anchorage sites.

alpha- and beta-spectrin
The major structural components of the matrix that provide 'skeletal' support for the structure of the cell.

Cross references
Abnormalities in some of these components of the membrane and cytoskeleton lead to haemolytic anaemia, and will be discussed in Chapter 6.

We discuss the full importance of the Band 3, CD47, LW, alpha- and beta-spectrin surface and membrane molecules in the *Transfusion and Transplantation Science* title in this series.

Cross reference
The osmotic fragility test is described in Chapter 6, Section 6.3: Tests of a weakened membrane.

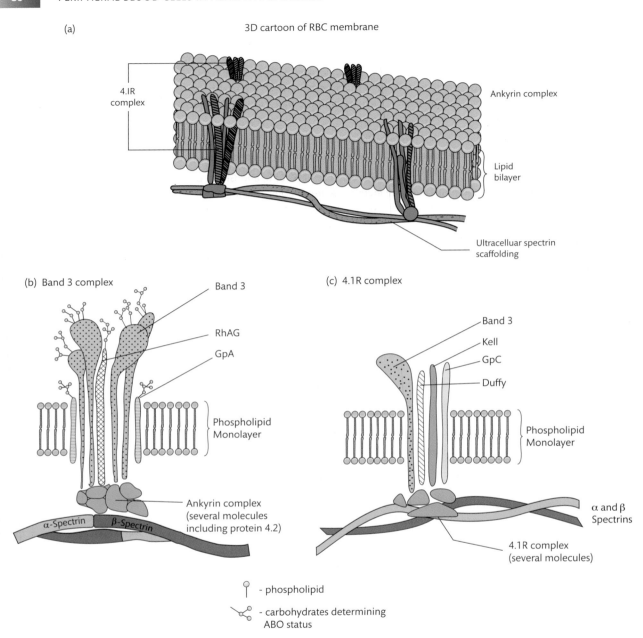

(a)   3D cartoon of RBC membrane

4.IR complex

Ankyrin complex

Lipid bilayer

Ultracelluar spectrin scaffolding

(b) Band 3 complex

Band 3

RhAG

GpA

Phospholipid Monolayer

Ankyrin complex (several molecules including protein 4.2)

α-Spectrin   β-Spectrin

(c) 4.1R complex

Band 3

Kell

GpC

Duffy

Phospholipid Monolayer

α and β Spectrins

4.1R complex (several molecules)

- phospholipid

- carbohydrates determining ABO status

FIGURE 4.4

The red cell membrane (see also box 4.2) (a) A schematic representation of the red cell membrane. (b) A representation of the ankyrin complex. Molecules such as RhAG, GPA, and Band 3 form a heterologous complex within the lipid bilayer. Some molecules span the membrane and interface with molecules of a sub-complex comprising protein 4.2, the enzyme aldolase, and ankyrin itself, which is in contact with the alpha and beta spectrins of the cytoskeleton. Not shown (for reasons of clarity) are molecules such as Rh C, D and E, LW, CD47, and GPB. (c) A representation of the 4.1R complex. This consists of molecules such as Duffy, Kell, Band 3, and GPC which span the membrane and link to a series of other molecules that collectively make up the 4.1R complex. This complex in turn links with other sections of the spectrin cytoskeleton that are apart from those complexed to the ankyrin complex. These cartoons are current representations and may be subject to re-interpretation, for new research on the structure and function of these molecules is often released. For example, some workers suggest Band 3 is a dimer in the Band 3/Rh macrocomplex, others suggest Band 3 is a tetramer.

BOX 4.2 The complex nature of the red cell membrane

A current model of the red cell membrane is of a diverse series of molecules (Table 4.2, Figs 4.4(b), (c)). These molecules cluster into two principal macromolecules—the ankyrin complex and 4.IR complex. These are named according to the molecules that anchor the cytoplasmic components to the intracellular cytoskeleton.

The 'ankyrin' complex consists of the Band 3, Rh, RhAG, CD47, LW, GPB, and GPA proteins, which together form a heterologous transmembrane supermolecule that contributes to the glycocalyx. Components of this complex span the membrane and in turn link with an intracellular subcomplex consisting of protein 4.2, the enzyme aldolase, and ankyrin itself within the cytoplasm. A notable component of this intracellular complex is the enzyme carbonic anhydrase. As this enzyme is involved in bicarbonate movement in and out of the red cell, it has been hypothesized that this macrocomplex has a role (or roles) in the passage of various ions across the membrane. However, the complex also forms a link to the major proteins alpha- and beta-spectrin, which make up the 'skeleton' of the red cell, suggesting a role in the shape of the red blood cell (Figure 4.4(b)). As ICAM-4 and CD47 have adhesive properties, they may be involved in an interaction with the endothelium of the capillary beds and so facilitate the exchange of oxygen and carbon dioxide.

The '4.1R' complex is a similar collection of other glycoproteins (including GPC, Kell, Duffy, and Glut-1), which link together with other molecules of Band 3 to form the extracellular component that also contributes to the glycocalyx. The intracellular parts of these molecules interact with a more comprehensive series of molecules that include dematin, adducin, P55, tropomysin, actin protofilament and tropomodulin, and 4.1R. Like the ankryin macrocomplex, the 4.1R complex also interacts with the internal skeleton of alpha- and beta-spectrin (Figure 4.4(c)). The structure/function aspect of this second complex are not as well developed as for the ankyrin macrocomplex, although there are some clues. For example, the Duffy molecule is a receptor for cytokines and Glut-1 is involved in the transport of glucose and I-dehydroascorbic acid.

deformability, and, ultimately, destruction in the spleen. This is the pathological basis of several other types of red cell defects that lead to anaemia, as will be explained in Chapters 5 and 6.

SELF-CHECK 4.3

What are the major components of the red blood cell membrane and what are their principal functions?

Key Points

The membrane of the red blood cell is unique. It needs to be relatively fragile to allow the free passage of oxygen and to enable the cell to deform and so flow along the finest capillaries. However, this high degree of specialization brings susceptibility to damaging factors that would not normally be a problem to the membrane of a nucleated cell.

4.3 The cytoplasm of the red blood cell

The function of the red blood cell is to transport oxygen. This is achieved by the highly specialized protein haemoglobin. However, while the transport of oxygen is essential to our survival, it is not without problems: high concentrations of oxygen within the cell can be toxic as it can form highly reactive chemical species (called free radicals), which can damage proteins, fats, and carbohydrates. Thus, the red cell must defend itself with antioxidants, principally using the complex amino acid **glutathione**.

glutathione
A metabolite that provides protection against toxic reactive oxygen species.

As the red cell has no mitochondria, it cannot use the oxygen it is carrying to generate energy. However, it can generate a limited amount of energy from the anaerobic (without oxygen) conversion of glucose to lactic acid.

Haemoglobin

As we have noted in Chapter 2, haemoglobin is an iron-containing protein synthesized by the blast cell precursors in the bone marrow, such as the erythroblast, that ultimately give rise to mature red blood cells. Each red cell contains approximately 640 million haemoglobin molecules. It is designed to absorb oxygen from areas of high oxygen content (that is, at the lungs) where it becomes **oxyhaemoglobin**, and then release it in areas were oxygen levels are low, which is likely to be the case in the body tissues. Emphasizing the importance of oxygen transport, haemoglobin molecules that are not carrying oxygen can often be described as **deoxyhaemoglobin**.

Cross reference
The minor subtypes of haemoglobin are also described in Chapter 2.

The structure of the haemoglobin molecule has two parts—a protein part (**globin**) and a complex non-protein part (**haem**). The haem group contains the iron and is where the oxygen is attached. The globin part consists of four individual subtypes of globin that come together to form a functional tetramer.

Haem

Haem is a complex molecule synthesized in the cytoplasm and mitochondria of developing red blood cell precursors (principally the erythroblasts and nucleated red blood cells). Several of the enzymatic reactions leading to the synthesis of haem require micronutrients that must be provided in the diet; these include iron, **vitamin B_{12}, vitamin B_6**, and **folate**. A shortage of iron is a common problem encountered in haematology and will be discussed shortly. Isolated vitamin B_6 deficiency is rare in the absence of certain drugs, which include the antituberculosis agent isoniazid, and pencillamine. However, deficiency of vitamin B_{12} and/or folate is relatively common and will be discussed in Chapter 5.

vitamin B_{12}, vitamin B_6, and folate
Micronutrients essential for erythropoiesis: their absence results in anaemia.

The initial step in the formation of haem is the synthesis of a protoporphyrin ring, an overview of which is given in Figure 4.5(a). The early steps in the mitochondria involve the carboxylation of propionyl-coenzyme A (propionyl-CoA, a three-carbon molecule and participant in the Krebs cycle) and so the formation of the four-carbon methylmalonic-CoA, often described as methylmalonic acid. The next step is an isomerization which results in the formation of succinyl-CoA. The enzyme which controls this reaction, methylmalonyl-CoA mutase, requires vitamin B_6 as a cofactor. Vitamin B_6 is also known as pyridoxine.

Succinyl-CoA and glycine, from the diet, are then converted into the five-carbon molecule aminolaevulinic acid (ALA) by the enzyme ALA synthase. This enzyme requires one of the forms of vitamin B_{12} (adenosylcobalamin) as a cofactor. A slightly different form of vitamin B_{12} (cyanocobalamin) is required for another essential metabolic step—that of the conversion of homocysteine and methyl-tetrahydrofolate (itself derived from dietary folate) into tetrahydro-folate (which is required for DNA synthesis) and methionine (needed for myelin synthesis and maintenance). We will revisit this metabolism in more detail in Chapter 5.

Later steps involve the generation of a series of complex metabolic intermediates in the cyto-plasm. Two molecules of laevulinic acid are dehydrated and condensed by the enzyme por-phobilinogen synthase to a ring structure of carbon and nitrogen atoms to form the pyrrole structure called porphobilinogen, itself the fundamental building block of haem.

Next, four porphobilinogen molecules are amalgamated to form hydroxymethylbilane, in which the ring structure is almost complete. Closure of this ring is effected with the forma-tion of uroporphyrinogen III. Subsequent steps are the conversion of uroporphyrinogen III to coproporphyrinogen III, which then moves into the mitochondria to become protopor-phyrinogen IX, and ultimately protoporphyrin IX. The final step is the action of the enzyme ferrochelatase, which controls the insertion of an atom of ferrous iron into the protoporphyrin ring to create haem. This pathway is summarized in Figure 4.5(b). However, the specificity of ferrochelatase for iron is not 100%, as it may also place an atom of zinc into the protopro-phyrin ring. (Zinc, like iron, is a divalent cation (that is, Zn^{2+}).) Thus, zinc protoporphyrin is an indirect marker of the levels of iron within the erythroblast: if levels of iron are low, zinc may be inserted instead. The next step is the folding of the globin molecules around the haem to give haemoglobin.

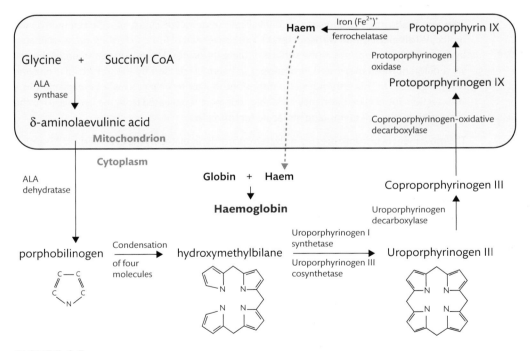

FIGURE 4.5
Biochemical steps in the formation of haem and haemoglobin. This process occurs in cells such as the erythroblast and nucleated red blood cell. Many of these steps occur in the mitochondria although the final assembly of haemoglobin takes place in the cytoplasm.

The synthesis of this protoporphyrin ring requires two important cofactors: vitamins B_6 and B_{12}. Lack of these micronutrients may result in defects in red blood cell maturation, as well as in other areas of metabolism. Furthermore, defects in the various enzymes responsible for the many complicated metabolic pathways in the synthesis of haem will also lead to red cell diseases, principally sideroblastic anaemia, megaloblastic anaemia, and porphyria, as will be discussed in Chapter 5. However, haem has important roles in other aspects of metabolism: it is present in myoglobin, in cytochrome, catalase and peroxidase enzymes, and has a place in tryptophan metabolism. Figure 4.6 shows the molecular structure of haem.

Cross reference

The importance of folate, vitamin B_6, and vitamin B_{12} as micronutrients, as demonstrated by their deficiency, is described in Chapter 5.

SELF-CHECK 4.4

Why are vitamins needed during erythropoiesis? Where in the red cell are they required?

Iron

The iron that is held at the centre of the porphyrin ring is the site in the haemoglobin molecule to which the molecule of oxygen reversibly binds. Like folate, vitamins B_6, and B_{12}, iron must also be provided in the diet. Absorption of iron from the diet, about 15 mg/day in the healthy adult, occurs in the duodenum and jejunum. Normally, only about 5–10% of dietary iron (that is, about 1–2 mg per day), is absorbed. The foods with the highest proportion of this mineral include liver, meat, eggs, and dried fruit. Iron already in the form of haem—as may be present in liver and meat, or in the ferrous (Fe^{2+}) state—is absorbed more rapidly than the other form of free inorganic iron found in vegetable matter, which is likely to be in the ferric (Fe^{3+}) state.

Free iron is absorbed by intestinal epithelial cells (enterocytes) via a specific cell membrane molecule (**divalent metal transporter-1**). The conversion of ferric to ferrous iron is facilitated by ferroreductase enzymes at the surface of the enterocytes. Haem appears to enter the cell via a different mechanism, and iron present in haem is released by the intracellular enzyme haemoxgenase-1. This enzyme is also important in iron recycling, as will be explained in a later section. Intracellular iron may be stored, but most is delivered from the cytoplasm to the circulation by the cell membrane molecule **ferroportin**.

divalent metal transporter-1, ferroportin, and hepcidin

Proteins involved in the absorption of iron and its delivery to the circulation.

The movement of iron into the plasma by ferroportin is regulated by the liver-derived 25-amino acid peptide **hepcidin**, coded for by the *HAMP* gene on chromosome 19. Interestingly, binding of the inflammatory cytokine interleukin-6 to its receptor on the hepatocyte cell membrane leads to a process that upregulates the transcription of *HAMP* and so the release of hepcidin. This hormone controls the expression of ferroportin, which in turn controls the

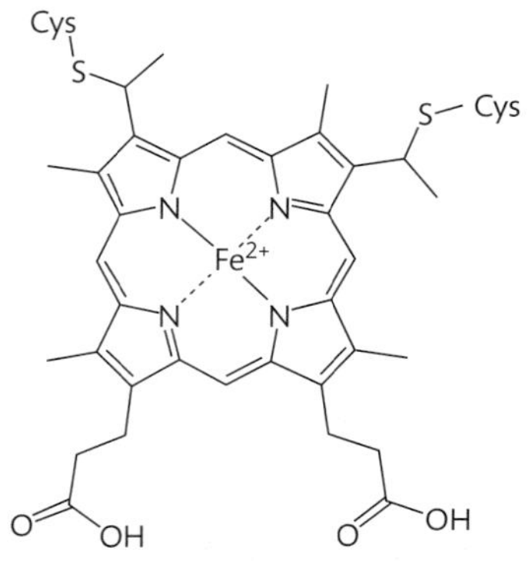

FIGURE 4.6

Molecular structure of haem. The atom of iron (Fe^{2+}) is held in place by four atoms of nitrogen. These atoms are in turn part of the complex porphyrin ring, which itself interacts with globin via two acid groups (-OOH) and two sulphur rich groups (-S-Cys).

export of iron from intestinal enterocytes, macrophages, Kupffer cells, hepatocytes, and placental cells. At the molecular level, when hepcidin binds to an extracellular aspect of ferroportin, the latter is internalized and degraded in lysosomes. A consequence of this is that iron is not moved out of the cell and into the bloodstream. So a feedback mechanism exists, which involves the enhanced release of hepcidin by a liver whose iron stores are full. Hepcidin also regulates the release of iron from macrophages by its inactivation of ferroportin. This regulatory system explains why the rate of absorption of iron is related to the demands of erythropoiesis (increased absorption when erythropoiesis is active) and of the amount of stored iron (increased absorption when stores are low). A raised hepcidin concentration is key to the development of anaemia of chronic disease (ACD) and its synthesis is also induced by bacterial infections as a protective mechanism.

Once in the circulation, free iron is collected from the intestinal cells by carrier proteins that are synthesized by the liver: these include albumin, lactoferrin, and **transferrin**. Although enterocytes preferentially absorb iron in the ferrous form, it is carried more efficiently in the ferric form. The copper-containing enzyme caeruloplasmin and membrane-bound ferro-oxidase enzymes convert ferrous iron to ferric iron to aid this transport. The most important of the carrier proteins is transferrin, a 76–80 kDa protein, which can carry two atoms of ferric iron. When free of iron it is called apotransferrin, and one gram of apotransferrin can carry 1.25 mg of iron. Transferrin delivers the iron to the bone marrow. The amount of iron being carried by transferrin can be a useful indication of the general iron status of the body, and levels can also be monitored as part of the clinical regulation of iron uptake. This is because the saturation (or binding status) of transferrin with high levels of iron will stimulate hepcidin release, which in turn will reduce the levels of iron passing from the intestines to the blood.

The iron–transferrin complex can only enter the developing red blood cell (such as the erythroblast) by binding to one of the 50 000 transferrin receptors on the surface of the cell. The **transferrin receptor** (TfR) can be shed from the surface of the erythroblast into the circulation, in which state it can be described as the soluble transferrin receptor (sTfR). Since levels of sTfR reflect levels of membrane-bound transferrin receptor, they may be used as a surrogate laboratory marker for increased activity of the erythroblasts and possibly of erythropoiesis itself. However, the transferrin receptor is also found on macrophages, rapidly dividing cells, and on activated lymphocytes.

Once inside the cell, ferrous iron is released from the transferrin molecule in response to a pH change, and the resulting apotransferrin is returned to the plasma from where it can travel back to the intestines to collect more iron. A second transferrin receptor, named TfR2, has been described and is present almost exclusively on liver cells. Its function has yet to be fully determined, but it could have a role in sensing iron levels and so may be a regulator of hepcidin.

Iron not channelled directly to the liver may instead be stored in organs such as the liver, pancreas, spleen, and bone marrow, in association with proteins **ferritin** and **haemosiderin**. Apoferritin, the form of ferritin that is free of iron, is a very large spherical molecule, with a relative molecular mass of 450–465 kDa. However, it can store up to 5000 atoms of ferric iron in the centre of the sphere, so that the mass of iron-replete ferritin may be increased by 35%. There is also evidence that ferritin supports iron absorption by cells of the intestinal enterocytes.

Haemosiderin is formed by the aggregation of partially digested ferritin, and is found in macrophages. Release of iron from haemosiderin is slow and therefore haemosiderin-complexed iron represents a long-term store that cannot readily be accessed. In this form it can be detected under light microscopy using a special stain, Perls' Prussian blue. This stain is particularly valuable in assessing iron stores in the bone marrow. Most body iron, generally 65% (the equivalent of maybe 3–4 g) is sequestered within haemoglobin, but a considerable proportion (approximately 30%) is stored in ferritin and haemosiderin. The remainder is in myoglobin (a form of globin present in muscles), in enzymes (such as cytochromes and catalase), and in complexes with transferrin. The passage of iron from the intestines, through the blood, to the cells is illustrated in Figure 4.7.

SELF-CHECK 4.5

Describe the process by which iron gets into the blood.

SELF-CHECK 4.6

Once absorbed, how does the iron get to the bone marrow and then into the developing red blood cell?

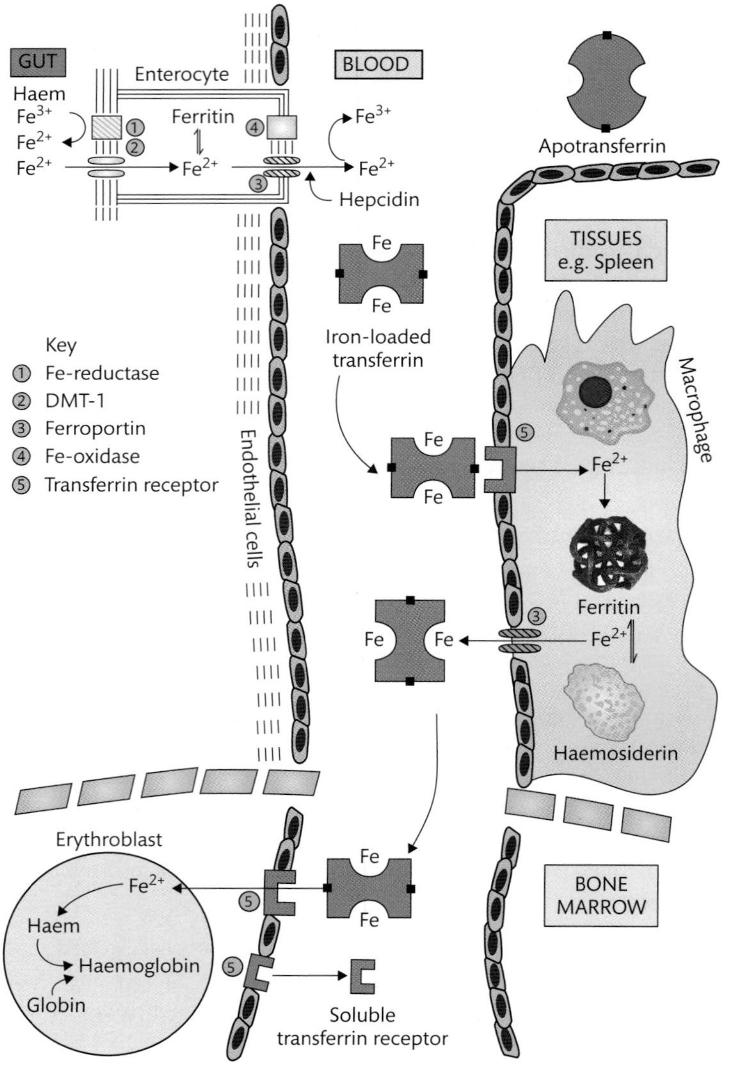

FIGURE 4.7

Iron: absorption, transport, storage and assimilation into haem. Iron must be provided in the diet, and is absorbed across the lumen of the intestines into enterocytes (top left). Some iron may be stored in ferritin, but most passes, via ferroportin, into the plasma. This process is regulated by hepcidin. Free ferric iron is collected by apotransferrin, and iron-loaded transferrin is carried in the blood to cells such as splenic macrophages (centre right) where ferrous iron may be stored in ferritin. Alternatively, transferrin may pass to the bone marrow (bottom right) where it is taken up by erythroblasts. The iron-loaded transferrin passes into cells via the transferrin receptor, which may be shed into the plasma as the soluble transferrin receptor.
Key: 1 = Fe-reductase, 2 = divalent metal ion transported (DMT) −1, 3 = ferroportin, 4 = Fe-oxidase, 5 = the transferrin receptor, Fe^{2+} = ferrous iron, Fe^{3+} = ferric iron.

> *Key Points*
>
> **The synthesis of haem relies on complex metabolic pathways. Key enzymes rely on vitamins as cofactors, so that deficiency of the micronutrients, as well as iron itself, can lead to the failure to produce a mature red blood cell and so to anaemia.**

Globin

Globin is a large globular protein with a relative molecule mass 16–17 kDa that exists in a number of slightly different forms. These subtypes of globin are coded for by different genes: two genes, for alpha- and a single zeta-globin gene, are on chromosomes 16; whilst the genes for epsilon-, beta-, delta-, and gamma-globin are on chromosome 11. These genes each produce specific messenger RNAs that in turn generate different types of globin protein molecules. For example, the alpha-globin chain contains 141 amino acids, whereas the beta-globin chain has 146 residues. The gene for gamma-globin has two subspecies, each coding for a globin molecule with slightly different amino acid compositions. The gamma-A gene produces a globin molecule with alanine at a certain position, whilst the globin molecule coded for by the gamma-G variant instead has glycine at that position. Synthesis of globin molecules in the cytoplasm for red blood cell precursors, such as the erythroblast and the nucleated red blood cell, occurs in parallel with the synthesis of haem: the two are then combined to form haemoglobin—commonly abbreviated to Hb.

The mature haemoglobin molecule is made up of four individual globin molecules, and so is called a **tetramer**—each single unit, or molecule of globin, is a monomer, and possesses one haem ring. Thus the entire molecule has a relative molecular mass of approximately 64–68 kDa. The different globin monomer molecules (alpha-, beta-, delta-, gamma-, etc.) all confer different oxygen-carrying properties on the mature haemoglobin tetramer at different times in the development of the individual.

The precise make up of the globin tetramer evolves from the embryo and fetus, via the neonate, to the adult, as illustrated in Figure 4.8. Embryonic haemoglobin exists for the first 12 weeks, and consists mostly of alpha-, zeta-, epsilon-, and gamma-globin chains—making up haemoglobins Portland, Gower I, and Gower II. (These three haemoglobins are made up of a 'mix' of the different globins, e.g. Portland Hb has two zeta- and two gamma-globin chains; see Figure 4.8.) Zeta chains are considered the embryonic equivalent of alpha chains. By contrast, fetal haemoglobin comprises alpha- and gamma-globin chains. The embryo and fetus is faced with the challenge of obtaining its oxygen not from its lungs but from the placenta, and thus ultimately from the maternal circulation. Hence embryonic, and subsequently fetal, haemoglobin must effectively take oxygen from the adult haemoglobin of the mother. It does this by having a considerably greater affinity for oxygen than does the maternal haemoglobin. The fetus and neonate face a similar challenge as it develops, which it partly solves by introducing delta-globin in the haemoglobin molecule in the place of gamma-globin. The major final switch from fetal to adult haemoglobin in the neonate occurs gradually some 3–6 months after birth as beta-globin slowly replaces delta- and gamma-globin when associating with alpha globin chains.

The dominant haemoglobin species in the adult, making up perhaps 96–98% of this protein, is HbA. This consists of two alpha-globin molecules and two beta-globin molecules. A minor form of HbA is HbA_2, which has two alpha-globin chains (as does HbA) but has two delta-globin chains in place of the beta-globin chains of the HbA. This second species

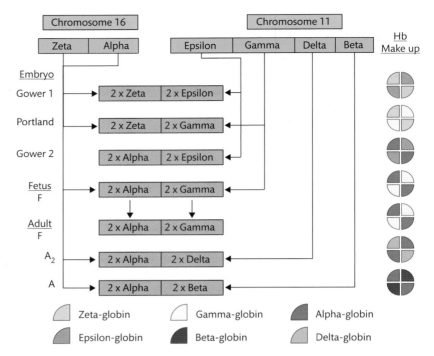

FIGURE 4.8

Ontogeny of haemoglobin. Changes in species of haemoglobin (Hb) in different stages of development. In the embryo, Gower 1 Hb is composed of two zeta-globin molecules and two epsilon-globin molecules. In Portland Hb the epsilon-globin is replaced by gamma-globin, whilst Gower 2 Hb is a tetramer of two alpha-globins and two episilon-globin molecules. In the fetus, fetal Hb consists of two alpha-globins and two gamma-globins. However, a trace of fetal Hb is present in the adult, where two other species are HbA$_2$ (a tetramer of two alpha-globins and two delta-globins) although the dominant species is HbA, consisting of two alpha-globin molecules and two beta-globin molecules.

makes up about 2% of all haemoglobin in the healthy adult. The remainder, HbF, comprises two alpha- and two gamma-globin chains, and makes up the remaining small fraction (less than 1%). Thus the healthy adult is still expressing genes that were most active in fetal and neonatal life. Notably, therefore, all adult haemoglobin consists of two alpha-globin molecules paired up with a second type of molecule, which can be either beta-, delta-, or gamma-globin.

Key Points

As the individual develops from embryo to fetus, neonate and adult, its oxygen sources and needs vary. Accordingly, the haemoglobin present at each of these steps also differs in order to maintain an optimum capture and carriage of oxygen.

Highly sophisticated techniques such as spectroscopy can detect several other minor species of haemoglobin. **Carboxyhaemoglobin**, **carbaminohaemoglobin**, **methaemoglobin**, and

sulphaemoglobin arise not from different genes for haemoglobin, but are caused by changes to haemoglobin once it has been synthesized and is within the red cell.

Carboxyhaemoglobin, which in normal subjects makes up a maximum of 2% of total haemoglobin, is formed by the attachment of carbon monoxide to haemoglobin. This attachment occurs at the same site of the haemoglobin molecule as oxygen, so that carbon monoxide effectively prevents the carriage of oxygen. This happens because the affinity of haemoglobin for carbon monoxide (that is, the readiness with which carbon monoxide binds) is over 200 times that of the affinity for oxygen, and results in decreased release of oxygen to the tissues. Increased levels of carboxyhaemoglobin are present in habitual tobacco smokers, where levels may rise to 5% of total haemoglobin. High levels of carboxyhaemoglobin can be reversed by hyperventilation with air, although this is quicker if pure oxygen is breathed. However, death occurs when levels of carboxyhaemoglobin exceed 80% of total haemoglobin, as may follow the prolonged inhalation of petrol engine exhaust.

The gaseous product of respiration is carbon dioxide, which must be transported from the tissues to the lung. A tiny fraction is carried in plasma as dissolved gas, but the greater proportion is carried in combination with water as bicarbonic acid, H_2CO_3. However, perhaps 10% of carbon dioxide is carried in a carbamino form, that is, as carbaminohaemoglobin.

Methaemoglobin is a variant of haemoglobin, characterized by the iron being in the oxidized ferric state instead of its usual reduced ferrous state. Methaemoglobin is continuously being formed in the red blood cell by metabolites of oxygen (oxidants), but it can be converted back to 'normal' haemoglobin or deoxyhaemoglobin. Under normal conditions, levels of methaemoglobin (which is essentially inert and does not carry oxygen) do not exceed 2% of the total haemoglobin pool. This is because oxygen does not bind to ferric iron. However, if the red blood cell lacks the ability to return the ferric iron of methaemoglobin to the ferrous state of haemoglobin, then levels of methaemoglobin will rise, and when such levels reach perhaps 10% of total haemoglobin, then clinical signs of headaches, breathing problems, and cyanosis can develop. Fortunately, both methylene blue and ascorbic acid can reverse high levels of methaemoglobin.

Sulphaemoglobin, an inert non-toxic form of haemoglobin, can be produced by the action of sulphur-containing drugs such as sulphonamides. In this form, oxygen can neither be carried nor delivered, and cyanosis results when levels are 3–5% of that of total haemoglobin. Unlike methaemoglobin, sulphaemoglobin cannot be converted back to haemoglobin.

As outlined in Chapter 2, the WHO recommended method for determining haemoglobin concentration can convert all but sulphaemoglobin to cyanmethaemoglobin.

Cross reference

Haemoglobin measurement was introduced in Chapter 2.

SELF-CHECK 4.7

What are the major types of globin proteins and how do they come together to form adult haemoglobin?

Red cell enzymes and metabolism

Whilst the major component of the cytoplasm is haemoglobin, there are also numerous enzymes with key roles in the physiology of the cell. These enzymes are also synthesized whilst the developing cell still retains a nucleus, that is, during the erythroblast and nucleated red blood cell stages in the bone marrow. They are mediators in metabolic pathways that generate ATP, provide defence from oxidants, and regulate the carriage of oxygen.

Metabolic pathways

As mature red blood cells lack mitochondria, they are unable to obtain energy by normal aerobic respiration (that is, obtaining energy by the use of oxygen). Energy is needed to enable the cell to maintain its shape and deformability, and to resist the toxicity of oxygen. However, the cell can obtain energy by anaerobic respiration (that is, obtaining energy in the absence of oxygen) by using the **Embden–Meyerhof glycolytic pathway**. The substrate for this pathway is glucose.

An early step in this pathway is the generation of glucose-6-phosphate. Most of the glucose-6-phosphate (perhaps 90%) proceeds along the glycolytic pathway to form two molecules of glyceraldehyde-3-phosphate. However, perhaps 10% of the glucose-6-phosphate is diverted to a subpathway, the pentose phosphate pathway, where an atom of hydrogen is transferred to NADP, to generate the hydrogen carrier NADPH. The glucose-6-phosphate is therefore transformed to 6-phosphogluconate, which can be further metabolized to phosphoglycerate. A further step involves the transfer of a hydrogen atom from glyceraldehyde-3-phosphate (which is converted to 1,3-diphosphoglycerate) to generate another hydrogen carrier (NADH). We will explain the importance of these hydrogen carriers shortly.

In many cells, such as those of the liver, 1,3-diphosphoglycerate is the substrate for enzymes that generate ATP, the product of which is phosphoenolpyruvate. A further step is the generation of additional ATP from phosphoenolpyruvate by the action of the enzyme **pyruvate kinase**. The final step in this pathway is conversion of pyruvate to lactate. However, the red blood cell has an abundance of an enzyme which can convert 1,3-diphosphoglycerate to **2,3-diphosphoglycerate (2,3-DPG)**, in the Rapoport–Luebering shunt. Although the synthesis of 2,3-DPG sacrifices the production of one molecule of ATP, it can be recycled back into the main metabolic pathway by other enzymes. (A more detailed discussion of the role of this 2,3-DPG will follow in a subsequent section on the carriage of oxygen by haemoglobin.)

Defence against oxidation

Apart from the enzymes involved in respiration, the red cell possesses a separate group of enzymes and other molecules designed to help protect it from the cytotoxic effect of oxygen and its metabolites, such as the **superoxide** radical. One of the principal protective systems is glutathione, a tripeptide of glutamine, cysteine, and glycine. In its reduced state, often denoted as GS-H, it is a buffer that can limit the potentially damaging effects of these reactive oxygen species within the cell by effectively donating hydrogen to the oxygen, so forming water. In this process, glutathione becomes oxidized, a state denoted by GS-, and with another molecule forms the dimer GS-SG. Alternatively, GS- can combine with a sulphur group on a bystanding protein (forming, for example, GS-S-protein). These oxidized glutathione species can then be converted back to reduced glutathione (GSH) by the enzyme glutathione reductase and the metabolic hydrogen donating intermediate, NADPH.

An important enzyme in the generation of this NADPH from glucose-6-phosphate and NADP is **glucose-6-phosphate dehydrogenase (G6PD)**. The substrate glucose-6-phosphate is converted into 6-phosphogluconate, which can be fed back into the metabolic pathway, or can move into another metabolic pathway. Therefore lack of G6PD leads to the impaired generation of NADPH, which in turns lead to a lack of GSH. Low levels of GSH leave the red blood cell open to the toxic effects of oxygen.

The interrelationships between these molecules and their metabolic pathways are summarized in Figure 4.9.

Embden-Meyerhof glycolytic pathway

A highly complex series of metabolic reactions whereby energy (in the form of ATP, NADH and NADPH) is generated from glucose.

pyruvate kinase

A metabolic enzyme of the glycolytic pathway involved in the generation of ATP.

2,3-diphosphoglycerate (2,3-DPG)

A red blood cell metabolite product of anaerobic respiration but which is also involved in oxygen carriage by haemoglobin.

superoxide

A toxic form of oxygen and powerful oxidizing agent that can attack and destroy many components of the red cell.

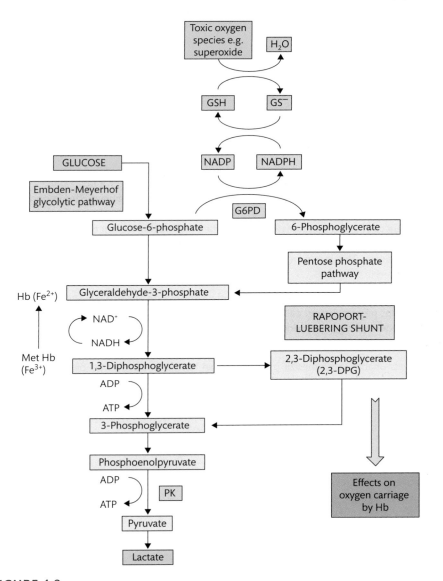

FIGURE 4.9

Biochemical pathways of the red blood cell. The major pathway for the anaerobic generation of energy (in the form of ATP, NADH and NADPH) is the Embden-Meyerhof glycolytic pathway (central spine). Glucose is first phosphorylated to glucose-6-phosphate (G6P) and is then converted to glyceraldehyde-3-phosphate. However, some G6P is converted via glucose-6-phosphate dehydrogenase (G6PD) to 6-phosphoglycerate. This pathway (top left) also generates NADPH from NAD, the former of which ultimately contributes, via glutathione, to the removal of toxic oxygen species. Further down the major pathway (mid-left), NADH is generated from NAD, which has the ability to convert methaemoglobin (Met-Hb) to haemoglobin (Hb). A subsequent pathway (mid-right) generates 2,3-DPG, which can influence oxygen transport by haemoglobin. Finally, the enzyme pyruvate kinase (PK) generates ATP from phosphoenolpyruvate, which results in pyruvate and ultimately lactate.

Key Points

The presence of oxygen is not always beneficial. Instead, it can cause cellular damage. The red blood cell protects itself with several molecules and metabolic pathways to contain these toxic oxygen effects. Loss of this protection leads to premature red cell destruction.

Clinical aspects of metabolism

There are numerous clinical consequences of errors in these pathways. The importance of G6PD is demonstrated by mutations in the gene that gives rise to the intact enzyme. The consequences of these mutations are twofold: the mutated G6PD is not only less efficient than the normal G6PD, but also has a shorter lifespan within the cell, giving rise to what is, in effect, G6PD deficiency. This is in turn manifested as a particular type of anaemia, details of which are presented in Chapter 6.

Other important antioxidant enzymes include **superoxide dismutase** and **catalase**. The former helps protect the red cell by converting oxygen radicals such as superoxide to hydrogen peroxide. Hydrogen peroxide is still toxic to the cell, but can be neutralized by the enzyme catalase, by glutathione, and by other molecules.

Individuals unable to synthesize pyruvate kinase have decreased levels of intracellular ATP, which leads to early destruction of the red cell and so to a different type of anaemia. Because pyruvate kinase effectively removes the metabolites of 2,3-DPG, a deficiency in pyruvate kinase activity may lead to an accumulation of 2,3-DPG in the cell, which could influence the way in which the haemoglobin molecule carries oxygen.

Cross reference

The consequences of the deficiencies of pyruvate kinase and G6PD (that is, anaemia) are explained in Chapter 6.

An additional example of the importance of these metabolic enzymes is in the conversion of methaemoglobin back to haemoglobin by NADH. Increased levels of methaemoglobin can be indicative of a deficiency in an enzyme that can use NADH to convert ferric iron to the ferrous iron of haemoglobin. Lack of this enzyme, NADH-linked methaemoglobin reductase, can be congenital and can lead to 10–20% of the total haemoglobin pool being methaemoglobin, a condition associated with mental handicap and cyanosis.

SELF-CHECK 4.8

What are the purposes of the metabolic pathways within the red blood cell?

SELF-CHECK 4.9

What are the dangers of oxygen within the cell? How do we describe dangerous oxygen-type molecules?

Oxygen transport and the oxygen dissociation curve

The physical and chemical properties of the haemoglobin molecule are such that it exhibits characteristic oxygen-binding properties. Haemoglobin (or, more accurately, deoxyhaemoglobin) needs to be able to pick up large amounts of oxygen at the lungs (where it is abundant) to become oxyhaemoglobin. The oxygen molecule is held in place by a complex non-covalent interaction with the atom of iron at the centre of the haem ring. Subsequently, the oxyhaemo-globin must be able to deliver this oxygen in those places where the gas is scarce (for example, in the tissues), whereupon it reverts to deoxyhaemoglobin. The key to understanding this process of uptake and release is the oxygen dissociation curve, a representation of the relationship between the amount of oxygen in the blood and the tissues, and the amount of oxygen carried by haemoglobin.

The amount of oxygen in the blood or tissues can be quantified in terms of partial pressure (denoted pO_2), which has the units of mmHg. At a high pO_2 (such as 90 mmHg) which we expect at the lungs, all the haemoglobin should be saturated with oxygen (so oxygen saturation is as close to 100% as is practicable). Each haemoglobin molecule can carry up to four molecules of oxygen, but the process of uptake is staggered. The uptake and binding of the first molecule of oxygen by deoxyhaemoglobin increases the affinity for the binding of the second molecule, a phenomenon called 'facilitation'. Similarly, once the first two oxygen molecules are bound, the uptake of the third and fourth molecules are increasingly easy. Indeed, the affinity of haemoglobin for the fourth molecule of oxygen is approximately 400 times that of the first.

This enhanced or cooperative uptake is called allosterism—an expression coined largely to explain the changes in the structure of an enzyme to facilitate an increase in its uptake of its ligand.

As the oxyhaemoglobin circulates from the lungs to the tissues, where oxygen levels are low (that is, a low pO_2 is present, such as 15 mmHg), the haemoglobin is forced by laws of chemistry to give up its oxygen, and so revert to deoxyhaemoglobin. This relationship between the uptake or release of oxygen and the amount of oxygen in the blood or tissues gives the oxygen dissociation curve its typical sigmoid shape which we can see in Figure 4.10.

A convenient measure of the ability of an individual person to carry oxygen is their P50. This is that particular partial pressure of oxygen at which 50% of their haemoglobin is oxygenated—that is, where there are equal proportions of oxyhaemoglobin and deoxyhaemoglobin. In health, this pO_2 is generally a little under 27 mmHg. However, this figure can vary with disease or other conditions, and is associated with a shift in the oxygen dissociation curve to the left or right.

- An increased P50 indicates a *shift to the right* and so a decreased affinity of the deoxy-haemoglobin for oxygen. In practice this means that it is more difficult for haemoglobin to bind oxygen, so that a larger pO_2 is required to maintain the 50% oxygen saturation. However, it also means that it is easier for oxyhaemoglobin to give up its oxygen to the tissues where it is needed, such as in cases of high metabolic activity.

- Conversely, if the P50 is low, we expect a *shift to the left* in the curve, which indicates increased affinity of the haemoglobin for oxygen and so a reduction in the amount of oxygen that is required to carry and maintain a 50% oxygen saturation. The practical consequences of this are that deoxyhaemoglobin can take up oxygen more easily, but that the oxyhaemoglobin is less willing to release it.

Factors influencing oxygen metabolism

Several factors influence the ability of haemoglobin to absorb and/or release oxygen. These can be explained in both left and right shifts in the oxygen dissociation curve.

Metabolic influences on the carriage of oxygen include the hydrogen ion concentration (as pH) inside the red cell. A decrease in pH (as occurs in acidosis) shifts the curve to the right, whilst

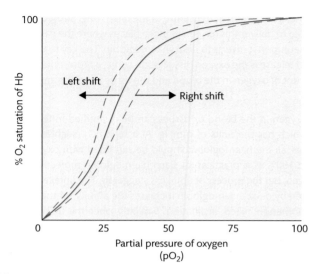

FIGURE 4.10

The oxygen dissociation curve. The normal relationship between the partial pressure of oxygen in the blood and the degree to which haemoglobin is saturated with oxygen is given by the solid line. It is convenient to refer to the degree of oxygen saturation where 50% of the haemoglobin is saturated (that is, the P50, where in theory each molecule of haemoglobin carries 2 molecules of oxygen from a maximum of 4 molecules). This equates to a partial pressure of oxygen (pO_2) of approximately 27 mmHg.

This particular partial pressure can be influenced by external factors which force the relationship between the P50 and the pO_2 to vary to the left (as in fetal haemoglobin, where the pO_2 may be, for example, 18 mmHg) or to the right (as in acidosis or high levels of 2,3-DPG, giving a pO_2 of maybe 40 mmHg)—hence the left shift and right shift.

an increase in pH (as in alkalosis) causes a left shift. However, this effect may be influenced by carbon dioxide and the subsequent formation of the bicarbonate anion and a proton. This is important in, for example, exercising muscles, as the metabolic effects of this exercise, which generate high levels of carbon dioxide and hydrogen ions, and hence low pH, act to shift the oxygen dissociation curve to the right so that for a given pO_2, more oxygen is released to the tissues.

Conversely, in the lungs, levels of carbon dioxide and hydrogen ions are both low, so the pH is high. This shifts the curve to the left so that more oxygen is absorbed by the deoxyhaemoglobin. An exercising muscle is also generally associated with increased local temperature and the generation of protons, the latter resulting in a low pH. These conditions act to move the curve to the right to enable the release of oxygen to that muscle. At the lungs, where ambient air temperature (which on a cool day may be 10°C) is generally lower than the body temperature of 37°C, a decrease in temperature shifts the curve to the left, enabling oxygen uptake.

In a preceding section we briefly examined 2,3-diphosphoglycerate (2,3-DPG), a metabolic product of anaerobic respiration in the glycolytic pathway (Figure 4.9). In the red cell, 2,3-DPG is generally present at a similar molar concentration as haemoglobin and can influence the ability of the haemoglobin molecule to carry oxygen. It binds to a specific site between the beta-globin molecules, separate from the oxygen-binding site, when the entire molecule is deoxygenated. In practice this means that high levels of 2,3-DPG shift the oxygen dissociation curve to the right, and so are associated with a reduced oxygen affinity. Conversely, low levels of 2,3-DPG favour oxygen carriage as the curve will be shifted to the left. This happens because 2,3-DPG has a greater binding affinity for deoxyhaemoglobin than it does for oxyhaemoglobin. When oxygen is given up to the tissues, which are at low oxygen tension, 2,3-DPG gains access to the sites in the haemoglobin molecule that carry oxygen and prevents reuptake of oxygen by haemoglobin in these tissues.

As we have already noted, a small amount of carbon dioxide may combine with haemoglobin to form carbaminohaemoglobin, which is associated with a leftward shift in the curve. However, carbon monoxide has a far more powerful effect, as it is bound by haemoglobin far more avidly than is oxygen, and in high concentrations also causes a left shift in the curve. The same leftwards shift is also seen in the presence of high levels of methaemoglobin.

Fetal haemoglobin is a complex of two alpha-globin and two gamma-globin molecules, whereas adult haemoglobin is composed of two alpha-globin and two beta-globin molecules (HbA) and two alpha-globin with two delta-globin molecules (HbA_2). The fetus survives in the uterus because fetal haemoglobin has an oxygen dissociation curve to the left relative to the maternal adult haemoglobin. The P50 of fetal haemoglobin is about 18 mmHg compared to about 27 mmHg in 'adult' haemoglobin. In practice, this means that it is easier for fetal haemoglobin to take up oxygen than it is for adult haemoglobin. This difference enhances the placental uptake of oxygen from the maternal circulation.

In addition, the placental microenvironment is associated with a high concentration of 2,3-DPG, assisting the release of oxygen from adult oxyhaemoglobin. The gamma-globin chains of fetal haemoglobin do not bind 2,3-DPG, so this metabolite does not promote oxygen release by the fetal oxyhaemoglobin.

It is therefore clear that the biochemistry of oxygen uptake by deoxyhaemoglobin and release by oxyhaemoglobin is complex and is influenced by several factors, some of which may be competing. However, these factors are not present in isolation but act together. In the tissues, the local pH, CO_2, 2,3-DPG, and temperature all act in concert to promote the release of oxygen. At the lungs the reverse is true as CO_2 is expelled and oxygen taken up. These effects are summarized in Table 4.3.

TABLE 4.3 **Factors influencing the oxygen dissociation curve.**

Physiological effect	Left shift	Right shift
O_2	Increases O_2 affinity, easier for Hb to bind O_2, harder for Hb to release O_2	Decreases O_2 affinity, harder for Hb to bind O_2, easier for Hb to release O_2
pH	High pH (alkalosis)	Low pH (acidosis)
Temperature	Low	High
Carbon dioxide	Low	High
Carbon monoxide	High	Low
2,3-DPG	Low	High
Haemoglobin	Fetal	(−)

2,3-DPG: 2,3-diphosphoglycerate. Hb: haemoglobin.

What is the significance of the left and right shift in the oxygen dissociation curve?

Key Points

The complex mechanics of the oxygen dissociation curve explain how haemoglobin can collect oxygen when local levels are high (as in the lungs), but can then release it when local levels are low (as in the tissues).

4.4 The death of the red cell

At the end of its 4-month lifespan, the red cell is destroyed and much of it is recycled. As the red cell has no DNA or ribosomes, it is unable to generate new enzyme molecules, such as G6PD and pyruvate kinase, and an important reason for the death of the cell is that these enzymes are eventually depleted. A consequence of this gradual depletion of enzymes is the loss of shape and flexibility, changes that are noted by phagocytic cells of the **reticuloendothelial system**, such as macrophages in the spleen. These cells then destroy the senescent red cells. As we shall see in Chapter 6, early and/or inappropriate loss of enzymes such as G6PD can also lead to premature red cell destruction and may therefore lead to anaemia.

The process that leads to the destruction of red blood cells, or to shortening of their lifespan of 120 days, is called **haemolysis**. When this process occurs in cells of organs such as the spleen and liver it is described as **extravascular haemolysis** (literally, haemolysis outside the blood vessels). When it happens within the circulation it is called **intravascular haemolysis** (haemolysis inside the blood vessels). Most of this red blood cell recycling (90%) is extravascular; the remaining 10% is intravascular.

When the haemoglobin molecule is degraded, possibly within phagocytic cells such as macrophages, all the proteins, lipids, and iron are recycled. However, the protoporphyrin ring from the haem molecule is too complex to be recycled, and is broken down to iron, carbon monoxide, and **biliverdin** by the enzyme **haemoxygenase**. This enzyme is also responsible for liberating iron from dietary haem absorbed by the enterocytes of the small intestine. The biliverdin is then converted to **bilirubin**, the major breakdown product of haem. The iron either complexes with ferritin, and may be converted to haemosiderin (if extravascular, such as in macrophages), or complexes with transferrin (if intravascular). Haemoxygenase may also be linked to other aspects of iron metabolism such as ferroportin. Furthermore, a patient deficient in haemoxygenase also has low hepcidin levels and high levels of the soluble transferrin receptor.

Most of the bilirubin binds to albumin and gives our plasma and serum its mildly lemon-yellow colour. In this form bilirubin is described as unconjugated, or indirect bilirubin. Upon its passage through the liver, bilirubin may be combined with glucuronic acid, whereupon it is described as conjugated, or direct bilirubin, and is then moved into the gall bladder. Conjugated bilirubin is then excreted via the bile duct and duodenum; it is this form that gives faeces its brown colour. Intestinal bacteria can convert some of this bilirubin to urobilin and urobilinogen. However, some intestinal conjugated bilirubin may be absorbed from the large intestines, and may be found in the circulation. In this form it may be excreted via the kidney, giving the urine its characteristic light-yellow colour.

If red cell destruction is intravascular, the majority of free haemoglobin is likely to form a complex with the plasma protein **haptoglobin**. This complex is removed by the macrophages

---

reticuloendothelial system

A collection of white blood cells (such as macrophages) present in organs such as the liver, spleen, and lymph nodes, with roles in immunology and phagocytosis.

biliverdin

A breakdown product of haem that is converted into bilirubin.

haemoxygenase

A key enzyme in the recycling pathway of the haem molecule that generates iron, carbon monoxide, and biliverdin.

bilirubin

The major breakdown product of haem which is not recycled.

of the reticuloendothelial system and so prevents iron being filtered by the kidney. Reduced plasma concentrations of haptoglobin may indicate intravascular haemolysis.

Excess circulating haem can form a complex with **haemopexin**, in which form it can also be cleared by the liver. Any free haem not bound to haemopexin may be broken down by plasma haemoxygenase into iron (which may be picked up by apotransferrin), carbon monoxide, and bilirubin, which can be carried by albumin. Figure 4.11 summarizes the fate of the products of the red blood cell.

haptoglobin and haemopexin
Plasma proteins that complex with, and thus remove, haemoglobin and free haem from the circulation.

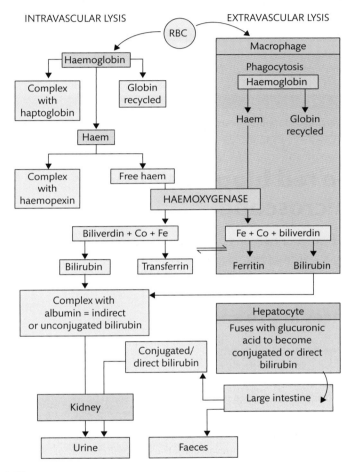

FIGURE 4.11

Breakdown of the red blood cell. The fate of the red blood cell is to be lysed either in the circulation (intravascular haemolysis) or in cells of the reticuloendothelial system (extravascular haemolysis, such as in macrophages). Intravascular haemoglobin may bind to haptoglobin or may be broken down to haem and globin (which is recycled). Haem may complex with haemopexin or be broken down further by haemoxygenase. Within the macrophage, extravascular haemolysis sees the globin being recycled and the haem being processed by haemoxygenase. The products of haem are iron, carbon monoxide, biliverdin, and bilirubin. The latter complexes with albumin (and is described as indirect or unconjugated), but in the liver it combines with glucuronic acid and is described as direct or conjugated bilirubin. The latter then passes into the gall bladder and bile into the intestines, where it may be converted to urobilin. However, some conjugated bilirubin may re-enter the blood and, with unconjugated bilirubin, be excreted by the kidney.

When healthy, the body is perfectly capable of clearing and recycling millions of senescent red blood cells each day. However, if there is excess red blood cell destruction (that is, pathological haemolysis) then the recycling processes of the liver and other organs can be overwhelmed. One consequence of this is a build up of bilirubin which, if deposited in tissues, may lead to the yellowing coloration of the skin, the condition we know as **jaundice** (from the French for yellow). This may also manifest itself as more heavily (yellow) coloured urine and plasma. Hence, clinically evident jaundice may be present in severe haemolyic anaemia and is a clear pathological sign. However, jaundice may also follow severe liver disease, such as obstructive cholestasis, liver cancer, or alcoholic cirrhosis, which does not directly reflect abnormal red blood cell turnover.

SELF-CHECK 4.11

What factors are associated with the destruction of the red blood cell?

SELF-CHECK 4.12

What is the major excretory product of the red blood cell and how is it removed?

4.5 The red blood cell under the microscope

The basic morphology of a red blood cell when viewed under a light microscope is of a disc, as with white blood cells. However, this very simple descriptor masks a great variety of different sizes, shapes, and colours of different populations of these cells, as can be seen in Fig. 4.12.

Differences in size and shape

The average red cell blood cell is generally taken to have a diameter of around 7 μm and to have a shape that is ideally perfectly round in two dimensions. However, this can vary somewhat according to various pathophysiological conditions. Variation in size is called **anisocytosis** (Figure 4.12(b)). Just as a human population will have some people who are tall and others who are short, then a red cell population will have some cells which are larger than others, and some which are smaller than others. The issues of 'large' and 'small' have been described in Chapter 2, and generally depend on the local reference range, which depends on age. (For example, a neonate has larger red blood cells than an adult.)

A large red cell is called a **macrocyte**, a small red cell a **microcyte**. A cell with an MCV within the reference range is a **normocyte**. (Figures 4.12(a)–(c)). The autoanalyser in the laboratory will automatically give the size of the average red blood cell (i.e. the mean cell volume, or MCV). However, this simple empirical result can mask some important pathology. The red cell distribution width (RDW) is the measure of the variation of the MCV as defined by the haematology autoanalyser. Consider a population of red cells with an 'average' MCV of 85 fL but with some slightly smaller (perhaps 81 fL) and others larger (such as 89 fL). Now consider a second population whose cells have the same 'average' MCV of 85 fL but whose cells show more variation in size, for example between 76 fL and 95 fL. The RDW of the first population will be considerably smaller than that of the latter. Thus the RDW is a *quantitative* method for describing anisocytosis. The greater the variation in red cell size, the greater the RDW. The RDW can be expressed as the standard deviation of the MCV, in femtolitres (fL), or as the coefficient of variation of RBC volume (%). We will examine the importance of this index in greater detail in Chapters 5 and 6.

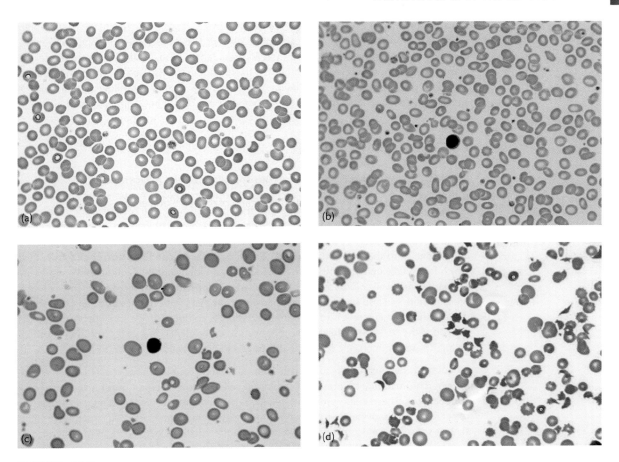

FIGURE 4.12

(a) Normal red cells (hence 'normocyte'): bi-concave discs, when stained showing a central area of pallor. Note the small variation in size and shape. The small purple bodies are platelets. (b) Microcytosis: red cells are smaller than normal; and anisocytosis: there is a variation in size of red cells—some are clearly much larger than others. The dark stained cell is a lymphocyte; the red cell to its right is a microcyte. (c) Macrocytosis: some red cells are larger than usual; and anisocytosis: there is a variation in size of red cells—some are clearly much larger than others. The dark stained cell is a lymphocyte; a macrocyte is present to its left. Compare this to the difference between the lymphocyte and the microcyte in Figure 4.12(b). (d) Polychromasia: some of the red cells are bluer (and larger) than usual and so are representative of young red cells. There are also numerous microcytes and several mis-shapen red blood cells, the significance of which we shall discuss in Chapter 6. (Magnification ×400.)

Macrocytes can be defined as those over a certain size, as defined by the laboratory's reference range, but taken by many to be more than 100 fL. The exact size that defines a macrocyte is generally determined by a senior haematologist, and can therefore be different in different hospitals. As we shall see in Chapter 5, a primary cause of a high MCV is to have a high intake of alcohol; another is to be pregnant; and a third is to be deficient in vitamin B_{12} or folate. However, it should be recalled that reticulocytes are slightly larger than mature erythrocytes, so that, overall, a raised MCV may be to do with a large number of these immature red blood cells (Figure 4.12(d)). The full significance of this will be developed in Chapters 5 and 6 on anaemia.

Cross reference

Sickle cell disease and an allied condition, thalassaemia, are discussed in Chapter 6.

sickle cell disease

A disease that follows from a mutation in a gene for one of the globin molecules.

Cross reference

As has been explained in Chapter 2, the definition of a normal MCV varies from laboratory to laboratory.

Similarly, microcytes may be those cells smaller than 80, 78, or 75 fL. Again, the exact definition of a microcyte depends on local conditions; thus the local reference range is of importance. Once more, this feature is not merely of academic value, as the most common cause of microcytes is iron deficiency; another is a haemoglobinopathy such as **sickle cell disease**. Therefore the size of the cell can become important as an index to allow certain types of anaemia to be identified. This and other issues will be explored in Chapters 5 and 6.

Differences in colour

Red blood cells readily take up dyes and so appear under the microscope as if coloured. As with variation in cell size, there is also a variation in this colour. As the stains are taken up by haemoglobin, the density or strength of the stain can help us to estimate the amount of haemoglobin inside the cell (haemoglobinization) and, hence, the ability of that cell to carry oxygen. Typically, red blood cells should contain an area of central pallor, which is approximately one third the size of the red cell. These cells are described as **normochromic**. Cells which fail to take up a lot of the dye (because they are deficient in haemoglobin), and so are not particularly well coloured, may be described as **hypochromic**. If there are many such cells present there will also be hypochromia. Several cells that are both microcytic and hypochromic are shown in Figure 4.12(d). In some cells there is colour only in a small band around the outside of the cell—the middle of the cell seems to be 'empty'. This is called 'the area of central pallor'. These hypochromic cells probably have a low MCH and MCHC.

By contrast, hyperchromia—too much colour—is rarely found in practice. However, a type of hyperchromia may be present if red blood cells lose their central pallor and appear as if **spherocytes**. These cells commonly reflect either an immune process directed against the red cells, or an abnormality in the cell membrane (generally a deficiency in structural proteins such as spectrin or ankyrin) and die prematurely, often in the spleen. This is frequently accompanied by anaemia, additional details of which will be presented in Chapter 6.

The combined term 'normocytic normochromic' is frequently used to describe the finding associated with the blood loss or anaemia of chronic diseases. As previously described, polychromasia refers to a bluish tinge associated with an immature red blood cell population—the reticulocyte. This is illustrated in Figure 4.12(d)—the large reticulocytes are clearly stained blue more strongly. As with variation in size, this characteristic of variation in colour, called anischromasia, is important in the diagnosis of different types of anaemia, as we shall see in Chapters 5 and 6.

Other morphological changes

Close examination of the shape of the red cell can provide a wealth of information regarding the likelihood of different diseases. Many of these will be discussed in Chapters 5 and 6. For example, sickle cell disease is so named for the curved shape that the red cell tends to form when deprived of oxygen. Figure 4.12(d) has many fragments or distorted red blood cells that indicate an active disease process.

Haematologists also recognize various other irregular shapes that red cells may adopt. These include burr cells (Figure 4.13(a)) and target cells (Figure 4.13(b)). Burr cells are characterized by having a 'spiky' appearance and are also known as acanthocytes (*akanthos* = thorny/spiky; *-cyte* = cell). Target cells have a darker area within the central area of pallor ('Mexican hat'). Variation in cell shape is called poikilocytosis. There are also changes that are not due to a particular pathology but due instead to laboratory artefacts, such as prolonged storage or

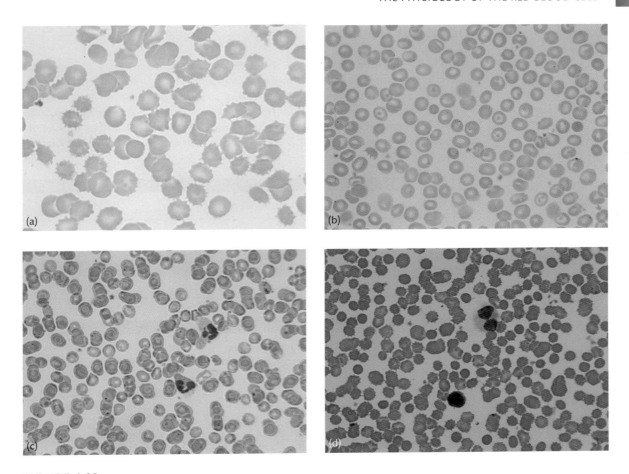

FIGURE 4.13

(a) Burr cells: many of these cells that are 'spiky'. (b) Target cells: these have darker areas within the central area of pallor ('Mexican hat'). There are two excellent examples close together on the right of the centre of the figure. (c, d) Storage and fixation changes. Samples taken into EDTA and stored incorrectly or for too long will undergo changes. These may be crenation (irregular, slightly spiky edges) of the red cells and deterioration of the white cells (loss of membrane and nuclear integrity). Poor drying and fixation results in trapped water within the cells and so a poor morphology. One of the white blood cells in 4.13(d) (a lymphocyte) has retained a normal morphology whilst the other, a neutrophil, is abnormal. (Magnification varies: ×400 to ×600.)

poor fixation. Figures 4.13(c) and (d) show typical artefactual changes to the morphology of both red blood cells and white blood cells—there are clear differences compared to cells in the other figures.

Key Points

Examination of a blood slide under a light microscope can give useful information about the integrity of the red blood cell, its size, how much haemoglobin it carries, and factors that can cause damage.

Inclusion bodies

Normally, the red blood cell when seen under the light microscope should be homogeneous with no unusual internal features. However, in various diseases and conditions, **inclusion bodies** can be seen within the cell that can be of considerable diagnostic value. Inclusion bodies may be parasites, deposits of iron, remnants of DNA, or denatured haemoglobin. Some of these inclusion bodies demand special techniques for visualization as they may not be detectable by conventional staining. More details of particular inclusion bodies will follow in Chapters 5 and 6 on diseases of the red blood cell. (Table 6.4, page 170)

SELF-CHECK 4.13

What is the importance of the red cell distribution width (RDW)?

SELF-CHECK 4.14

What are the correct haematological terms for red blood cells that are larger or smaller than normal?

SELF-CHECK 4.15

What is meant when a red cell is described as being hypochromic?

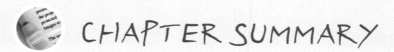

CHAPTER SUMMARY

- The development of the red cell (erythropoiesis) occurs in the bone marrow: precursors such as the proerythroblast and erythroblast give rise to the reticulocyte and the mature erythrocyte.

- The red blood cell is highly specialized for the carriage of oxygen.

- A consequence of this specialization is the lack of a nucleus and cell organelles.

- The cell membrane is also highly specialized, with a series of structural proteins providing shape and flexibility.

- The cytoplasm contains haemoglobin, metabolites, and enzymes.

- Haemoglobin consists of protein (globin) and non-protein (haem) components.

- There are various types of globin that vary throughout the life of the subject and that have a differing capacity to carry oxygen.

- Haem is a complex molecule, with an atom of iron at its centre.

- Intracellular enzymes are required to provide energy and resist the toxic effects of oxygen.

- Upon the death of the cell, globin proteins, lipids, and iron are recycled. However, once the iron has been extracted from the haem, the remaining pyrrole/porphyrin ring is degraded to bilirubin and excreted.

■ Anisocytosis describes the variation in size of red blood cells—cells larger than the top of the reference range are macrocytes, cells below the bottom of the reference range are microcytes, whilst those whose size is within the reference range are normocytes.

■ Polychromasia, anisochromasia, and hypochromia describe variation in the 'colour' of different red blood cells.

■ Red cells may contain one or more different types of inclusion body, which often indicate a particular metabolic problem.

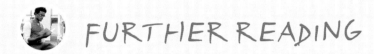

FURTHER READING

● An X, Mohandas N. **Disorders of red cell membrane.** *British Journal of Haematology* 2008:**141**;367–75.

● Andrews NC. **Forging a field: the golden age of iron biology.** *Blood* 2008:**112**;219–30.

● Blau CA. **Erythropoietin in cancer: presumption of innocence?** *Stem Cells* 2007;**25**:2094–7.

● Chasis JA, Mohandas. **Erythroblastic islands: niches for erythropoiesis.** *Blood* 2008:**112**;470–8.

● Daniels G. **Functions of red cell surface proteins.** *Vox Sanguinis* 2007:**93**;331–40.

● Manwani D, Bieker JJ. **The erythroblastic island.** *Current Topics in Developmental Biology* 2008:**82**;23–53.

● Mohandas N, Gallagher PG. **Red cell membranes: past present and future.** *Blood* 2008:**112**;3939–48.

● Phrommintikul A, *et al*. **Mortality and target haemoglobin concentrations in anaemic patients with chronic kidney disease treated with erythropoietin: a meta-analysis.** *Lancet* 2007:**369**;381–8.

Answers to self-check questions, case study questions, and discussion questions are provided in the book's Online Resource Centre, visit www.oxfordtextbooks.co.uk/orc/moore

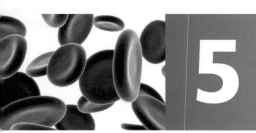

5

The pathology of the red blood cell: Part 1

Andrew Blann and Sukhjinder Marwah

The pathology of the red blood cell is a broad field comprising a range of diverse topics. As such, we will split our coverage into two chapters. This chapter will examine the major disease of red cells (anaemia) and look at some of the different pathways by which it may arise. These include problems with the bone marrow, problems with micronutrients (iron and vitamins), and how disease in other organs can lead to anaemia. In the chapter that follows we will look at the remaining causes of anaemia, and at other red blood cell disease.

Learning objectives

After studying this chapter you should confidently be able to:

- Appreciate that the principal diseases of red blood cells can involve both low red blood cell levels/numbers (leading to anaemia) and high red blood cell levels/numbers (leading to erythrocytosis and polycythaemia).

- Explain how anaemia can arise from changes within the bone marrow.

- Describe the consequences of abnormal iron metabolism.

- Describe the consequences of the poor supply of vitamins B_{12} and B_6, and folate to the bone marrow.

- Outline how disease in different body organs can lead to anaemia.

- Suggest how the laboratory can diagnose these conditions.

5.1 Diseases of the red blood cell

Having established the basics of red cell function in Chapter 4, we are now in a better position to understand the dysfunction of this cell. Broadly speaking, the pathology of red blood cells considers the two polar extremes of the reference range. However, as we have discussed in Chapter 2, having a result within the reference range is no guarantee of health just as having a result marginally outside the reference range does not automatically mean ill health. Low numbers of red cells, and/or low levels of haemoglobin generally lead to the clinical condition called anaemia. Considerably less common is the reverse of anaemia, whereby the red blood cell count and haemoglobin are high and are also likely to lead to illness. This situation is present in two closely related conditions—polycythaemia and erythrocytosis.

Anaemia

When there are too few red blood cells in circulation, or there is a problem with their function, then we consider the major pathology of red blood cells, anaemia. The problem may arise because of the poor supply of the building blocks of red blood cells, such as iron, or problems with the part of the body where they are being produced (the bone marrow). Alternatively, there may be mutations in certain genes (such as those of haemoglobin, components of the cell membrane, or metabolic enzymes) that can lead directly to anaemia. Many of these changes can lead to the early destruction of the red blood cell. This destructive process is called haemolysis.

Cross reference
Red blood cell function is described in Chapter 4.

Anaemia is the primary pathological condition of red blood cells. However, despite its importance, there is a surprising lack of consensus as to how it should be defined. For example, one textbook defines anaemia (in the adult) as a level of haemoglobin in the blood of less than 14 g/dL in adult males, or less than 12 g/dL in adult females; in another textbook a result of less than 13.5 g/dL in men or 11.5 g/dL in women defines the condition. The World Health Organization, taking a global view, defines the state of anaemia to arise when haemoglobin is less than 13 g/dL in men and 12 g/dL in women (11 g/dL if pregnant). Others characterize the disease as abnormalities in red blood cells that, alongside appropriate symptoms, call for treatment—a definition that does not specify the level of haemoglobin or the sex of the subject. It follows from this point of view that someone whose haemoglobin is 9 g/dL, but is asymptomatic, may not be anaemic. Some authorities have proposed that age (in age-ranges of 20–49 years and 50+ for women, and of 20–59 years and 60+ for men), and race (white European, black Afro-Caribbean) should also be considered when formulating a reference range. Others suggest degrees of anaemia can be further quantified, such as being mild (haemoglobin >10 g/dL) or moderate (haemoglobin 8.5–10 g/dL).

It is again important to emphasize that the practitioner must take note of their local reference range, which may be different not only in actual values, but also in the units for haemoglobin. Many laboratories are moving towards reporting haemoglobin in units of g/L instead of the g/dL unit described above.

Recognition and management of anaemia in an individual is also complicated by the variety and severity of signs and symptoms in different people as set out in Table 5.1, few of which are fully sensitive enough (that is, are present in a large number of people with the condition) or are specific enough (that is, are found only in those people with the condition) to be reliable in practice.

A widespread understanding of anaemia is also frustrated by the different methods of classification of the different subtypes of this condition, such as those based on the size of the red blood cell (i.e. **the mean cell volume, MCV**) or based on the condition of the bone marrow. For example, if there is anaemia, and the red blood cells are small (with a low MCV, perhaps 70 fL), then the anaemia can be described as **microcytic**. Conversely, the anaemia associated with large red cells (where, for example, the MCV may be 105 fL), is termed **macrocytic**. When the red blood cells are of normal size *and* the subject is anaemic then the term **normocytic** anaemia is used.

mean cell volume (MCV)
The volume of the 'average' red blood cell.

Other classification systems focus on clinical signs and symptoms, others on genetic considerations. However, the system about to be presented relies on aetiology, that is, how the condition came about (Table 5.2). The key considerations here are the bone marrow, problems with micronutrients (such as iron, vitamin B_{12}, and folic acid), haemoglobin, the cell membrane, and metabolic enzymes. There are, of course, other less common causes of anaemia.

TABLE 5.1 Signs and symptoms of anaemia.

Signs	Pallor (especially of the conjunctiva)
	Tachycardia (pulse rate over 100 beats per minute)
	Glossitis (swollen and painful tongue—reasonably specific for vitamin B_{12} deficiency)
	Koilonychia (spoon nails—reasonably specific for iron deficiency)
	Dark urine (in haemolytic anaemia)
Symptoms	Decreased work capacity
	Fatigue, lethargy
	Weakness
	Dizziness
	Palpitations
	Shortness of breath (especially on exertion)
	'Tired all the time'
	Rarely: headaches, tinnitus, taste disturbance
More severe disease	Jaundice
	Splenomegaly
	Hepatomegaly
	Angina
	Cardiac failure
	Fever

TABLE 5.2 An aetiological classification of anaemia.

The bone marrow	• Suppression
	• Infiltration
Problems with iron	• Deficiency at the bone marrow
	• Excess absorption
	• Ineffective incorporation into haem
Lack of vitamins	• Vitamin B_{12}
	• Folic acid
Anaemia associated with disease in other organs	• Liver
	• Kidney
	• Reproductive organs
	• Connective tissues
	• Thyroid
Haemolysis	• Due to antibodies
	• Due to drugs
	• Infections
Anaemia arising from gene mutation	• Haemoglobinopathy
	• Membrane defects
	• Enzyme defects

The first four topics are explained in this chapter, the last two topics in Chapter 6.

Erythrocytosis and polycythaemia

The polar extreme from the low red blood cell count often found in anaemia is when the red blood cell count is above the top of the reference range. The reason for the elevation in red blood cell count is generally due to one of two different causes: these are termed erythrocytosis and polycythaemia. The former is used when there is an increase in red cells alone, the latter when there are also increased numbers of other blood cells—white blood cells and/or platelets. An increased red blood cell count is considerably less common than anaemia, and is fundamentally different in nature. For example, there are many different types of anaemia, but relatively few causes of erythrocytosis and polycythaemia. However, all conditions may arise from disorders in the way that red blood cells develop in the bone marrow—the process of haemopoiesis. We shall leave the discussion of erythrocytosis and polycythaemia for Chapter 6.

Despite the discussion above, the competent practitioner will be aware that the presence of a result outside the reference range does not always confer a label of anaemia or erythrocytosis/polycythaemia. For a particular subject, small red blood cells or large red blood cells (i.e. with many microcytes or macrocytes respectively, so that the MCV is outside the reference range) may be entirely normal and therefore acceptable. For example, it may be quite normal for a pregnant woman to have red blood cells which are larger than before the pregnancy began—but she would hardly be described as having a disease! Similarly, the red cells of newborns and infants are larger than in the adult, so that in these situations an MCV of 108 fL may not be pathological.

The first aspects of red cell disease (the bone marrow, problems with micronutrients, and disease in other organs) will be discussed in the present chapter. Anaemia due to haemolysis and to gene mutation (causing haemoglobinopathy, membrane defects, and lack of enzymes), as well as erythrocytosis and polycythaemia, will be explained in the chapter that follows.

SELF-CHECK 5.1

What is the basis of the major types of disease of the red blood cell?

BOX 5.1 *The definition of anaemia*

As has been mentioned, the traditional approach to the definition of anaemia is essentially numerical—a level of haemoglobin lower than a particular value, dependent on age and sex, regardless of signs and symptoms. Perhaps the most authoritative source of a definition of anaemia is the World Health Organization, which defines the disease as haemoglobin <13 g/dL in men, <12 g/dL in women, or <11 g/dL if pregnant.

However, an alternative definition positions anaemia as a disease, linked with a set of symptoms and abnormalities in red blood cell biology, that needs to be treated. It follows that an elderly woman with an Hb of 11.7 g/dL, who is asymptomatic, may not, on clinical grounds, be treated. In which case it could be argued that she is not anaemic.

The reference range for haemoglobin for this textbook is 133–167 g/L (13.3–16.7 g/dL) for men and 118–148 g/L (11.8–14.8 g/dL) for women. This in no way invalidates or criticizes any other reference range, and vice versa. Each practitioner must act on their local reference range. Other reference ranges for this textbook are given in Table 1 at the front of this book (page xiii).

How do we classify anaemia according to the size of the red blood cell?

5.2 Anaemia arising from changes in the bone marrow

The bone marrow is an excellent place to start our examination of diseases of the red blood cells as this is the site of their production. This production process, erythropoiesis, has been described in Chapter 4. Interference with this process can lead to a reduction in the numbers of red blood cells being produced, with no change in the production of other blood cells—the white blood cells and platelets. The most common condition that leads to this reduction in red cell numbers alone is described as **pure red cell aplasia**.

However, in many cases, one or more factors that reduce red cell numbers will also lead to a reduction in white blood cells and platelets as these are also made by the bone marrow. This feature, **pancytopenia**, meaning 'low levels of all types of blood cells', often arises when the bone marrow is invaded by cancer originating in other organs. Alternatively, the bone marrow is very sensitive to external factors such as drugs (whether medicinal, environmental, or industrial) and infectious agents (bacteria and viruses), all of which can lead to pancytopenia. The anaemia associated with pancytopenia is called aplastic anaemia.

Cross reference
Erythropoiesis is discussed in Chapters 3 and 4.

Selective reduction in red blood cells

The key to this group of diseases is the major red blood cell precursor—the erythroblast. There are two major variants of this condition. In the first, there is a severe reduction, or even an absence, of erythroblasts. In the second, erythroblast numbers are increased.

Pure red cell aplasia (PRCA) is the most common form of red cell aplasia due to absent or reduced numbers of erythroblasts. It may appear as a congenital condition, or it could arise as an acquired syndrome. Arguably, the most common congenital form of PRCA, which is generally apparent during the first year of life, is **Diamond–Blackfan anaemia** (also called congenital hypoplastic anaemia), having an incidence of only 4–7 per million live births. A family history of anaemia is common and inheritance appears to be autosomal-dominant. However, an alternative diagnosis for anaemia between the ages of 1 and 5 years is transient erythroblastopenia (that is, lack of erythroblasts) of childhood, which usually develops in the second year of life without a family history of anaemia.

Cross reference
Diamond–Blackfan anaemia is discussed in the context of malignancy in Chapter 9.

Acquired PRCA can be classified as primary (idiopathic—where no clear cause can be identified) or secondary (acquired as the result of exposure to a clear pathogenic agent, such as a drug or a virus). The list of known causes of acquired PRCA is considerable (Table 5.3).

The congenital dyserythropoietic anaemias (CDAs) include several conditions resulting from increased numbers of erythroblasts (that is, erythroid hyperplasia). Erythropoiesis is ineffective and the anaemia is generally mild. Red blood cells from the best-characterized and most common variant (Type II) are susceptible to lysis by acidified serum. The molecular basis of this appears to be lack of an enzyme necessary for the correct processing of certain cell membrane proteins, which renders the cell fragile.

TABLE 5.3 Causes of red cell aplasia.

Congenital	Diamond–Blackfan syndrome, congenital dyserythropoietic anaemia
Infections	Viruses: parvovirus B19, hepatitis B virus, Epstein–Barr virus, mumps, cytomegalovirus, human immunodeficiency virus Bacteria: meningococcal and staphylococcal species
Malignancy	Solid tumours (such as cancer of the thymus, stomach, breast, lung, thyroid and kidney) Haematological tumours (leukaemias, lymphomas, myeloma, myelofibrosis, essential thrombocythaemia, Waldenström macroglobulinaemia)
Autoimmune disease	Systemic lupus erythematosus, rheumatoid arthritis and auto-immune haemolytic anaemia, Sjögren's syndrome, autoantibodies to red cell progenitors, autoantibodies to erythropoietin, T-cell mediated recognition of red-cell progenitors.
Other causes	Drugs and chemicals (notably azathioprine, methotrexate, gold, chloramphenicol, recombinant human erythropoietin and co-trimoxazole) Pregnancy, severe renal failure

N.B. Many of these also cause pancytopenia and so aplastic anaemia.

Pancytopenia

Unlike PRCA, where only red cell production is suppressed, pancytopenia is characterized by low levels in the blood of all three types of blood cell—red cells, white cells, and platelets. The accompanying anaemia is called aplastic anemia. The causes of this reduction in cell numbers can be classified as being congenital, acquired, or idiopathic.

The principal *congenital* cause of pancytopenia (accounting for two-thirds of cases) is **Fanconi's anaemia**, an inherited autosomal-recessive condition with abnormalities in several genes. Apart from pancytopenia, there are also likely to be skeletal, renal, and neurological abnormalities alongside short stature and upper limb abnormalities (such as the absence of thumbs). At the nuclear level the disease is characterized by chromosomal fragility, with breaks in the DNA; a late consequence of this disease is an increased risk of malignancy, including leukaemia and myelodysplasia. Other rare congenital causes of pancytopenia include the Schwachman–Diamond syndrome and dyskeratosis congenita.

Like PRCA, there are many causes of acquired pancytopenia, and several are common between the two (such as viral hepatitis and systemic lupus erythematosus) (Table 5.4). Although many of the remaining causes of pancytopenia and aplastic anaemia are idiopathic, they often have an immunological basis. Indeed, it has been argued that the aplastic anaemia following pregnancy and viral infections is in fact a direct consequence of an aberrant immune response. This theory is supported by the observation of immune-mediated, T-lymphocyte destruction of bone marrow cells, and that this can be reversed by immunosuppression with anti-thymocyte globulin and ciclosporin.

Cross reference

Fanconi's anaemia is discussed in greater detail in Chapter 9.

SELF-CHECK 5.3

What are the two most common forms of congenital reduction in the number of red blood cells?

TABLE 5.4 **Causes of pancytopenia.**

Congenital	Fanconi's anaemia
Acquired	Chemotherapy (e.g. chloramphenicol, phenylbutazone, gold)
	Infections (e.g. viral hepatitis, parvovirus B19)
	Other defined bone marrow disease (e.g. myelofibrosis, myelodysplasia)
	Other defined disease (e.g. hypersplenism, systemic lupus erythematosus)
	Severe vitamin B_{12} deficiency
Idiopathic	Frequently shown to be immune mediated

The anaemia of haemopoietic cancer

The bone marrow is simply a place of production, perhaps a factory, whose products are blood cells. Any factory whose work space is taken over by external forces or objects, and is thus at a reduced work capacity, will clearly be unable to produce goods. In this respect, the bone marrow is no exception. The major invader is cancer, which can spread from its original site (such as the breast or prostate) to invade other tissues. However, there may also be cancer arising within the bone marrow itself. In both cases, the pathological basis of the disease is that the cancer tissue invariably grows and slowly takes over normal bone marrow tissue. If this is the case then erythropoiesis will suffer and so anaemia may result.

Cancer of the bone marrow includes the haemoproliferative diseases of leukaemia and myeloma. Leukaemia is characterized by a failure of the bone marrow to correctly regulate the number of white blood cells it produces, such that it makes too many. Not only are too many white blood cells produced, but in addition they are unable to provide support to the body in defending itself from attack by microorganisms. In the early stages of the disease, these cancerous white blood cells remain in the bone marrow, but as the disease develops they pass into the blood. Ultimately, the number of these cancerous white blood cells rises so that the peripheral white blood cell count itself will become elevated.

Myeloma is also a disease of white blood cells, which sees them multiply in an inappropriate manner. In this case, however, the tumour of these abnormal cells generally remains inside the bone marrow until the terminal stages of the disease, when abnormal cells can be found in the blood.

A third white blood cell tumour, **lymphoma**, is centred on the lymph node. Like myeloma and leukaemia cells, lymphoma cells can also spread from their site of origin (that is, a particular lymph node) and invade other lymph nodes and other organs, notably the spleen, liver, and bone marrow. Thus when lymphoma cells, which may also be found in the blood, invade the bone marrow they may displace those stem cells responsible for producing red blood cells and so cause anaemia.

Myelodysplastic Syndrome is a collection of disorders characterized by the clonal proliferation of multipotential haemopoietic stem cells (that is, stem cells that give rise to different types of blood cells such as granulocytes and monocytes), whereby these cells are disordered and inefficient. Many cells die in the bone marrow, leading to ineffective haemopoiesis and a reduction in the numbers of all circulating blood cells. In a significant proportion of patients, the development of the disease is preceded by chemotherapy and/or radiotherapy for other neoplasia. As perhaps 25% of patients will convert into developing acute myeloid leukaemia, myelodysplasia has been described as 'preleukaemia' or 'smouldering acute leukaemia'.

Myelofibrosis is a condition where, like leukaemia and myeloma, the initial problem is with the cells of the bone marrow itself. However, unlike leukaemia and myeloma, the proliferating cell is not haemopoietic (that is, it is not a stem cell). Instead, the bone marrow becomes overgrown with fibroblasts. These cells are not directly involved in haemopoiesis but normally have a supporting role. The fibroblasts are often driven to proliferate and produce collagen by inappropriate responses to growth factors produced by other cells such as monocytes, macrophages, and megakaryocytes. Like cancer, this inappropriate growth of fibroblasts is progressive and eventually leads to deterioration in haemopoiesis and thus to anaemia.

Cross reference

Tumours of the bone marrow and of lymph nodes (leukaemia, myeloma, and lymphoma) are described fully in Chapters 9–12. The importance of stem cells has been discussed in Chapters 3 and 4 and in relation to malignancy in Chapter 9.

Chemotherapy

An important component of modern medicine is **chemotherapy** (treatment using drugs). While the common usage of the term 'chemotherapy' is taken to imply the use of drugs in the treatment of cancer, it actually applies to the administration of *any* drug. An important source book widely available in hospitals in the UK is the *British National Formulary* (BNF), which lists all drugs licensed by Government agencies for the treatment of precise disorders. Each drug has notes regarding its mode of action, dose, and also side-effects. Entries include those drugs that are perceived to be supposedly innocuous, with few side-effects, such as aspirin (although even aspirin can lead to gastrointestinal upsets in some subjects). Other drugs, such as antibiotics, can cause side-effects such as allergy. However, the most dangerous diseases call for the more severe forms of chemotherapy, as are demanded in certain cancers. One of the most frequent side-effects of the many different classes of drug used in the treatment of cancer is suppression of the bone marrow. Fortunately, bone marrow suppression is almost always reversible upon cessation of use of the particular drug.

A standard treatment for many conditions including cancer is the administration of drugs such as methotrexate, cyclophosphamide, busulphan, and vinblastine, which act to destroy the tumour. Notably, many of these drugs may be used to treat haematological neoplasia such as leukaemia. However, a problem is that the cytotoxic drugs themselves can be relatively indiscriminate in terms of the cells they attack, so that effectively any cell in the body can be damaged by chemotherapy. This is particularly true of the bone marrow: it is a highly active tissue, which is very susceptible to cytotoxic drugs of this type. Nevertheless, even supposedly benign and commonly used classes of drugs such as antibiotics (for example, chloramphenicol) and non-steroidal anti-inflammatory drugs (NSAIDs; for example, phenylbutazone) can also suppress the bone marrow.

Together, medication drugs cause 15–25% of cases of bone marrow suppression. Indeed, a frequent cause of both PRCA and pancytopenia (and therefore also aplastic anaemia) is chemotherapy (Tables 5.3 and 5.4). Various non-medication drugs and chemicals can also attack the bone marrow; examples include industrial hydrocarbons such as benzene, and agricultural drugs such as pesticides.

Cross reference

The role of benzene in the development of malignancies is discussed in Chapter 9.

SELF-CHECK 5.4

What are the principal types of haematological cancer that can lead to anaemia?

Treatment of anaemia resulting from disease of the bone marrow

Treatment of bone-marrow derived anaemia very much depends on the aetiology and the clinical severity of the particular disease. Where the cause of the anaemia is evident—for example, where it is being caused by a particular drug—then the disease should be reversible upon withdrawal of the drug. Equally, the aplastic anaemia of pregnancy generally resolves after delivery of the neonate. By contrast, congenital diseases such as Fanconi's anaemia are curable only by bone marrow transplantation, although androgens may help stimulate erythropoiesis.

Some cases of acquired or idiopathic pure red cell aplasia may be successfully treated by immunosuppression with ciclosporin or corticosteroids (for example, prednisolone 1 mg/kg per day). Unfortunately, the treatment of most haematological malignancies is with agents that will also further suppress erythropoiesis (including cytotoxic drugs and radiotherapy). However, growth factors such as erythropoietin and GM-CSF can be given to help the recovery of the red cell count.

In other circumstances, treatment will be palliative—red cell transfusion for incapacitating or life-threatening anaemia, platelet transfusion for severe thrombocytopenia, and prophylactic antibacterials and antivirals if the numbers of white blood cells are profoundly low. Intravenous immunoglobulins may be used for active viral infections. If there is iron overload because of hypertransfusion then iron chelation (the process of the chemical removal of iron) may be necessary.

The role of the laboratory in the investigation of anaemia following bone marrow changes

The initial signs of PRCA are likely to be those of general anaemia—that is, a reduced red cell count and haemoglobin. The haematocrit is unlikely to be below the lower end of the reference range unless the red cell count is considerably reduced. By definition, white cells and platelets will be within the reference range. Consequently, a full blood count is essential. However, key investigations also involve examination of the bone marrow—which in PRCA is normocellular with respect to leucocyte precursors and megakaryocytes, but will reveal grossly reduced or absent erythroblasts.

In Diamond–Blackfan anaemia, the anaemia is often moderate to severe (haemoglobin 20–100 g/L) but the MCV often exceeds the top of the reference range (that is, there is likely to be a macrocytic anaemia). Notably, fetal haemoglobin may be increased, possibly as an adaptation to the anaemia. This is in contrast to the transient erythroblastopenia of childhood where the MCV is within the reference range and the expression of fetal haemoglobin is normal. In the peripheral circulation there is mild to moderate anaemia (haemoglobin 80–110 g/L) with mild macrocytosis, anisocytosis, and **poikilocytosis**, although in some forms acanthocytes and

poikilocytosis
A variation in the shapes of the red cell population. Causes include abnormal erythropoiesis and myelofibrosis.

other bizarre red cells may be present. If a bone marrow examination is thought necessary, PRCA is characterized by low or absent erythroblasts, whereas the CDAs are characterized by increased numbers of erythroblasts.

The anaemia that follows from leukaemia is perhaps the easiest to detect, as a high white blood cell count (and possibly a thrombocytopenia) is often present. The anaemia is most likely to be normocytic and normochromic. A bone marrow aspiration will inevitably be performed and should find all the erythroid precursors (including reticulocytes) to be present but in reduced numbers. The bone marrow in myelodysplasia is usually hypercellular often with enlarged and abnormal erythroid precursors (such as multinucleate normoblasts), although there may be abnormalities in the precursors of all cell lineages. However, a hallmark of the bone marrow in myelodysplasia is the presence of **ring sideroblasts**. These will be described more fully in the section on iron that follows.

ring sideroblasts
Abnormal erythroblasts with iron granules arranged in a ring around the nucleus.

The definition of pancytopenia is a reduction in the numbers of red cells, white cells, and platelets. Consequently, it should be relatively simple to diagnose from a full blood count. Generally, the (aplastic) anaemia should be normochromic and normocytic. The bone marrow will be hypoplastic, with the normal haemopoietic tissues being grossly reduced and replaced by fat cells and other non-haemopoietic tissues. However, deviations from this picture occur in Fanconi's anaemia and in acquired aplastic anaemia where the red cells may be macrocytic. The bone marrow in myelofibrosis will show increased collagen and fibroblasts alongside reduced haemopoietic precursors.

Generally speaking, the reticulocyte count, normally 0.5–2.5% of the red cell count (absolute count 25–125 $\times$ 10^9 cells/L), should be raised in most cases of chronic anaemia as a physiological response to the inability of the depleted red cell mass to supply the tissues with sufficient oxygen for its physiological needs. However, in those anaemias where the bone marrow and erythropoiesis is compromised (as in PRCA and aplastic anaemia) then reticulocytes should be low or even absent from the peripheral blood and grossly reduced in the bone marrow.

Further details of the use of bone marrow analysis in leukaemia and other neoplasia are presented in Chapter 10.

Key Points

The bone marrow is a very active and a very sensitive organ. Generating millions of cells daily, it can be influenced by many conditions not allied directly to haematology, and also by many drugs and other treatments. Consequently, it is not surprising that even the slightest adverse effect could lead directly to changes in blood cell numbers and so to illness.

5.3 **Iron-related disease**

In this section we examine the consequences of insufficient iron and of excess iron. The essential micronutrients iron, vitamins B$_{12}$ and B$_6$, and folic acid are required for various aspects of human physiology, including haemopoiesis. Chapter 4 has indicated the steps in the development of red blood cells that require the vitamins and folate as cofactors for key enzymes in the metabolism of haem. The same chapter has also explained the need for iron. These micronutrients are obtained from the diet, so that inadequate nutrition (that is, malnutrition) is likely to cause different types of anaemia. However, an apparently adequate diet may still lead to disease: essential micronutrients may fail to be absorbed due to abnormalities of the intestines (that is, malabsorption).

Each molecule of haemoglobin must have an atom of iron to which oxygen can (transiently) bind and so be carried from the lungs to the tissues. Thus, a lack of iron leads directly to impaired carriage of oxygen. Indeed, iron deficiency, when due to malnutrition and/or malabsorption, is the most common cause of anaemia in the developed and developing world. The World Health Organization estimates that 30% of the world's population (some 2 billion people) is anaemic, and within this group the most common is **iron-deficiency anaemia**, which results from insufficient iron being delivered to the bone marrow. In turn, the most common cause of this deficiency is poor nutrition. However, iron deficiency does not lie behind all anaemias: a numerically minor aspect of iron-related disease is **sideroblastic anaemia**, another being iron overload. We will consider both of these conditions shortly.

sideroblastic anaemia
An anaemia that results from impaired inclusion of iron into haem, and thus into haemoglobin.

Iron requirements

The total iron load of an average adult is in the region of 3–5 g (towards the lower end of the range in the female) and is distributed in different molecules, cells, and tissues. The majority of iron is found in haemoglobin (generally two-thirds of total body iron) and deposits in stores in the liver, bone marrow, and elsewhere (as ferritin and haemosiderin; 25% of total body iron). The remainder occurs as trace amounts in cells and tissues where, for example, the iron may be needed as a cofactor for metabolic enzymes such as catalase and the cytochromes. Almost all total body ferritin is in the cytoplasm, but a small fraction is present in the plasma at a concentration of 20–300 µg/L.

Approximately 1–2 mg of iron a day is lost in urine, in shed epithelial cells of the skin and intestines (the latter in faeces), and in sweat; all of these losses must be recovered from the diet. However, daily iron requirements vary with age, sex, and pregnancy (Table 5.5). This requirement of 1 mg a day is relatively easy to achieve in a Western diet, which provides approximately 15 mg of iron each day.

Iron-deficiency anaemia

Whilst the biological basis of this anaemia seems clear, the aetiology is diverse, and deficiency can occur at any point in the path of iron from the diet to the erythroblast in the bone marrow.

TABLE 5.5 Daily iron requirements.

Infant and adult male	1 mg
Adolescent	2–3 mg
Menstruating adolescent	3–4 mg (loses 20–25 mg per menstruation)
Menstruating adult	2–3 mg (loses 20–25 mg per menstruation)
Pregnancy	3–4 mg (500–1000 mg required overall)
Lactation (thus amenorrhea likely)	1.5–2.5 mg (but is also required to repopulate stores)
Post-menopausal female	1 mg

Although, as an element, iron is relatively abundant, it is not present in all foodstuffs. Thus, an iron-poor diet may be unable to supply enough of this micronutrient. As a result, a clinically evident iron deficiency may develop whose aetiology is malnutrition. Indeed, the fortification with iron of common processed foodstuffs (such as bread) has been advocated as one method to alleviate the iron deficiency of malnutrition.

Chapter 4 has outlined the key steps in the absorption of iron from the intestines (summarized in Figure 4.7 in that chapter). These steps require: the acid environment of the stomach; the passage of iron from the lumen of the intestines into the cells of the intestine (enterocytes); the subsequent movement from the enterocyte into the blood; and its carriage to the bone marrow. It follows that, if certain steps in this process are impaired, then iron will fail to be absorbed, and will so fail to be provided to the bone marrow, leading to the development of anaemia.

Ferrous iron (Fe^{2+}) is readily absorbed by a transmembrane protein, the divalent metal transporter-1 (DMT-1), which is found on the luminal surface of enterocytes of the duodenum and upper jejunum. However, although ferric iron (Fe^{3+}) is poorly absorbed it can be converted to ferrous iron by the luminal enzyme iron-reductase. This functions best at low pH, an environment promoted by ascorbic acid and by acid secretions from the stomach. However, disease, or surgery to the stomach and intestines, can also lead to the malabsorption of iron (Table 5.6). Indeed, this aspect will be revisited in the section on vitamin B_{12} that follows.

Once imported by the enterocyte and subsequently exported in the circulation, iron must be picked up by its transport protein, apotransferrin, whereupon the two form transferrin. This protein is produced mainly by the liver, and so plasma levels may fall in the face of hepatic dysfunction such as that caused by alcoholic liver disease, cirrhosis, primary biliary sclerosis, and hepatoma.

Finally, upon arrival at the bone marrow, iron-loaded transferrin passes into red cell precursors such as erythroblasts by binding to transferrin receptors on the surface of the cell. Once inside the cytoplasm, the iron is uncoupled from the transferrin and moves to the mitochondria for incorporation into haem. The iron-free apotransferrin leaves the erythroblasts for the plasma where it picks up iron again, so repeating the process. However, plentiful iron in the diet, a healthy intestine, and good carriage to the bone marrow may be to no avail if the bone

TABLE 5.6 Intestinal factors contributing to reduced iron absorption.

The stomach	Achlorhydria
	Gastric atrophy
	Gastritis
	Alcoholism
	Gastric carcinoma
Upper and lower digestive tract	Duodenitis
	Coeliac disease
	Ulceration
	Crohn's disease
	Other inflammatory bowel diseases
Surgery	Resection of any of the above tissues

marrow is unable to present the iron to erythrocyte progenitors, as may be the case in diseases such as myclodyplastic syndrome and leukaemia.

Sideroblastic anaemia

Sideroblastic anaemia is characterized not by a lack of iron but by its failure to be incorporated into haem in red blood cell precursors such as the erythroblast. Figure 4.5 in Chapter 4 outlined the key steps in the synthesis of haem, one of the first being the synthesis of succinyl coenzyme-A from propionyl coenzyme-A, a process that requires vitamin B_{12}. The step which follows is the fusion of succinyl coenzyme-A with glycine to form delta-aminolaevulinic acid (ALA). This step is governed by the enzyme ALA-synthase and requires vitamin B_6 (as pyridoxal-6-phosphate) as a cofactor. A mutation in the gene for this enzyme means that haem synthesis is impaired: iron cannot be incorporated into the protoporphyrin ring but instead builds up in the mitochondria of the erythroblast. The gene for ALA-synthase is found on the X-chromosome, leading to a sex-linked variant of sideroblastic anaemia, which predominantly affects males.

There are numerous other forms of sideroblastic anaemia (and, indeed, non-sideroblastic anaemia) that are the consequence of mutations or deletions in other genes coding for mitochondrial and non-mitochondrial enzymes. For example, lack or malfunction of the enzyme ferrochelatase (which is responsible for the insertion of iron into the protoporphyrin ring) leads to reduced bone marrow iron availability and thus a mild microcytic anaemia.

A consequence of the failure to incorporate iron into the portoporphyrin ring is the intramitochondrial accumulation of the iron, as noted above, which becomes deposited in the iron-storage protein ferritin. These iron-rich mitochondria form a ring around the nucleus of the erythroblast, and as such the cells are described as sideroblasts. These ring sideroblasts give the disease, sideroblastic anaemia, its name. In some cases, red cells can still be produced, but these red cells may contain iron granules: such cells are called siderocytes, and the iron inclusion granules are called **Pappenheimer bodies**. These iron deposits can be detected using Perls' stain.

Although the most common form of inherited sideroblastic anaemia is due to a mutation in the X-linked gene that codes for the enzyme delta-ALA, it may also be acquired, as in the case of myelodysplasia, myelofibrosis, myeloma, myeloid leukaemia, rheumatoid arthritis, and haemolytic anaemia. However, there are also other types of sideroblastic anaemia caused by defects in other genes involved in the production of haem, such as for the enzyme pseudo-uridine synthase. Sideroblastic anaemia may also be caused by drugs such as alcohol, isoniazid, and chloramphenicol, by a lack of copper (as it is a cofactor for other enzymes involved in haem synthesis), and by excess ingestion of zinc (as it inhibits the absorption of copper in the intestines).

Further, lead poisoning is linked (but not directly related) to sideroblastic anaemia: it interferes with several steps in protoporphyrin synthesis (such as inhibition of the enzyme pyrimidine-5′-nucleotidase) and blocks the placement of iron into the centre of the protoporphyrin ring. However, the anaemia is a relatively late complication of systemic pathology that includes constipation and peripheral neuropathy.

In most cases, the treatment of inherited sideroblastic anaemia is with oral vitamin B_6, which should be effective in one-third of patients. Severe cases may need to be transfused but this may lead to iron overload, although chelation therapy may be effective in reducing inappropriately high iron stores caused by the failure to utilize iron appropriately. Treatment of acquired cases may require the removal or replacement of the causative agent, such as a different antibiotic in place of chloramphenicol.

What are the principal causes of iron deficiency?

Iron overload

The presence of too much iron can be just as problematic as iron deficiency. The body has no effective mechanism for actively eliminating iron, so absorption must be carefully regulated. When this mechanism fails, iron stores rise, causing problems for the tissues where it is stored or deposited (Table 5.7). Iron overload can be classified as primary (hereditary) or secondary (acquired) depending on whether it is a consequence of a primary defect in the regulation of iron balance or is secondary to genetic or acquired disorders, or their treatment.

A key regulator of iron absorption is the HFE protein, coded for by the *HFE* gene, which is present on chromosome 6, close to the genes for the HLA molecules. The mature molecule is present on the surface of cells from a variety of tissues—including the duodenum, liver, pancreas, placenta, kidney, and ovary—and on macrophages. Its precise function is unclear but several possible roles have been proposed. The first is that the HFE protein associates with the transferrin receptor and decreases its affinity for iron-loaded transferrin. A second is that HFE blocks the cellular export of iron from macrophages, whilst a third is of an impaired regulation of the hepcidin gene.

Hereditary haemochromatosis (HH) is the most common genetic cause of iron overload, and perhaps 83% of cases of HH are caused by a mutation (named C282Y) in *HFE*. (Thirty other variants in *HFE* have also been described.) The genetic cause of C282Y is a G→A transition at nucleotide position 845, which leads to the insertion of tyrosine instead of cysteine at position 282 in the mature HFE protein (hence: C282Y). The second most common mutation results in another mutation in the mature HFE molecule, His-63→Asp

TABLE 5.7 **Iron overload.**

Causes	• Mutations in key genes (for example, C282Y causing hereditary haemochromatosis)
	• Repeated red blood cell transfusions
	• Increased dietary uptake of iron
	• Ineffective erythropoiesis (beta-thalassaemia, sideroblastic anaemia)
Consequences: damage to:	• The liver (present in 30% of men and 7% of women with iron overload, causing cirrhosis and possibly carcinoma)
	• The heart (arrhythmia and heart failure)
	• Skin (rash, pigmentation and dermatitis)
	• Joints (arthralgia, osteoarthritis)
	• Endocrine organs (diabetes (present in 2–5 %) and hypopituitarism)

(H63D), and a significant proportion of patients with HH who are heterozygous for C282Y also have the H63D mutation.

C282Y is present in Europeans in its heterozygous form in perhaps 9.2% of people, although this figure varies greatly with region—ranging from approximately 1% in Southern Europe, to 12% in the Netherlands, to 25% in Ireland. Heterozygotes do not have an increased risk of clinically evident HH, although iron levels may be raised in perhaps 25%. African, Middle Eastern, and Australian populations have a prevalence of perhaps 0–0.5%. In its homozygous form HH is present in 0.4% of Europeans and inevitably has clinical consequences.

The consequence of the C282Y mutation is that malfunctioning HFE protein is present at the surface of the cell. If the proposed physiology is correct, then the mutated HFE protein promotes high levels of body iron by being unable to inhibit the uptake of iron-loaded transferrin by the particular cell, and by being unable to block the export of iron from intracellular stores in macrophages. Several reports support a role for hepcidin in HH. HFE-related haemochromatosis is characterized by low messenger RNA for the hepcidin gene in the liver and low serum hepcidin. Thus, in this setting low levels of hepcidin would be unable to regulate (in this case, inhibit) the absorption of iron, resulting in the hyperferraemia (in excess of iron in the blood) which is a characteristic of HH. Although serum hepcidin is low in both those heterozygous and homozygous for the C282Y mutation, hepcidin levels are strongly related to levels of ferritin in homozygotes for C282Y.

The dominant form of HH, caused by mutations such as C282Y in *HFE*, may be classified as Type 1 HH. Four other types of genetic variants have been described:

- Haemojuvelin-associated HH (Type 2A) is due to a mutation in the gene for the poorly understood molecule haemojuvelin. Consequences include the loss of regulation of hepcidin, which leads to increased iron absorption.
- Type 2B HH is due to a mutation in the hepcidin gene, which results in no or inactive hepcidin.
- Type 3 HH is associated with a mutation in the gene for the transferrin-receptor 2, which also leads to low levels of hepcidin.
- Ferroportin disease (Type 4 HH) differs from other HH disease as the defect is autosomal-dominant, and leads to reduced ability to transport iron, and an accumulation of iron in reticuloendothelial cells. There are also rare patients with defects in more than one gene responsible for iron metabolism.

Secondary iron overload can be due to a number of factors: the indirect effect of excessive iron consumption, a particular condition (such as sideroblastic anaemia or severe liver disease), or as consequence of treatment (Table 5.7). Regarding the latter, patients with severe haemoglobinopathy or myelodysplastic syndrome are likely to require regular blood transfusions and, as a consequence, develop iron overload. One unit of transfused blood contains approximately 200–250 mg of iron, and, although blood transfusion may ameliorate anaemia, a consequence may well be iron overload. Generally, after the transfusion of 10–20 units, patients become overloaded. Consequently, iron chelation therapy is recommended after approximately 12 months of blood transfusion, but the figures vary markedly between patients. Transfusional iron overload can have serious clinical consequences and, unless body iron is seriously controlled, patients may suffer significant morbidity and mortality.

In patients with iron overload, cardiac failure is a major, life-threatening complication. After about 100 units of blood transfusion, the deposition of excess iron in the heart muscles leads to myocarditis and cardiac fibrosis, which eventually causes severe arrhythmias or heart failure. Without treatment, these patients survive less than a year. Other complications include

Cross references

The role of hepcidin in the regulation of iron homeostasis is outlined in Chapter 4.

Haemoglobinopathy is explained in detail in Chapter 6.

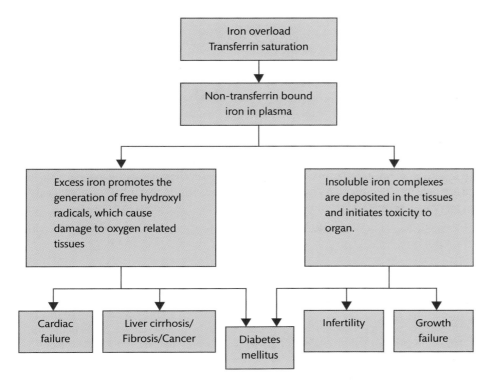

FIGURE 5.1
Clinical consequences of iron overload.

the deposition of iron in the liver, which may lead to fibrosis, cirrhosis, or cancer and diabetes mellitus as a result of B-cell destruction secondary to iron overload in the pancreas. Iron deposits in the pituitary gland may lead to growth failure and infertility (hypogonadism) due to reduced gonadotropin levels. The relationships between excess iron, biochemistry, and the clinical complications of iron overload are summarized in Figure 5.1.

SELF-CHECK 5.6

What are the principal causes of excess body iron?

Treatment of iron overload

Since the introduction of iron chelating therapy, deaths from iron overload have significantly decreased in patients who receive regular treatment. Iron chelators are usually administered by subcutaneous infusion, and the treatment should be started after 10–15 units of blood transfusion or when ferritin is over 2000 ng/ml. The most widely available iron chelating agent is desferrioxamine, and the success of treatment is monitored through the assessment of ferritin levels. Desferrioxamine reduces the amount of iron in the liver and also labile plasma iron. In addition, desferasirox shows potential in protecting cells from the damaging effect of intracellular oxidative stress.

An alternative to active iron chelation therapy is to simply bleed the patient from a vein in the arm as if they were a blood donor (venesection), and is the preferred method in hereditary haemochromatosis. Venesection should proceed regularly (perhaps each month) until

BOX 5.2 Why does excess iron cause disease?

The principal theory linking iron and clinically evident disease involves the generation of reactive oxygen species such as the hydroxyl radical. In normal healthy individuals, transferrin is only 30% saturated with iron and so has a large reserve capacity to take up further iron. However, in patients with iron overload, transferrin saturation may reach 100% and so the ability of transferrin to absorb further iron is exceeded. This leads to 'free iron' or non-transferrin bound iron (NTBI) which circulates in the plasma. NTBI is not only directly toxic to cells but is also indirectly toxic, in that it has the potential to generate free hydroxyl radicals that propagate oxygen-related tissue damage.

NTBI catalyses the Fenton reaction to generate free hydroxyl radicals ($^{\bullet}$OH) in the two following steps:

$$Fe^{3+} + O_2^{\bullet -} \qquad\qquad Fe^{2+} + O_2$$

$$Fe^{2+} + H_2O_2 \qquad\qquad Fe^{3+} + OH^- + HO^{\bullet}$$

(Note: The hydroxyl radical is generated (i.e. is a product) and so goes on the right hand side of the second equation. The superoxide radical $O_2^{\bullet}$ is on the left hand side of the first equation and so is a substrate. H_2O_2 is hydrogen peroxide and $HO^{\bullet}$ is the hydroxyl ion.)

Fortunately, a series of metabolic pathways exists (involving glutathione) to limit their effect (see Figure 4.9). The importance of this pathway is illustrated by the lack of an enzyme (glucose-6-phosphate dehydrogenase) that helps generate glutathione. The consequences of this deficiency often include a haemolytic anaemia.

---

ferritin levels are at the lower end of the reference range (perhaps 50 μg/L). Furthermore, the response of the FBC and iron indices to phlebotomy provides an essential assessment of the severity of the iron overload. Dietary advice is to minimize foodstuffs with a high iron content.

Porphyria

porphyria

Disease caused by abnormalities in the production of haem characterized by anaemia and, in the laboratory, by increased iron.

Porphyria is the collective noun for a number of diseases that follow from defects in the biosynthesis of haem, which lead to the overproduction of porphyrins and/or associated precursors such as aminolaevulinic acid and protoporphyrin. The aetiology of these conditions can be genetic (such as loss- or gain-of-function mutations in genes for the numerous biosynthetic enzymes), or (less frequently) can be caused by lead intoxication or drugs. Examples of the latter include barbiturates and certain antibiotics, which may cause an intermittent porphyria. Porphyria can also be the product of sideroblastic anaemia.

The consequences of porphyria depend on the nature of the biochemical lesion. For example, a sign of excess uroporphyrin is pink urine (red if severe), which can be easily distinguished from haematuria and haemoglobinuria. A hypochromic haemolytic anaemia is common and is likely to be associated with splenomegaly, hyperbilirubinaemia, and thus jaundice. Other signs include psychiatric changes, photosensitivity, stained teeth, abdominal pain, and neuropathy.

The role of the laboratory in iron-related pathology

The laboratory investigation of anaemia and iron overload demands a full blood count, which provides six red cell indices. These are haemoglobin, the red cell count, haematocrit, mean cell haemoglobin (MCH), mean cell haemoglobin concentration (MCHC), and mean cell volume (MCV). Of these, the MCV is of particular value as it is likely to be reduced in the face of iron deficiency, whereby red cells may be described as microcytic. It follows that an anaemia associated with microcytes is a microcytic anaemia (Figure 5.2). However, not all cases of microcytic anaemia are due to iron deficiency—an alternative cause may be haemoglobinopathy.

In addition to a reduced MCV, iron deficiency is generally associated with a reduced MCH and MCHC. If this is the case, then the red cells are said to be hypochromic. Furthermore, some autoanalysers can report the proportion of red cells that they consider to be hypochromic—a proportion greater than 2% is generally considered suggestive of iron deficiency. An additional feature of iron-deficient anaemia is the reduction, or even the absence, of stored iron (as ferritin and haemosiderin) in macrophages of the bone marrow, liver, and spleen. Indeed, it is likely that bone marrow stores of iron become depleted before there is evidence of iron deficiency from the red cell indices.

Several laboratory measurements are important in assessing iron-deficient anaemia. These include serum ferritin (the level of which is generally reduced: male <20 μg/L, female <12 μg/L), decreased iron (male <50 μg/dL, female <40 μg/dL), reduced transferrin saturation (<20%), and levels of the soluble transferrin receptor (levels often elevated). However, over-reliance on plasma ferritin may lead to error because, as an acute-phase reactant, levels may be raised in acute or chronic inflammation or in other acute disease or trauma. This can be a great frustration as anaemia is present in many chronic diseases, as we shall discuss in a subsequent section. Nevertheless, in the absence of illness or inflammation, body stores of iron can be assessed by levels of ferritin. Equally if the ferritin concentration is low, regardless of inflammation, this is highly suggestive of iron deficiency. The blood film from an iron-deficient subject will show microcytic hypochromic cells with pencil cells and occasional target cells.

The importance of the acid environment of the stomach is underlined by the high rate of iron-deficiency anaemia in patients with autoimmune gastritis, a disease characterized by failure of the stomach wall to produce acid. This condition may also lead to vitamin B_{12} deficiency, to be elaborated in a section that follows. Indeed, deficiency of both micronutrients can coexist.

Sideroblastic anaemia is diagnosed from an examination of bone marrow where greater than 15% of erythroblasts are ring sideroblasts. However, a small number of ring sideroblasts may

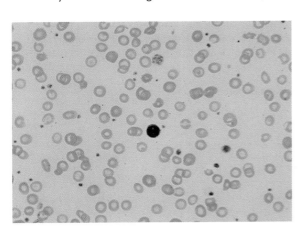

FIGURE 5.2

Iron deficiency, as is characterized by hypochromic microcytes—the cells seem to be 'empty', with a lack of staining in the centre of the cell. There is often anisocytosis (variation in cell size). A lymphocyte is also present. (Magnification ×400.) The red cells are significantly smaller than the nucleus of the small lymphocytes.

be present in other conditions such as myelodysplasia and copper deficiency, also diagnosed by examination of the bone marrow. The blood film of X-linked sideroblastic anaemia is characterized by microcytic anaemia, in the bone marrow by ineffective erythropoiesis, and in the tissues by iron overload. The key laboratory test is **Perls' stain** (also known as Perls' Prussian blue).

The sign of lead poisoning in a blood film is the appearance of basophilic stippling of red blood cells. This is due to denatured RNA. There may be ring sideroblasts in the bone marrow and the related anaemia may be hypochromic and/or haemolytic. Occasionally, a dimorphic picture of a hypochromic/microcytic population in conjunction with a normochromic/normocytic population may be present.

In iron overload, the role of the laboratory is different. The liver is the prime site for iron storage, with more than 90% of all excess body iron being deposited as intracellular ferritin and haemosiderin. Liver biopsy is the best method for assessing iron stores and is quantitative, specific, and sensitive. However, it is an invasive and painful procedure that carries the risk of sampling error, especially in a patient with liver damage. Fortunately, as mentioned, serum ferritin levels give a good indication of the status of iron stores, but this test is subject to a major

> **Perls' stain**
> The principal stain of blood, or bone marrow or tissues such as of the liver for deposits of iron

TABLE 5.8 Major laboratory features of iron related haematological disease.

Iron deficient anaemia	**Full blood count** Reduced haemoglobin, MCV, MCH and MCHC. RBCC may be normal but haematocrit more often than not is low (recall that haematocrit is the mathematical product of the RBCC and the MCV). Increased number of hypochromic red blood cells.
	Blood film Increased reticulocytes, following iron replacement therapy. Presence of microcytes (hence reduced MCV), often hypochromic. A population of elliptocytes called pencil cells, is commonly present.
	Bone marrow Examination not usually indicated. However, iron may be reduced and there may be evidence of increased erythropoiesis as the bone marrow attempts to remedy the low red cell mass with compensatory hyperactivity.
	Serology Low serum ferritin (but beware false positive effects of the acute phase response), low transferrin saturation. Increased soluble transferrin receptors (evidence of increased erythroblast activity).
Iron overload/ Sideroblastic anaemia	**Full blood count/film/bone marrow** MCV often raised in acquired cases but low in inherited variants: bone marrow sideroblasts (Perls' stain) and possibly siderocytes on the blood film, presence of Pappenheimer bodies. Dimorphic red cell population of hypochromic/microcytic cells in conjunction with normochromic/normocytic cells.
	Serology High serum iron and ferritin, high transferrin saturation (possibly 100%). Low soluble transferrin receptor levels
	Other investigations Liver biopsy, and possibly bone marrow aspirates, demonstrate high iron stores (Perls' stain). Refer for genetic screening if HH considered. If treatment by phlebotomy, FBC and iron studies must be performed before and after to monitor the expected fall in iron levels.

confounding influence: inflammation. Consequently, interpretation must be made with caution in the presence of infections and in inflammatory diseases such as rheumatoid arthritis.

If transferrin saturation exceeds 45% and there is raised ferritin (>300 µg/L in men and >200 µg/L in women), then HH may be suspected. Increased liver function tests (such as raised transaminase enzymes) imply the involvement of (and damage to) this organ. If this damage is severe there may be raised serum bilirubin and the classical sign of jaundice.

In the investigation of porphyria, reference laboratories are likely to measure enzymes such as aminolaevulinic acid dehydratase and synthetase, and urobilinogen synthetase in parallel with their particular substrates and products. They may also conduct molecular biology studies to demonstrate mutations in relevant genes.

Table 5.8 summarizes the role of the laboratory in the investigation of iron-related disease, whilst Figure 5.3 illustrates the pathways of iron cycling. However, the laboratory is not only required for diagnosis, but also to monitor treatment. One of the treatments of iron-deficient anaemia is the provision of iron. This is likely to lead to a burst in erythropoiesis with new, fresh erythrocytes of normal size appearing in the blood. However, this burst of new erythrocyte production may outstrip folate stores so cells may be folate-deficient. Thus a dimorphic picture may be present on a blood film, consisting of 'old' microcytes alongside 'new' normocytes, as is illustrated in Figure 5.4. Figures 4.12(b) and (d) also illustrate microcytes.

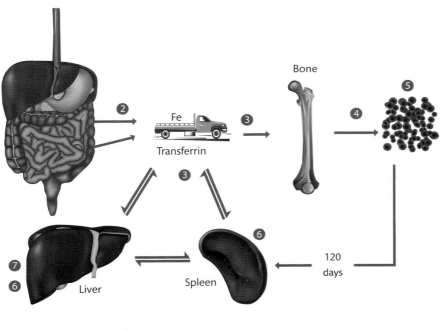

1 Ingestion   4 Erythropoiesis   7 Disposal of bilirubin by excretion, e.g. into bile

2 Absorption   5 Red blood cells

3 Transport   6 Destruction in the spleen and liver

FIGURE 5.3
Pathways of iron cycling.

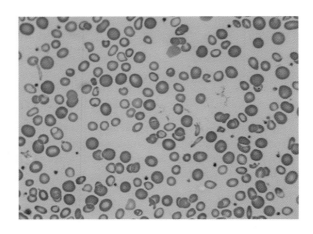

FIGURE 5.4

Following treatment for iron deficiency, or post transfusion, there may be two distinct populations: one of normal and another of abnormal cells leading to anisocytosis (variation in size) and anisochromasia (variation in colour). Note in this photograph that the majority of smaller cells (microcytes) are also pale (hypochromic), whilst the larger cells (normocytes, new cells having responded to oral iron, or perhaps transfused cells) have a good colour. (Magnification ×400.)

METHOD *Staining for iron*

The key stain for iron is Perls' stain, developed by the German pathologist, Max Perls. Samples of bone marrow or peripheral blood spread out on glass slides are air-dried and then fixed with methanol for 10–20 min. When dry, they are exposed to acidified potassium ferrocyanide for a further 10 min, washed with tap water and then distilled water, and then exposed for around 10–15 s to a second stain such as aqueous neutral red or eosin as a counterstain. (Iron stain 56 °C for 10 min or 30 min at room temperature). Following a final wash and air-dry, slides may be examined by light microscopy. If present, any iron-containing (siderotic) material or haemosiderin is converted to the blue-coloured product, ferriferrocyanide. Consequently, the stain is also known as Perls' Prussian blue.

A modification of the technique can be used in the histopathology laboratory to stain body tissues or biopsies. Neither ferritin nor apoferritin take up Perls' stain. However, ferritin undergoes degradation to generate haemosiderin, which can be detected in tissue macrophages of the liver (Kupffer cells) and spleen.

When the body is overloaded with iron, it may also be found in other tissues, including cardiac tissue. Siderotic material can also be detected by Romanowsky dyes as basophilic granules, which are a mixture of protein and iron. Such granules are called Pappenheimer bodies.

Figures 5.5 and 5.6 illustrate Perls' staining of a blood and bone marrow sample, respectively.

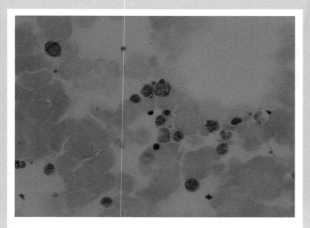

FIGURE 5.5

Perls' stain for iron in a blood film. The blue material is iron, the red-pink materials are counterstained nuclei of white blood cells.

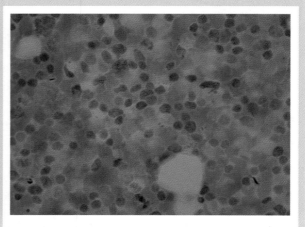

FIGURE 5.6

Perls' stain for iron in a sample of bone marrow. Note the greater density of cells than in the blood film. The blue material is iron, the red-pink materials are counterstained nuclei of white blood cells.

What are ring sideroblasts and what can they tell us?

Case study 5.1 is illustrative of the consequences of iron deficiency.

CASE STUDY 5.1 Consequences of iron deficiency

A 50-year-old woman with long-term Crohn's disease, on various treatments and with a history of surgery to the abdomen, had the following test results following a GP visit where she complained of tiredness, some lethargy, fevers, and diarrhoea.

This case		Reference range (page xiii–xiv)
Haemoglobin	105 g/L	118–148
MCV	70 fL	77–98
WCC	6.1×10^9/L	3.7–9.5
ESR	26 mm/hour	<10
Platelets	350×10^9/L	143–400
Fibrinogen	3.5 g/L	1.5–4.0

The low haemoglobin was followed up with an assessment of micronutrient status, reporting serum iron 5.4 µmol/L (reference range 10–37) and serum vitamin B_{12} 227 ng/L (normal range 160–925).

■ Can you make a preliminary diagnosis based on the FBC and ESR? What are the abnormalities?

■ Are you able to modify this diagnosis in view of the iron and vitamin B_{12} results?

■ What are your next steps?

Key Points

Iron is clearly a very important micronutrient, required not only for haem but also for certain enzymes. However, it is also a double-edged sword, because too much iron can be as disabling as too little iron.

5.4 **Anaemia arising from lack of vitamins**

Section 4.3 indicated the importance of vitamins B_{12} and B_6, and folate in the development of red blood cells, although they have other roles in other aspects of metabolism (such as in maintaining the integrity of nerves). Much of the metabolism and pathology of the vitamins have parallels with those of iron: all are micronutrients that must be obtained in the diet, so that deficiency may be the consequence of a poor diet. In addition, since absorption demands a healthy intestine, active intestinal disease or abdominal surgery is a likely contributor to anaemia.

Vitamin B_{12}, vitamin B_6, and folate

Vitamin B_{12}

Physiology

The crystalline structure of vitamin B_{12}, the largest of all vitamins with a molecular weight of 1355 Da, was elucidated in 1948. It is composed of a ring of four pyrrole units (similar to haem), with an atom of cobalt at its centre. This leads some to describe the vitamin as **cobalamin** (abbreviated to Cbl) or, if complexed to a cyanide group, as cyanocobalamin. Other forms active in haematological metabolism are methylcobalamin and deoxyadenosylcobalamin.

The daily requirement of this vitamin is in the region of 1 µg, which should be easily satisfied by a mixed diet providing about 10–30 µg per day, of which perhaps 2–3 µg are absorbed. However, others suggest the recommended daily allowance should be higher at 2.5 µg/day and up to 3 µg/day if pregnant. Unlike iron, these requirements are independent of age or sex. Also unlike iron, vitamin B_{12} is almost absent from the plant kingdom—it is synthesized only in certain bacteria (such as *Streptomyces* species) and concentrates in the tissues of higher predatory organisms near the top of the food chain.

Like iron, the liver (and kidney) can store vitamin B_{12} in milligram quantities. Such quantities are sufficient to meet the needs of the body even if it is deprived of an external source of the vitamin for several years. Consequently, there may be a considerable period between a failure to consume sufficient quantities of the vitamin, or to absorb it, and the onset of clinical signs of the deficiency.

To be absorbed, the vitamin B_{12} present in a foodstuff must first be liberated and extracted by the combination of the proteolytic enzyme pepsin and the acid environment of the stomach. Free vitamin BR then binds to an R-binder - a glycoprotein secreted into saliva which enters the stomach. Specialist **gastric parietal cells** synthesize and release **intrinsic factor** (IF), which then binds the free vitamin B_{12} (the latter was once known as extrinsic factor) in the upper duodenum, following the release of vitamin BR from the R-binder facilitated by the proteolytic action of pancreatic trypsin. A 45-kDa molecular weight glycoprotein, IF is a carrier transport protein that delivers the vitamin B_{12} to the large intestine, although perhaps 1–5% of free vitamin B_{12} is absorbed along the entire intestine by passive diffusion. Factors such as histamine and gastrin stimulate the release of IF into the gastric juice.

Absorption of the IF/vitamin B_{12} complex occurs in the distal/terminal ileum, and requires the IF to dock to its receptor on the luminal surface of the enterocyte. This receptor has three components: cubilin, megalin, and amnionless. In the post-enterocyte circulation, vitamin B_{12} binds the specific carrier molecules **transcobalamin** I (TC-I, described by some as haptocorrin, which has a half-life of 9–10 days) and transcobalamin II (TC-II, with a half-life of 1.5 hours) as transcobalamin III. Radioactive tracer experiments established that vitamin B_{12} first binds to TC-II and then to

cobalamin
The chemical 'template' for vitamin B_{12} and related molecules.

gastric parietal cells
Cells of the luminal wall of the stomach which synthesize and secrete the intestinal vitamin B_{12} carrier molecule **intrinsic factor (IF)**, which is essential for the absorption of the vitamin across the gut wall.

transcobalamin
The molecule that carries vitamin B_{12} in the blood. It is present in three forms—transcobalamin I and transcobalamin II and III.

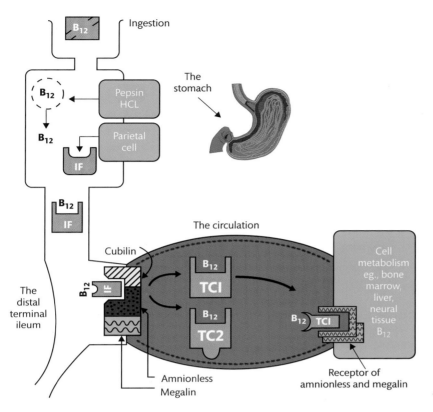

FIGURE 5.7
Absorption and transport of vitamin B$_{12}$.

TC-I. At the surface of the receiving cell, perhaps the erythroblast or the hepatocyte, the complex of vitamin B$_{12}$/TC-II binds to a heterodimer of megalin and the TC-II-receptor. Once inside the cell, lysosomal degradation of TC-II and the release of vitamin B$_{12}$ allow the latter to participate in metabolism in the cytoplasm and in the mitochondria. These steps are summarized in Figure 5.7.

Vitamin B$_{12}$ is an essential cofactor for two enzymes. The first enzyme takes methylmalonic acid/propionyl-coenzyme A as a substrate and converts it to succinyl coenzyme A (succinyl-CoA) using vitamin B$_{12}$ as a cofactor. This is a key early step in the synthesis of haem. In the second process, homocysteine is converted to methionine by using vitamin B$_{12}$ and folate as cofactors. Therefore, a lack of vitamin B$_{12}$ leads not only to the absence of the products succinyl-CoA and methionine, but also to the build up of the two substrates for these reactions, which are methylmalonic acid and homocysteine (Figure 5.8).

SELF-CHECK 5.8

Why is the stomach important for the absorption of vitamin B$_{12}$?

Deficiency of vitamin B$_{12}$

The complex steps in the passage of vitamin B$_{12}$ from the diet to the cell give rise to many possible causes of deficiency. It is widely distributed in animal material (such as fish, meat, eggs, and dairy products). Consequently, perhaps the only form of deficiency arising from malnutrition is in those who follow a strict vegan diet, and is relatively rare.

In addition, a very small number of well-characterized functional mutations in the genes for various plasma carriers (IF, TC-I, TC-II) and receptors (at the luminal surface of the enterocyte—cubilin, amnionless—and at the surface of the receiving cell) also result in deficiency of the

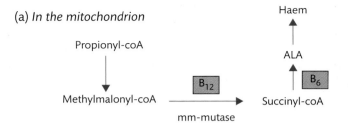

(a) *In the mitochondrion*

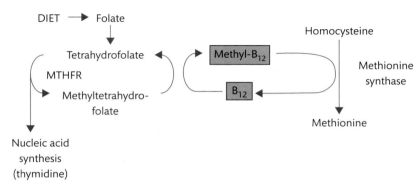

(b) *In the cytoplasm*

FIGURE 5.8
Metabolic pathways of vitamins B$_6$, B$_{12}$ and folate.

MTHFR = Methyltetrahydrofolate reductase, ALA = aminolaevulinic acid,
MMA = methylmalonic acid

vitamin at the bone marrow. Low or absent levels of TC-I can be detected by immunoassay, a test likely to be offered by a Reference laboratory.

However, the leading cause of vitamin B$_{12}$ deficiency (>90% of cases) is autoimmune gastritis, being present in up to 2% of the population, a rate that increases with age (up to 10% of those in their eighth decade) and in those with other autoimmune disease. The principal serological aspect of the disease is the presence of circulating autoantibodies to gastric parietal cells and to their product, IF. The presence of these autoantibodies defines the disease as **pernicious anaemia** (PA). How do these antibodies arise? It has been suggested that the initial pathogenic stimulus is an inappropriate response to *Helicobacter pylori*. The autoantibodies direct chronic autoaggression towards the gastric proton pump, resulting in parietal cell destruction and decreased gastric juice secretion. (Any gastric juice that is present is not necessarily acidic.) Notably, this lack of acid may also lead to iron-deficient anaemia, which is present in 20–40% of PA patients.

pernicious anaemia
The anaemia defined by the autoimmune destruction of gastric parietal cells and/or IF, and which cause vitamin B$_{12}$ deficiency.

However, the pathological basis of PA in patients with acquired hypogammaglobulinaemia cannot be an autoantibody. In such cases, abnormal cell-mediated immunity can generally be demonstrated. This is supported by the high frequency of leukocyte infiltrations in stomach biopsies of patients with PA.

Another frequent serological finding is an elevation in the levels of plasma gastrin (>300 ng/L) and/or pepsinogen. It should be stressed that the vitamin B$_{12}$-deficient PA should be regarded as the long-term consequence of the autoimmune destruction of the parietal cells. A further long-term consequence is an increased (tenfold) rate of gastric tumours. Other forms of non-immune gastric damage (alcoholism, gastric atrophy, non-specific gastritis, surgery, carcinoma) may also lead to a failure to generate acid and/or IF, ultimately leading to vitamin B$_{12}$ deficiency. The increasing therapeutic use of proton-pump inhibitors (designed to reduce gastric acid) and histamine H$_2$-receptor blockers are an additional possible cause of this disease.

The metabolic pathways reliant on vitamin B_{12} are widely distributed, so that there may be several pathological consequences of vitamin B_{12} deficiency for the body. Non-haematological consequences of vitamin B_{12} deficiency include a swollen and painful tongue (glossitis), peripheral neuropathy/polyneuritis (possibly manifesting as poor motor coordination (ataxia), loss of sensation, tremor, or tingling), and consciousness and personality changes (which may range from simple confusion and irritability, to depression, loss of memory, and even psychosis).

Vitamin B_6

This vitamin (also known as pyridoxine) is an essential cofactor for the conversion of succinyl-CoA and glycine into aminolaevulinic acid (ALA) by the enzyme ALA synthase (Figure 5.8(a)). It is also important in many metabolic processes, including those of amino acids, sphingolipids, and glyconeogenesis. Vitamin B_6 is common in many foodstuffs (fruit, vegetables, cereals, and meat) and easily passively absorbed in the jejunum and ileum, so that the recommended daily requirement of 0.5–2.0 mg (towards the higher end if lactating or pregnant) is easy to achieve.

Folate

The intestinal absorption of folate is less complex than that of vitamin B_{12} and occurs in the duodenum and upper small intestine. General dietary folates are then transported to the liver, becoming methyltetrahydrofolate. The daily requirement of folate is approximately 100–200 mg; this should be adequately provided for through a mixed diet, which is able to provide 200–300 mg per day. The importance of folate (and vitamin B_{12}) in other aspects of pathology is demonstrated by the fact that most cases of spina bifida and neural tube defects result from maternal deficiency in these micronutrients during the periconceptual period. This may be related to an increased incidence in pregnant women who are more likely to become folate-deficient as stores last only a few months, whereas vitamin B_{12} stores are generally sufficient for over a year. Studies in the USA, where foodstuffs are fortified with folate, demonstrate a significant reduction in the rates of cleft palate, pyloric stenosis, and upper limb reduction defects. The metabolic requirement for folate stems from its role as a substrate for thymidine and thus DNA (Figure 5.8(b)).

The leading genetic cause of low serum folate is a loss-of-function mutation in the enzyme methylene-tetrahydrofolate reductase, which also results in increased homocysteine and low methionine (Figure 5.8(b)). However, this mutation does not lead to megaloblastic anaemia, and may or may not lead to low folate, but almost always leads to hyperhomocysteinaemia. Hereditary folate malabsorption has been described but is extremely rare.

SELF-CHECK 5.9

What are the primary causes of vitamin B_{12} deficiency?

Treatment of vitamin and folate deficiency

The cause of the deficiency should always be defined and remedied for its complete resolution. However, in the short term, the standard treatment is replacement therapy. For vitamin B_{12} deficiency this is likely to be regular injections of vitamin B_{12}. Common regimes include a loading dose of perhaps 100–1000 µg/day intramuscular for a week, followed by a fortnightly dosing, then a lower maintenance dose of once a month to once every three months. The success of this regime should be sought with an improvement in symptoms, which can be monitored with the appropriate blood testing. Many regard this as an improvement over the original treatment of 100–300 g of raw beef liver, to be taken orally, which provided folate and iron in addition to vitamin B_{12}. This regime produced a peak rise in reticulocytes 5–7 days after treatment began, alongside an acceleration in the maturation of megaloblasts. Notably, a diet of raw beef muscle fails to elicit this response. However, the approach of providing parenteral vitamin B_{12} is not always successful. For example, certain cases are caused by loss-of-function mutations in genes coding for enzymes that convert 'raw' vitamin B_{12} into deoxyadenosylcobalamin (in the mitochondrion) or into methylcobalamin (in the cytoplasm). Treatment in the latter cases is with systemic hydroxocobalamin. The autoimmune form (that is, PA) may be treated with immunosuppression (generally steroids). Folate deficiency is treated with oral supplements.

The successful treatment of vitamin or folate deficiency should be evaluated with FBC and blood film and reticulocyte counts 10–14 days after the start of treatment. This should reveal a rising haemoglobin and falling MCV. Bone marrow examination at this stage is rarely necessary. All indices should have returned to normal after 8 weeks. A failure to respond in this way suggests inadequately low levels of supplements or an incorrect diagnosis.

Table 5.9 summarizes the main causes of vitamin B_{12} and folate deficiency.

The role of the laboratory in the investigation of anaemia following lack of micronutrients

As with iron-related pathology, laboratory investigation of vitamin B_{12} deficiency centres on a full blood count and blood film. The principal finding in the FBC is that the MCV becomes elevated in both vitamin B_{12} and folate deficiency, hence the red cells may be described as macrocytic, leading to a diagnosis of macrocytic anaemia. In addition to increased MCV, vitamin

TABLE 5.9 Causes of vitamin B_{12} and folate deficiency.

Vitamin B_{12}	Folate (serum and red cells)
Pregnancy	Alcohol, pregnancy
Strict veganism	Anticonvulsants
HIV infection	Vitamin B_{12} deficiency
Myeloma	Malabsorption
Folate deficiency	
Sjögren's syndrome	
Use of proton-pump inhibitors or other acid antagonists	
Loss of function mutation in genes for receptors and carrier proteins	
Ileal disease	
Gastric surgery and other disease	
Pernicious anaemia	
Bacterial overgrowth in the intestines	
Pancreatic insufficiency	
Tropical sprue	
Tapeworm infestation	
Unknown causes (present in perhaps 10% of patients)	

B_{12} and folate deficiency is often associated with elevated MCH, in which case the red cells are said to be hyperchromic.

Although the macrocyte is important in the diagnosis of vitamin B_{12} deficiency, two points must be made. The precise definition of this cell depends on local conditions, as some describe the upper limit of the reference range to be, for example, 98 fL, whereas others may put this limit at 100 fL. It follows that in some laboratories, a red blood cell with an MCV of 99 fL may be a macrocyte, but in others the same cell may be a normocyte. Consequently, the practitioner must refer to his or her own local reference range. The second point refers to the specificity and sensitivity of the macrocyte in defining vitamin B_{12} deficiency: a large number of drugs and conditions are associated with macrocytosis, but not all of these are associated with an anaemia. Consequently, alternative and differential diagnoses must be addressed when considering a diagnosis of macrocytosis and vitamin B_{12} deficiency (Table 5.10). A key physiological cause of macrocytosis is pregnancy. Macrocytes are shown in Figure 5.9.

Similarly, the aware practitioner will be avoid the pitfalls in the interpretation of the blood film with a raised MCV, such as 110 fL. The presence of oval macrocytes, anisocytosis, and poikilocytes suggest vitamin B_{12} deficiency, whereas round macrocytes are commonly seen in numerous chronic diseases, such as hepatitis, obstructive jaundice, and those conditions listed in Table 5.9. An additional consideration, although rare, is marked reticulocytosis (such as >10% of the total red blood cell count). This should be considered if there is evidence of haemolysis, polychromasia, nucleated red blood cells, spherocytes, or schistocytes.

In the bone marrow, a consequence of the shortage of vitamin B_{12} is that erythroblasts become enlarged and oval shaped, and are referred to as megaloblasts (literally, large blasts). This finding gives the disease an additional and perhaps more scientific name—**megaloblastic anaemia**. Progenitors of other lineages are also abnormal, with the presence of giant metamyelocytes. These abnormalities are caused by defects in DNA synthesis, which retards proliferation and maturation, and the entire marrow is hypercellular. In very severe deficiency this may lead to haemopoietic arrest and thus pancytopenia.

The phenomenon of increased size continues as the erythroid cells develop within the bone marrow, and is the basis of increased numbers of large erythrocytes (macrocytes) in the bone marrow and in the peripheral blood. These DNA defects also explain **hypersegmented neutrophils** present in peripheral blood, and are an established feature on a blood film (Figure 5.10).

hypersegmented neutrophil
A principal blood film sign of vitamin B_{12} deficiency: the nucleus of the normal neutrophil may have perhaps three or five lobes; in vitamin B_{12} deficiency the number of lobes may rise to seven or eight.

TABLE 5.10   Causes of macrocytosis.

Drugs	Chemotherapy: cyclophosphamide, hydroxycarbamide, methotrexate, azathioprine
	Antimicrobials: pyrimethamine, trimethoprim, zidovudine
	Anticonvulsants: phenytoin, primidone, valproic acid
	Others: metformin, sulfasalazine
Pathology	Vitamin B_{12} and or folate deficiency
	Alcoholism, hypothyroidism, multiple myeloma, liver disease
	Myelodysplasia, aplastic anaemia, acute leukaemia
	Reticulocytosis, hyperglycaemia, marked leukocytosis, cold agglutinins

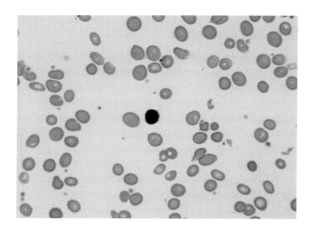

FIGURE 5.9

Macrocytosis may be present in patients deficient in vitamin B$_{12}$, vitamin B$_6$ or folate. If so, the macrocytes are often oval and may be accompanied by schistocytes and anisocytosis. Note that a macrocyte is larger than the nearby lymphocyte. Contrast this with Figure 5.2, where the microcytes are notably smaller than the lymphocyte. (Magnification ×400.)

A further consequence of ineffective erythropoiesis is a low reticulocyte count and intramedullary haemolysis, which may lead to raised lactate dehydrogenase and bilirubin levels. Because many of these changes are also present in myeloid leukaemia and myelodysplasia, interpretation must be cautious. An additional aspect of megaloblastic anaemia on the blood film is basophilic stippling, although several other conditions (such as lead poisoning) also cause this sign (Figure 5.11).

The ultimate definition of vitamin B$_{12}$ deficiency is obviously serum levels below the local reference range. However, the tests for levels of this vitamin demonstrate poor sensitivity and specificity, poor agreement between laboratories regarding a reference range, and, hence, the definition of a lower limit of a reference range. This can be crucial, as a 'high' lower limit of the reference range will, of course, define fewer cases of deficiency than a 'low' lower limit of the reference range, which will find more cases. The patient will continue with the same signs

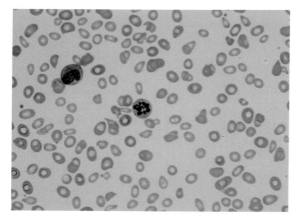

FIGURE 5.10

Hypersegmented neutrophils are a sign of vitamin B$_{12}$ deficiency and are the consequence of abnormal DNA synthesis. Neutrophils normally have 3-5 nuclear lobes, but if hypersegmented there may be seven or more lobes, as in the cell in the centre of this figure. This can be compared with Figure 5.11, where the normal neutrophil has few lobes. (Magnification ×400.)

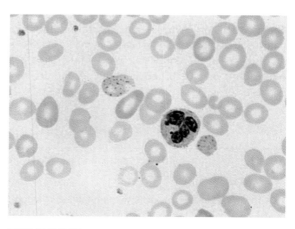

FIGURE 5.11

Basophilic stippling of red cells, but also called punctate basophilia, as may be seen in megaloblastic anaemia. However, it is also seen in many other conditions, including lead poisoning, myelodysplasia, haemoglobinopathy and haemolytic anaemia. This slide shows two excellent examples either side of a neutrophil; note also that two red blood cells are not only oval shaped but have a more blue coloration than others (polychromasia). (Magnification ×600.)

and symptoms regardless of the laboratory findings, underlining the importance of the symbiosis between the laboratory and the clinic.

These issues have led to the adoption of a second round of testing, for methyl-malonic acid (MMA) also known as methylmalonyl CoA (Figure 5.8). The rationale for this is that lack of the vitamin results in poor activity of the enzyme MMA-mutase which normally transforms MMA into succinyl-CoA. Thus, lack of the activity of this enzyme leads to high (unused) levels of its substrate (that is, MMA). This is illustrated in Figure 5.12. However, MMA may be reduced in acute or chronic renal failure, and very rarely in defects in enzymes involved in the generation of MMA. As such a cautious approval to interpreting MMA results in patients with renal disease should be adopted.

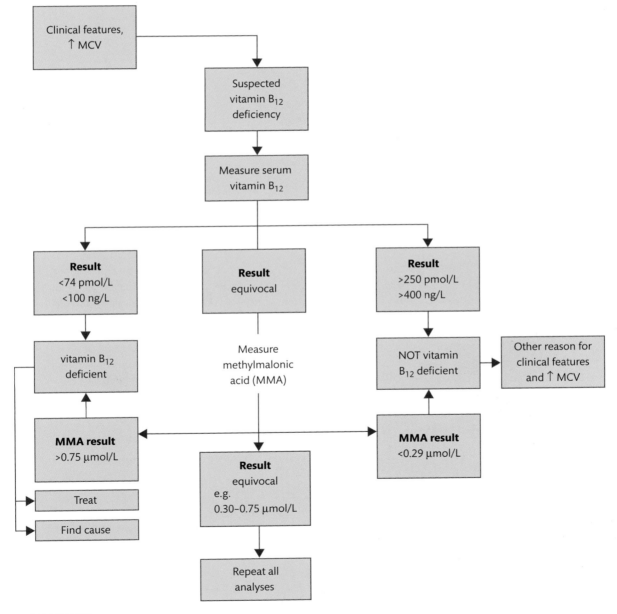

FIGURE 5.12
Schematic for the use of vitamin B_{12} and methylmalonic acid in the diagnosis of vitamin B_{12} deficiency.

Rarely, if the combination of vitamin B_{12} and MMA assay is equivocal, then measurement of homocysteine may be necessary. This exploits the requirement of methylcobalamin as an essential cofactor for methionine synthase, which takes homocysteine as a substrate (Figure 5.8(b)). A growing body of opinion suggests that measuring TC-II could be valuable in circumstances where vitamin B_{12} could be falsely elevated, such as in cases of renal failure and myeloproliferative disease. In myeloproliferative diseases TC-I and TC-III are released in large quantities from the abnormal grabulocytes. These compete with TC-II when binding vitamin B_{12}, resulting in a failure to provide tissues with bioavailable B_{12}. Notably, the assays of MMA and homocysteine may also be useful in a different setting. High levels of the former will be present in deficiency of the deoxyadenosylcobalamin variant of vitamin B_{12}, whereas hyperhomocysteinaemia will be a consequence of the failure to generate the methylcobalamin variant of the vitamin.

Once proven to be present, the aetiology of vitamin B_{12} deficiency, if caused by autoantibodies to gastric parietal cells and/or IF, is defined in the laboratory as PA. The presence of these autoantibodies is relatively easy to detect in the immunology laboratory by standard serological techniques such as indirect immunofluorescence, although an enzyme-linked immunosorbent assay (ELISA) may also be used. In addition, anti-IF antibodies may be found in gastric juice. The laboratory may also offer a test for levels of plasma gastrin or pentagastrin, which are likely to be high in PA. Furthermore, vitamin B_{12} deficiency may be due to low levels (<35 pmol/L) of the plasma carrier protein, TC-II, which can also be determined by immunoassay.

The (auto)immunological basis of PA is supported by relationships with other autoimmune diseases. In one study, 9% of patients with autoimmune thyroid disease also had PA, compared with 0.1% in the general population. Conversely, thyroid autoantibodies are present in the serum of 55% of patients with PA. The disease is ten times more common in type-1 diabetes than in type-2 disease. Indeed, it is regarded as prudent to prospectively test such patients for autoantibodies perhaps annually, whilst endoscopic surveillance for tumours at five-yearly intervals has been recommended.

An alternative test to help define the nature of the deficiency is of the absorption of vitamin B_{12}. In this test, developed by Schilling, the patient is presented with an oral dose of radiolabelled vitamin B_{12} and a large excess of injected unlabelled cyanocobalamin. The urine and/or blood can then be probed for labelled and unlabelled vitamin to determine the proportion of each type of the vitamin which has been absorbed. A variant of this test is to measure the absorbance of the vitamin in the presence and absence of oral IF. However, the Schilling test has fallen out of favour because of the inherent safety issue associated with radioisotopes, its complex nature, difficulties with its interpretation (such as in renal disease), and the improved performance of alternative assays. Table 5.11 summarizes major laboratory features of vitamin B_{12}-deficient anaemia.

Case study 5.2 is illustrative of the consequences of vitamin B_{12} deficiency.

TABLE 5.11 Major laboratory features of vitamin B_{12} deficient anaemia.

Full blood count	Reduced haemoglobin, increased MCV, MCH and MCHC
Blood film	Presence of macrocytic red cells, anisocytosis, occasional nucleated red cells. Increased number of hyperchromic red blood cells. Hypersegmented neutrophils
Bone marrow	Presence of megaloblasts (thereby defining megaloblastic anaemia)
Serology	Presence of autoantibodies to gastric parietal cells and to intrinsic factor (if present, these define pernicious anaemia). Low levels of serum vitamin B_{12}, often with reduced serum and red cell folate

CASE STUDY 5.2 Consequences of vitamin B₁₂ deficiency

A 75-year-old woman complains of slowly developing fatigue so that she has difficulty getting out of the house. On examination, she has a swollen and painful tongue, and she complains of becoming forgetful, with occasional 'tingling' of her fingertips, and numbness in her toes. Routine bloods were:

This case		Reference range (page xiii–xiv)
Haemoglobin	96 g/L	118–148
WCC	5.7×10^9/L	3.7–9.5
Platelets	198×10^9/L	143–400
MCV	108 fL	77–98
ESR	15 mm/hour	<10
Haematocrit	0.45	0.33–0.47

In view of her signs, symptoms, and history, additional bloods were requested. The results of these were serum iron 11.6 µmol/L (reference range 10–37), serum vitamin B₁₂ 102 ng/L (reference range 160–925).

- Can you make a preliminary diagnosis based on the FBC and ESR? What are the abnormalities?
- Are you able to modify this diagnosis in view of the iron and vitamin B₁₂ results?
- What are your next steps?

SELF-CHECK 5.10

What are the primary FBC, blood film, and bone marrow abnormalities to be expected in vitamin B₁₂ deficiency?

Because vitamin B₆ is abundant and easily absorbed, a deficiency in this vitamin is extremely rare. However, if present, deficiency (probably defined by serum levels <10 nmol/L of pyridoxal phosphate) can be treated with oral vitamin B₆ 50–200 mg/day. The elderly, those on dialysis, and alcoholics are at risk. Inadequate levels of vitamin B₆ may cause reduced haem synthesis and thus a haemolytic, sideroblastic and megaloblastic anaemia, a picture similar to that of vitamin B₁₂ deficiency.

Deficiency of folate is also rare. However, measuring serum folate is problematical because of its liberation from stores and transiently increased levels after a meal. Consequently, red blood cell folate is regarded as being a more reliable determinant as levels are constant throughout the life of the cell. Low red cell folate levels are very common in PA (>50%), possibly because vitamin B_{12} is required for the transfer of methyltetrahydrofolate from the plasma into the red cell. Other causes of low folate are listed in Table 5.9.

Key Points

The aetiology and pathology of pernicious anaemia (PA) is well understood, and its many links make it a classic of disease unravelling. However, one of its major laboratory signs—macrocytosis—is also found in several other pathological and healthy conditions.

5.5 Anaemia of chronic disease (ACD)

This heterogeneus condition brings together numerous different aetiological aspects, several of which we have already addressed. However, a common feature is an impairment of erythropoiesis and the hypoproliferative anaemia which follows. Key components of the pathology of this general condition are inflammation (which may suppress erythropoiesis) and erythropoietin (low levels of which will result in anaemia), although these processes do not apply to all subtypes of the anaemia.

The liver

Cross references

Full details of the role of erythropoietin and erythropoiesis are presented in Chapter 4.

Liver function tests are fully explained in the *Clinical Biochemistry* volume of this series.

The functions of this complex organ include the storage of iron and the synthesis of iron-related molecules. Therefore both these factors impact upon anaemia. Part of the body's iron stores are carried in hepatocyte and liver macrophages (Kupffer cells) as ferritin and haemosiderin. A failing liver (as may be present in hepatoma, cirrhosis, or hepatocellular carcinoma) will therefore be unable to synthesize these proteins and thus to adequately store and transport iron. This situation can lead to (or at least contribute to) a microcytic anaemia. Severe damage to hepatocytes is associated with acanthocytosis. Alcoholism may not simply lead directly to liver disease and atrophy, but may also develop into malnutrition and malabsorption, with deficiencies in vitamin B_{12} and folate, which in turn may promote megaloblastic anaemia. However, alcohol abuse can cause macrocytosis in the absence of vitamin B_{12} or folic acid deficiency.

Inflammation, in the form of the acute-phase response, may induce increased levels of ferritin and transferrin. Such inflammation may be the secondary response to a distant infection, to an autoimmune disease (such as rheumatoid arthritis), or to active inflammation of the liver itself (that is, hepatitis). The anaemia associated with inflammation is generally normocytic. Actual damage to the liver (as may be caused by cytotoxic chemotherapy) may liberate iron-rich ferritin from intracellular stores. Consequently, levels may appear normal or even high, erroneously suggesting plentiful iron stores. Hypercholesterolaemia, whether the result of obstructive jaundice or genetic-type familial hypercholesterolaemia, can lead to macrocytosis and target cells; in contrast, hepatocellular damage, as may be caused by toxins (such as heavy metals or the hepatitis B virus) is associated with acanthocytosis. Macrocytes are also present in other forms of liver disease.

If there is severe liver disease it is likely that liver function tests such as alkaline phosphatase, bilirubin, and gamma glutamyl-transferase will also be abnormal. This illustrates an additional reason why the experienced biomedical scientist will be aware of issues outside his or her immediate discipline—in this case, in biochemistry.

The kidney

The kidney produces the red blood cell growth factor erythropoietin, which is required for effective erythropoieisis. Thus patients with chronic renal failure, and possibly on dialysis, are at risk of becoming anaemic. Such anaemia is generally normocytic. The normal inverse relationship between erythropoietin and haemoglobin is lost when serum creatinine rises above 135 μmol/L, and the degree of hypoxia required to stimulate release of the hormone rises considerably. Fortunately, recombinant erythropoietin can be prescribed to treat anaemia of this aetiology, although this is not always as beneficial in the long term. Rarely, in frank and serious renal damage—as may be present in trauma or disease such as glomerulonephritis—there may be blood loss into the urine (haematuria). If this is heavy and persistent, a normocytic anaemia may follow.

Measurement of serum erythropoietin may be useful in assessing significant anaemia. However, the level of erythropoietin cannot be taken as a measure of oxygenation because many conditions (such as hyperviscosity, cancer, and pregnancy) suppress erythropoietin production independently of the effects of hypoxia.

In parallel to severe liver disease, severe renal disease may be assessed by the biochemistry blood tests of urea and electrolytes (U&E).

Cross reference
Urea and electrolytes are fully explained in the *Clinical Biochemistry* volume of this series.

Gastrointestinal disease

Sections 5.3 and 5.4 have discussed how disease of the digestive tract can lead to microcytic and macrocytic anaemia because of the malabsorption and consequent deficiency of iron and vitamin B_{12}, respectively. However, anaemia may also arise from other disease of the intestines, such as the physical loss of blood from bleeding lesions. Such anaemia is generally normocytic. These diseases may be present in the upper section of the intestinal tract, and include oesophagitis and oesophageal varices.

In the lower section of the intestines, blood may be lost from haemorrhagic ulcers, or as a consequence of colorectal cancer, inflammatory bowel disease (such as duodenitis, colitis, and Crohn's disease), or haemorrhoids. Indeed, occult bleeding is an early sign of gastrointestinal cancer and may lead to normocytic anaemia. However, if chronic blood loss persists, of whatever aetiology, and iron stores become depleted, then the anaemia may become microcytic.

Reproductive organs

Increased haemoglobin, haematocrit, and red cell numbers in men compared to women is the result of testosterone acting on the bone marrow as a growth factor. Loss of the testes to trauma or disease is associated with a reduction in the red cell indices to those of healthy women. Healthy women lose blood approximately each month as part of their menstrual cycle, and this also contributes to their lower haematology indices. However, excessive blood loss (**menorrhagia**) can lead to a normocytic anaemia.

Endocrine disease

Anaemia is often present in patients with anterior pituitary failure, chronic adrenal insufficiency, and primary hyperparathyroidism, whilst haematological abnormalities are present in both an overactive and underactive thyroid. The anaemia of hypothyroidism may be masked by a reduced blood volume, but acanthocytosis and macrocytosis may be present—the latter generally responding to replacement therapy with thyroxine, which is believed to stimulate erythropoiesis. Conversely, microcytosis is common in hyperthyroidism, even if there is no anaemia; moreover, an increase in plasma volume can mask an increased red cell mass possibly driven by high levels of thyroxine, which has the capacity to overstimulate erythroblasts. Recall also that an abnormal profile may be caused not by the disease process but by its drug treatment.

Systemic inflammatory disease

The most common diseases in this group are rheumatoid arthritis (RA) and systemic lupus erythematosus (SLE), both of which are related to a normocytic anaemia. Indeed, anaemia is the most common non-connective tissue pathology associated with SLE. However, many diverse inflammatory diseases are associated with anaemia and we have already noted several (such as thyroiditis, glomerulonephritis, Crohn's disease, and hepatitis). This has been described as anaemia of inflammation, and, in addition to a normocytic anaemia, is associated with low serum iron (hypoferraemia), low serum iron-binding capacity, and normal to elevated ferritin concentrations. A key driver of this process may be the pro-inflammatory cytokine interleukin-6 (IL-6). Increased levels of this cytokine induce the synthesis of hepcidin, high levels of which may inhibit the entry of iron into the blood. Hepcidin is also regulated by bacterial lipopolysaccharide (LPS) and bone morphogenetic proteins.

Cancer

Several aspects of anaemia in cancer must be considered. One is a direct effect of the tumour on erythropoiesis, which may be present in many malignancies: either in suppressing renal erythropoietin production or by having a direct effect on the bone marrow that is likely to produce a normocytic anaemia. An alternative aspect is the secondary effect of the tumour. Examples of this include the chronic loss of blood from a bleeding gastrointestinal cancer (which can be detected by testing for faecal occult blood), and the effects of liver cancer. A third aspect is treatment. As we have seen in the opening section of this chapter, anti-tumour chemotherapy is a common cause of pure red cell aplasia, pancytopenia, and aplastic anaemia. Finally, many malignancies have an inflammatory component and this too may lead to anaemia, as has been discussed in the section on liver disease. Increased numbers of platelets are also often present, and this many be due directly to the malignancy or indirectly, via the response of the body to the malignancy.

Table 5.12 summarizes the various routes by which chronic disease can cause anaemia. Case study 5.3 illustrates an anaemia of chronic disease.

SELF-CHECK 5.11

What is the pathological basis of the anaemia of chronic disease?

Key Points

The proficient haematologist not only needs a deep understanding of the mechanics of his or her subject, but also an awareness of the whole body and how other organs influence the blood, both in health and disease.

TABLE 5.12 **The anaemia of chronic disease.**

The liver	Failure to store iron and synthesize carrier proteins (e.g. transferrin)
The kidney	Failure to produce erythropoietin
Gastrointestinal disease	Failure to absorb micronutrients: occult blood loss from bleeding tumours
Reproductive organs	Menorrhagia: failure of testes to produce testosterone
Endocrine disease	Anaemia associated with hypothyroidism
Systemic inflammatory disease	Suppression of erythropoiesis and hypoferraemia, both potentially due to inflammatory cytokines
Cancer	Suppression of the bone marrow by the metastatic process: effects of chemotherapy

The laboratory in the anaemia of chronic disease

Many (and, crucially, not all) cases of the anaemia of chronic disease are inflammatory. A key regulator of iron, hepcidin, is itself regulated by iron availability, hypoxia, erythropoietin,

CASE STUDY 5.3 *An anaemia of chronic disease*

An 82-year-old man complains of being tired and lethargic. On examination, he has a distended and painful abdomen. He also complains of periodic diarrhoea and constipation, and recalls that he has lost perhaps a stone in weight in the past year. Routine bloods were as follows.

This case		Reference range (page xiii–xiv)
Haemoglobin	106 g/dL	133–167
WCC	6.3×10^9/L	3.7–9.5
Platelets	268×10^9/L	143–400
MCV	88 fL	77–98
ESR	15 mm/hour	<10
Haematocrit	0.38	0.35–0.53

■ Can you make a preliminary diagnosis based on the FBC and ESR? What are the abnormalities?

■ What are the potential causes of the diagnosis?

■ What are your next steps?

inflammatory cytokine IL-6, and LPS, but also by the hormone growth-differentiation factor 15 (GDF 15), the latter a member of the TGF-beta superfamily. GDF15 is strongly expressed in beta thalassaemia, and blocks hepcidin. Both the anaemia of chronic disease and iron deficiency anaemia are characterized by low haemoglobin and MCV, but other serum levels of these molecules may be useful in differentiating those cases of the anaemia of chronic disease that have an inflammatory component (such as a chronic infection or an auto-immune disease) from cases of (non-inflammatory) iron deficiency anaemia (Table 5.13). It is possible that, like soluble transferrin receptor, measurement of hepcidin and GDFI5 may enter a clinical service.

TABLE 5.13 **The laboratory in anaemia of chronic disease (ACD) and iron deficiency anaemia (IDA).**

	IDA	ACD
Haemoglobin	↓	↓
MCV	↓	N
Iron	↓	↓
Ferritin	↓	↑↑
Transferrin	↑	↓
Transferrin saturation	↓↓	↓
Soluble transferrin receptor	↑↑	↑
IL-6	N	↑↑
CRP	↑	↑↑
Erythropoietin	↑↑	↑
Hepcidin	↓	↑
Growth-differentiation factor 15.	N	↑

Key: ↑ = increased relative to health; ↑↑ = markedly increased relative to health; ↓ = reduced relative to health; ↓↓ = markedly reduced relative to health; N = equivalent to health. MCV: mean cell volume; IL-6: interleukin-6; CRP-reactive protein. Table modified by permission from Theurl. I, Finkenstedt A, Schroll A et al. Growth differentiation factor 15 in anaemia of chronic disease, iron deficiency anaemia and mixed type anaemia. *British Journal of Haematology* 2010:**148**; 449–55.

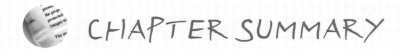

CHAPTER SUMMARY

- The principal diseases of red blood cells involve insufficiency (leading to anaemia) and excess (that is, erythrocytosis and polycythaemia).

- Anaemia may result from invasion of the bone marrow (for example, by cancer cells) or suppression (by drugs such as chemotherapy).

- Lack of vital nutrients such as iron and certain vitamins can lead to anaemia.

- Excessive body iron can also lead to disease.

- Disease in other organs (such as the liver, kidney, intestine, and reproductive organs) can also lead to anaemia.

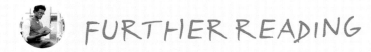

FURTHER READING

- Aslinia F, Mazza JJ, Yale SH. Megaloblastic anaemia and other causes of macrocytosis. *Clinical Research Medicine* 2006:**4**;236–41.

- Ballas SK. Iron overload is a determinant of morbidity and mortality in adult patients with sickle cell disease. *Seminars in Hematology* 2001:**381**(1, Suppl. 1);30–6.

- Beutler E, Waalen J. The definition of anaemia: what is the lower limit of normal of the blood haemoglobin concentration? *Blood* 2006:**107**;1747–50.

- Camaschella C. Recent advances in the understanding of inherited sideroblastic anaemia. *British Journal of Haematology* 2008:**143**;27–38.

- Chanarin I. A history of pernicious anaemia. *British Journal of Haematology* 2000:**111**;407–15.

- Kell DB. Iron behaving badly: inappropriate iron chelation as a major contributor to the aetiology of vascular and other progressive inflammatory and degenerative diseases. *Biomedical Central Genomics* 2009:**2**;2. http://www.biomedcentral.com/1755-8794/2/2

- Marsh JCW, Ball SE, et al. Guidelines for the diagnosis and management of aplastic anaemia. *British Journal of Haematology* 2009; 147: 43–70.

- Piperno A. Classification and diagnosis of iron overload. *Haematologica* 1998;**83**:447–55.

- Porter JB. Practical management of iron overload. *British Journal of Haematology* 2001:**115**;239–52.

- Spivak JL. The blood in systemic disorders. *Lancet* 2000:**355**;1707–12.

- Wallace DF, **Subramaniam VN**. Non-HFE haemochromatosis. *World Journal of Gastroenterology* 2007:**13**;4690–8.

- Young NS, Calado RT, Scheinberg P. Current concepts in the pathophysiology and treatment of aplastic anaemia. *Blood* 2006:**108**;2509–19.

- http://www.who.int/topics/anaemia

- Quadros EV. Advances in the understanding of cobalamin assimilation and metabolism. *British Journal of Haematology* 2010:**148**;195–204.

- Theurl I, Finkenstedt A, Schroll A, et al. Growth differentiation factor 15 in anaemia of chronic disease, iron deficiency anaemia and mixed type anaemia. *British Journal of Haematology* 2010:**148**;449–55.

- Sieff CA, Yang J., Merida-Long LB, Lodish HF. Pathogenesis of the erythroid failure in Diamond Blackfan anaemia. *British Journal of Haematology* 2010:**148**;611–22.

Answers to self-check questions, case study questions, and discussion questions are provided in the book's Online Resource Centre, visit www.oxfordtextbooks.co.uk/orc/moore

6

The pathology of the red blood cell: Part 2

Andrew Blann and Sukhjinder Marwah

Having established the basics of red cell function in Chapter 4, and having described some aspects of diseases of red blood cells in Chapter 5, we now move to complete our study of the principal diseases of erythrocytes by looking at the remaining causes of anaemia. Whilst some of the different types of anaemia we examined in Chapter 5 were due to a shortage of essential factors (such as iron), in this chapter we focus on the destruction of red blood cells, a process called haemolysis. We will conclude our study of the disease of red blood cells by looking at conditions in which there are too many red blood cells (essentially the reverse of anaemia), namely polycythaemia and erythrocytosis.

Learning objectives

After studying this chapter you should confidently be able to:

- Understand the meaning of haemolysis.
- List the different causes of the inappropriate destruction of red blood cells.
- Explain the relationship between gene mutation and anaemia.
- Describe the major features of the haemoglobinopathies.
- Outline how mutations in genes for membrane components and enzymes can lead to anaemia.
- Appreciate that high numbers of red blood cells and increased haemoglobin levels (polycythaemia and erythrocytosis) can lead to disease.
- Suggest how the laboratory can diagnose these conditions.

Broadly speaking, the pathology of red blood cells considers the two polar extremes of the reference range, although, as we have discussed in Chapter 2, having a result well within the reference range is no guarantee of health, just as a result marginally outside the reference range is no guarantee of disease. When there are too few red blood cells, or the cells that are present are not functioning as they should, we consider the major pathology of red blood cells—**anaemia**. Anaemia may stem from the attack and destruction of perfectly good red cells by an outside agent or agents—so called *extrinsic* defects. Alternatively, there may be *intrinsic* defects within the red blood cell itself that lead to its premature destruction. The **haemolytic anaemias** (that is,

haemolytic anaemia
Anaemia that follows the destruction (lysis) of red blood cells.

TABLE 6.1   **A classification of haemolytic anaemias.**

An extrinsic pathological process acting on a healthy red cell	Antibodies • autoantibodies • alloantibodies
	Mechanical destruction
	Drug induced haemolysis
	Infections: malaria
Intrinsic defect of the red cell	The haemoglobinopathies • sickle cell disease • thalassaemia • compound haemoglobinopathy
	The membrane • spherocytosis • elliptocytosis • paroxysmal nocturnal haemoglobinuria
	Enzymes • glucose-6-phosphate dehydrogenase deficiency • pyruvate kinase deficiency

anaemia due to (premature) destruction of the cell) are generally caused by a shortening of the lifespan of the red cell and failure of the bone marrow to be able to compensate for this reduced life-span. If bone marrow production matches the rate of red cell destruction this is called compensated haemolytic disease. The causes of the destruction of the red cell may, in turn, be due to one or two broadly different processes.

• In the first, there is nothing fundamentally wrong with the red blood cell itself, but it is destroyed because of some external pathological process, such as drugs, toxins, an auto-antibody, or an infection.

• In the second, red blood cells are destroyed because there is something intrinsically wrong with them. This may be due to damage to, or loss of integrity of, the red cell membrane, the absence of certain enzymes, or perhaps to an abnormal type of haemoglobin (Table 6.1).

Whatever the aetiology, these damaged cells are detected and removed by cells of the reticu-loendothelial system, mostly in the spleen, although this can also occur in the bone marrow and liver. Alternatively, cells may be destroyed whilst in the blood. In the laboratory, haemolysis is investigated by assessing the red blood cells themselves, and also by looking for evidence of an increased rate of their destruction in the blood.

Cross reference

Red blood cell function is described in Chapter 4, haemopoiesis in Chapter 3.

6.1 Immune-mediated and other 'extrinsic' causes of haemolytic anaemia

Anaemia occurs when the body is unable to compensate for either a reduced production of red cells or an increase in their rate of destruction. Any condition shortening the red cell life span to less than 120 days is called *haemolysis*. In the previous section, haemolytic anaemias were subdivided according to type. In this section we will specifically discuss immune-mediated and other extrinsic mechanisms of haemolysis.

Immune haemolysis can occur as a consequence of the presence of two main types of antibody. *Alloantibodies* are produced in response to the immune recognition of foreign red cells that have been introduced either via a blood transfusion or due to pregnancy (classically following the mixing of maternal and fetal blood at delivery). *Autoantibodies* are found when a patient's immune system produces antibodies that recognize their own red cells as foreign and mediate their destruction. These two processes cause *alloimmune* and *autoimmune* haemolysis respectively.

Alloimmune haemolysis

The introduction of foreign red cells into an individual may initiate an immune response. In the first instance, a primary response may occur, producing large, pentameric IgM antibodies against the stimulating 'foreign' red cell antigen. The concentration of these antibodies is usually rather low and the immune response slow, thus the initial influx of foreign red cells does not have any significant clinical consequences. However, any subsequent immunising event (via transfusion or pregnancy) that involves the re-introduction of red cells expressing the same foreign antigen, will result in a secondary immune response that rapidly produces high levels of IgG antibodies. These IgG antibodies attach to their corresponding antigen and coat the 'foreign' red cells, a process called *sensitization* or *opsonization*. The classical complement system may also be activated and **complement** components may also coat the 'foreign' red cells.

Both of these events facilitate the premature removal of these red cells by the reticuloendothelial system. Macrophages of the reticuloendothelial system, in particular, express receptors on their cell surface, which recognize the IgG and the complement components covering the sensitized cells, thus enabling the process of phagocytosis to occur. In the first instance, portions of the sensitized red cell membrane are removed, reducing the surface area of the red cells whilst maintaining their volume. This process results in the formation of spherocytes. These spherocytes become prone to increased sequestration in the spleen which leads to their shortened life-span. This type of premature destruction is called extravascular haemolysis.

Most frequently, alloimmune haemolysis occurs in response to antigens of the Rh and Kell Blood Group system (in cases of Haemolytic Disease of the Newborn) or antigens of the Duffy and Kidd Blood Group system in cases where the 'foreign' antigens are expressed on donor cells following blood transfusion.

However, it is important to recognize that any red cell antibody can cause haemolysis when it combines with its respective antigen *in vivo*. Indeed, the most clinically significant cases of alloimmune haemolysis, which can cause major morbidity and even a fatal outcome, are the result of red cell transfusions where the ABO blood groups of the donor and recipient are incompatible. This is a situation unique to this Blood Group System because of the unexpected presence of potent pre-formed antibody in most individuals, depending on their blood group. This type of alloimmune haemolysis involves IgM antibody, complement activation and red cell destruction in the vascular system itself. Premature destruction in this case is called *intravascular haemolysis*.

In order to avoid immune-mediated haemolytic transfusion reactions, which inevitably result in the extravascular or intravascular lysis of donor red cells, compatibility testing procedures should be performed in the Transfusion laboratory. A number of steps are involved, including the matching of particular blood group types, checking of historical

complement
A series of defensive proteins that normally assemble on the surface of pathogens such as bacteria, helping to cause their destruction.

Cross reference
Blood group systems, complement components and their role in haemolysis are discussed further in the *Transfusion and Transplantation Science* text in this series.

BOX 6.1 Cold autoantibodies and the local environment

Our core temperature is considered to be 37°C, although variations in temperature are recorded throughout the body. The most peripheral areas of the body, such as the ears, armpits or mouth have a lower temperature reading than the rectum. The core temperature, which refers to the temperature of the liver—the metabolic powerhouse of the body, is considered 1°C higher than that of the rectum, the site from which the core temperature is measured. These variations in body temperature can impact upon the way in which cold autoantibodies bind to red cells and lead to haemolysis. Cold autoantibodies, which are IgM in nature, react optimally at 4°C but have a thermal amplitude ranging up to 30–32°C. A low environmental temperature, as frequently seen in the winter months in the UK, will cause cold autoantibodies to bind to the patient's own red cells within the cooler peripheral circulation of the nose, fingertips and ears and start to fix complement. As the coated red cells move centrally towards higher 'internal' temperatures, the IgM dissociates leaving complement components attached to the red cell surface. These components form membrane attack complexes leading to intravascular lysis of red cells.

In the Haematology laboratory it is essential to maintain blood specimens from patients with known or suspected cold autoantibodies at 37°C prior to performing a full blood count analysis. Failure to do so will lead to red cell agglutination within the specimen and abnormal FBC results. The FBC will show a low red cell count, a normal or raised MCV and a raised MCH and MCHC. The blood film will contain red cell agglutinates. In the blood transfusion laboratory, strong cold autoantibodies may cause ABO typing anomalies in which case tests may need to be performed at 37°C to confirm ABO type and antibody identification.

records, and screening for the presence of alloantibodies. If antibodies are detected, their specificity will have to be identified and a serological crossmatch performed. This final stage involves incubating donor red cells with recipient serum or plasma in the presence of antihuman globulin (AHG) at 37°C and then assessing for agglutination. (See below and Fig 6.1 for further details of this technique.) The observation of agglutination indicates that the recipient's serum or plasma contains antibodies directed against an antigen expressed on the donor blood cells. This is an incompatibility and the unit of donor red cells should not be transfused.

direct antiglobulin test (DAT) and indirect antiglobulin test (IAT)
Laboratory tests to search for an antibody on the surface of red blood cells or finding patients plasma respectively. Commonly used in the diagnosis of AIHA.

The detection and identification of red cell antibodies and the final crossmatch itself are achieved by using an **indirect antiglobulin test (IAT)**. The IAT is the 'benchmark' technique and is performed by a number of different methods (e.g. 'gel', tube or microplate methods). However, the principles are the same regardless of the method adopted, and involve first incubating patient plasma or serum with red cells. In the case of antibody detection/identification, the patient plasma or serum is incubated with a panel of reagent red cells (the antigenic makeup or 'phenotype' of which is known); in the case of a crossmatch, the patient plasma or serum is incubated with donor red cells, as indicated above. Incubation will be performed at body temperature (37°C) to ensure that any antibody detected is clinically relevant. If antibody is present during the incubation phase it will effectively coat the reagent or donor red cells. However, clinically significant antibody is invariably of the smaller IgG type which cannot directly cause red cell agglutination and thus be observed.

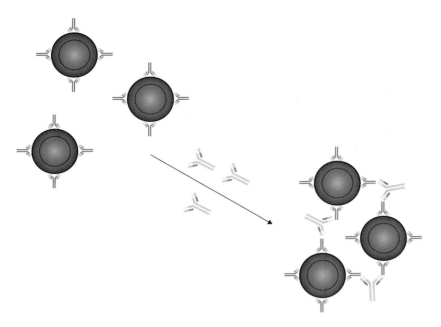

FIGURE 6.1

A case of *in vivo* red cell sensitization. This is where the patient's own red cells are coated by IgG antibodies. These antibodies are unable to agglutinate red cells without an enhancement technique. Sensitized red cells can be detected by the Direct Antiglobulin Test (DAT). Patient red blood cells are obtained (left hand image) and are mixed with antihuman globulin (AHG) reagent, depicted in green. *In vivo* sensitized red cells agglutinate in the presence of AHG (right hand image), through the formation of complexes between the sensitized red cells and the AHG, which acts as a bridge.

Consequently, observation is achieved by the addition of AHG. (A washing phase may be required before this addition, depending on the method used.) Polyspecific AHG is routinely used, and is composed of two main ingredients: anti-IgG, which attaches to any IgG antibody that has coated the test red cells, and anti-C3d, which will attach to the main complement component that may be present on the red cells if the antibody has also activated complement. AHG effectively acts as a bridge to allow IgG-coated red cells to link together, causing visible agglutination. This can now be observed *in vitro* and the antibody detected (see Fig. 6.1).

The IAT is also important for assessing the presence of antibodies associated with haemolytic disease of the fetus and newborn (HDFN), and can also be used to identify the specificity of autoantibodies in a patient's plasma. This will be further discussed in the next section.

Autoimmune haemolysis

Patients who are shown to possess within their plasma autoantibodies that are directed against their own red cells antigens and who have a reduced haemoglobin concentration are considered to have autoimmune haemolytic anaemia (AIHA). Approximately 80% of patients with AIHA possess warm-reactive IgG autoantibodies that react optimally at 37°C and, as such,

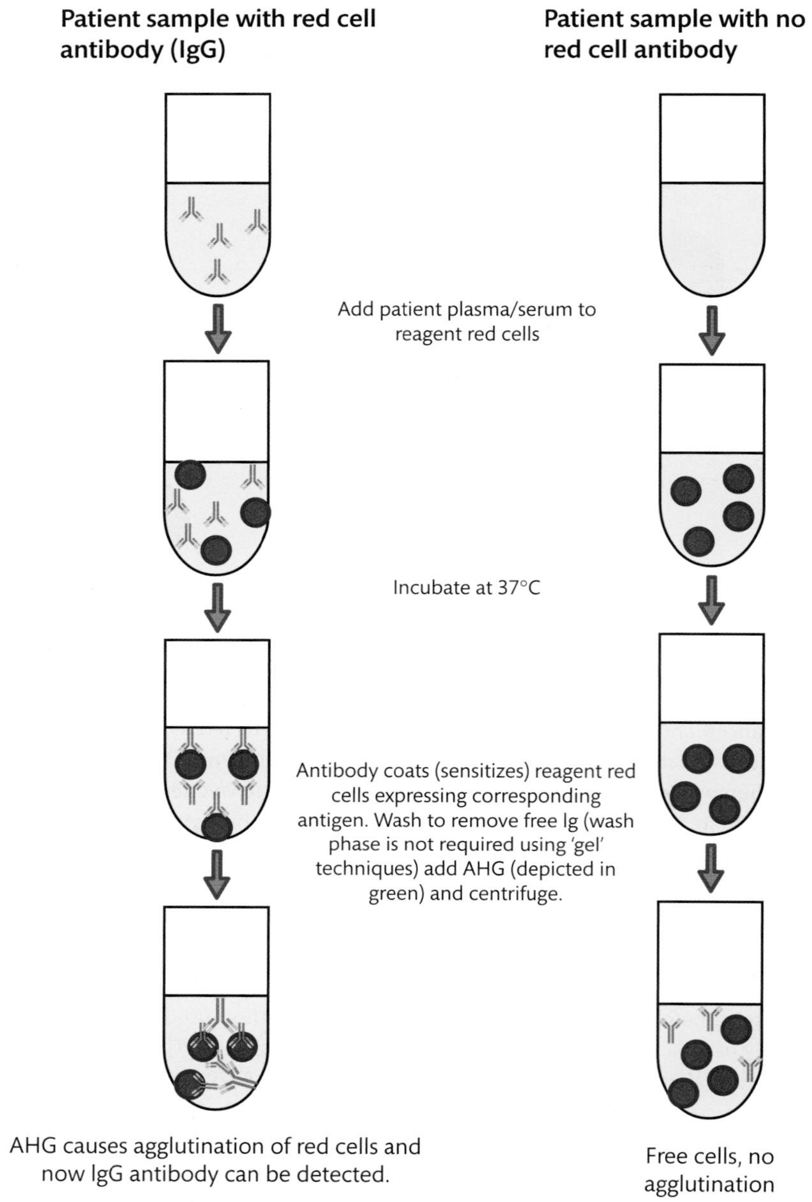

Patient sample with red cell antibody (IgG)

Patient sample with no red cell antibody

FIGURE 6.2

The Indirect Antiglobulin Test (IAT) is used to detect IgG red cell antibodies in a patient's blood sample. Serum or plasma is separated from a patient's sample and incubated at 37°C with reagent red cells. If specific antibody is present, sensitization of the reagent red cells exhibiting the corresponding antigen will occur *in vitro* . The antibody can now be detected by the addition of AHG which leads to agglutination of reagent cells (left panel). By looking at the reaction pattern with a range of reagent red cells of known antigenic phenotype, the antibody specificity can be determined. Agglutination does not occur in the absence of IgG red cell antibodies (right panel). Depending upon the technique used, a washing phase may be required prior to the addition of AHG to remove free Ig which would otherwise neutralize the AHG leading to false negative results.

Add patient plasma/serum to reagent red cells

Incubate at 37°C

Antibody coats (sensitizes) reagent red cells expressing corresponding antigen. Wash to remove free Ig (wash phase is not required using 'gel' techniques) add AHG (depicted in green) and centrifuge.

AHG causes agglutination of red cells and now IgG antibody can be detected.

Free cells, no agglutination

are classified as having warm AIHA. The reminder exhibit cold-reactive autoantibodies. These are generally of an IgM type, which reacts optimally at 4°C. Characteristically, however, these antibodies have a wide thermal amplitude, still being able to react at temperatures of 30–32°C. Those patients that exhibit cold-reactive antibodies are classified as having cold AIHA.

Autoimmune haemolytic anaemias have a wide variety of causes. Those with unknown causes are called *primary* or *idiopathic* conditions, whereas those attributable to an identifiable cause are called *secondary* conditions. Both warm and cold AIHA can be secondary to lympho-proliferative conditions such as chronic lymphocytic leukaemia (CLL) or lymphoma. These are both discussed in detail in chapter 12. Warm AIHA may also be seen in other systemic autoimmune diseases such as systemic lupus erythematosus (SLE) or ulcerative colitis, in solid

BOX 6.2 Nomenclature

Although the naming of particular processes, diseases, and conditions seems to be a mystery to many students, there is in fact logic in the system which can be decoded by breaking down the formal name into its constituent parts. For example:

Autoimmune haemolytic anaemia (AIHA)—'auto' means 'one's self', 'immune' implies an antibody, 'haem' = 'of red blood cells', 'lytic' means 'bursting' or 'breaking', and 'anaemia' is essentially low levels of haemoglobin. Hence AIHA = low levels of haemoglobin caused by bursting of red blood cells, itself caused by an antibody made by the patient themselves.

The closely related *alloimmune haemolytic anaemia*—where a patient has developed an antibody following exposure to red cells from somebody else (allo- means a different member of the same species).

Microangiopathic haemolytic anaemia (MAHA)—describes anaemia resulting from red blood cell destruction (= haemolytic), which involves disease (= pathic, from pathology) of the small (= micro) blood vessels (= angio).

Paroxysmal cold haemoglobinuria (PCH)— paroxysmal means intermittent, or every now and then; cold is fairly obvious; haemoglobinuria mean haemoglobin in urine. Put it all together and PCH becomes a condition where every now and then, when it is cold, the urine goes red because of the presence of haemoglobin. The abbreviation PCH seems to be close to another: *paroxysmal nocturnal haemoglobinuria (PNH)*—which translates to occasional red urine (because of the haemoglobin) during the night. However, both these pictures may also be due to some kinds of renal disease.

non-haemopoietic tumours, or following the use of drugs such as α-methyldopa. Cold AIHA may be secondary to infections such as *Mycoplasma pneumoniae* or infectious mononucleosis (Epstein Barr virus).

Both warm and cold AIHA result in the reduction of the red cell lifespan. Warm AIHA is accompanied by spherocytes and polychromasia on the peripheral blood film, and hyperbilirubinaemia. Cold AIHA is accompanied by red cell agglutination on the peripheral blood film, a raised mean cell volume (MCV) and mean cell haemoglobin concentration (MCHC) in the full blood count. Clinically, patients will demonstrate signs and symptoms consistent with anaemia and jaundice. Usually patients with Cold AIHA do not demonstrate splenomegaly or hepatosplenomegaly, although these are prominent features in warm AIHA.

To diagnose a patient with AIHA, typical clinical features accompanied by a positive direct antiglobulin test (DAT) and the detection of auto antibodies in the serum or plasma should be demonstrated. The DAT is used to confirm that the patient's own cells have been sensitized by autoantibody *in vivo*. The DAT is performed by mixing washed patient cells with AHG and centrifuging. An incubation phase is not necessary. The observation of red cell agglutination demonstrates that the red cells are already coated with autoantibody. Confirmation of the presence of autoantibody in the serum or plasma is then accomplished using the IAT, as described above. Usually a specificity cannot be identified: the antibody is described as 'non-specific' or 'pan-specific'. This IAT will be accompanied by an 'auto', in which patient plasma is incubated with patient red cells. A positive result with the 'auto' is expected in these cases.

We should now consider the mechanisms of red cell destruction in warm and cold AIHA, and mechanisms of treatment.

Warm AIHA

Warm AIHA is associated with the production of autoantibodies of the IgG class. As a reminder, these autoantibodies recognize 'self' antigens expressed on the red cell surface, leading to red cell sensitization and removal by the reticuloendothelial system. The reduction in red cells leads to reduced oxygen delivery to the tissues, and a corresponding rise in erythropoietin synthesis and secretion by the peritubular cells of the kidney. This increased erythropoietin drive results in increased red cell production and release from the bone marrow, resulting in reticulocytosis, with polychromasia apparent on the peripheral blood film. In symptomatic patients, red cell transfusion may be required to maintain oxygen delivery to the tissues. However, the compatibility testing of these patients is often difficult and requires specialised serological techniques to uncover any alloantibodies that could potentially cause haemolytic transfusion reactions but are being masked by the patient's autoantibody.

Patients may also be administered glucocorticoid corticosteroids to try to improve their red cell lifespan. These glucocorticoids reduce the expression of IgG specific receptors on macrophages of the reticuloendothelial system, thereby reducing phagocytosis of these sensitized cells. As a consequence, sensitized cells are retained for a shorter period in the splenic vasculature and can contribute to oxygen delivery to systemic tissues. Glucocorticoids induce remission in approximately 80% of patients, although this remission is maintained in only 20–35% of patients.

As a second line therapy, splenectomy is considered for the management of these patients and can induce a response in 50% of patients. The removal of the organ primarily responsible for the destruction of these sensitized cells will increase red cell survival. However, splenectomy is not without its risks. Primarily, patients are at increased risk from infection by encapsulated organisms, and patients should be vaccinated against pneumococcus, *Haemophilus influenzae* b, and meningococcal serogroup C, and should be prescribed lifelong penicillin or erythromycin.

Other immunosuppressive agents including azathioprine and cyclophosphamide may be indicated although some, such as cytotoxic drugs, should be used with caution as their usage is associated with the development of secondary malignancies. In other patients, a monoclonal antibody specific for the B-cell antigen (CD20) called rituximab (anti-CD20) may be indicated. Rituximab is often used for the treatment of B-cell malignancies but can be used in AIHA by removing the B-cells that produce the autoantibody. At present, this is a non-routine strategy. Removal of these B-cells will improve red cell survival as the production of red cell autoantibodies is inhibited.

Cold AIHA

Cold AIHA is mostly associated with the development of red cell autoantibodies of the IgM type and the patient is described as having Cold Haemagglutinin Disease (CHAD). These autoantibodies can be of very high levels and are almost monoclonal-like in nature. They are characterized by having a wide thermal range such that they can often still react just above 30°C (but not at 37°C). However, they do not cause a major problem for patients providing the patients are kept warm. By contrast, patients suffer symptoms in cold conditions, where the temperature of the peripheral areas of the body, such as the finger tips, nose, and ear lobes, may drop to a level that allows the IgM autoantibody to bind to the red cells in these regions and to activate complement. Red cell agglutination may cause some vasculature occlusion in these areas leading to acrocyanosis. When the red cells return to the core body temperature from the extremities, the sensitizing IgM antibodies dissociate from the red cell surface. However, as the IgM autoantibodies have been effective at binding complement components to the red cell surface, and as complement is most active at body temperature, the completion of this chemical cascade can occur, resulting in the formation of membrane attack complexes (MAC) and intravascular haemolysis of the red cell. As a result, the patient may experience bouts of haemoglobinuria, haemosiderinuria and possibly jaundice following exposure to the cold. Some extravascular haemolysis will also occur.

The other rarer type of cold AIHA is called Paroxysmal Cold Haemoglobinuria (PCH). This transient condition is mostly associated with childhood viral infections and is caused by an unusual 'biphasic haemolysin' complement binding IgG autoantibody (the Donath Landsteiner antibody). In this case, the antibody normally has an anti-P specificity. The mechanism of red cell destruction is similar to above: when exposed to cold conditions the patient will often experience acute episodes of intravascular haemolysis. The haemolysis is self-limiting but may require transfusions to correct the resulting anaemia.

Other 'extrinsic' causes of haemolytic anaemia

These types of anaemia cover a broad spectrum of pathologies, including mechanical and drug-mediated, and those caused by infections and animal toxins. Red blood cells may also be destroyed as a consequence of other diseases. Examples of the latter include thrombotic thrombocytopenic purpura, malignant hypertension, haemolytic–uraemic syndrome, and pre-eclampsia/eclampsia. Red cells may also be adversely affected by high levels of urea (that is, uraemia) and of bilirubin (that is, hyperbilirubinaemia). Microangiopathic haemolytic anaemia (MAHA) is associated with physical damage to red cells either on abnormal surfaces (such as an artificial heart valve) or by damage caused by red cells travelling through fibrin strands deposited in capillary microvessels. These blood vessel problems may also be caused by **disseminated intravascular coagulation** (DIC), probably the most severe and acute coagulopathy.

Cross reference

Disseminated intravascular coagulation will be discussed in depth in Chapter 14.

Mechanical damage

Mechanical causes of haemolytic anaemia include prolonged and/or unaccustomed exercise or physical activity, such as may be present in soldiers after a long route march (hence, the term 'march haematuria') or endurance sports such a running a marathon. The same effect can be caused by a malfunctioning artificial heart valve. But whatever the cause, otherwise healthy red blood cells are destroyed by a physical force.

Drug-induced haemolytic anaemia

Haemolytic anaemia can occur as a result of a particular drug being potentially toxic, possibly by accidental or deliberate overdosage, and also by the induction of a hypersensitivity response. Drug effects are moderately common precipitants, accounting for 10–20% of haemolytic anaemias. Mechanisms may include direct chemical destruction of the membrane, or perhaps the generation of an increased oxidative stress, which may lead, for example, to lipid peroxidation and oxidation of sulphydryl groups of the membrane and to the oxidation of ferrous iron in haemoglobin forming methaemoglobin.

Another cause is the development of an antibody that is directed against a drug, such as penicillin, cephalosporin, and tetracycline. The mechanism for cell destruction is such that if the drug binds or otherwise sticks to the cell membrane, this will be recognized and bound by the antibody, which will then render the entire cell more susceptible to haemolysis by the body's immune system. This mechanism may also be called 'neoantigen', or 'immune complex'.

An alternative type of drug-induced immune haemolytic anaemia occurs when the drug itself stimulates the production of an autoantibody to a component of the normal red cell membrane, but the drug itself does not directly take part in the reaction. Perhaps the best example of such a drug that induces this type of haemolytic anaemia is alpha-methyldopa.

Alternatively, the drug itself may bind directly to the red blood cell, and this combination induces the production of an antibody towards the combination of the drug and the red cell. Examples of drugs which induce these antibodies include the blood pressure drug hydrochlorothiazide, the antibiotic rifampicin, levodopa, and procainamide. It could rightly be argued that this is really antibody-mediated haemolysis, but it is clearly primarily a drug reaction, and the direct antiglobulin test is generally positive.

Infections

Infection can lead to haemolytic anaemia via several routes. A good example of this is *Clostridium perfringens* septicaemia, which is associated with acute haemolysis.

A high temperature, such as may be present in response to influenza, may also cause red cell destruction. This is likely to be semi-physiological as a small number of red cells (perhaps those that are aged) are likely to be more sensitive to brief adverse changes in temperature, such as that associated with a fever. This explains the frequent reports of more yellow-coloured urine during and shortly after an episode of influenza.

Severe infections with the red cell parasite of malaria plasmodium are also likely to precipitate a haemolytic anaemia, in addition to other laboratory and clinical changes, such as a raised ESR and fevers, respectively. These occur partly because the parasite-loaded cell is detected as being abnormal, and so is eliminated. Haemolytic anaemia can also develop as the new red cells lyse releasing merozoites, facilitating the spread in parasites between adjacent red cells. This is the subject of Chapter 7.

Key Points

Antibodies constitute a crucial and efficient aspect of our defence against microorganisms such as bacteria. However, if misdirected, they can cause considerable harm, as in the case of antibody-mediated haemolysis. Red blood cells are more susceptible to this type of damage as they have a highly specialized yet delicate membrane.

The role of the laboratory in haemolytic anaemia

A full blood count, reticulocyte count, and blood film are essential initial investigations in haemolytic anaemia. There is likely to be a reduced haemoglobin and, if the reticulocyte count is grossly raised, there may also be a raised MCV. Increased numbers of reticulocytes reflects increased bone marrow activity, and on the blood film these larger cells may be more blue-tinged and so contribute to **polychromasia**. If the disease is severe and prolonged, there may be an additional reaction from the bone marrow. This can be demonstrated by the presence of nucleated red blood cells, reflecting (like reticulocytosis) a reactive increase in **erythropoiesis**. Bone marrow examination is infrequently required but, if so, it is likely to demonstrate erythroid hyperplasia.

The pathological basis of haemolytic anaemia is the destruction of red blood cells. This is often reflected on the blood film by red cell fragments called **schistocytes.** However, the damage to the red cell may leave the cell intact but instead change its characteristic discoid shape to that of a sphere—identifiable on the film as **spherocytes**. The blood film may give other clues

polychromasia
A finding on blood film that translates as 'many colours'. In practice there will be red blood cells of a normal colour, but others (reticulocytes) with a blue tinge.

erythropoiesis
The process of the development of blood cells.

schistocytes
Fragments of red blood cells that are evidence of haemolysis.

spherocytes
Acquired or inherited disorder invalid red cells have lost their discoid shape to become spheroid.

as to the cause of the haemolytic anaemia. For example, a raised white blood cell count in leukaemia or low platelets in idiopathic thrombocytopenic purpura are both diseases where autoimmune haemolytic anaemia may occur. Figures 6.3, 6.4, and 6.5 illustrate changes in the blood film that are commonly found in haemolytic anaemia.

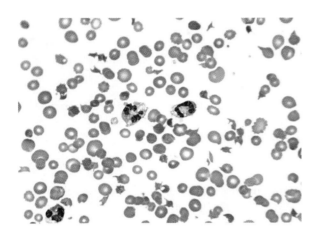

FIGURE 6.3

Schistocytes and marked polychromasia. Destruction of red blood cells in haemolytic anaemia produces fragments—schistocytes. If the anaemia is prolonged, the bone marrow may respond by increasing the release of reticulocytes—juvenile red cells markedly larger than mature cells. The blue tinge of reticulocytes leads to the descriptive term polychromasia. There are also three neutrophils present. (Magnification ×400.)

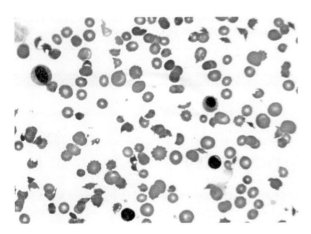

FIGURE 6.4

Schistocytes, polychromasia, and a nucleated red blood cell. This film from a patient with disseminated intravascular coagulation illustrates many features of haemolytic anaemia with schistocytes, polychromasia, burr cells, spherocytes, and a nucleated red cell (upper right quadrant). There are also two lymphocytes and, on the left, a metamyelocyte. (Magnification ×400.)

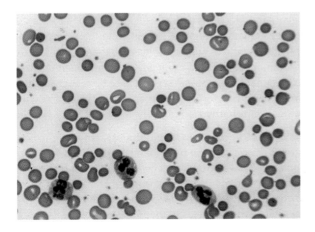

FIGURE 6.5

Spherocytes. This film from a patient with autoimmune haemolytic anemia exhibits spherocytosis. Some cells are very small, that is, are microspherocytes. There is also a modest degree of polychromasia alongside three neutrophils. (Magnification ×400.)

Since all these haemolytic diseases are characterized by the destruction of red blood cells, the results of this destruction should be detectable in the circulation. However, in many cases, the red blood cell destruction may occur within organs such as the spleen (that is, it is extravascular). If so, there may not necessarily be a great deal of evidence of red cell destruction in the blood, although the spleen itself may be enlarged (that is, it exhibits splenomegaly). However, in intravascular haemolysis, there should be abundant evidence of red cell destruction, such as schistocytes.

In Chapter 5 we learned of the fate of the red blood cell and how one sign of this is bilirubin, which (broadly speaking) makes our plasma and urine yellow(ish) and our faeces brown. Thus, in haemolysis, increased unconjugated bilirubin, haemoglobin, and haptoglobin in the plasma, and increased urobilinogen in the urine, are all likely. In severe cases there may also be free haemoglobin in the urine. In cases of chronic intravascular haemolysis, haemosiderin is stored in the tubular cells of the kidney when these cells are sloughed off, haemosiderin may be detected in the urine when stained with Perls stain.

Haemolytic uraemic syndrome (HUS) is characterized by acute renal failure, thrombocytopenia, and a microangiopathic haemolytic anaemia that is DAT-negative. Some cases of HUS are associated with diarrhoea and may be due to a toxin from *E.coli* or other pathogens. Atypical HUS is often characterized by dysregulation of complement components: the latter may be measured in an immunology laboratory.

SELF-CHECK 6.1

What are the different types of antibody-mediated haemolytic anaemia?

SELF-CHECK 6.2

What non-antibody factors external to the red cell cause haemolytic anaemia?

6.2 Haemoglobinopathy

A second (and much larger) group of haemolytic anaemias arise from mutations in various genes. These mutations can be classified as those that act on haemoglobin, on the molecules that make up the cell membrane, and on intracellular enzymes. Whilst it is certainly the case that the vast majority of these conditions have a hereditary component, they may also arise in the newborn of parents who are themselves subsequently shown to be healthy.

Chapter 3 has highlighted the genetics and structure of haemoglobin. In the adult, globin genes code for different variants of globin proteins such as alpha-globin and beta-globin. In health, the different variants of globin molecules lead to different types of haemoglobin, such as HbA, HbA_2, and HbF. However, mutations in the genes give rise to different types and amounts of haemoglobin, which are the cause of a certain type of anaemia. This type of haemoglobin abnormality is called **haemoglobinopathy**.

The principal two haemoglobinopathies (**sickle cell disease** and **thalassaemia**) are almost always inherited, and, to date, hundreds of variants have been identified. Both types of haemoglobinopathy result from the mutation of a healthy globin gene, with a consequent alteration in the amino acid composition of, or the amount of, a particular globin chain. This, in turn, influences the ability of that haemoglobin to transport oxygen. It is this failure to provide the tissues with sufficient oxygen for their needs that leads to the clinical consequences such

sickle cell disease

This is a qualitative haemoglobin disorder that is characterized in the laboratory by a chronic haemolytic anaemia, and in the clinic by infection and microvascular occlusion.

thalassaemia

A quantitative haemoglobinopathy caused by a mutation in alpha, beta, or both genes that leads to a reduction, or even abolition, in the expression of alpha- or beta-globin.

as venous ulceration and the symptoms of anaemia. Some of these haemoglobin variants are asymptomatic, while others may severely affect the quality of life of patients.

The common haemoglobinopathies include *qualitative* abnormalities in beta-globin, such as HbS (leading to sickle cell disease), HbD, HbC, and HbE. These are essentially due to a single change in the DNA, and of the amino acid that the DNA encodes. Importantly, there is no shortage of globin protein itself; the abnormality lies with its component amino acids.

Another type of haemoglobinopathy represents a *quantitative* defect—the thalassaemias alpha (α) and beta (β) being good examples. These are called quantitative because there is a reduced mass of globin protein produced: dozens (and perhaps hundreds) of amino acids are missing.

Both types of haemoglobinopathy can be found all over world, but there are areas of increased prevalence. Sickle cell disease is of greatest prevalence in West Africa, the Caribbean, the eastern Mediterranean, the Middle East, and South-East Asia. Thalassaemia is also found in those individuals who originate from the Mediterranean, the Middle East, and throughout South-East Asia, and also in Southern China and Thailand (Figure 6.6). However, the link between the genetics of the disease and problems with quality of life that the person may have is complicated. Nevertheless, we can classify everyone with a haemoglobinopathy by the number and type of genes that are abnormal. Recall that we all have four genes for alpha-globin and two genes for beta-globin (as explained in Chapter 4). If, for example, both beta-globin genes carry a mutation (such as may cause sickle cell disease) then the person is said to be **homozygous**. By contrast, someone with only one mutated gene, but a normal second gene, is said to be **heterozygous**. These heterozygotes are often called 'carriers', and the condition a 'trait'; such subjects typically have less severe clinical disease. It is also possible to have a combination of mutated genes, such as one mutation in a gene for alpha-globin and also a mutation in a gene for beta-globin, or

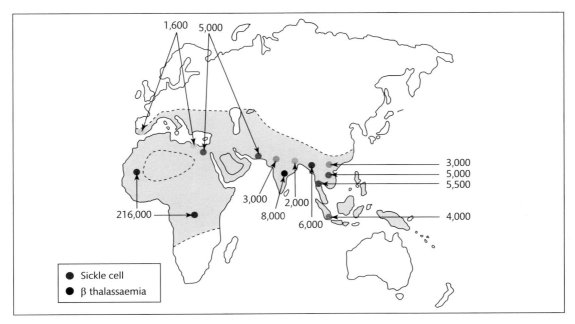

FIGURE 6.6
Worldwide distribution of haemoglobinopathy. Reproduced by permission from document EB118/5, *Thalassaemia and other haemoglobinopathies*. Report by the Secretariat. © World Health Organization, 2006.

perhaps a different mutation in each of the two beta-globin genes. These points will be revisited in detail in the sections that follow.

SELF-CHECK 6.3

What are the principal differences between the two major types of haemoglobinopathy?

Sickle cell anaemia

Sickle cell disease, the most frequent haemoglobinopathy, was first described by Herrick in Chicago a century ago. It is so named because of the characteristic sickle shape of the red blood cells when viewed by light microscopy on a blood film, or in a wet (unfixed and unstained) preparation of blood (Figure 6.7). Disease follows because these abnormal cells do not flow normally through capillaries, they carry oxygen poorly, and are detected and removed from the circulation, leading to anaemia. The characteristic change in shape occurs at low oxygen tension (that is, during a state of hypoxia) during dehydration and with fever. Re-oxygenating blood can lead to the reversal of a sickled cell back to its normal state. Subsequent research determined the disease to be attributable to characteristics of the globin molecule, described as haemoglobin S (HbS); the phenotypic differences that characterized a sickle-shaped cell were ultimately attributed to mutations in the beta-globin gene.

Epidemiology

Haemoglobin S (sickle haemoglobin) is the most common haemoglobinopathy worldwide. The frequency of the HbS gene (including both heterozygotes and homozygotes) is found in different racial, geographical, and ethnic groups as follows: West African 1:5, Afro-Caribbean 1:10, Asian 1:50, Mediterranean and the Middle East 1:100. Areas where HbS is common run parallel with areas where falciparum malaria is endemic, leading to the hypothesis that HbS had been selected for in evolutionary terms as a protective mechanism against malaria. In the UK more than 12 500 people have a clear sickle cell disorder. Over 240 000 are seemingly 'healthy' carriers, and each year 1 in 200 neonates are born with sickle cell disease. In the USA, perhaps 8% of African-Americans are heterozygous for this mutation.

Pathophysiology

The genetic basis of the most common form of the disease is a mutation in the beta gene for one of the major protein components of haemoglobin, that is, beta-globin. Mutations in the

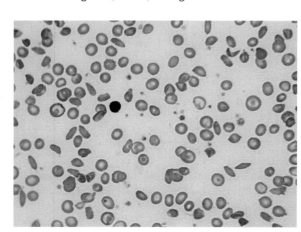

FIGURE 6.7

Sickle cell disease. There are numerous cells that are not round but instead are oblong or oval shaped. These are sickle cells: a striking example is in the top right corner. There are also several target cells, and a lymphocyte. (Magnification ×400.)

alpha gene leading to abnormal alpha-globins are rare. So what is the nature of these mutations at the molecular level? Normally, a triplet of nucleotide bases in the globin gene (guanine, adenine, and guanine: GAG) codes for a globin molecule with the amino acid glutamine at position six. However, in sickle cell disease the beta-globin gene is mutated by the substitution of a thymine for the adenine, so the triplet becomes guanine, thymine, guanine: GTG. Consequently, the amino acid valine is substituted at position 6 in the globin chain instead of glutamine. This gives the beta-globin molecule, and so the whole haemoglobin molecule, a different shape and, hence, a reduced ability to carry oxygen. This is illustrated in Figure 6.8.

Under normal oxygenation conditions (such as in well-oxygenated arterial blood, especially near the lungs), HbS is fully oxygenated and the haemoglobin remains in the soluble form. However, after deoxygenation, perhaps in the tissues where oxygen is given up, HbS loses its solubility, and becomes polymerized into long rigid chains that distort the red cell into the characteristic sickle shape seen under the microscope. Conditions that predispose to sickling include hypoxia, acidosis, and increased temperature. Polymerization of haemoglobin S is reversible and, after re-oxygenation, the sickled red cell may revert to a normal red cell shape. However, after numerous cycles of oxygenation and deoxygenation, the red cell eventually becomes irreversibly sickled.

These permanently damaged elongated rigid red cells contribute to vaso-occlusion and obstruct small blood vessels so that other red cells cannot deliver oxygen to the tissues, leading to infarction. Further obstruction to blood vessels is caused by the accumulation of reticulocytes, each of which expresses high levels of cell-adhesion molecules on its surface. The binding of these to the vascular endothelium leads to a narrowing of the blood vessel lumen at the site where the reticulocytes adhere. Sickle cells not only lose deformability but also develop increased 'stickiness', which promotes adhesion to the endothelial cells and increases the risk of thrombosis. These red cell changes lead to a chronic haemolytic anaemia, because

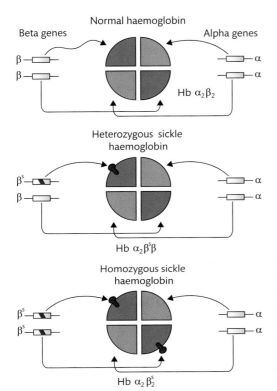

FIGURE 6.8

Relationship between beta-globin gene mutations and haemoglobin S. In health (top panel), alpha and beta genes each produce globin molecules that combine to form normal haemoglobin ($\alpha_2\beta_2$). In heterozygous sickle cell disease (middle panel), one beta gene carries a mutation that generates sickle globin (β^s). The other beta gene generates normal beta globin, resulting in ($\alpha_2\beta^s\beta$). In homozygous sickle cell disease (lower panel), two beta genes each carry a mutation that generates sickle globin, resulting in ($\alpha_2\beta^s_2$).

the sickled cells are detected as abnormal and so are eliminated by the reticuloendothelial system, most often through the activity of macrophages in the liver and spleen.

In heterozygotes (that is, those with haemoglobin AS; HbAS), the presence of a residual amount of normal haemoglobin (such as HbF and HbA$_2$) moderates not only the extent of the polymerization, but also its reversal. Thus, sickle cell carrier status leads to a clinical picture that is generally asymptomatic, although there are reports of occasional renal disturbances, and painful crises may occur at times of physiological stress, such as in unpressurized aircraft and during anaesthesia. HbAS red cells do not sickle unless the oxygen saturation is <40%, a level rarely achieved in the circulation.

Clinical features

Patients with sickle cell anaemia present with a very broad phenotype—ranging from no clinical complications to severe crises, even as infants—and they may require blood transfusion. The symptoms of anaemia are mild in relation to the low haemoglobin levels, and this is due to a right shift in the oxygen dissociation curve (that is, when HbS releases oxygen to tissues more readily when compared to normal HbA). We will discuss the oxygen dissociation curve in a section that follows. Disease severity is not simply a matter of the number of mutated genes present (two genes in the case of homozygous disease HbSS, one gene in the case of heterozygous disease HbAS) as the clinical consequences of the disease vary considerably between patients. The major clinical aspects of sickle cell disease are:

- *Painful vaso-occlusive crises*: During a crisis, irreversibly sickled cells cause blockage of blood vessels, which in turn initiates tissue hypoxia, and leads to ischaemia with bone and muscle pain. This debilitating process can occur in a variety of organs including bone (hips, shoulders and vertebrae), the lungs, and the spleen. These complications may be further enhanced by infection, exposure to cold temperature, hypoxia, strenuous exercise, dehydration, emotional disturbances, and pregnancy. The most serious vaso-occlusive crisis is of the brain (a stroke—which occurs in 7% of all patients) or spinal cord. The 'hand and foot' syndrome is one of the first presentations of the disease in young children and may lead to the formation of digits of varying lengths.

- *Visceral sequestration crisis*: Sickling of red cells in the liver, spleen, and sequestration in the lungs is partly responsible for the acute chest syndrome, although infection and infarction may exacerbate the condition.

- *Aplastic crises*: This may occur as a result of folic acid deficiency or parvovirus infection and is characterized by a sudden drop in haemoglobin level, resulting in the patient requiring a blood transfusion.

- *Haemolytic crises*: These present with an elevated rate of haemolysis with a fall in haemoglobin, and an increase in the reticulocyte count.

Other clinical features commonly include lower leg ulcers, which occur as a result of vascular stasis and local ischaemia. The spleen is often enlarged in infancy and early childhood due to trapping of sickle cells, but is later reduced in size as a result of infarcts. Other clinical complications include retinopathy, priapism, chronic liver damage, gall stones, kidney damage, and osteomyelitis.

Other qualitative beta-globin gene disorders

Haemoglobin E disease

Haemoglobin E (HbE) disease is the second most common haemoglobinopathy worldwide, and is commonly found in South-East Asia (including Cambodia, Laos, Malaysia, and Thailand) where the frequency varies from 8% to 50%. This variant is caused by replacement of glutamic acid by lysine at position 26 on the beta-globin chain. This haemoglobin also has a higher incidence in malarial areas, leading to the suggestion that HbE heterozygotes may also have some protection from this disease. Homozygous HbE disease results in a mild haemolytic anaemia with target cells, and a compensatory erythrocytosis. The heterozygous state is asymptomatic, but the film shows microcytosis.

Haemoglobin C disease

Haemoglobin C (HbC) is the third most common qualitiative haemoglobinopathy. Like haemoglobin S, it is also caused by a mutation in the beta gene, which leads to a different amino acid at position 6 of the globin protein chain. However, in HbC, the amino acid lysine is substituted for glutamic acid, leading to a different type of abnormality. Perhaps the highest frequency of this haemoglobin worldwide is in parts of West Africa, such as Ghana, where the incidence may reach 20%. Approximately 2–3% of African-Americans are heterozygous carriers, such that 1 in 5000 live births in this population will be homozygotes.

Haemoglobin C has a lower solubility, resulting in a crystalline structure that in turn decreases red cell deformability. In the homozygous state (that is, HbCC) there is an enlarged spleen, and a mild haemolytic anaemia. Like haemoglobin E, the blood film is dominated by target cells, but these are small, and there may also be some microspherocytes. In the heterozygous (carrier) state (that is, with HbAC) the full blood count generally reports normal haemoglobin and only a few target cells.

Haemoglobin D disease

Haemaglobin D (HbD) disease may be described as a collection of different mutations in the beta-globin gene. The variant with the highest frequency occurs in the western (Punjab) region of India and Pakistan (hence, it is often described as haemoglobin D$_{Punjab}$) and is caused by substitution of glutamine for glutamic acid at the 121 position on the beta-globin chain. In the homozygous state, there is a mild haemolytic anaemia with target cells, but haematological abnormalities are generally absent in the heterozygous HbAD form.

Other haemoglobinopathies

Several hundred mutations in alpha and beta genes, all of which give rise to abnormal alpha- and beta-globin, have been described. One such mutation, haemoglobin G Philadelphia, results from a mutation in an alpha gene, but generally does not have clinical implications. The vast majority of this group are family-specific and, as such, have less impact upon public health. Table 6.2 summarizes key aspects of the qualitative beta gene haemoglobinopathies.

SELF-CHECK 6.4

What are the molecular determinants of the different qualitative beta-globin haemoglobinopathies?

Thalassaemia

This group of diseases is characterized by the reduced synthesis of either or both globin chains (hence 'quantitative' defect), and consequently results in a serious abnormality in the intact

TABLE 6.2 Major aspects of the common haemoglobinopathies.

Sickle cell disease	Thalassaemia syndromes	
The most common haemoglobinopathy, and also the most common single-gene defect worldwide	Can be quantitative or qualitative defects in alpha- or beta-globins. Can be heterozygous or homozygous, and appear in different forms:	
	Molecular nature of defect	**Clinical syndrome**
A qualitative defect in beta-globin that leads to an abnormality in the red cell under hypoxic conditions and so a change in shape to that of a sickle	Homozygous alpha-thalassaemia major fetalis. (Complete lack of alpha-globin)	Hb Bart's/hydrops Incompatible with life
	Homozygous beta or doubly Severe heterozygous thalassaemia major (complete or almost complete lack of beta-globin)	Thalassaemia major or moderate clinical disease
Can be heterozygous (HbAS) or homozygous (HbSS) Other beta-globin abnormalities include haemoglobins C, D, and E	Milder beta gene defects than in thalassaemia major, increased gamma-globin chains or reduced alpha-globin chains.	Thalassaemia intermedia. Moderate or mild clinical disease
	Heterozygous alpha- or beta-thalassaemia, that is, one altered globin protein alongside a normal globin protein.	Thalassaemia carrier. Generally asymptomatic

haemoglobin molecule, which leads to poor oxygen transport and, ultimately, the clinical signs and symptoms associated with this disease. In contrast to sickle cell disease, those red cells carrying the abnormal haemoglobin do not go markedly out of shape. However, they are still detected as defective and so are removed from the blood, leading to anaemia. Subsequent research defined the disease at the level of the globin molecule, with the shortening of alpha- or beta-globin molecules, or even their absence altogether. In turn, this was traced back to defects in the genes for these molecules.

Epidemiology

Thalassaemia is predominantly found in the eastern Mediterranean region, the Middle East, the Indian subcontinent, and South East Asia—all regions where sickle cell disease is also highly prevalent. Like sickle cell disease, this reinforces the notion that thalassaemia carriers are protected against malaria. Alpha-thalassaemia is frequently present in Chinese people, whilst beta-thalassaemia is often found in Cypriots, Asians, Chinese, and Afro-Caribbeans. In south Italy and Greece, 5–10% of the population is heterozygous for beta-thalassaemia, whereas in Thailand, the gene frequency for the various forms of alpha-thalassaemia reaches 25%.

Pathophysiology

The thalassaemias can be classified as alpha (α)-thalassaemia, in which alpha-globin chain synthesis is reduced (or completely absent), and beta (β)-thalassaemia, in which there is a reduced level of beta-globin chain synthesis (or synthesis is entirely absent). Rarely, there can be defects in both beta and delta genes. Serious clinical disorders result only when two or more of the various genes are affected. Thalassaemia major is the most severe clinical form of the disease and patients inevitably require regular blood transfusions in order to survive. In contrast, thalassaemia carrier status is the mild form of the disease and many patients are asymptomatic, such that they do not generally require a blood transfusion. Between the two are a collection of conditions described as thalassaemia intermedia (Table 6.2).

The alpha-thalassaemias

Chromosome 16 carries two alpha-globin genes. Consequently, as we each carry two copies of chromosome 16, we have four alpha-globin genes overall. Single point mutations (as can cause sickle cell disease) in particular sections of alpha-globin genes are rare. Instead, the vast majority of mutations are deletions. If both alpha genes are malfunctioning, no alpha-globin chains are produced (α^0-thalassaemia), whereas if only one of the pair of genes is aberrant the synthesis of globin chain is reduced (α^+-thalassaemia). The clinical severity of any particular thalassaemia depends on the total number of aberrant genes; in many cases, the genes have simply become deleted altogether.

- A *one* gene mutation, represented by $-/\alpha/\alpha/\alpha$, in which alpha-globin output is 75% of normal, is generally clinically silent and without an anaemia. However, this carrier status may give rise to more serious disease if an individual has a child with another such carrier.

- Mutations in *two* genes, either $-/-/\alpha\alpha$ or $-/\alpha/-/\alpha$, may arise from deletions of the two alpha genes from the same chromosome whilst the two genes of the other chromosomes are intact (that is, $-/-/\alpha\alpha$). An alternative form is present when one of the two alpha genes on each chromosome has become deleted, leaving the remaining gene functional (that is, $-/\alpha/-/\alpha$). This is described as alpha-thalassaemia minor, or as alpha-thalassaemia carrier. In both cases, alpha-globin production is 50% of normal.

- Deletion or functional inactivity of *three* of the four alpha-globin genes, that is, $-/-/-\alpha$, is Haemoglobin H disease. It presents clinically as a type of thalassaemia intermedia and is characterized by levels of alpha-globin 25% of normal.

- Complete loss of all *four* alpha-globin genes ($-/-/-/-$, thus no alpha-globin) results in haemoglobin Bart's, also called hydrops fetalis syndrome, where the fetus is unable to make either normal fetal (α_2/γ_2) or adult A (α_2/β_2) haemoglobin. Hb Bart's is incompatible with life, and death usually occurs *in utero* or soon after birth.

Cases involving both delta- and beta-globin, and complexes of gamma-, delta-, and beta-globin, do occur but are rare. Impaired alpha-globin leads to excess gamma-globin and beta-globin chains, which form unstable and physiologically afunctional tetramers. In haemoglobin Bart's this becomes gamma (γ_4), whilst in haemoglobin H the tetramer is of beta-globin (β_4). Although almost all alpha-thalassaemia is caused by gene defects, it has been established that it may also be a consequence of a chronic myeloid disorder, usually the myelodysplastic syndrome.

The beta-thalassaemias

There are more than 200 different mutations of the beta-globin genes (present on chromosome 11) which result in the reduced or absent synthesis of beta-globin chains. There is also a consistent synthesis of gamma-globin chains, which leads to increased levels of fetal haemoglobin (HbF, $\alpha_2\gamma_2$). These mutations may be within the gene complex or on nearby promoter or enhancer regions. As with alpha-thalassaemia, the severity of the disease, at both clinical and laboratory levels, depends on the number and character of the abnormal genes. Three broad categories of disease are recognized:

- *Thalassaemia major* is a consequence of the inheritance of two different mutations, which lead to interference with β-globin chain production, and includes both β^0-thalassaemia (where the globin chains are absent) and β^+-thalassaemia (where globin chains are

Cross reference
Globin chains were discussed in Chapter 4, Section 4.3: Haemoglobin–Globin and Figure 4.8.

Cross reference
Myelodysplastic syndromes are discussed in depth in Chapter 11.

partially present). In homozygous beta-thalassaemia either no beta-globin chain exists (β^0), or only small amounts (β^+) are synthesized, leading to severe anaemia. Hypertrophy of the ineffective bone marrow is associated with skeletal changes, and there is hepatosplenomegaly.

- *Thalassaemia intermedia* may be caused by a variety of genetic defects, and so is often classified clinically, as opposed to genetically or haematologically. In one manifestation there is homozygous β-thalassaemia, but effects of the anaemia are countered by a greater synthesis of haemoglobin F than usual. In another form there are mild defects in the synthesis of beta chains. The coexistence of alpha-thalassaemia carrier status improves the haemoglobin levels by decreasing the degree of chain imbalance.

- Heterozygotes for beta-thalassaemia are generally asymptomatic. As such, they are described as *thalassaemia minor (or trait)*, which includes β^0-thalassaemia carrier, and β^+-thalassaemia carrier status. These conditions are not associated with anaemia because the remaining non-mutated β-globin gene is able to synthesize sufficient beta-globin to permit oxygen carriage. Consequently, clinical presentations are mild. This picture is also seen in α-thalassaemia.

Table 6.2 summarizes these aspects of thalassaemia.

Clinical features

Medical care in all cases of thalassaemia focuses on disease severity, regardless of genotype. Deletions in one or two alpha genes are asymptomatic. Deletions in three alpha genes, giving rise to HbH, leads to jaundice, hepatosplenomegaly, leg ulcers, gall stones, and folate deficiency. Most patients will not need blood transfusions, although iron overload can be a problem, probably due to increased intestinal absorption.

In β-thalassaemia major, anaemia dominates after the age of 3 months when the switching from γ- to β-chain synthesis occurs. However, in milder forms, there may be no symptoms up to the age of 4 years. Children generally fail to thrive, show recurrent infections, pallor, and mild jaundice. Enlargement of the liver and spleen is due to trapping of the excessively damaged red cells. To compensate for the anaemia, extramedullary haemopoiesis becomes dominant. Expansion of the bones caused by intensive marrow hyperplasia leads to thalassaemic facial features such as bossing (swelling of the bone of the jaw) leading to enlarged maxilla, a 'hair on end' appearance on X-ray, and thinning of the cortex of the bones, leading to easy fractures.

In a severe thalassaemia, causing a profound anaemia, blood transfusions are necessary to maintain quality of life, or even life itself, and may be required every six weeks. However, a major complication of these repeated transfusions is the build-up of iron in organs such as the liver, heart, and endocrine organs, which can lead to irreversible damage to these organs, although fortunately there are treatments to remove this excess iron. This is developed in more detail in a section that follows. During infancy, the anaemic child is prone to bacterial infection from *Pneumococcus*, *Haemophilus*, and *Meningococcus* species, amongst others. Transfused patients are at risk from virus transmission associated with blood transfusion, such as hepatitis C and B. However, overall, beta-thalassaemia carrier status provides a benign and a generally asymptomatic condition.

Compound and other haemoglobinopathies

It is clear that different haemoglobin gene mutations can occur in various different combinations, and that these different combinations effectively create hybrids of quantitative and qualitative defects, or indeed two different quantitative defects such as in alpha- and beta-thalassaemia. Given the overlapping geographical areas where these mutations are endemic, these associations are to be expected, and arise because of the asymptomatic nature of many types of heterozygous disease.

Combined qualitative defects include those arising from the combination of haemoglobin S and haemoglobin C (that is, HbSC), and of haemoglobin S with haemoglobin D (HbSD). The compound heterozygosity of HbSC may be designated $\alpha_2\beta^s$ β^c. Combined quantitative and qualitative defects may also be present, such as a combination of beta-thalassaemia and sickle cell disease. Indeed, both HbS/β^0 and HbS/β^+ are known. Because of the dominance of the sickle haemoglobin, all of these are clinical sickling conditions, and the clinical picture resembles homozygous sickle cell disease (for example, with splenomegaly). The heterozygous disease of combined haemoglobin E and β^0-thalassaemia resembles homozygous β^0-thalassaemia both clinically and haematologically, and so is managed in the clinic as thalassaemia major.

In some cases, deletion of β gene(s), δ and β genes, or δ, β or γ genes occurs. In rare conditions, unequal crossing-over of globin genes leads to the production of haemoglobin Lepore. This hybrid has globin chains of δ-globin at one end fused with β-globin at the other end. If present in both sets of genes (that is, as a homozygous state) the clinical presentation is of thalassaemia intermedia, whilst the heterozygous state is less severe and is clinically akin to a carrier status.

Another form of mutation in both delta and beta genes leads to impaired production of both species of globin molecules, hence $\delta\beta$-thalassaemia. However, fetal haemoglobin (HbF, $\alpha_2\gamma_2$) is increased, giving at least some (limited) capacity to carry oxygen, and the production of alpha- and gamma-globin is generally unaffected. Indeed, in homozygous $\delta\beta$-thalassaemia, only haemoglobin F is synthesized. This leads to the syndrome termed 'hereditary persistence of fetal haemoglobin' (HPFH), and presents clinically as thalassaemia intermedia. However, there are other forms of HPFH caused by deletions, point mutations, or cross-over of beta and gamma genes. Indeed, measurement of the level of HbF can be very informative (Table 6.3). Figure 6.9 illustrates globin molecule interactions in thalassaemia and HPFH.

SELF-CHECK 6.5

What are the laboratory differences between the alpha- and beta-thalassaemias?

TABLE 6.3 **HbF levels in haemoglobinopathy (Table modified from *Dacie & Lewis, by permission*).**

Hb F level	Indicative clinical picture
<1%	Normal result
1–5 %	Present in approximately 30% of beta-thalassaemia carriers. Many other conditions, for example, compound haemoglobinopathy
5–20 %	Some cases of beta-thalassaemia trait, compound heterozygotes, some cases of heterozygous HPFH, $\delta\beta$-thalassaemia
15–45 %	Most cases of heterozygous HPFH, some cases of beta-thalassaemia intermedia
>45%	Beta-thalassaemia major, some cases of beta-thalassaemia intermedia, neonates
>95%	Homozygous HPFH, some neonates (especially if premature)

HPFH, hereditary persistence of fetal haemoglobin.

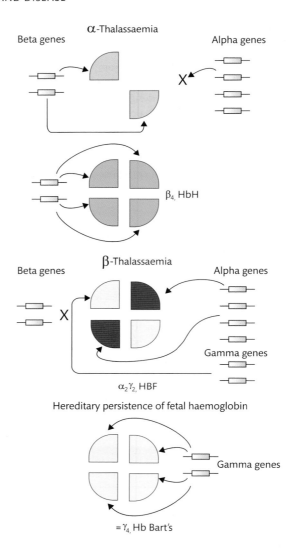

FIGURE 6.9

Molecular variants of haemoglobins in thalassaemia and hereditary persistence of fetal haemoglobin. In the most severe form of alpha-thalassaemia (top panel), the four alpha genes fail to produce alpha-globin; the beta genes are unaffected, but the product ($0_2\beta_2$) is incompatible with life. However, the two normal beta genes can produce sufficient beta-globin to combine to form a homogeneous haemoglobin (β_4) called HbH.

In β-thalassaemia (third panel), beta genes fail to produce beta-globin. However, functioning alpha genes and gamma genes still produce alpha-globin and gamma-globin which together form functional haemoglobin F (HbF, $\alpha_2\gamma_2$), which retains oxygen-carrying capacity.

Hereditary persistence of fetal haemoglobin is present when all alpha and beta genes fail to produce alpha- and beta-globin. The gamma genes are intact and functioning, and generate sufficient gamma-globin to form a haemoglobin molecule where the only globin component is gamma-globin (γ_4).

Laboratory tests in haemoglobinopathy

As in the investigation of any anaemia, a full blood count (including reticulocytes) and blood film are essential, and many also find the ESR useful. However, a range of other tests are specific for the haemoglobinopathies, many of which are based on properties of the abnormal globin molecules, and of the genes themselves. These are essential in confirming a preliminary diagnosis, in monitoring treatment, and also have a place in screening at-risk populations. Dedicated haemoglobinopathy methods include two 'wet' preparations, electrophoresis (capillary, cellulose, alkaline, and acid), microcolumn analysis for HbA_2, high performance liquid chromatography (HPLC), estimation of HbF (Betke method), immunoassay, and DNA analysis.

Wet preparations

These tests are so named because they are performed directly on whole blood. They are also very quick, cheap (in terms of reagents), and require simple equipment (a light microscope or a water bath). However, they are prone to error.

The simplest test relies on the way that phenotypically normal-looking red cells adopt the sickle phenotype when hypoxic (as they would in the circulation). The test relies on a reducing agent that effectively lowers the oxygen content of a sample of whole blood. A small volume of blood is mixed with an equal volume of the oxygen-consuming reducing agent (such as sodium metabisulphate) in a physiological buffer and is immediately placed in a counting chamber for viewing under a light microscope. As the reducing agent reduces the oxygen levels, cells carrying haemoglobin S will adopt the characteristic sickle shape. The test must be performed with positive and negative controls—respectively, a blood sample known to be from a patient with sickle cell disease, and the proband's blood mixed with simple buffer alone (which should not induce hypoxia).

A similar test is of the solubility of sickle cells. Under deoxygenated conditions, sickle haemoglobin becomes insoluble in phosphate buffer supplemented with saponin as a haemolyser and sodium dithionite as a reducing agent. A subject's blood is again mixed with the buffer, then incubated for a short period, and placed in front of a grid with defined lines. As the red cells lyse, the solution becomes clear, implying a negative result for sickle cell disease. However, if the blood solution is opaque or turbid (due to the red cells being intact and in suspension), as defined by an inability to see the lines through the test tube, then the result is deemed positive (Figure 6.10).

This test can be extended by centrifugation of the tubes at 1200 g for five minutes. In the presence of sickle haemoglobin, the buffer solution gives a clear dark-red or purple coloration at the top of the tube, with a thin 'scum' of precipitated protein and red cell stroma, whilst the solution below will be pink or colourless. In the absence of sickle haemoglobin, there is no

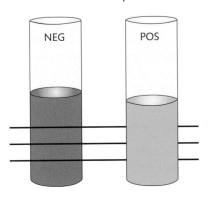

FIGURE 6.10
The sickle solubility test. When sickle positive blood is mixed with saponin and a reducing agent, the resultant solution is cloudy, whereas with normal blood the solution is clear. This property is used to define sickle status.
NEG = Negative for sickle status
POS = Positive for sickle status

such coloured ring. False-positives may be due to red cell debris, erythrocytosis, increased paraprotein, and unstable haemoglobin(s). This can be corrected by washing the red cells.

A false-negative may be due to deterioration of the dithionite, unstable saponin, anaemia, and a post-transfusion sample. High levels (10–20%) of HbF, which counter the polymerization of the sickle haemoglobin, can also give a false-negative. Accordingly, the test is unreliable in neonates during the first few months of life.

Electrophoresis

The separation of proteins can be achieved by exploiting the way they carry a net charge. If a sample is placed in an electric field, it will migrate, with its final resting position being dependent on the charge it carries. This process of movement in an electric field is called electrophoresis.

Haemoglobin has a net positive charge, as conferred by the particular combination of amino acid side chains that are present in the molecule. However, different haemoglobin variants are composed of different amino acids, and so carry slightly different electrical charges. As a result, these variants will migrate to different positions on a gel. Different types of electrophoresis (for example, those employing different pH, or using different physical supports such as cellulose acetate or agarose) can be employed to detect different haemoglobin species.

Cross reference
We learn more about electrophoresis in the *Biomedical Science Practice* volume in this series.

An additional electrophoresis method (using a different buffer and urea, and at pH 6.3 or pH 8) can be used to separate different alpha- and beta-globin chains. Of course, haemoglobin is found within red cells, not in plasma. Therefore the haemoglobin must be released from the red cell by lysis, creating a lysate.

Alkaline (pH 8.4–8.7) electrophoresis

When performed on cellulose acetate, this method is simple, reliable, and rapid. Within this pH range, haemoglobin in the red cell lysate is negatively charged and will move towards the anode. However, different types of haemoglobin will separate from haemoglobin A, and form their own line of identity. At the practical level, with each set of samples, there must be a control sample containing haemoglobins A, F, S, C, D, and Punjab. However haemoglobins C and E co-migrate to the same position, as do haemoglobins S, D, and G. Haemoglobin Lepore has an electrophoretic motility similar to that of haemoglobin S. Consequently, these haemoglobin variants cannot be differentiated, so that other techniques are demanded. The separation pattern of common haemoglobin variants, and some unknowns, is shown in Figure 6.11.

Acid (pH 6.0–6.3) electrophoresis

The broad principle of acid electrophoresis is the same as that for alkaline electrophoresis, but it is best performed on agarose. At an acidic pH the different haemoglobin variants migrate to different positions than they do at an alkaline pH, giving the opportunity to distinguish between alternative phenotypes. For example, haemoglobins S and D co-migrate at alkaline pH, as do haemoglobins C and E, but at acid pH they migrate to different positions. Consequently, acid electrophoresis is effectively a back-up method. As before, known positive controls must be run as part of each assay.

HbA₂ estimation by microcolumn chromatography

HbA_2 is a tetramer of two alpha-globin molecules and two delta-globin molecules (hence $\alpha_2\delta_2$), and comprises around 2% of total adult haemoglobin. Estimation may be called for in the investigation of a suspected thalassaemia. The most common method is of anion exchange chromatography whereby negatively charged haemoglobin is adsorbed to a positively charged

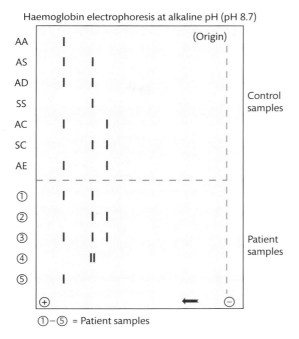

Haemoglobin electrophoresis at alkaline pH (pH 8.7)

① – ⑤ = Patient samples

FIGURE 6.11

Haemoglobin electrophoresis patterns. Samples of haemoglobin are placed on the right hand (anode) edge of the electrophoresis plate, and are driven over to the left hand side (towards the cathode) by the electrical change. The migration distance depends on their overall physicochemical make up, and so differs between different types of haemoglobin. This figure consists of control samples and patient samples. The topmost trace, AA, is of normal haemoglobin A, which migrates to a fixed position as a single band. Other traces show different patterns according to their composition—HbAS shows two bands, one of the A globin, and the other of the S globin. Thus the trace of HbSS (that is, indicative of homozygous sickle cell disease) is of a single line. Other bands indicate haemoglobins AD, AC, SC, and AE by combinations of different individual lines. The lower traces, 1–5, are the subject of Case Study 6.2 on page 176.

resin. A mobile phase with different pH is applied to the resin to elute HbA_2, with the developer passing through the column. Normal haemoglobin and Hb variants retained on top of the column are then eluted with a second buffer of different pH. The two fractions are collected separately and the absorbance of the eluate is measured on a spectrophotometer. This allows the amount of HbA_2 present to be expressed as a percentage of total haemoglobin.

The definition of the reference range for this test is crucial and must be defined locally. In β-thalassaemia carrier status, the HbA_2 level is elevated (perhaps 5%) compared with reference values (which may be up to 3.0%). However, in severe iron deficiency this may be lower at, for example, 3.5%. It is also possible to modify the procedure to allow measurement of HbA_2 in the presence of sickle haemoglobin. Modified columns are available commercially for this purpose. HbA_2 may also be estimated by cellulose acetate electrophoresis and by HPLC.

Detection of haemoglobin variants by immunoassay

Commercially prepared kits known as HemoCards are available for the detection of common haemoglobins S, C, D, E, and A_2 with sensitivity down to 5–10%. However, the use of the

HemoCard kit in the laboratory is limited due to availability, unreliability, and the poor quality of kits. By contrast, HbF can be measured by immunodiffusion and by enzyme-linked immunosorbent assay (ELISA).

HbF quantitation

Fetal haemoglobin (HbF) is a tetramer of two alpha-globin molecules and two gamma-globin molecules (that is, $\alpha_2\gamma_2$). A dominant variant in the fetus, levels fall in the initial few months of life, such that it is present as perhaps 0.5–0.8% of total adult haemoglobin. However, increased levels are present in various haemoglobinopathies and as such are an aid to diagnosis and the monitoring of treatment (Table 6.3).

HbF levels below 12% can be accurately quantified by HPLC or the alkali denaturation method (also called the Betke method, developed 50 years ago). These have replaced the traditional acid elution method of Kleihauer. Although Betke's alkali method is accurate down to 0.1%, it is labour-intensive, and involves handling a cyanide reagent and an open blood sample. HbF greater than 12% should be confirmed by alternative method.

One of the disadvantages of these tests is that they measure total HbF in a collection of cells, not in individual cells. Consequently, they are unable to distinguish the HbF of a $\delta\beta$-thalassaemia carrier—in which the distribution of HbF is usually heterocellular (that is, is present or absent from particular cells)—from hereditary persistence of fetal haemoglobin (HPFH) in which the distribution is pancellular (that is, is present in every single cell). Instead, these two patterns can be determined by staining a blood film with an antibody to HbH, and then staining with a second antibody conjugated to a visualizing signal such as fluorescein isothiocyanate. The qualitative and quantitative differences in the distribution of HbF can be detected by an appropriate microscope set up for fluorescence. HbF-bearing cells can also be detected by flow cytometry.

High-performance liquid chromatograpy (HPLC)

This method is quite possibly the 'gold standard' technique for determining haemoglobin variants. Although the capital investment and running costs are considerable when compared to electrophoresis, the method can be automated (giving high throughput), is frugal of sample (requiring as little as 5 μL of blood), and is accurate, rapid (perhaps 5 minutes), reproducible, and reliable. The method is particularly suited to a high throughput laboratory that may be required to perform antenatal screening for haemoglobinopathy.

The use of HPLC for the determination of haemoglobin variants relies on the different ionic properties of different haemoglobins. Positively charged haemoglobin within the red cell lysate is separated by adsorption on to a negatively charged stationary phase in the column, typically an amino acid coated onto a silica particle resin. The mobile phase (such as a salt solution), featuring an increasing concentration of cations, detaches the bound haemoglobin protein from the anionic binding amino acid, and the optical density of the eluted solution (which carries the haemoglobins) is measured spectrophotometrically. This result is converted into a chromatogram that shows all the haemoglobin peaks in a particular sample. Each type of haemoglobin molecule carries a distinctive net charge (as we noted above). Consequently, each haemoglobin exhibits a unique retention time on the column, which can be exploited to facilitate haemoglobin identification. This is illustrated in Figure 6.12.

As with gel or cellulose acetate electrophoresis, positive controls of known haemoglobin variants must be present in each batch. An additional aspect of this technique is that it can also provide levels of glycosylated haemoglobin (HbA_{1C}).

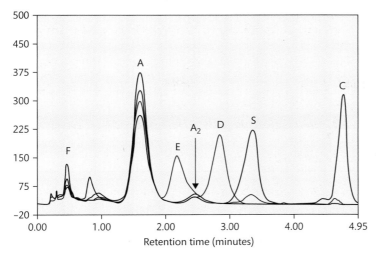

FIGURE 6.12

HPLC chromatograms. HPLC is an additional tool to investigate a presumed haemoglobinopathy. The principle is allied to that of electrophoresis, where different types of globins can be identified by their combined physical and chemical properties. The figure is a composite of a collection of different globins illustrating how each can be found along the spectrum from left to right. The 'height' of the peak is proportional to the amount of the particular globin present in a sample.

Isoelectric focusing (IEF)

This technique, related to electrophoresis, also relies on the different electrical properties of haemoglobin variants. IEF plates are made from either polyacrylamide or agarose and both contain amphoteric molecules with various isolectric points. These molecules are used to establish a pH gradient in the gel, generally running between pH 6 and pH 8.

Isoelectric focusing exploits the way that different proteins have different isoelectric points— that is, the pH at which they carry no net charge. As we noted earlier when discussing electrophoresis, a charged protein will migrate when placed in an electric field. If this migration occurs through a pH gradient, however, the protein will stop moving once it reaches the point in the gel at which it carries no net charge.

Different haemoglobins have different net charges, with the result that different haemoglobin molecules have unique isoelectric points on the gel (that is, they will migrate to different extents). Once completed, the gel can be stained and the position of the various haemoglobin species can be quantified by densitometry. The densitometry peaks can be superimposed on traces of known variants to assist in the diagnosis.

Like HPLC, IEF demands capital investment, but advantages include the ability to separate many different variants, clear demarcation due to sharp bands, the ability to separate haemoglobins D and G from S, and the requirement for only a small blood sample, so that it is suitable for neonatal haemoglobinopathy investigation and screening.

DNA analysis

This specialized method, inevitably found in a reference laboratory, is used for the confirmation of haemoglobin variants, alpha (^{0})-thalassaemia carriers, and prenatal diagnosis of serious disorders of haemoglobin synthesis. It can also be used for fetal diagnosis of haemoglobin-opathy. The general area of molecular genetics is intensely technical and so very demanding of skilled scientists, who are very likely to be based in regional referral laboratories. The basic technique of DNA analysis may be modified according to the mutations expected given the particular ethnicity of the patient, and are used to define the exact nature of a particular gene mutation predominantly in sickle cell disease, beta-thalassaemia, and alpha-thalassaemia.

SELF-CHECK 6.6

What laboratory tests can give the most precise and comprehensive information about the protein nature of a suspected haemoglobinopathy?

Laboratory findings in haemoglobinopathy

The essential tests for studying haemoglobinopathy are the full blood count and blood film. The consistent finding from the full blood count in haemoglobinopathy is a reduced haemo-globin and a reduced MCV, indicating a microcytosis. If the patient is symptomatic, this makes the diagnosis of microcytic anaemia. However, the sensitivity and specificity of a reduced MCV is poor as a common alternative diagnosis is iron deficiency, which should be considered and excluded, either by iron studies (such as serum ferritin, iron, transferrin, transferrin saturation) or additional haemoglobinopathy testing.

A reactive erythrocytosis may also be present as the bone marrow attempts to maintain the ability of the blood to deliver oxygen to the tissues. Further evidence of this stress erythropoi-esis is a reticulocytosis. These cells are larger than mature erythrocytes, and are certainly larger than microcytes. Consequently, the MCV (a global score of red cell volume) may not be far below the bottom of the reference range. Thus an increased RDW may be present, and this should be detected and reported by the haematology autoanalyser.

Sickle cell disease

Simple screening of this disease is most rapidly achieved by the sickling test, although this will need to be defined with other tests such as HPLC. Patients with sickle cell anaemia have a haemolytic anaemia, with a broad range of haemoglobin concentration in the range 60–90 g/L and elevated reticulocyte count of perhaps 10–20%. The haematocrit ranges between 0.18 and 0.30 L/L.

Haemoglobin electrophoresis of homozygous sickle cell disease (HbSS) will report >80% HbS, with variable levels of HbF (5–15%) but a normal (trace) amount of HbA_2. In HPLC the chromatogram shows a small peak at the HbF retention time and a large peak in the HbS window. In heterozygous disease (HbAS) there is generally an excess of HbA (50–60%) compared to HbS (perhaps 35–45%). This picture can be contrasted with the relatively common combined defect, sickle/β-thalassaemia, wherein electrophoresis reveals that 60–90% of the haemoglobin is HbS, whereas 10–30% is HbF. However, if the patient retains some alpha gene activity then HbA may be present. Haemoglobin A_2 is generally moderately elevated in sickle/β-thalassaemia disease.

Thalassaemia

General hospital haematology laboratories do not have one single test to confirm an α-thalassaemia carrier. Instead, multiple investigation data together with patient ethnic data are used to indicate probable α-thalassaemias. The same aspects of screening and preven-tion apply to other haemoglobinopathies, such as HbS, C, D, E, Lepore, and thalassaemia.

In α-thalassaemia carrier status (when one or two alpha genes are deleted), the haemoglobin may be normal but produced at slightly reduced levels, providing an asymptomatic phenotype. The MCV (<77 fL)) and MCH (<25 pg/) may both be reduced, but the red cell count may be raised (>5.5 × 10^{12}/L). Measurement of the relative rates of α- and β-synthesis may support a diagnosis of α- thalassaemia.

When three alpha genes are deleted, HbH disease is present. Haemoglobin is typically 60–110 g/L. In the neonate, electrophoresis or HPLC shows Hb Bart's (γ_4) up to 25%, the remainder being HbA ($\alpha_2\beta_2$) and HbF ($\alpha_2\gamma_2$) with a small amount of HbH (β_4). As the γ-chain production switches to β-chain synthesis, HbH (β_4) gradually replaces Hb Bart's, and HbF also disappears. In adults, the haemoglobin pattern is HbA and HbH, which may range from 5 to 25%. HbA_2 levels are slightly decreased and the HbF level is normal or slightly increased. The high levels of beta-globin can form deposits or precipitates within the red cell, and this can be detected on a blood film using a supra-vital stain such as Brilliant cresyl blue.

Overall, the beta-thalassaemias demonstrate a broad range of clinical and haematological variability due to the heterogeneous nature of the molecular defects that affect beta-chain production. Heterozygotes for beta-thalassaemia (carriers) are generally asymptomatic, but have microcytic, hypochromic red cells, reduced MCV (typically 65–75 fL), reduced haemoglobin (90–110 g/L), and reduced MCH (20–22 pg/). There is also likely to be raised HbA_2 (>3.5%).

Patients with thalassaemia intermedia present with a very broad phenotypic picture, ranging from symptomless to the requirement of blood transfusions, and subsequent iron chelation therapy. Patients with haemoglobin ranging from 60 to 100 g/L generally do not require blood transfusion. The red cells are very microcytic and hypochromic, and there is increased erythropoiesis. These patients may demonstrate some bone deformity, enlarged spleen and liver, and features of iron overload.

Severe beta-thalassaemia major is associated with a profound anaemia (haemoglobin 20–60 g/L), reduced MCV (<65 fL) and MCH, and raised reticulocyte count. Investigation of the bone marrow is generally unnecessary (unless a differential diagnosis needs to be excluded) but, if performed, should show hypercellularity with erythroid hyperplasia. Haemoglobin electrophoresis or HPLC demonstrates the absence (in β^0-thalassaemia) or almost complete absence (β^+-thalassaemia) of normal adult haemoglobin (HbA) with almost all the circulating haemoglobin being fetal haemoglobin (HbF) and varying level amounts of HbA_2, ranging from low to slightly raised. Globin-chain synthesis studies show no synthesis of the β-chain.

The blood film in haemoglobinopathy

The blood film provides two sets of clues that are useful in diagnosis: the specific and the non-specific. The only finding on a blood film specific for haemoglobinopathy is the sickle cell, inevitably present in hypoxic blood from a person with homozygous sickle cell disease (Figure 6.7). However, the intracellular changes brought about by abnormal haemoglobin in severe thalassaemia may also induce the cells to adopt the sickle phenotype.

There are many non-specific aspects of abnormal red cell morphology in the haemoglobinopathies. The presence of schistocytes—see Figures 6.3 and 6.4—is evidence of red cell destruction, the hallmark of many haemolytic anaemias, and so are not specific for haemoglobinopathy. Similarly, microcytes are present in both haemoglobinopathy and in iron-deficient anaemia. Other non-specific morphological changes in haemoglobinopathy include anisocytosis, poikilocytosis, and basophilic stippling, the latter also being found in lead poisoning (Figure 5.11). Target cells are a common finding in haemoglobinopathy (especially in HbC disease), but are also likely to be present in iron deficiency, in liver disease, and following splenectomy. An additional finding following splenectomy, and also in splenic atrophy, are Howell–Jolly bodies. Appearing as a small dot within the red cell (Figure 6.13), Howell–Jolly bodies are an example of an **inclusion body**—a pathological finding within a red blood cell. Other inclusion bodies are described in Table 6.4.

The more severe the disease is, then the more marked these changes can be. For example, in severe beta-thalassaemia major, the blood film demonstrates marked morphological changes with anisocytosis, hypochromic microcytic cells, basophilic stippling, and nucleated red blood cells (normoblasts) (Figure 6.14). Nucleated red blood cells indicate a hyperactive or stressed erythropoiesis, although these cells are also found in numerous conditions, such as a myeloid malignancy. Conversely, in mild conditions such as sickle cell trait, there should be no abnormalities on a blood film.

Non-specificity and other haemoglobinopathies

A common theme of this section is the clustering of various laboratory findings (such as a low MCV and target cells) in the different haemoglobinopathies, even if compound. For example, both HbS/β-thalassaemia and HbSC are associated with prominent target cells, basophilic stippling, and a microcytosis. Furthermore, the electrophoresis and HPLC pattern in compound HbS/thalassaemia may resemble HbSS, as both will lack HbA. Target cells and spherocytes are also commonly found in both homozygous and heterozygous HbC and E diseases. In all cases there will be microcytosis and hypochromia. These two variants co-migrate on cellulose-acetate electrophoresis gels but can be separated using acid-citrate agar electrophoresis. In compound HbSF, 70% of the haemoglobin

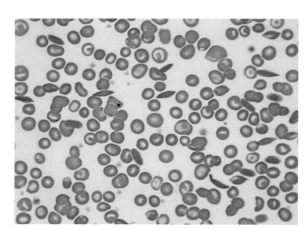

FIGURE 6.13

Sickle cells, target cells, and a Howell–Jolly body (left of centre). This film is from a patient with compound haemoglobin S and thalassaemia. There are abundant sickle cells, many target cells, and a single Howell–Jolly body. The latter implies splenic atrophy or post splenectomy. (Magnification ×400.)

TABLE 6.4   Red blood cell inclusion bodies.

Basophilic stippling	Denatured RNA
Heinz bodies	Oxidized denatured haemoglobin
Howell–Jolly bodies	Formed from DNA remnants and often found after splenectomy
Nuclei	Nucleated red blood cells
Pappenheimer bodies	Particles of iron-rich protein found in siderocytes
Parasites	As are present in malaria

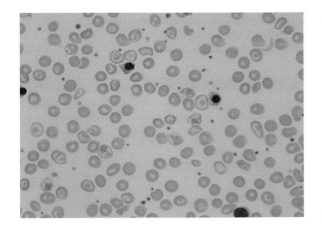

FIGURE 6.14

Target cells and nucleated red blood cells. The anaemia in this case of severe beta thalassaemia is so profound that the overactive bone marrow has released nucleated red blood cells into the circulation. Compare the density of the nuclear staining in these red cells with that of the lymphocyte on the lower margin. (Magnification ×400.)

is HbS, 30% HbF. However, a notable feature of HbC disease is of intracellular crystals of the abnormal haemoglobin, which become more prominent in a hypertonic solution.

Although not generally considered classical haemoglobinopathies, a number of other haemoglobin variants justify a mention. A small number of variants readily take up oxygen but are reluctant to give it up at the tissues. These are called high-oxygen affinity variants. The consequences of these mutants are tissue hypoxia, and a reactive raised red cell count in response. Conversely, in low-oxygen affinity variants, oxygen is taken up poorly, and haemoglobin tends to dissociate into its subunits, again resulting in poor oxygen distribution. Despite the rarity of these conditions, they provide the opportunity to probe the relationships between oxygen uptake, erythropoietin, and erythropoiesis.

Haemoglobin M has a tendency to form methaemoglobin, the molecular basis of which stems from substitutions in either alpha- or beta-globins. The biochemical consequence of this is that the iron remains in the ferric form and so cannot bind oxygen, leading to cyanosis in the patient. However, methaemoglobin may also be found in red cell enzyme deficiency diseases, and in the presence of certain drugs (such as antituberculosis agents and sulphonamide antibiotics), and chemicals (such as silver nitrate and amyl nitrate). Although detectable on electrophoresis, HbM can also be determined by spectrophotometry.

Iron

In order to maintain a haemoglobin level of 90–100 g/L in those with severe disease, regular transfusion of concentrated red cells is required, possibly at a rate of 2–4 units of red cells every 4–6 weeks, but this is very variable and is driven symptomatically. Each 500 ml of transfused blood contains 200–250 mg of iron and, since the human body has a very limited means to excrete iron, regular blood transfusion eventually leads to iron overload. After the patient has received about 10–15 units of blood and the serum ferritin level exceeds 1000 µg/L, iron chelation therapy needs to be seriously considered. Although serum ferritin is the marker of choice, it is an acute-phase protein and is raised in viral hepatitis and other inflammatory disorders. Therefore, caution in interpretation is required. Removal of iron normally involves overnight infusion of an iron chelating agent such as desferrioxamine, together with vitamin C, to increase iron excretion, on 5–7 nights per week. Deferiprone, an orally active chelator, may be administered in conjunction with desferrioxamine to remove iron from the organs. Combined treatment is more effective than deferiprone alone in reducing serum ferritin. Treatment is also required for iron overload-associated complications such as of the heart, liver, and endocrine systems.

SELF-CHECK 6.7

What are the principal findings in the FBC from a patient with a haemoglobinopathy?

SELF-CHECK 6.8

What are the principal findings in the blood film from a patient with a haemoglobinopathy?

Management of haemoglobinopathy

There is no simple effective treatment of sickle cell disease. Generally, the patient should avoid known precipitants of sickle cell crisis, such as dehydration, infection, anoxia, and the cooling of the skin surface. During sickle cell crises the patient will need to take rest, keep warm, and rehydrate with oral fluids or (if seriously dehydrated) intravenous normal saline. Analgesia should be given to reduce pain, and oxygen should be provided if there is tissue hypoxia. Red blood cell transfusion should be considered for severe anaemia, whilst exchange transfusion should be considered for severe sickling or sequestration. With this treatment the level of HbS could be reduced to <30%.

Oral hydroxycarbamide (hydroxyurea) is a common choice to reduce both the frequency and duration of sickle cell crisis. This drug increases HbF synthesis, decreases intracellular HbS levels by increasing the mean cell volume (MCV), lowers the white cell count, and reduces the adhesiveness between the sickle cell and the endothelium. Erythropoietin is also used to promote HbF levels. Increased platelet activation in sickle cell disease and thalassaemia brings a risk of venous thromboembolism and thus requires attendance at an oral anticoagulation clinic.

Vaccinating patients against pneumococcal and meningococcal organisms may reduce the frequency of infection, whilst oral penicillin is recommended to compensate for splenic atrophy. A vaccination against hepatitis B is also given, since these patients may require blood transfusion at some stage. Splenectomy is considered at the age of 5 years to reduce the blood requirement, and is followed by oral penicillin therapy for life as subjects are susceptible to infections. A consequence of splenectomy (often offered to prolong the life of the abnormal red cell) is the appearance on the blood film of Howell–Jolly bodies within red cells, although these bodies (being nuclear remnants) may also be present in any splenic pathology, and so are common in the haemoglobinopathies.

In both types of haemoglobinopathy, bone marrow transplantation, perhaps from an HLA-matching sibling, may offer the prospect of a permanent cure if carried out early in life. The success rate is over 80% in well-chelated young children, provided that liver complications do not arise.

Prenatal diagnosis and prevention of haemoglobinopathy

The severity of many haemoglobinopathies has prompted initiatives aimed at their prevention. Almost all sickle cell disease and thalassaemias are genetically inherited conditions, and the affected patients (carriers) are at risk of transmitting the disease to their descendants.

Under the current NHS guidelines, hospitals within a high-prevalence area perform universal haemoglobinopathy screening for all antenatal attenders (when a first pregnancy), regardless of ethnic or racial origin. Mothers who are tested positive for significant haemoglobinopathy are invited to call the father for screening. If both parents are carriers for a haemoglobinopathy there is a 25% chance that the newborn may have the homozygous disease during each pregnancy (Figure 6.15). Such couples, with appropriate genetic counselling, would be given the informed choice for investigation and termination.

If a couple is diagnosed with haemoglobinopathy then there is a one in four chance that the fetus is homozygous, or doubly heterozygous, and a one in two chance that the fetus is a carrier. In at-risk couples, prenatal diagnosis is offered using either DNA (from a chorionic villous or amniotic fluid sample) or fetal blood. The fetal DNA is amplified by using polymerase chain reaction (PCR) and the DNA mutation(s) are detected. In homozygous disease of the fetus, the couple should be counselled and, if appropriate, termination may be offered.

Key Points

The epidemiology, molecular and cell biology, and the pathology of the haemoglobinopathies are well characterized. However, less well understood is the impact that the disease has upon the haematology and clinical course of the disease for each individual. Both these phenotypic aspects can differ widely in two individuals with apparently the same genotype, indicating that there is still much we have to learn.

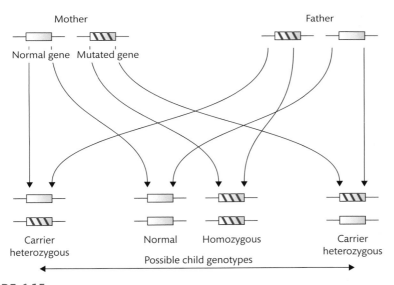

FIGURE 6.15

Simple inheritance of a single gene defect. Inheritance of a haemoglobinopathy (such as sickle cell disease) obeys simple Mendelian genetics. Each parent has two genes, but in the present illustration, each has a normal gene and a mutated gene that gives rise to an abnormal haemoglobin. Thus each parent is a heterozygote and so is a carrier of the disease. Either parent can pass on only one of their genes to their offspring, which then has two genes, one from each parent.

On the far left, the child has inherited a normal gene from the mother and an abnormal gene from the father. Thus, like its parents, it is also a heterozygote and a carrier of the disease. To the right, the offspring has inherited a normal gene from each parent and so is a (normal) homozygote. The offspring third from the left has inherited two mutated genes, one from each parent, and so is a homozygote and will fully express the genotype (such as sickle cell disease). On the right, the offspring has inherited a normal gene from the father and an abnormal gene from its mother, and so is a heterozygote carrier.

CASE STUDY 6.1

A 20-year old female has recently moved, with her family, to the UK from the Far East. Following a few weeks' acclimatization and recovery from jet lag, it became clear to her family that she was consistently tired and lethargic, more so than her siblings. On examination she had no symptoms of infection (e.g. a fever, sweating) or aches and pains, and did not report heavy menstrual bleeding. The full blood count and ESR were as follows.

How should this subject be investigated?

	This case	Reference range (female)
Haemoglobin	105 g/L	118–148 g/L
RCC	6.0×10^{12}/L	$3.9–5.0 \times 10^{12}$/L
MCH	17.5 pg	26–33 pg
MCV	55 fL	77–98 fL
MCHC	318 pg/L	330–370 pg/L
Hct	0.33	0.33–0.47
Reticulocytes	150×10^{9}/L	$25–125 \times 10^{9}$/L
ESR	15 mm/hour	<10 mm/hour

CASE STUDY 6.2

Haemoglobin electrophoresis is a useful tool in determining the phenotype of various haemoglobinopathies. Consider Figure 6.11. The top section consists of patterns from subjects with known haemoglobin patterns—they, therefore, are the positive controls. The lower five samples are from patients with a suspected haemoglobinopathy. Study the patterns of these five samples, and compare them with the patterns of the positive controls. In this way you can determine the haemoglobin phenotype of the five patients.

6.3 Membrane and enzyme defects

The three principal causes of haemolytic anaemia relating to abnormalities in the red blood cell membrane are hereditary spherocytosis, hereditary elliptocytosis, and paroxysmal nocturnal haemoglobinuria. The principal enzyme defects are of glucose-6-phosphate dehydrogenase and pyruvate kinase. There are, of course, literally dozens of minor membrane and enzyme defects that also cause haemolysis.

Principal membrane defects

Hereditary spherocytosis (HS)

This is the most common hereditary haemolytic anaemia in North Europeans and is inherited in an autosomal-dominant manner, with variable clinical presentations ranging from a severe neonatal haemolytic anaemia to an asymptomatic state. Several mutations are known to cause HS. The link is that the particular gene defect affects the proteins involved in the vertical interaction between the skeleton membrane and lipid layer of the red cell (such as ankyrin, alpha- and beta-spectrins, Band 3, and protein 4.2). The relationships between these molecules is described in Chapter 4, where Fig. 4.4 is relevant. Notably, HS cells present increased Lu glycoprotein to laminin in blood vessel walls, thus promoting adhesion. The molecular basis of this may result from failure of the intra-cellular portion of Lu interacting with spectrin.

Part of the membrane that is not supported by skeleton is lost, causing the cells to lose sections of membrane and become more and more spherical. These abnormal red cells have a considerably reduced lifespan (between 6 and 20 days, compared to 120 days in health), and are unable to pass through the splenic microcirculation. Consequently, they are eliminated.

Clinical features include anaemia and jaundice. These features may be present at any age throughout the lifespan but can be compounded if associated with Gilbert's disease, a heritable enzyme defect associated with bilirubin metabolism. Patients with spherocytic anaemia benefit from splenectomy, which may increase their haemoglobin level to normal. Patients are further supported by folic acid supplement to avoid folate deficiency.

The full blood count from an HS patient can be expected to show an increased reticulocyte count (5–20%), low haemoglobin (for example, 70 g/L), reduced MCV, raised MCH, and raised MCHC (such as 360 g/L). The blood film shows dense microspherocytes, with no central pallor, as shown in Fig. 6.16. However, recall that spherocytes may also be present in other disease, such as AIHA (Figure 6.5). The laboratory can differentiate between these two manifestations of spherocytosis as the direct antiglobulin test will be positive in AIHA but negative in HS. Other special tests in HS include impaired spectrin phosphorylation and decreased red cell deformability due to membrane-bound calcium. Polyacrylamide gel electrophoresis of a preparation of red cell membranes will display an absence of particular spectrins.

Hereditary elliptocytosis (HE)

In its classical form, this red cell abnormality is most frequently found in Europeans and is inherited as an autosomal-dominant characteristic. On a blood film the phenotype shows a broad spectrum of abnormal red cell morphology, ranging from slightly oval cells to extreme elliptocytosis. Most patients do not have a haemolytic anaemia and there is no correlation between haemolysis and the degree of elliptocytosis. The underlining membrane abnormality is a deficiency of protein 4.1 leading to the failure of spectrin heterodimers to assemble into

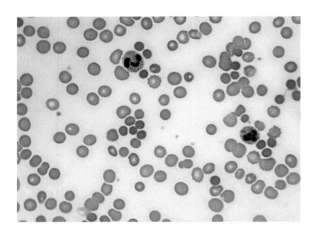

FIGURE 6.16

Hereditary spherocytosis. There is considerable variation in the sizes of the red cells in this film (anisocytosis), with many cells being small. These are not microcytes, but spherocytes, as they are well stained and so have a high component of haemoglobin. There are also two neutrophils, and a burr cell slightly below and to the right of the upper neutrophil. Note also the lack of schistocytes. (Magnification ×400.)

heterotetramers. However, the same elliptoid phenotype is also present in some defects of alpha-spectrin, beta-spectrin, and glycophorin C.

Most cases of elliptocytosis are heterozygous with no haemolysis, but a few cases of homozygous hereditary elliptocytosis present with a severe haemolytic anaemia. The full blood count may show a normal to slightly low haemoglobin, whilst the blood film may show typically that 80% of cells are oval, as are present in Figure 6.17. However, in cases where numbers are not large, an alternative diagnosis such as acquired elliptocytosis (such as that seen in iron deficiency) may be considered (Figure 6.18).

A variant of this disease is South-East Asian ovalocytosis, commonly found in Indonesia, the Philippines, and Malaysia, where the prevalence may be 30%. The abnormal red cell shape is caused by mutations that lead to errors in membrane component Band 3. This molecule is both a component of the cytoskeleton and also the chloride–bicarbonate anion exchanger.

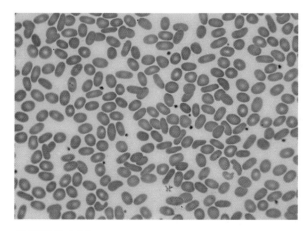

FIGURE 6.17

Hereditary elliptocytes. Well over half of the cells in this film are elliptical—hence elliptocytosis. (Magnification ×400.)

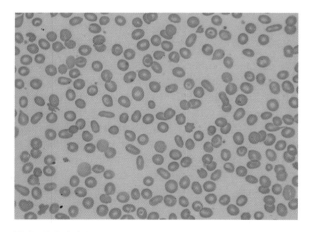

FIGURE 6.18

Iron deficiency with elliptocytes. There are many excellent examples of elliptocytes, but relatively few compared to Figure 6.17 in iron deficiency we tend to refer to these elliptocytes as pencil cells. Note also several target cells and microcytes, as may be expected in this condition. (Magnification ×400.)

As a consequence, the red cell is exceptionally rigid, a characteristic that is detected by cells of the reticuloendothelial system (as for HS cells), leading to their elimination, often in the spleen. Like many hereditary membrane, enzyme, and haemoglobin diseases, the high frequency in this part of the world may have arisen as a protection against malaria.

Tests of a weakened membrane

Perhaps the simplest and most physiological test of a weak membrane, such as that seen with HS and HE, is an increased osmotic fragility. Equal volumes of blood are added to a series of buffered hypotonic sodium chloride solutions, ranging from 0.1% to 0.9% (the latter being physiological). The suspensions are allowed to stand for 30 minutes at room temperature, during which time some cells (the weakest) will lyse. The degree of haemolysis in each test tube is recorded spectrophotometrically and is expressed as a percentage of haemolysis at each sodium chloride concentration when compared to the positive control (that is, distilled water). Interpretation relies on the marked increased fragility of the red cell population in HS and HE; the test can also be useful in other red cell diseases (Figure 6.19). Extension of the incubation test to 24 hours can also be useful in defining other pathologies.

In an alternative test, the acidified-glycerol lysis test, red cells are suspended in a slightly acidified phosphate-buffered sodium chloride–glycerol reagent and the time taken for 50% haemolysis to occur is measured. Interpretation relies on a shortened haemolysis time in HS compared to normal red cells. The cryohaemolysis test employs a similar principle—namely, to stress the cells and observe the result. The stress in this case is to warm the cells to 37 °C,

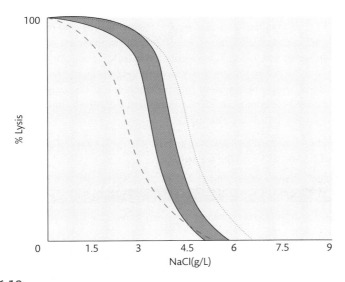

FIGURE 6.19
Osmotic fragility. Red blood cells are suspended in different concentrations of sodium chloride for 30 minutes at 37 °C, during which time the weakest will lyse in the most hypotonic saline solutions. The profile of normal red cells, and most enzymopathies, is present as the solid bar. Red cells in sickle cell disease, thalassaemia and iron deficiency show a left shift (dashed line), those from hereditary spherocytosis show a right shift (dotted line). In hereditary elliptocytosis the pattern is slightly right shifted. The figure is modified from *Dacie and Lewis*.

then to transfer them promptly to an ice bath for an additional incubation, at which point weakened cells, such as those from a patient with HS, will lyse.

The fluorescent probe eosin-5-maleimide binds to normal red cells, and may be detected by a flow cytometer, but does so less avidly if there are abnormalities in membrane components spectrin, protein 4.2, or Band 3. Consequently, the test may be useful in the diagnosis of HS and SE Asian ovalocytosis.

Paroxysmal nocturnal haemoglobinuria (PNH)

Paroxysmal nocturnal haemoglobinuria is caused by a rare acquired mutation in the *PIG-A* gene (present on the X-chromosome) in haemopoietic stem cells, leading to the defective synthesis of glycosyl phosphatidylinositol (GPI) on the cell surface. This molecule is an anchor that supports the integrity of several proteins, including two molecules, CD55 and CD59, which are important in resisting the activation of complement. As a consequence, the red cells become sensitive to complement-mediated intravascular haemolysis. The result of this sensitivity is the constant clinical feature of haemoglobinuria. This can give rise to iron deficiency, which may exacerbate the anaemia. Since CD55 and CD59 are also present on platelets and white cells, other clinical features include recurrent thrombosis of large veins, with intermittent abdominal pain. Thus laboratory findings include anaemia (ranging from mild to severe), leucopenia, and thrombophilia (for which anticoagulants (such as warfarin) may be required).

The typical full blood count from a patient with PNH demonstrates mildly reduced haemoglobin, with an increase in reticulocytes, mild leucopenia ($<2.5 \times 10^9$/L), and thrombocytopenia ($<50 \times 10^9$/L). Consequently, PNH should be excluded in patients with pancytopenia.

A number of diagnostic tests are available. The acidified-serum lysis test (Ham test) involves suspending red cells in normal serum which has been acidified to pH 6.5–7.0, followed by incubation at 37 °C, and subsequent examination for haemolysis. This red cell destruction will be induced by activation of the alternative pathway of complement activation. Similarly, for the sucrose haemolysis test, red cells are incubated in isotonic solutions of low ionic strength with a small amount of serum present in the mixture. Lysis is induced by activation of the classical pathway of the complement system. Interpretation of <5% haemolysis is inconsequential, 5–10% haemolysis is borderline, but >10% is consistent with PNH. For both these tests, good positive and negative controls are essential.

Diagnosis may be confirmed by flow cytometry, which relies on the absence of membrane components CD55 and CD59 on the cell surface.

Cross reference

The importance of CD55 and CD59 in the pathology of PNH is also described in Chapter 4. Flow cytometry and immunophenotyping are considered in detail in Chapter 10.

SELF-CHECK 6.9

How would you go about distinguishing between hereditary spherocytosis and hereditary elliptocytosis?

Other membrane defects

Hereditary stomatocytosis (HSt) describes several autosomal-dominant conditions where the transport of cations (notably sodium and potassium) is impaired. It is characterized on a blood film by stomatocytes, often with an oblong bar of central pallor. The lesion is generally due to abnormalities in membrane components, those of Band 3 being the most common. However, some cases of HS and South-East Asian (SEA) ovalocytosis also have defects in this molecule. Red cells are large and osmotically fragile with a low MCHC, which leads to a mild to moderate anaemia.

Hereditary pyropoikilocytosis is a rare autosomal-recessive disorder characterized on the blood film by microcytes and bizarre poikilocytes with marked red cell fragmentization (schistocytes). These cells, with a defect in alpha-spectrin, show exceptional heat sensitivity, and their spectrin cytoskeleton denatures at a lower temperature (45–46 °C) instead of the expected 49 °C.

Principal enzyme defects

G6PD deficiency

The enzyme glucose-6-phosphate dehydrogenase is responsible for removing hydrogen from its substrate, the metabolic intermediate glucose-6-phosphate, which becomes 6-phosphogluconate. The hydrogen is received by NADP, which becomes NADPH. In turn, NADPH passes the hydrogen to oxidized glutathione (abbreviated as GS⁻), which is con- verted to reduced glutathione (GSH). Reduced glutathione is a crucial antioxidant which counters the damaging and toxic effects of oxygen within the red cell by effectively neu- tralizing or quenching it with the hydrogen. This short metabolic pathway is illustrated in Figure 6.20.

In patients with G6PD deficiency, the hydrogen is unavailable to regenerate levels of GSH, which subsequently decrease, leading to a fall in the antioxidant capacity of red cells. The practical consequences are that the red cells are more susceptible to oxidant stress leading to increased levels of methaemoglobin, damage to the membrane, and ultimately to haemolysis.

The gene for G6PD is found on the X-chromosome and so the inheritance is sex-linked. The condition affects up to 1% of the world's population, but is considerably higher (13%) in those of West African descent. The gene has a number of isoforms, some of which are loss-of-function mutations, leading to G6PD deficiency. This condition shows marked clinical heterogeneity, with symptoms including sensitivity to different drugs. The most common consequence of G6PD deficiency is drug-induced haemolysis.

The oxidant drugs that can cause haemolysis include antimalarials (such as primaquine), anti- biotics (chloramphenicol), analgesics (aspirin), and antihelminths (nitrodazole). The ingestion of fava beans also precipitates acute crises of haemolytic anaemia, with haematuria and pain. In contrast to these acute crises, in 'steady state' G6PD deficiency there is chronic haemolytic anaemia and therefore jaundice. Treatment for G6PD deficiency is to treat the cause: avoid- ance of the precipitating factor(s) (stopping the ingestion of fava beans and agents that pro- mote haemolysis), resolution of an infection, and in severe cases, the consideration of a blood transfusion. There is no replacement therapy.

In the absence of haemolytic crisis, the FBC is normal, although during acute intravascular exacerbations, the blood film demonstrates features of haemolysis, such as red cell ghosts (without haemoglobin—'bite' and 'blister' cells) and polychromasia. Heinz bodies (haemoglo- bin denatured by the high levels of oxidants) may be seen in reticulocytes.

Commercial screening and assay kits are available for the assessment of G6PD deficiency, and these tests are based on the measurement of the levels of NADPH. In the presence of G6PD, NADP is reduced to NADPH, which fluoresces under long-wave ultraviolet light. Specimens from normal healthy individuals fluoresce brightly, indicating a normal G6PD activity. However, specimens from G6PD-deficient samples show reduced or no fluorescence. Intermediate degrees of fluorescence indicate a specimen from heterozygotes, or patients with a mild G6PD variant. Reticulocyte cells demonstrate higher G6PD activity.

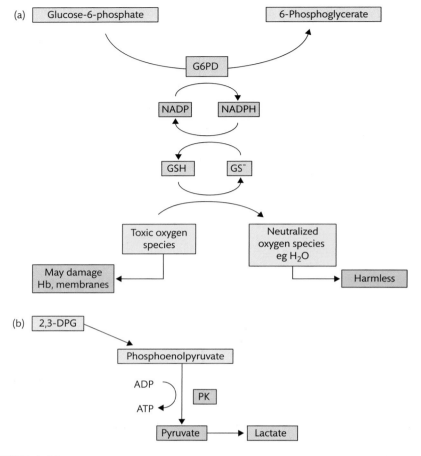

FIGURE 6.20

Biochemical pathways Illustrating the effects of glucose-6-phosphate dehydrogenase (G6PD) deficiency and pyruvate kinase (PK) deficiency. The upper panel shows the role of G6PD in generating NADPH from NADP and its substrate, glucose-6-phosphate. Lack of the enzyme, i.e. G6PD deficiency, leads to failure to generate NADPH, and so failure to reduce GS– to GSH. Hence no GSH is available to defend against toxic oxygen species, leading to cell and molecular damage. The lower panel shows how PK is required to mediate the transfer of a phosphate group from phosphoenolpyruvate (PEP) to ADP, thus generating ATP and pyruvate. However, note that PEP is itself derived from 2,3-DPG. Thus once the metabolic processes involving PEP are saturated, then levels of 2,3-DPG are likely to rise.

Pyruvate kinase (PK) deficiency

Pyruvate kinase (PK) participates in the generation of ATP by transferring a phosphate group from the metabolic intermediate phosphoenolpyruvate to ADP. Consequently, a lack of activity of this enzyme leads to reduced intracellular ATP, this failure most likely being due to a loss-of-function mutation in the relevant gene. Deficiency of pyruvate kinase is inherited in an autosomal-recessive manner, and is the most common enzyme deficiency in the Embden–Meyerhof pathway. Reduced levels of ATP lead to a mild to moderate chronic non-spherocytic haemolytic anaemia (haemoglobin is typically 40–100 g/L) with spleno-megaly and an increased reticulocyte count. The blood film shows poikilocytes, and a reticu-locytosis is common. Reduced red cell survival and chronic haemolysis result in increased iron turnover—increased ferritin is found in 60% of untransfused PK-deficient patients and there is low hepcidin, which correlates with haemoglobin.

A further consequence of PK deficiency is that—as the substrate phosphoenolpyruvate is not consumed—levels rise, and, in turn, cause a rise in levels of another metabolite in the meta-bolic pathway, 2,3-diphosphoglycerate (2,3-DPG). In Chapter 4 we discussed the importance of this molecule in the movement of oxygen in and out of the red cell in the lungs and in the tissues. Thus, in PK deficiency, high levels of 2,3-DPG shift the oxygen dissociation curve to the right, which effectively reduces the clinical symptoms of anaemia in comparison to the haemoglobin concentration.

The laboratory confirmation of PK deficiency relies on the ability of PK to convert its substrate (phosphoenolpyruvate) to its products, pyruvate and ATP, in the presence of ADP. Lactate dehydrogenase (LDH) catalyses the reduction of pyruvate to lactate with the oxidation of NADH to NAD; this reaction can be monitored by measuring the change in fluorescence at 340 nm. Specimens from healthy individuals demonstrate reduced or no fluorescence. In con-trast, PK-deficient samples show bright fluorescence.

The PK pathway is shown in Figure 6.20, whilst Table 6.5 summarizes the pathology and labo-ratory aspects of membrane and enzyme defects.

Key Points

The small number of well characterized membrane and enzyme defects provide the haematologist with an excellent opportunity to link a gene defect with a cellular abnor-mality and thus a clinical syndrome.

TABLE 6.5 Common membrane and enzyme defects leading to haemolysis.

Condition	Nature of the pathology
Hereditary spherocytosis	Defects in the internal cytoskeleton leading to abnormal cell shape
Hereditary elliptocytosis	Defects in the internal cytoskeleton leading to abnormal cell shape
Paroxysmal nocturnal haemoglobinuria	Failure to anchor key protective molecules to the cell membrane
Glucose-6-phosphate dehydrogenase deficiency	Poor regeneration of reduced glutathione results in increased oxidant activity
Pyruvate kinase deficiency	Reduced ability to generate ATP

6.4 **Erythrocytosis and polycythaemia**

We complete these two chapters on the pathology of red blood cells with an examination of polycythaemia and erythrocytosis. In contrast to the pathologies in the previous chapter and elsewhere in this chapter, where we considered low levels of haemoglobin and low numbers of red cells, here we look at *high* levels of haemoglobin and *raised* numbers of red cells. Both these conditions are characterized by an increase in the total red cell mass of the body, and also a high haematocrit. However, recall that the haematocrit is in fact the mathematic product of the red cell count and the MCV, so that inaccuracies may be present and could confuse the diagnosis. An increased red cell mass brings hyperviscosity, and so a stress on the heart and cardiovascular system, which may precipitate a stroke.

Cross reference

Red cell mass is discussed in detail in Chapter 11.

Erythrocytosis and polycythaemia, and their consequences, are the product of very dissimilar pathologies. Although the naming of particular processes, diseases, and conditions seems, to many students, to be a mystery, there is in fact logic in the system which can be decoded by breaking down the formal name into its constituent parts, as we saw earlier in this chapter. For example, erythrocytosis describes the number of red blood cells (erythrocytes) being raised in the blood (-osis). (Similarly, recall that leucocytosis means white blood cells (leucocyt-) being raised in the blood (-osis).) By contrast, polycythaemia means an increase (poly-) in cells (-cyth-) in the blood (-aemia)—it does not specify which cells are increased, but is taken to be all blood cells. The aetiology of this could be primary, whereby a genetic mutation in the bone marrow promotes erythropoiesis without an increase in physiological demand.

Erythrocytosis

At the simplest level, erythrocytosis is defined by a red cell count being above the top of the reference range. It follows that haemoglobin and haematocrit are also likely to be increased. Indeed, one guideline suggests a haematocrit >0.52 in males and >0.48 in females, which must be present for at least two months for erythrocytosis to be confirmed. The World Health Organization focuses on a haemoglobin >185 g/L in males and >165 g/L in females. An additional test is to estimate the total mass of red cells within the body.

Pathology

There are a number of possible reasons for erythrocytosis, and we can focus on four such causes. The most simple (Type 1) is a reduction in the volume of plasma, as may be present in dehydration. If this is the case, the root pathology lies elsewhere, perhaps as the consequence of renal failure. If so, the condition is not primarily of haematology. The term 'relative erythrocytosis' should be reserved for this pathology. Alternatively, 'apparent erythrocytosis' (Type 2) is applicable in those whose red cell mass is within the reference range but who have an increased haematocrit. Furthermore, 'idiopathic erythrocytosis' (Type 3) describes the situation in which no clear mechanism can be identified.

Cases of the fourth type of erythrocytosis, absolute erythrocytosis, can be classified as being congenital or acquired (Types 4A, B, and C). A principal cause of Type 4A erythrocytosis is an abnormal haemoglobin (such as those with a high affinity for oxygen), or in cases of congenitally low levels of 2,3-DPG. However, most causes of Type 4 erythrocytosis are acquired and are generally reactive to a state of hypoxia. Table 6.6 summarizes this classification system.

TABLE 6.6 Erythrocytosis and polycythaemia.

Erythrocytosis (an isolated increase in red cells)	Type 1: relative (e.g. due to dehydration)
	Type 2: apparent (raised haematocrit but normal red cell mass)
	Type 3: idiopathic (no clear cause)
	Type 4: absolute
	A: congenital: e.g. high–affinity haemoglobin, 2,3-DPG abnormality, erythropoietin receptor abnormality, Chuvash polycythaemia
	B: acquired, as a secondary response to hypoxia, e.g. due to chronic obstructive pulmonary disease, severe cyanosis, cyanotic heart disease, renal disease, altitude
	C: acquired: as a secondary change due to pathology in a particular organ, e.g. erythropoietin production by a tumour
Polycythaemia vera (increased red cells, but also increased platelets and/or leucocytes)	*JAK2 V617F* mutation positive, giving a 95% likelihood of polycythaemia vera
	JAK2 V617F mutation negative: other mutations and/or causes possible

One of the functions of the kidney is to sense levels of oxygen. When such hypoxia occurs, the kidney will increase its release of erythropoietin to stimulate the bone marrow to produce more red cells. Peripheral hypoxia can be assessed by measuring the arterial oxygen saturation, most easily achieved with a pulse oximeter. However, this technique can also give misleading results. Another cause of hypoxia causing Type 4 erythrocytosis may be lung pathology such as congestive obstructive pulmonary disease (COPD). Erythrocytosis may also arise from cyanotic congenital heart disease.

Although not strictly a pathology, the erythrocytosis of high altitude (as may be found in the Andes and Himalayas) is inductive. The increased red cell count and other indices are a required physiological response to the atmospheric hypoxia, and are therefore entirely normal in this setting. When the subject descends to sea level, the erythrocytosis (as it is at 'normal' atmospheric oxygen levels) is an unnecessary burden and slowly resolves. It follows that those unaccustomed to high altitude need weeks of acclimatization to allow their bone marrow to generate a high red cell mass, and is the basis of altitude training by athletes. Type 4C erythrocytosis is most frequently caused by pathological generation of erythropoietin as may be present in certain renal neoplasias.

The laboratory in erythrocytosis

In addition to changes in red cell indices (raised haemoglobin, red cell count, haematocrit), there is also likely to be a neutrophilia and a thrombocytosis (for reasons which are unclear). However, smokers may have a neutrophil leucocytosis, possibly the result of chronic pulmonary inflammation. Bone marrow examination is rarely required but may be called on to exclude polycythaemia. Estimation of red cell mass requires the use of radioisotopes and is therefore reserved for specialist centres. However, estimation of erythropoietin is probably the most useful diagnostic tool, and although levels are typically raised in erythrocytosis secondary to hypoxia, they may also be increased in polycythaemias of various aetiologies.

Management of erythrocytosis

The first step in the management of erythrocytosis is to identify and treat, where possible, contributing factors such as smoking, alcohol, and treatments of hypertension that are based on fluid elimination by diuretics. The standard treatment is venepuncture to reduce the red cell mass, and is generally considered if the haematocrit exceeds 0.54. Patients having had a thrombosis, or who are deemed to be at risk (perhaps by virtue of thrombocytosis and/or hyperviscosity) may require anticoagulation. In this high-risk group, venesection may be called for at a lower haematocrit, such as 0.45, especially in the presence of diabetes or hypertension.

Polycythaemia

The aetiology of this disease is completely different from that of erythrocytosis, in that it is primarily the consequence of molecular changes in the genes involved in responses to hypoxia. The disease also extends from red cells to other blood cells and can transform into myelofibrosis, essential thrombocythaemia or acute myeloid leukaemia.

Pathology

The key to a diagnosis of polycythaemia is the relationship between erythropoietin and its receptor (the EpoR), which activates a cytoplasmic protein tyrosine kinase. This intermediate, named Janus kinase 2 (JAK2), in turn activates other intracellular messengers, which ultimately results in the transcription of various genes within the nucleus of the erythroid precursor (such as the erythroblast). Therefore failure of this system, whether through lack of erythropoietin or through a loss-of-function mutation in the *EpoR* gene, will result in a failure to stimulate the erythroblast, resulting in falling red cell numbers. JAK2 is also allied to the thrombopoietin receptor messenger pathway, suggesting a link with platelets and so thrombosis. Interestingly, *JAK1* mutations are present in 18% of certain leukaemias.

However, the most important mutation in the *JAK2* gene (*JAK2 V617F*) confers on erythroblasts an increased sensitivity to erythropoietin and so an overactivity that results in erythrocytosis.

Cross reference

Polycythaemia is discussed in detail in Chapter 11.

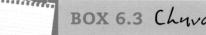

BOX 6.3 *Chuvash polycythaemia*

This condition is an interesting endemic congenital polycythaemia, which is present in an ethnically homogenous population of a part of Russia. Although described in the literature as polycythaemia, almost all the pathology is based on the red cell, so it should really be described as an erythrocytosis. The disease results from a mutation in the von Hippel–Lindau tumour suppressor gene (*VHL598C-T*) and its protein product, which effectively fails to switch off a hypoxia-sensing mechanism. Consequently, the cell continues to behave as if hypoxia is present. This ultimately results in high levels of erythropoietin (up to ten times the normal level) and so a raised haemoglobin of perhaps 180 g/L. Interestingly, the levels of ferritin and soluble transferrin receptor are also elevated, and the frequency of varicose veins (which would seem to be the product of venous congestion) and thrombosis is also increased. The mutation is found very rarely outside this ethnic group.

Furthermore, this condition can develop into a full-blown, multi-cell lineage pancytosis with increased platelets (thrombocythaemia) and leucocytes. Accordingly, this disease is described as polycythaemia vera (where 'vera' derives from 'true'). *JAK2 V617F* also results in the increased phosphorylation and expression of red cell membrane Lu that increases red cell adhesiveness. This may be, in part, related to the increased frequency of thrombosis in polycythaemia vera.

The laboratory in polycythaemia

Proposed criteria for the diagnosis of polycythaemia vera include raised red cell mass, or a haematocrit greater than 0.60 in males and 0.56 in females; the absence of a firm alternative cause of secondary erythrocytosis; thrombocytosis (platelets $>400 \times 10^9$/L); and a neutrophil leucocytosis (neutrophils $>10 \times 10^9$/L in non-smokers, $>12.5 \times 10^9$/L in smokers). Low serum ferritin and raised vitamin B_{12} may also be found, the latter possibly reflecting transcobalamine release from an increased granulocyte mass. As with erythrocytosis, the primary specific laboratory test is for levels of erythropoietin.

A regional molecular laboratory is likely to be able to offer advice on identification of the *JAK2 V617F* mutation, and the presence of this mutation considerably influences the diagnosis. Bone marrow examination is not crucial in simple unequivocal polycythaemia, but may be necessary to determine transformation to a more severe multi-lineage disease. It may also serve as a baseline for subsequent investigations, and an aspirate is expected to demonstrate marked erythroid hyperplasia with mild to moderate hyperplasia of granulocyte precursors and megakaryocytes. Iron stores are likely to be low or absent. Cytogenetic abnormalities (such as trisomy of chromosomes 8 and 9) are found in 10–20% of patients and are a strong risk factor for progression to acute leukaemia.

Management of polycythaemia

As presenting signs include thrombosis, haemorrhage, and splenomegaly, the aims of treatment include reducing the risk of these events, such as is possible through the use of aspirin. Polycythaemia vera describes a clinical sign—the ruddy complexion which is a likely consequence of the high red cell mass. Venesection will reduce the red cell mass (as monitored by the haematocrit, aiming at less than 0.45) and therefore reduce the risk of cardiovascular complications, but will not alleviate the root cause of the disease. Accordingly, bone marrow suppression with radiotherapy, radioactive phosphorus, and chemotherapy (principally anagrelide, busulphan, chlorambucil, hydroxycarbamide, and interferon) is advocated. Figure 6.21 shows an algorithm using levels of erythropoietin to drive diagnosis, whilst Table 6.6 summarizes erythrocytosis and polycythaemia.

SELF-CHECK 6.10

What are the principal differences between erythrocytosis and polycythaemia?

Key Points

Despite a commonality in increased numbers of red blood cells, there are fundamental differences between erythrocytosis and polycythaemia. These include aetiology, laboratory findings, and prognosis.

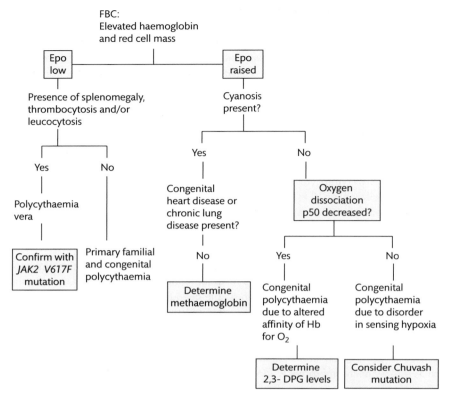

FIGURE 6.21

Role of the laboratory in erythrocytosis and polycythaemia. This figure provides a possible algorithm for the investigation of erythrocytosis and polycythaemia. An initial full blood count is likely to report a raised haemoglobin (and perhaps other indices such as Hct), and, using other methods, an increased red cell mass may be noted. The first step will be measurement of erythropoietin (Epo). Low levels (left hand side) are followed up with a physical examination for an enlarged spleen, and in the full blood count for raised platelets and white blood cells. If present, polycythaemia may be confirmed by the presence of the JAK2 V617F mutation.

Alternatively, on the right hand side, if Epo is raised, the presence or absence of cyanosis drives further investigation. If present, it may be due to heart and/or lung disease, and may trigger the determination of methaemoglobin. In the absence of cyanosis, alteration in the oxygen dissociation curve will trigger additional investigations, such as for levels of 2,3-DPG or the presence of the Chuvash mutation. Figure modified from Gordeuk _et al_.

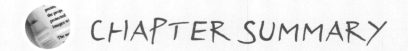 CHAPTER SUMMARY

We complete our study of diseases of low levels and numbers of red cell indices (when due to haemolysis), and examine the two conditions where increased numbers of red cells are present.

Low levels and numbers of the red cell indices:

■ Antibody-mediated haemolytic anaemia may be classified as being caused by autoanti-bodies or alloantibodies.

■ External causes of haemolytic anaemia include drugs and mechanical processes.

■ The principal haemoglobinopathy conditions are sickle cell disease and thalassaemia.

■ Defects in the red cell membrane, as in hereditary spherocytosis, hereditary elliptocytosis, and PNH all cause haemolysis.

■ The principal enzyme defects leading to haemolysis are G6PD deficiency and PK deficiency.

High levels and numbers of the red cell indices:

■ Erythrocytosis describes an increase in the number of red cells, the haematocrit, and haemoglobin.

■ In polycythaemia, there is also a rise in red cell indices, but in addition there are raised platelets and/or white cells and a risk of malignancy.

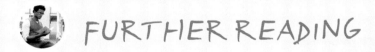

FURTHER READING

● Ataga KI, Cappellini MD, Rachmilewitz EA. Beta thalassaemia and sickle cell anaemia as paradigms of hypercoagulability. *British Journal of Haematology* 2007:**139**;3–13.

● Beutler E. Glucose-6-phosphatase deficiency: a historical perspective. *Blood* 2008:**111**;16–24.

● Flatt JF, Bruce LJ. The hereditary stomatocytoses. *Haematologica* 2009:**94**;1039–41.

● Gordeuk VR, Stockton DW, Prchal JT. Congenital polycythaemias/erythrocytosis. *Haematologica* 2005:**90**;109–16.

● Hankins J, Aygun B. Pharmacotherapy in sickle cell disease—state of the art and future prospects. *British Journal of Haematology* 2009:**145**;296–308.

● Lewis SM, Bain BJ, Bates I (ed). *Dacie and Lewis—Practical Haematology*, 9th edn. Churchill Livingstone, London, 2001.

● McMullin MF, Bareford D, Campbell P, *et al*. Guidelines for the diagnosis, investigation and management of polycythaemia/erythrocytosis. *British Journal of Haematology* 2005:**130**;174–95. (Amendment 2007:**138**;812–13.)

● Packman CH. Hemolytic anemia due to warm autoantibodies. *Blood Reviews* 2008:**22**;17–31.

● Parker C, Omine M, Richards S, *et al*. Diagnosis and management of paroxysmal nocturnal haemoglobinuria. *Blood* 2005:**106**;3699–709.

● Spivak JL, Silver RT. The revised World Health Organization diagnostic criteria for polycythaemia vera, essential thrombocytosis, and primary myelofibrosis: an alternative proposal. *Blood* 2008:**112**;231–9.

Answers to self-check questions, case study questions, and discussion questions are provided in the book's Online Resource Centre, visit www.oxfordtextbooks.co.uk/orc/moore

7

Blood-borne parasites

Gary W. Moore

In this chapter you will be introduced to the major blood-borne parasites and their life cycles. You will see how morphological characteristics are important for accurate diagnosis and meet other laboratory tests available to biomedical scientists for the detection of blood parasites.

Learning objective

After studying this chapter you should confidently be able to:

- Name the main blood-borne parasites that cause disease in humans.
- Understand parasite life cycles.
- Appreciate the importance of the recognition of parasite morphology.
- Describe the appearances of parasites in Romanowsky-stained blood films.
- Describe additional laboratory tests for parasite detection.

7.1 Introduction

symbiosis
Close interaction between different species.

endoparasite
A parasite that lives within the body of the host.

ectoparasite
A parasite that lives on the body of the host.

Cross reference

Eosinophilia in response to certain parasitic infections is discussed in further detail in Chapter 8.

Parasitism is a form of **symbiosis** where the parasitic organism benefits from the association to the detriment of the host organism. The other forms of symbiosis are mutualism, where both organisms benefit, and commensalism, where one organism benefits but the other is unaffected.

The main types of **endoparasite** organisms that affect humans are protozoa and helminth worms. Although they commonly infect the intestines, they also infect other sites such as the blood, brain, eyes, liver, and kidneys. In this chapter we will be concerned only with parasites that have life cycle stages detectable in peripheral blood. Biomedical scientists play a crucial role in the detection and identification of blood-borne parasites, which is integral to their practice of assessing stained peripheral blood films for morphological abnormalities. Arthropods such as head lice and scabies mites are **ectoparasites**; the most likely haematological effect of infection with these parasites is eosinophilia.

Like many parasites, blood-borne parasites target specific organs and species for different stages of their life cycles. The nature of each life cycle and the target organs involved dictate the clinical symptoms of each infection. The main blood-borne parasitic organisms of humans and the resultant diseases are outlined in Table 7.1.

TABLE 7.1 Blood-borne human endoparasites.

Phylum	Species	Resultant disease
Protozoa	*Plasmodium falciparum* *Plasmodium vivax* *Plasmodium malariae* *Plasmodium ovale* *(Plasmodium knowlesi)*	Malaria
	Babesia bovis *Babesia microti* *Babesia divergens*	Babesiosis
	Trypanosoma brucei gambiense *Trypanosoma brucei rhodesiense*	African trypanosomiasis (sleeping sickness)
	Trypanosoma cruzi	American trypanosomiasis (Chagas disease)
	Leishmania donovani *Leishmania infantum*	Leishmaniasis (Kala-azar)
Nematoda	*Wucheria bancrofti* *Brugia malayi* *Brugia timori*	Lymphatic filariasis
	Loa loa	Loa loa filariasis
	Mansonella perstans *Mansonella ozzardi*	Mostly asymptomatic

7.2 Malaria

Malaria is a serious and sometimes fatal vector-borne infectious disease, the vector being mosquitoes. Rarely, malaria infection occurs through transfusion of parasitized blood, transplantation of infected bone marrow, or by placental transmission (congenital malaria). It is widespread in tropical and subtropical areas, including areas of Africa, Asia, and the Americas. Between 300 and 500 million cases of malaria are diagnosed every year, of which between 1 and 3 million will die from the disease. The majority of deaths are of young children in Sub-Saharan Africa.

There are four species of protozoa from the *Plasmodium* genus which cause malaria in humans: *P. falciparum*, *P. vivax*, *P. malariae*, and *P. ovale*. A fifth species, *P. knowlesi*, predominantly causes fatal malaria in long-tailed macaques (*Macaca fascicularis*) but has been known to infect humans. Infection by *P. falciparum* accounts for approximately 80% of all cases. *P. falciparum* malaria is more severe than the other forms and is the cause of 90% of deaths from this disease.

Key Points

Only female mosquitoes of the *Anopheles* genus can act as vectors to transmit malarial parasites to humans. There are more than 450 known species of *Anopheles* mosquitoes, of which approximately 100 can transmit malaria to humans. *Anopheles gambiae* is the best known because of its significant role in the transmittance of *P. falciparum*.

Life cycle of malarial parasites

When taking a blood meal from a human, an infected anopheles mosquito injects thousands of motile, spindle-shaped cells called **sporozoites** into the circulation. The life cycle is illustrated in Figure 7.1. The sporozoites are the stage of the parasite life cycle resulting from sexual reproduction in the midgut of the mosquito. The sporozoites infect the blood for a maximum of a few hours before they migrate to the liver. Those that are not destroyed by phagocytes infect the parenchymal cells of the liver (hepatocytes). The sporozoites divide and mature into **schizonts** by an asexual reproductive process of multiple fission called 'pre-erythrocytic **schizogony**'.

Over the next 1–2 weeks multiplication occurs inside each schizont such that each will contain thousands of the next phase of the life cycle, the **merozoite**, which consists of a single nucleus and a narrow ring of cytoplasm. The merozoites exit the hepatocytes contained within structures called **merosomes**, which consist of hundreds of merozoites encased in host membrane. Inside the merosome, the merozoites are protected from phagocytic attack. The merosomes travel to the lungs where they lodge in pulmonary capillaries and the membranes disintegrate over the next 4–6 days. This liberates parasites into the bloodstream where they begin the process of erythrocyte invasion by attaching to specific receptors on red cell membranes:

- *P. falciparum* binds to glycophorins A, B, and C.
- *P. vivax* and *P. knowlesi* bind to the Duffy antigen.
- The receptors for *P. malariae* and *P. ovale* are unknown.

Merozoites initially attach to red cells via any point on the merozoite surface, a process involving their surface-coat filaments. You can see in Figure 7.2 that the merozoite then reorientates to bring its apical pole into direct contact with the red cell membrane. Remarkably, the red cell membrane itself cooperates in this reorientation by partially 'wrapping round' the merozoite to facilitate the re-positioning.

Once orientated, a closer membrane-to-membrane adhesion forms between the two cells, which is called a tight junction. At this point, a slight indentation in the red cell membrane appears, into which the apical cone of the merozoite is inserted. Unlike the initial membrane contacts, this adhesion is irreversible and the merozoite is now committed to entering this red cell.

A series of molecular events then occur in order for the merozoite to gain entry into the red cell. The adhesion zone around the tight junction moves to cover the entire merozoite surface

BOX 7.1 *Dormant malaria*

In *P. vivax* and *P. ovale* some sporozoites differentiate into **hypnozoites** as well as **merozoites**. Hypnozoites can remain dormant in hepatocytes for up to 30 years. Once 'reactivated' (by an, as yet, undetermined mechanism), they grow and undergo exo-erythrocytic schizogony to generate a wave of merozoites that invade the blood and produce a clinical relapse. Recent reports have suggested that *P. falciparum* and *P. malariae* may occasionally have a dormant stage.

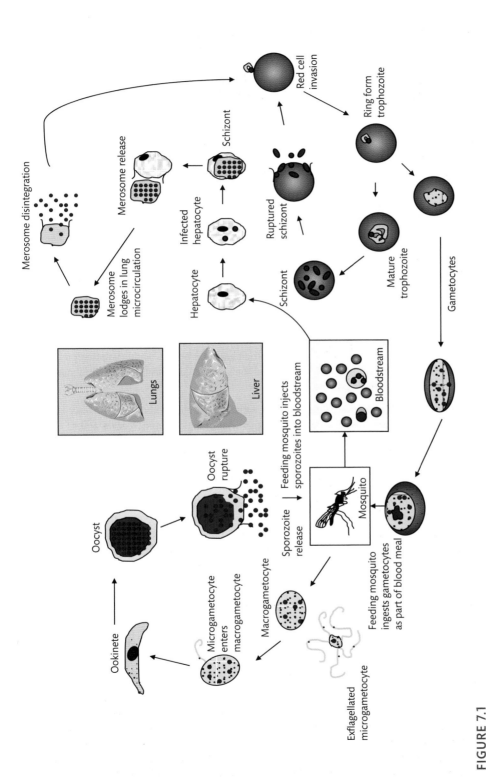

FIGURE 7.1

Life cycle of malarial parasites. An infected mosquito injects sporozoites into the bloodstream of the human host. The sporozoites migrate to the liver and invade hepatocytes whereupon they enter shizogony and multiply to form merozoites. The merozoites exit the hepatocytes encased in a merosome which travels to the lungs and lodges in the lung microcirculation. The merosome membrane disintegrates, liberating merozoites to invade host red blood cells and progress through the trophozoite stages and then enter schizogony. Rupture of the schizont releases merozoites which infect further red cells. Some trophozoites transform into gametocytes which are ingested by another mosquito when it feeds on the infected human host. The microgametocytes exflagellate and then fertilize the macrogametocytes to form the ookinete which embeds in the gut wall and develops into an oocyst. Multiple cell divisions occur in the oocyst to generate sporozoites which are released from the oocyst to travel to the mosquito's salivary glands and are injected into another human host to perpetuate the life cycle.

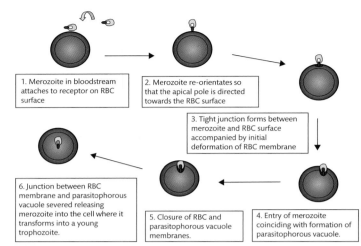

FIGURE 7.2

Red cell invasion by a malarial merozoite.

1. Merozoite in bloodstream attaches to receptor on RBC surface

2. Merozoite re-orientates so that the apical pole is directed towards the RBC surface

3. Tight junction forms between merozoite and RBC surface accompanied by initial deformation of RBC membrane

4. Entry of merozoite coinciding with formation of parasitophorous vacuole.

5. Closure of RBC and parasitophorous vacuole membranes.

6. Junction between RBC membrane and parasitophorous vacuole severed releasing merozoite into the cell where it transforms into a young trophozoite.

so facilitating its entry into the red cell. Merozoites contain an organelle called the **rhoptry**. The contents of the rhoptries are released to interact with inner membrane red cell lipids. Local alteration of the red cell membrane architecture follows which produces an invagination to create the **parasitophorous vacuole membrane** (PVM). You can see in Figure 7.2 that the PVM then surrounds the merozoite to form the **parasitophorous vacuole** (PV) which remains attached to the red cell membrane via the junction at the posterior end of the PV. The red cell membrane and PVM close and the parasite is now locked inside the red cell. The junction then fuses with the PVM and severs the connection with the red cell membrane so that the parasite is free inside the red cell.

Dense bodies inside the merozoite then fuse with the plasma membrane of the merozoite and release their contents into the PV, which triggers flattening of the merozoite and its transformation into the next stage of the life cycle, the **trophozoite**. The trophozoites are the feeding stage of the life cycle and ingest haemoglobin and other contents of the red cell cytoplasm. Plasmepsin enzymes degrade up to 80% of the haemoglobin in the red cell, but the parasite only uses about 15% of the amino acids derived from this digestion for protein synthesis. The parasites create new transport pathways to export the excess amino acids from the red cell to prevent rupture of the red cell and thus death of the parasites before they are sufficiently mature to enter the next stage of the life cycle. Digestion of the haemoglobin generates a characteristic brown pigment called **haemozoin** which accumulates as the parasites mature.

On Romanowsky-stained blood films, young trophozoites appear inside red cells as characteristic ring forms with a chromatin dot, which you can see in Figure 7.3. They develop into large trophozoites whose cytoplasm has a more amorphous amoeboid shape (Figure 7.4).

Most large trophozoites undergo multiplication by erythrocytic schizogony to form schizonts containing merozoites. When mature, the schizonts rupture and break open the red cell to

haemozoin

Product of haemoglobin digestion by malarial parasites comprising polymerised insoluble haem residues.

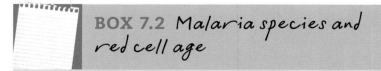

BOX 7.2 *Malaria species and red cell age*

P. vivax and *P. ovale* are commonly found in young or immature red cells. *P. malariae* tends to be found in ageing red cells, whilst *P. falciparum* is non-specific.

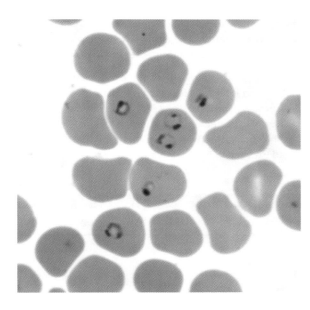

FIGURE 7.3
Ring-form trophozoites of
P. falciparum on a Giemsa-stained
thin film (×500 magnification).

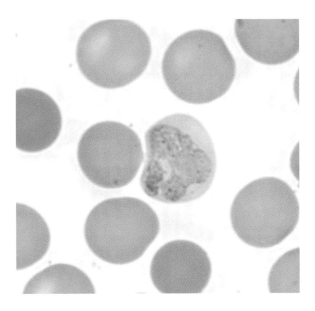

FIGURE 7.4
Large trophozoite of *P. vivax* on
a Giemsa-stained thin film
(×500 magnification).

release the merozoites, which then infect further red cells to perpetuate the erythrocytic cycle. The release of merozoites from red cells tends to be synchronized and is responsible for the cyclical nature of fevers associated with malarial infections. The period between fevers varies between species and is usually in the region of 2–3 days.

After several generations, some of the trophozoites develop into male **microgametocytes** or female **macrogametocytes**, which are typically oval or banana-shaped. You can see gametocytes in stained blood films in Figure 7.5. If the infected human is then bitten again by a mosquito vector, it takes up gametocytes in its blood meal which travel to the mosquito's stomach to undergo the sporogenic or sexual phase of the life cycle. Within 20 minutes of

zygote

Derived from the Greek for 'joined', it is the unicellular product of joining male and female genetic material—the product of fertilization.

arriving in the stomach, the alteration in pH stimulates the microgametocytes to extend up to eight slender flagella in a process called **exflagellation**. The exflagellated microgametocytes then fertilize the macrogametocytes to form elongated motile **zygotes** called **ookinetes**.

The ookinetes that survive the immune response penetrate and escape the midgut and then embed themselves in the gut wall close to the exterior. A few even migrate onto the surface. Once embedded, they develop into **oocysts**, which are the spore phase of the life cycle. Multiple cell divisions occur in the oocysts to generate large numbers of small, elongated **sporozoites**. Oocyst rupture releases the sporozoites which migrate to the mosquito's salivary glands where they are injected into the human host at the mosquito's next meal to perpetuate the life cycle.

SELF-CHECK 7.2

Outline the malarial parasite life cycle.

BOX 7.3 *Artefactual finding of exflagellated microgametocytes in blood*

Exflagellated microgametocytes are usually only found within the mosquito and are not seen in blood films made from fresh non-anticoagulated blood. However, if the blood sample is exposed to air for several minutes the pH rises as the CO_2 level falls to equilibrate with the surrounding air and *in vitro* exflagellation can occur. Blood samples collected into EDTA that are left unstoppered and unmixed can attain a high enough pH to precipitate exflagellation. Although it is of no clinical significance to find exflagellated microgametocytes in peripheral blood there is the possibility that they could be mistaken for other flagellated parasites such as *Trypanosoma cruzi*.

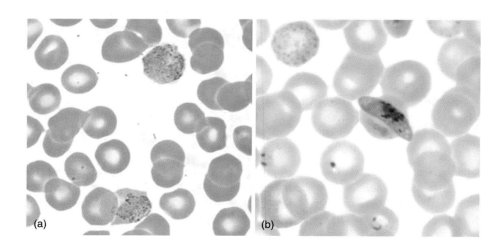

FIGURE 7.5

Gametocytes of *P. vivax* and *P. falciparum* (Giemsa-stained thin films; x500 magnification). (a) Gametocytes of *P. vivax*, (b) Gametocyte of *P. falciparum*.

(a)   (b)

Clinical features of malaria infection

The incubation period between the time of initial infection by a mosquito bite and the appearance of clinical symptoms and appearance of parasites in the peripheral blood varies between species. This is due to differences in the length of the erythrocytic and pre- and exo-erythrocytic cycles and the degree of **parasitaemia**. The typical incubation period for *P. falciparum* is 7–14 days, *P. vivax* and *P. ovale* 12–17 days and *P. malariae* 18–40 days.

The symptoms of malaria infection are not always severe and dramatic and are easily dismissed as relatively trivial. However, if the infection is not treated, sudden and drastic deterioration can occur as the parasites rapidly invade the bloodstream. Common symptoms are:

parasitaemia
Quantitation of the number of parasitized red blood cells (normally expressed as a percentage).

- Influenza-like symptoms including fever and sweating
- Headache
- Weakness
- Dizziness
- Nausea and vomiting
- Anaemia

The only species associated with complicated and severe disease is *P. falciparum* which can induce additional symptoms, such as:

- Neurological signs—delirium, coma, convulsions, focal signs
- Intense muscle spasms
- Oliguria (low urine output), renal failure
- Pulmonary oedema (fluid on the lungs), laboured breathing, cough
- Jaundice, liver failure
- Hypoglycaemia
- Diarrhoea
- Circulatory collapse

The first-line prophylaxis and treatment for malaria for many years has been chloroquine, and prior to that, quinine. Parasites are increasingly developing resistance to chloroquine and newer drugs are being used, such as proguanil, atovaquone, mefloquine, and doxycycline. No antimalarial drug is 100% effective and it is not uncommon to prescribe a combination of drugs. Different drugs may be prescribed for prophylaxis depending on the area someone is travelling to; for instance, if the area is known to have chloroquine-resistant strains of parasite, mefloquine may be prescribed instead. A drug called primaquine can be effective against hypnozoites.

 BOX 7.4 *Worldwide malaria monitoring*

The World Health Organization reports on the current malaria status of countries throughout the world and on the sensitivity of malarial parasites to particular anti-malarial drugs. Travel clinics and doctors can then use these data to provide the most appropriate prophylaxis for travellers.

Haematological and other features of malaria

The anaemia of malaria

The periodic release of merozoites from schizonts within infected red cells together with the accompanying red cell rupture causes a haemolytic anaemia, which can be life-threatening. In fact, malaria is the most common cause of haemolytic anaemia in humans. However, the degree of anaemia cannot be explained by this alone and malarial anaemia has multiple aetiologies.

reticuloendothelial system
Contains phagocytic cells located in reticular connective tissue, lymph nodes, and spleen that are able to ingest bacteria, immune complexes, and other foreign bodies.

splenomegaly
Enlarged spleen.

dyserythropoiesis
Abnormal red cell development.

pro-inflammatory cytokines
Regulatory cellular-communication signalling molecules that favour and promote inflammation.

The **reticuloendothelial system** removes parasitized red cells from the circulation by extravascular phagocytosis. The process of *pitting* in the spleen where red cell parasites (and other red cell inclusions such as Heinz bodies) are removed results in loss of red cell membrane in the area where the inclusion is removed. Although this does not necessarily result in the immediate destruction of the red cell it does reduce its lifespan. Parasitized red cells have reduced deformability that can lead to enhanced clearance by the spleen. Increased reticuloendothelial and splenic function can lead to enhanced clearance of non-parasitized red cells. It is a normal function of the spleen to remove senescent, or ageing, red cells from the circulation and the **splenomegaly** arising from malaria infection exaggerates this normal function.

A low reticulocyte response to severe haemolytic anaemia is often a remarkable finding in the severe malarial disease of *P. falciparum* infection. This inadequate response to anaemia arises from **dyserythropoiesis** which occurs due to the presence of **pro-inflammatory cytokines**, such as tumour necrosis factor-α (TNF-α) and interleukin-12 (IL-12), and suppression of erythropoiesis by haemozoin. Dyserythropoiesis can be seen in infections with the other *Plasmodium* species and can persist for some weeks after the acute phase of the infection.

Malaria occurs in many areas where chronic nutritional anaemias and haemoglobinopathies are endemic so it often exacerbates a coexisting anaemia. The anaemia of malaria itself is normocytic and normochromic, but the classic morphological appearances of a nutritional anaemia or haemoglobinopathy do not exclude the possibility of coexistent malaria infection.

BOX 7.5 Blackwater fever

Patients with *P. falciparum* malaria who have previously been infected with that species can present with sudden intravascular haemolysis followed by fever and haemoglobinuria, a syndrome termed **Blackwater fever**. It is commonly seen in non-immune individuals who have been in malarious countries for less than a year and have had inadequate doses of quinine for prophylaxis and/or treatment. Quinine itself can be a precipitating factor and Blackwater fever almost disappeared after 1950 when quinine was replaced by chloroquine as the treatment of choice. The syndrome reappeared in 1990 when quinine was reintroduced due to chloroquine resistance. More recently, cases have been described associated with newer drugs similar to quinine, such as halofantrine and mefloquine. Other factors that may precipitate an attack of Blackwater fever are cold, sun exposure, trauma, fatigue, pregnancy, and X-ray treatment of the spleen.

It is thought that the haemolysis occurring as a result of schizogony stimulates the formation of haemolysin antibodies that destroy red cells. The patients become hypersensitized as a result of repeated *P. falciparum* infection such that a subsequent heavy infection and administration of quinine, together with other precipitating factors, generates a sudden and massive output of haemolysin antibodies which cause severe, acute intravascular haemolysis. Patients present with pallor due to rapidly developing anaemia, nausea, jaundice, fever, renal failure due to tubule necrosis and haemoglobin deposition in the tubules, and urine that is black or dark red in colour from the excretion of free haemoglobin. Individuals with glucose-6-phosphate dehydrogenase (G6PD) deficiency are more likely to develop Blackwater fever as a complication of malaria infection.

SELF-CHECK 7.3

What are the causes of the anaemia of malarial infection?

Other haematological changes

The white cell count can be raised in severe malarial infection but it is often within the reference range. Some patients develop a leucoerythroblastic picture whilst others may have neutrophilia, atypical lymphocyte morphology, monocytosis, eosinopenia, or a reactive eosinophilia during the recovery phase.

Mild thrombocytopenia is common in malaria infection, resulting from a combination of platelet activation, increased pooling / clearance in the spleen, and reduced platelet lifespan due to immune responses. The platelet count can drop to around 100×10^9/L and sometimes below 50×10^9/L in severe disease. In addition, blood coagulation can be activated in malaria infection, particularly with P. *falciparum*, as a result of the following:

- The main reason is the cytokine storm produced in response to the infection which can activate blood clotting mechanisms.
- Alterations to the red cell membrane so that coagulation-promoting phospholipids are expressed on the surface.
- Adherence of parasitized red cells to deep tissue capillary endothelium which damages the endothelial cells and leads to activation of blood coagulation.

Reduced synthesis and increased activation of blood coagulation factors can lead to mild elevations of the prothrombin time and activated partial thromboplastin time. Fibrinogen concentration can be reduced, normal, or elevated. Factor XIII, which is responsible for stabilizing fibrin clots, and antithrombin, a regulator of blood coagulation, can both be reduced in malaria due to their consumption.

Cross references

You can find explanations of white cell abnormalities in Chapter 8.

You were introduced to blood coagulation in Chapter 2 and will meet more details about its activation in Chapter 13.

Cerebral malaria

Only P. *falciparum* invades the central nervous system to cause **cerebral malaria**. It is an acute, widespread disease of the brain accompanied by fever and can be fatal within 24–72 hours if not treated. It is caused by adherence of both parasitized and non-parasitized red cells to the cerebral microvasculature leading to blockage of cerebral blood flow. It is also hypothesized that a malarial toxin is released that stimulates macrophages to release cytokines which induce uncontrolled production of nitric oxide in the brain. The nitric oxide diffuses through the blood–brain barrier and affects nerve cell function in a similar way to anaesthetics and alcohol, resulting in a state of reduced consciousness. Children are more vulnerable to cerebral malaria than adults.

Cerebral malaria has three key symptoms:

1. Impaired consciousness with non-specific fever.
2. Generalized convulsions and neurological abnormalities.
3. Coma that persists for 24–72 hours, in which the patient is initially rousable and then unrousable.

Immediate treatment is necessary and includes chemotherapy with quinine to interfere with the parasite's digestion, antipyretics to reduce fever, and anticonvulsants.

Knob formation

Knobs are conical protrusions of the membranes of red cells infected by *P. falciparum*, *P. ovale*, and *P. malariae* and are not visible by light microscopy. Most of the research has been done on *P. falciparum* infected cells. The knobs are involved in mediating the cytoadherance of *P. falciparum* infected red cells to the vascular endothelium and the rosetting of non-infected cells around the adhered infected cells. The knobs form junctions between red cell and endothelial cell membranes. Cytoadherence may be a mechanism for *P. falciparum* to avoid destruction in the spleen.

A number of *P. falciparum* proteins occur on the red cell surface or associated with the red cell cytoskeleton in relation to knob formation. Table 7.2 lists the proteins and their functions.

TABLE 7.2 *P. falciparum* knob-associated proteins.

Protein	Abbreviation	Function
Histidine-rich protein 1*	HRP-1	Critical for structural formation of the knob
Histidine-rich protein 2	HRP-2	Released into plasma to suppress lymphocyte function
P. falciparum erythrocyte membrane protein 1	PfEMP 1	Expressed on knob surface; cytoplasmic region interacts with HRP-1
P. falciparum erythrocyte membrane protein 2**	PfEMP 2	Anchor for PfEMP 1
P. falciparum erythrocyte membrane protein 3	PfEMP 3	Probably involved in knob formation via interaction with red cell cytoskeleton
Ring-infected erythrocyte membrane surface antigen	RASA	Cytoskeleton binding
Sequestrin	–	Recognition protein for CD36 on endothelial membrane
Rosettin	–	Binds endothelial receptors and ABO antigens

* HRP-1 is also known as knob-associated histidine-rich protein (KAHRP)
** PfEMP 2 is also known as mature erythrocyte surface antigen (MESA)

BOX 7.6 Airport malaria

Mosquitoes have been known to enter aeroplanes and be transported to parts of the world where malaria does not occur naturally, and then infect someone at the airport who did not actually travel to a malarial region. In favourable climatic conditions, the mosquito may travel beyond the airport and infect people further afield. Mosquitoes can survive in baggage and infect someone when released from the baggage, not necessarily the person who had travelled.

Genetic protection from malaria

Genetic defects of haemoglobin and red cells are common in all parts of the world where malaria is prevalent, mainly because carriers are afforded a degree of protection from *P. falciparum* infection. These defects include: haemoglobinopathies such as haemoglobins S, C, E, and thalassaemias; red cell membrane defects such as Southeast Asian ovalocytosis (SAO) and some forms of elliptocytosis; and metabolic abnormalities such as G6PD deficiency. It is thought that natural selection has been responsible for elevating and maintaining their gene frequencies where malaria is endemic, and is probably why haemoglobinopathies are the most common single-gene disorders in the human population.

Sickle cell trait is the commonly quoted example of genetic protection from malaria. A variety of mechanisms have been proposed to explain the protective effect against *P. falciparum* infection, such as attenuating the infection by reducing intracellular oxygen tension, or targeting parasite-infected cells for splenic clearance due to reduced deformability of cells containing haemoglobin S and parasites. It is clear though that HbAS-containing cells are just as likely to be infected as cells containing HbAA. It has been proposed that red cells of homozygous haemoglobin C individuals resist lysis at the merozoite release stage.

More recently, atypical display of PfEMP1 has been reported on cells in patients heterozygous and homozygous for haemoglobin C and with sickle cell trait, leading to reduced cytoadhesion and rosetting and thus protection from cerebral malaria. Cytoadhesion can occur in other organs. The existence of variant malarial surface antigens may also precipitate an enhanced immune response and affect the early development of naturally acquired immunity.

Red cells of patients with thalassaemia and G6PD deficiency are highly sensitive to oxidant stress and provide a poor environment for *P. falciparum* parasites. Modified surface-antigen expression may also operate in some thalassaemias.

SAO is a hereditary disorder of red cell structure due to a deletion in the Band 3 gene that is widespread in parts of Southeast Asia. The ovalocytic red cells are rigid and resistant to invasion by various malarial parasites.

Absent or mutant Duffy antigens on red cell surfaces provide protection against *P. vivax* because it binds the Duffy antigen at the red cell invasion stage of the life cycle via its Duffybinding-like erythrocyte-binding protein (DBL-EBP). The same is not generally considered to be true for *P. falciparum* because it can use more than one red cell antigen as a receptor and the parasite has four DBL-EBPs. However, about 10% of Melanesians living in the northern provinces of Papua New Guinea are negative for the Gerbich antigen located on glycophorin C, and there is evidence to suggest that it may provide some degree of protection against *P. falciparum* infection.

Cross reference
You will find more detail about haemoglobinopathies in Chapter 6.

Malaria prevention

Anopheles mosquitoes feed at night and only one bite is needed to infect the human host. Some 90% of malaria cases occur in Sub-Saharan Africa with young children at greatest risk because they have yet to develop natural immunity, which can take up to 10 years.

Education is key to engendering the appropriate lifelong behaviours to reduce infection. Sleeping under nets suspended above a bed can be an effective barrier against the mosquitoes reaching humans to feed on, although the nets need to be maintained and used properly to be effective. More recently, nets impregnated with pyrethroid insecticides have become available. The insecticide is either incorporated within or bound around the net fibres. As well as providing a physical barrier, insecticide treated nets (ITN) deter mosquitoes from feeding and even drive them from their indoor resting places. A treated net with large holes can provide protection as effective as an intact, properly used untreated net. However, the insecticide does not last indefinitely and the nets need to be re-dipped in insecticide every six months. Long-lasting insecticidal nets (LLIN) are now available that remain effective for about three years but they are inevitably more expensive, albeit more cost-effective in the long term. Unfortunately, neither nets nor insecticides are sufficiently widely available or affordable, and less than half the people in Africa who need them have access.

Another strategy to prevent being bitten by mosquitoes in the home is indoor residual spraying (IRS), which involves covering the internal walls with an insecticide that kills and repels mosquitoes. Whilst nets and IRS can be very effective, it is important to remember that some *Anopheles* mosquitoes only bite outdoors. Even those that will bite indoors may enter the house, feed, and leave without resting on any of the indoor walls. The insecticide dichlorodiphenyltrichloroethane (DDT) has been used as an outdoor residual spraying strategy, but it affects other wildlife and DDT resistance is now common in mosquitoes.

A different approach to reducing malaria has been to target the aquatic but air-breathing larval stage of the mosquito's life cycle. In 1897, Major Ronald Ross discovered that *Anopheles* mosquitoes were the vectors for malaria. He initiated attempts to reduce mosquito numbers by coating the surfaces of ponds and marshes with oil to prevent the larvae from taking in air through their breathing tubes. Water has been treated with chemicals that can prevent larvae from metamorphosing into adults, impair **chitin** synthesis, or disrupt nerve function. Not surprisingly, there are problems with toxicity to other wildlife and humans. Some habitats lend themselves to the reduction of larvae numbers by introducing predatory fish into the water, such as the Common Carp (*Cyprinus carpio*) in rice fields and the Killifish (*Aphanius dispar*) into man-made containers. Introduction of *Bacillus thuringiensis israelensis* and *Bacillus sphaericus* bacteria into the water kill the larvae because toxins on the bacterial spore coat poison the larvae's stomach. Predatory fish and pathological bacteria can reduce larvae population density by up to 98–100%, but the fish are only effective for between 2 weeks and 1 year and the bacteria for a maximum of 10 weeks.

chitin
The principal component of arthropod exoskeletons.

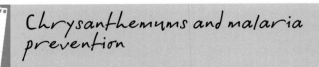

Chrysanthemums and malaria prevention

Pyrethroids are a group of man-made insecticides similar to the natural pesticide pyrethrum, which is derived from the dried flowers of *Chrysanthemum cinerariaefolium*. So-called pyrethrum daisies have been used as an insecticide for over 2000 years; the generic name for the six active compounds derived from them is pyrethrin. Since it is naturally produced it decomposes rapidly in sunlight and is considered one of the most environmentally safe insecticides, with very low mammalian toxicity.

BMJ Best Practice

Getting started guide

Follow these steps to get started.

Access to BMJ Best Practice is provided by Health Education England to all NHS staff in England through OpenAthens.

1. Visit **bestpractice.bmj.com** and click **'Log in'**.

2. You will be presented with an **'Access through your institution'** button.

3. When selected, you will be asked to search for your institution. Please type and select **'NHS in England'** , and then log in using your OpenAthens username and password.

4. Now create your **personal account**. This will allow you to sign in directly using these details. Your personal account also allows you to log in to the app and to track your CPD/CME activity and download certificates.

 To register for an OpenAthens account, go to **openathens.nice.org.uk** or contact your local NHS library and knowledge service through **www.hlisd.org**.

d help?

any questions, please do not hesitate to contact our support team at
i.com or +44 (0) 20 7111 1105.

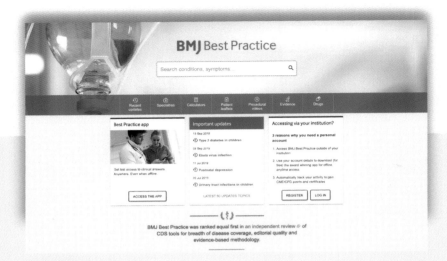
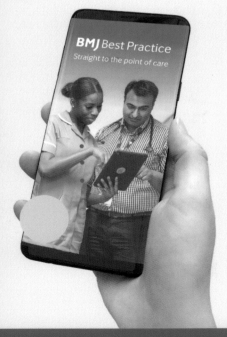

BOX 7.7 *What does 'malaria' mean?*

The word 'malaria' is derived from the Italian words *mala* and *aria* meaning bad air. Before the discovery that malaria is caused by a parasitic infection, it was believed that breathing in the foul smelling air from swamps and latrines was responsible for the disease. It was a mere coincidence that the stagnant water that provided a breeding ground for mosquitoes also frequently contributed to bad air.

Expanded polystyrene beads have been used in man-made reservoirs such as water tanks and wells. They form a floating layer on the water surface that blocks oviposition (egg laying). However, the beads can blow away if exposed to wind and it has been known for local people to collect the beads to manufacture into jewellery.

Environmental modification can contribute to a reduction in malaria infection. Strategies include siting housing away from breeding sites, raising houses on poles because the mosquitoes tend to fly low, covering windows and doors with screening and being vigilant in repairing cracks in walls, restricting outdoor human activity to between sunrise and sunset, and diverting vectors to other mammalian hosts (zooprophylaxis).

An important dimension to environmental manipulation is water management. Strategies include flushing streams and canals because larvae prefer still water, intermittent irrigation in agricultural fields, flooding or temporarily de-watering man-made or natural wetlands, or altering salinity. Planting trees can contribute to draining marshy land.

Pharmaceutical malaria prevention

You met examples of the main drugs for prophylaxis and treatment earlier in this chapter. The development of drug-resistant parasites and insecticide-resistant mosquitoes is causing an increased burden on health services and even the economic stability of the countries that are worst affected. Alternatives to current treatments and prevention strategies are badly needed. An area that attracts considerable attention is that of a vaccine for malaria which would be of particular value in individuals who have yet to develop natural immunity, such as young children, travellers, pregnant women, and people who live in endemic areas but are not now regularly exposed to the infections.

Development of vaccines to malaria has proven difficult to date because the parasites are very good at evading the immune response. The parasites enter human cells very quickly and are effectively hidden from the immune response for most of their time inside the human host. As you have seen, they express certain antigens which are recognizable by the immune system, and thus vaccines, but they have the ability to vary their antigen expression. The many different life cycle stages mean that a vaccine to just one stage will be ineffective. Because it is difficult to make a vaccine that targets the entire organism, most attempts at vaccine production have been directed at subunits.

It has proven difficult to create a vaccine that will precipitate an effective immune response. Some vaccines have been shown to generate antibody formation but the subsequent processes of the immune response were not initiated. Natural immunity builds up through early life as individuals encounter and develop resistance to different strains of parasite, so people in endemic areas are not effectively immune until adulthood. Therefore it is clearly possible to be immune to malaria, but developing a single vaccine remains elusive. Interestingly, natural immunity doesn't completely destroy the parasites as they can still grow in people who are clinically immune.

Laboratory detection of malaria

Detection of malarial parasites in peripheral blood and species identification is achieved primarily by light microscopy of Romanowsky-stained blood films. This approach has been the mainstay of malaria detection for decades and remains the 'gold standard'. Supplementary assays are available to affirm microscopical findings or for use as initial screening tests.

Light microscopy

Thick and thin blood films should be prepared, stained, and examined for all cases being investigated for malaria. Thin films are conventional wedge films. Thick films are prepared on a separate slide by spreading a drop of blood in a circular motion to cover an area with a diameter of about 1 cm. The films should be made with minimal delay because morphological alteration of parasites occurs in stored EDTA-anticoagulated blood.

Thin films can be stained with a conventional Romanowsky stain such as Leishman's or May Grünwald/Giemsa, although the pH of 6.8 does not permit sufficiently intense staining of some important structures that aid species identification, such as **Schüffner's dots**. Therefore, use of pH 7.2 stains is recommended. Some laboratories stain thin films with their usual preparation as it is usually adequate to demonstrate malarial parasites, and then follow-up with Leishman's or Giemsa staining of a separate slide at pH 7.2 if necessary.

Schüffner's dots are multiple, small, brick-red dots inside red cells infected with *P. vivax* or *P. ovale*. The dots are composed of invaginations of the red cell membrane called caveolae complexed to vesicles, forming structures called caveola–vesicle complexes. The dots may not be present in red cells containing the smaller, young ring-form trophozoites. The dots can be darker in *P. ovale* infection and are referred to as **James's dots**.

Thick films are not fixed so that when stained with **Field's stain**, the haemoglobin elutes from the red cells. It is crucial that the film is perfectly dry otherwise unfixed cellular material will flake off during staining. Giemsa stain can also be used for thick films. Thick and thin films are shown in Figure 7.6.

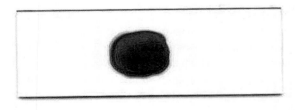

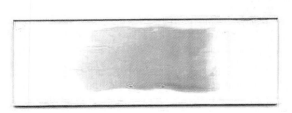

FIGURE 7.6
Stained thick film (top) and thin wedge film (bottom). Royal Perth Hospital, Government of Western Australia.

TABLE 7.3 Morphological differentiation of human malarial parasites.

Life cycle stage/ other morphology	P. falciparum	P. vivax	P. malariae	P. ovale
Ring-form trophozoite	Delicate small rings with scanty cytoplasm Can have double chromatin dots Older rings may be stippled (Maurer's clefts/dots) Trophozoites are sometimes found at the periphery of the RBC and are referred to as accolé forms	Rings can be ⅓ to ½ of the diameter of the RBC Heavy chromatin dot Thin, faintly stained cytoplasm	Rings can be ⅓ to ½ of the diameter of the RBC Heavy chromatin dot Thick, deeply stained cytoplasm	Rings can be up to ½ of the diameter of the RBC Heavy chromatin dot Thick, deeply stained cytoplasm
Large trophozoite	Not normally seen	Amoeboid vacuolated	Compact or band shaped Scattered dark granules	Band forms rare Scanty, dark brown granules
Mature schizont	Occasionally seen in peripheral blood 16–30 merozoites Numerous chromatin masses	Parasite can fill entire RBC 12–24 merozoites in a rosette Fine, central pigment Numerous chromatin masses	Parasite can fill entire RBC 6–12 merozoites in a rosette Central, coarse clump of pigment Few chromatin masses	8–12 merozoites in a rosette Few chromatin masses
Gametocytes	Crescent or sausage-shaped Central nucleus surrounded by darkly pigmented granules	Round or oval-shape Fills entire RBC Evenly distributed pigment	Round or oval-shaped Scattered pigment	Round or oval shaped Smaller than P. vivax
Stages present in peripheral blood	Ring-form trophozoites Gametocytes Occasionally schizonts	All stages	All stages	All stages
Schüffner's dots	Not present	Can be seen in all stages except early ring-form trophozoite	Not present	Can be seen in all stages except early ring-form trophozoite
Multiply-infected RBC	Common	Occasional	Rare	Rare
RBC size and shape	Normal	Up to 2 times larger than normal Normal or oval-shaped	Normal or smaller size Normal shape	RBC usually normal size or slightly enlarged RBC frequently oval Fimbriated (ragged) edges often seen

Microscopical examination of the thick film is used as the first screening tool because the larger volume of blood used increases the likelihood of finding the parasites, especially in scanty infections. Parasite density can be as low as 1 infected cell per 100 000 red cells and would take in the region of an hour to detect on a thin film, whereas a five-minute examination of a thick film would examine the equivalent amount of material. The limitation of thick films is that the red cell lysis distorts parasite morphology and so thin films are needed to determine the species and assess parasitaemia.

It is crucial to differentiate the species because *P. falciparum* infection can lead to complications and be fatal. Species are identified based mainly on trophozoite appearances, merozoite numbers in schizonts, gametocyte morphology, size and shape of infected red cells, and the presence of Schüffner's dots. Fortunately, a number of morphological features are either specific for *P. falciparum* infection or very rare in other infections. These features are:

- Smaller ring forms than in other species.
- Double chromatin dots can be present in ring forms.
- Multiply-infected cells are more common.
- Schüffner's dots are not present.
- Maurer's clefts/dots can be present.
- It is the only species whose gametocytes may be crescent-shaped.

Table 7.3 describes the important morphological features of the four main malarial parasites of humans. It is important to bear in mind that mixed infections do occur and clear identification of the presence of one species does not preclude the presence of another. The most commonly encountered stages are the ring-form trophozoites which appear as a ring of blue cytoplasm with red to purple chromatin. The larger trophozoites often contain malaria pigment.

Maurer's clefts appear as irregular red/mauve dots inside red cells infected with *P. falciparum*. Figure 7.7 demonstrates that Maurer's clefts are larger and fewer in number than Schüffner's dots. They are newly constructed clefts in the red cell cytoplasm that are continuous with the PVM. Maurer's clefts are involved in protein/antigen sorting and trafficking.

SELF-CHECK 7.4

What are the main morphological features that allow differentiation between *Plasmodium* species on Romanowsky-stained blood films?

Estimation of parasitaemia

The percentage parasitaemia must be estimated when *P. falciparum* infection is detected because the severity of the infection can affect treatment decision-making. Quantification is performed by counting the number of parasitized cells examined from different areas of a thin film from a minimum of 1000 cells and converting to a percentage. Only asexual stages should be counted and it is important to note that it is the percentage of parasitized cells that is being estimated and not the number of parasites per 100 red cells. A parasitaemia of >5% is considered to be a severe infection and a medical emergency.

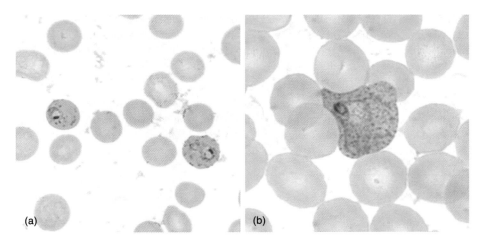

FIGURE 7.7
Maurer's clefts and Schüffner's dots (Giemsa-stained thin films; ×500 magnification).
(a) Maurer's clefts in P. *falciparum* infected red cells, (b) Schüffner's dots in a P. *vivax* infected red cell.

If the parasite count is less than 1 in 1000 cells on the thin film the parasitaemia can be quantified from the thick film in relation to the white cell count. The thick film is scanned and the number of parasites encountered when 200 white cells have been counted is recorded and entered into the calculation below. If fewer than ten parasites are encountered, 500 white cells should be counted.

(Number of parasites × WCC per µL)/(Number of white cells counted) = Number of parasites/µL

Limitations of malaria detection by light microscopy

Whilst marked infections can be immediately apparent when examining a blood film, scanty infections are easily missed. Separate thick and thin films should be examined by two biomedical scientists. A minimum of 200 oil-immersion fields with a × 100 objective should be examined in the thick film, which will take an experienced scientist up to 10 minutes. Less experienced staff should aim to take longer than this. The residual stroma in thick films can make the detection of parasites difficult. Where uncertainty exists, the entire thin film should be examined with a × 100 objective, which will take in the region of 30 minutes per operator.

Key Points

Cells containing parasites are inevitably heavier than non-parasitized cells so it is worth looking at the tails and edges of a thin film where larger and heavier cells can predominate.

Despite these precautions, false-negative reports will inevitably occur and it is good practice for at least three separate films taken during episodes of fever to be examined. Even if all three are negative, a diagnosis of malaria cannot be entirely excluded, particularly if the patient has taken antimalarial drugs. Conversely, a positive finding does not prove that symptoms are due to malaria or malaria alone because asymptomatic malaria is not uncommon in adults from endemic areas.

Malaria pigment can persist in peripheral blood mononuclear cells, which can be a useful diagnostic indicator where parasites cannot be found but the clinical suspicion is high. White cell differential histograms on automated analysers can exhibit abnormal patterns in this scenario and indicate the need for evaluation of white cell morphology.

Key Points

Sequestration of *P. falciparum* in deep capillaries can render the peripheral blood 'temporarily negative', which is another reason for taking a repeat sample of blood for the detection of malarial parasites. If an infection is present, parasites will be released into the blood after schizongony and potentially be detected in a repeat sample.

In scanty infections where very few parasites can be found it may not be possible to determine the species with certainty, in which case it is best that the patient is treated as for *P. falciparum* infection. Examining 1000 rather than 200 high-power fields increases the chances of finding more parasites and reduces the chances of false-negatives.

Care must be exercised during the apparently straightforward process of staining as parasites can be washed off, particularly *P. falciparum* gametocytes. Staining slides in bulk can even result in the transfer of parasites from one slide to another.

Artefacts on a stained blood film can lead to reporting false-positive results. A common problem is that platelets superimposed onto red cells can appear to be inside the red cell rather than on it. Moving the microscope stage up and down slightly is a good way of trying to differentiate between objects on red cells or within them. If an object is intracellular it will be in the same focal plane as the red cell, and therefore both will be in focus or out of focus together. If an object is on top of a cell, the red cell and the object will not be in the same focal plane, and therefore will not be in focus together. Platelets can be confused for trophozoites because they are a similar size and colour. Precipitated stain superimposed onto red cells can also lead to misidentification, as can other chromatoid body inclusions resulting from severe anaemia.

Key Points

Films from all positive cases should be sent to a reference laboratory for confirmation of species identification.

SELF-CHECK 7.5

What are the main limitations of detecting malarial parasites by light microscopy?

Supplementary assays

Alternatives to microscopy for malaria detection serve a variety of purposes. They can be useful when an individual is relatively inexperienced at microscopy, or an entire department lacks significant experience because their geographical location generates low demand. Work pressures, such as a biomedical scientist working alone on-call, can prevent adequate time being spent on microscopy. Outside of pathology laboratories where malaria is diagnosed 'in the field', simple and rapid tests that do not require microscopes, staining equipment, or sophisticated analysers can be extremely valuable.

Rapid and simple to perform, lateral-flow immunochromatographic techniques that detect parasite antigens have been available since the early 1990s. They are available in a variety of formats (such as dipsticks, strips, cards, wells, and cassettes), but all operate to the same basic principle. The blood sample can be anticoagulated whole blood, plasma, or direct from a fingerprick—which is ideal for testing 'in the field'. The blood is added to a buffered solution containing a haemolysing agent and one or more antibodies against malaria antigens that are labelled with a marker which can be visualized by the naked eye, such as colloidal gold. The antibodies complex with their target antigens if present, then migrate by capillary action along the test strip until they encounter separate immobilized capture antibodies directed against each target antigen in specific sections of the strip. There is a further antibody directed against the labelled antibody which is the final antibody in the sequence, acting as a control to indicate that the procedure itself has worked. The strip is washed with buffer to remove haemoglobin. You can see in Figure 7.8 that any malaria antigens that have been labelled and captured will manifest as coloured lines. The tests are qualitative and cannot assess parasitaemia.

Antibodies are used that target proteins specific for *P. falciparum*, such as HRP-2 (PfHRP-2), or pan-malaria proteins present in all species, such *Plasmodium* aldolase or *Plasmodium* lactate dehydrogenase (pLDH), which are enzymes in the glycolytic pathway of *Plasmodium* species. *P. falciparum* LDH (PfLDH) specific antibodies are also available.

Although the rapid immunochromatographic tests appear relatively straightforward in their design and operation they are not without their limitations and cannot be considered a replacement for microscopy. False-positives can occur for the following reasons:

- Cross-reacting antibodies such as rheumatoid factor.
- PfHRP-2 can cross-react with non-falciparum malaria.
- PfHRP-2 can persist after parasites have been cleared from the blood.
- Persistent viable asexual-stage parasitaemia undetectable by light microscopy.

False-negatives can occur for the following reasons:

- Genetic heterogeneity of PfHRP-2 expression.
- *HRP-2* gene deletions.
- Antibodies that block immune-complex formation.
- **Prozone** effect.
- Unknown causes.

> **prozone**
> Concentration of antibody or antigen is so high that the optimal concentration for maximal reaction with antigen is exceeded and binding is reduced or does not occur.

Clearly, the rapid tests are not totally reliable in detecting falciparum and non-falciparum malaria, although neither is microscopy. Some studies have demonstrated >95% sensitivity, although this has been in patients with high parasitaemia. Sensitivity to the presence of malaria is reduced when the parasitaemia is below 100 parasites per µL of blood. The rapid tests are, therefore, a useful adjunct to malaria detection in diagnostic laboratories and have a place in the field where malaria may otherwise be diagnosed on clinical symptoms alone.

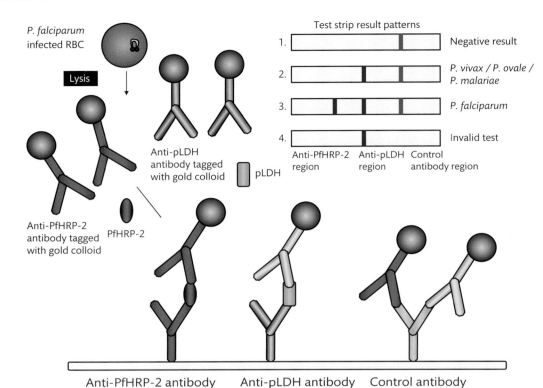

FIGURE 7.8

Immunochromatography for detection of malarial antigens. The patient in this example is infected with *P. falciparum*. Lysis of the red blood cells releases the *P. falciparum* specific antigen PfHRP-2 and the antigen that is present in all human-infecting species, pLDH. The lytic buffer also contains antibodies to PfHRP-2 and pLDH labelled with colloidal gold. The antibodies complex with their target antigens and migrate by capillary action along the test strip until they encounter separate regions of immobilized capture antibodies directed against each target antigen. An antibody directed against the labelled antibodies is present at the end of the strip as a control to ensure the antibodies have fully migrated. You can see that test strip 1 is negative because there is no colour formation in the regions of PfHRP-2 and pLDH antibodies. The band of colour in the control region indicates that the assay had worked. Test strip 2 has a band of colour in the pLDH region but not the PfHRP-2 region indicating non-falciparum malaria but it cannot differentiate between the other species. Test strip 3 has bands in all three positions and indicates *P. falciparum* infection. Although there is a band of colour in the pLDH region of test strip 4, the lack of colour in the control region indicates that the test may not have worked and should be repeated.

Another type of assay that is used as a screening test backed up by microscopy is the **quantitative buffy coat** (QBC) method. Capillary blood is taken into a glass haematocrit tube containing acridine orange (to stain parasite DNA) and potassium oxalate (as an anticoagulant). A cylindrical float is inserted into the tube which is then centrifuged to separate the cells according to their densities so that they form the discrete bands you can see in Figure 7.9. The bands would normally be small but the presence of the float, which occupies 90% of the bore of the tube, forces the blood components to the periphery thus significantly enlarging the

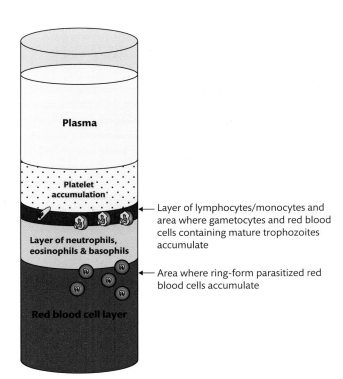

Layer of lymphocytes/monocytes and area where gametocytes and red blood cells containing mature trophozoites accumulate

Area where ring-form parasitized red blood cells accumulate

FIGURE 7.9

Distribution of blood components and parasites in the glass haematocrit tube of the quantitative buffy coat technique for detection of malaria.

areas occupied by each band. The tube is then placed on a holder and examined under a light microscope with an ultraviolet light adapter. Red cells do not contain DNA but red cells containing parasites will fluoresce because the parasite DNA takes up the acridine orange stain. Red cells containing parasites are less dense than unparasitized cells so they form a discrete band between the non-infected red cells and the white cell layer. The parasite nuclei appear as bright specks of green light and the cytoplasm as yellow-orange against a background of non-fluorescing red cells.

However, there are limitations to the QBC assay: it is almost impossible to differentiate between species, quantification is not possible, filarial worms can be misidentified as malaria, and visual artefacts can lead to false-positive reporting by inexperienced operators.

Polymerase chain reaction (PCR) techniques have been described to detect and differentiate malarial parasites. They are tenfold more sensitive than microscopy and more reliable in species differentiation, but are not suitable for rapid diagnostics.

Assays are available that detect antibodies against malarial parasites produced by the immune response of the infected patient. The antibodies can persist in the circulation for several months after the infection is over so the tests do not necessarily demonstrate a current infection.

SELF-CHECK 7.6

What tests are available to supplement peripheral blood microscopy in the detection of malaria and what are their main uses?

BOX 7.8 *Malaria as a medicine?!*

Before the widespread availability of penicillin in the 1940s there was no drug available to cure syphilis. Every patient with the disease died once it entered the terminal stage affecting the brain. The Austrian psychiatrist Julius Wagner von Jauregg received a Nobel prize in 1927 for his work on curing syphilis with pyrotherapy. He discovered that patients whose disease had progressed to neurosyphilis could be cured by being infected with a mild strain of malaria. The prolonged high fevers and elevation of body temperature associated with malaria infection were able to kill the causative spirochaete bacterium of syphilis, *Treponema pallidum*. Patients underwent about 10 bouts of fever before their malaria was subsequently treated with quinine. The results were remarkable, with many patients being completely cured of the physical and mental effects of their illness and returned to normal life. Understandably, the advent of widespread penicillin availability made 'treatment' with malaria obsolete.

7.3 **Babesiosis**

Babesiosis is an intraerythrocytic non-tropical parasitic infection predominantly described in the USA and Europe. It is caused by protozoa of the genus *Babesia* and transmitted by bites from the Deer or Blacklegged tick (*Ixodes scapularis*) in the USA, which is also the vector for the bacterial infection Lyme disease, and the Sheep or Castor bean tick (*Ixodes ricinus*) in Europe. *Babesia* organisms have been known to be transmitted from human to human by blood transfusion and via the placenta.

Babesiosis in Europe is mainly due to infection with *B. divergens*, and in the USA, *B. microti* and *B. duncani*.

Life cycle of babesiosis parasites

The main host of *Babesia* species is the white-footed mouse (*Peromyscus leucopus*), where the life cycle is similar to malaria in humans apart from the lack of a hepatic phase. An infected tick vector injects sporozoites into the mouse bloodstream when it takes a blood meal whereupon the sporozoites invade red blood cells and undergo trophozoite formation. Unlike malarial parasites, invading parasites are not encased in a parasitophorous vacuole. Asexual reproduction occurs to form more merozoites which lyse the red blood cells when released to infect other red cells. When another tick ingests infected cells most

BOX 7.9 *Another name for babesiosis*

In Northern USA, babesiosis occurs mostly in Long Island and the islands off the coast of Massachusetts where it is sometimes called the Malaria of the Northeast.

of the parasites are destroyed in its gut, but some differentiate into Ray bodies which divide to form four gametes. Male and female gametes fuse to form a motile zygote called a kinete. In some species the kinetes invade tick ovaries and are transmitted transovarially to the next generation of ticks. Sporogony occurs in the salivary glands to allow infection of the next host by the tick nymphs. Transovarial transmittance does not occur in *B. microti*. Instead, immature ticks are infected whilst feeding on a parasitized host, the parasites invade the ticks' salivary glands, multiply, and are then passed on to the next host at feeding.

Humans are occasional hosts to *Babesia* species. A feeding tick introduces sporozoites into the bloodstream which then invade red blood cells and undergo asexual reproduction by binary fission. Multiplication and release are responsible for the clinical manifestations of infection, but there is little, if any, transmission to ticks that feed on parasitized humans.

Clinical features of babesiosis

Many patients with *Babesia* infections are asymptomatic or have mild influenza-like symptoms, which are ignored and the infection resolves spontaneously. More severe cases present within 1–4 weeks of exposure with symptoms similar to malaria, such as fever, shaking, chills, fatigue, and (haemolytic) anaemia. The haemolytic anaemia is not as severe as malaria because *Babesia* species do not demonstrate periodicity as their release from red blood cells is not synchronized. Babesiosis commonly presents between May and September as a 'summer flu' because this is the period of nymph feeding. It is important that clinicians ascertain if the patient has visited tick-infested areas, such as those in the USA where there is a significant deer population. Patients rarely report a tick bite because the nymph stage of *Ixodes scapularis* is very small and mistaken for a small freckle. Severe and more persistent cases, which can lead to respiratory distress syndrome and death, tend to occur in very young children, the elderly, immunocompromised patients, and individuals who have had their spleen removed. Cases of babesiosis in Europe mainly involve splenectomized patients in whom the disease is far more severe, with >50% of patients dying. The clinical presentation can be complicated by coexisting Lyme disease and its own typical symptoms such as erythema migrans skin rash.

Laboratory detection of babesiosis

The parasites are detected on thick and thin Giemsa-stained blood films. The erythrocytic ring forms adopt oval, round, or pear-shaped rings and are easily mistaken for *P. falciparum* early trophozoites. Similarities with *P. falciparum* include normal red cell size, multiply-infected cells, small rings, and the absence of Schüffner's and James's dots. The main diagnostic criterion to differentiate *Babesia* species from *P. falciparum* is the presence of groups of pear-shaped rings forming tetrads that are referred to as **Maltese Cross formations**, which you can see in Figure 7.10. Other clues are a lack of schizonts, gametocytes, Maurer's clefts, and pigment.

Serological tests to identify antibodies against *Babesia* organisms are available and can detect low-level infections that may be missed by microscopy. They can also aid differentiation between malaria and babesiosis in patients who may be at risk of contracting both infections. *Babesia* organisms can also be detected using PCR techniques.

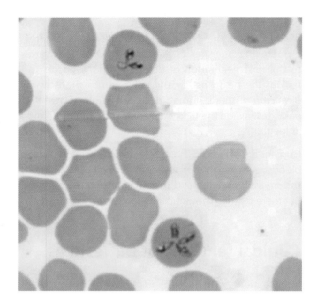

FIGURE 7.10
Red cells infected with *B. microti* (Giemsa-stained thin film; ×500 magnification). Note the tetrad of four pear-shaped ring forms forming the characteristic Maltese Cross formation.

SELF-CHECK 7.7

Compare and contrast the human-infective stages of the life cycles of malarial and babesiosis parasites.

7.4 Trypanosomiasis

Human **trypanosomiasis** is a vector-borne parasitic infection caused by haemoflagellate protozoa of the genus *Trypanomsoma*. There are two types of the disease in humans, African and American trypanosomiasis, which are fatal if left untreated.

African trypanosomiasis (sleeping sickness)

In Africa, *T. brucei gambiense* and *T. brucei rhodensiae* are transmitted by the tsetse fly (*Glossina* species). The distribution of African trypanosomiasis is determined by the ecological limits of tsetse flies and covers most of Sub-Saharan Africa, although the two trypanosome subspecies have more specific distributions.

T. brucei gambiense is found in the central and western regions of Africa and causes a chronic infection lasting years, referred to as West African trypanosomiasis. *T. brucei rhodensiae* is found in southern and eastern regions and causes an acute illness lasting several weeks, referred to as East African trypanosomiasis.

Metacyclic
A biochemical term for the extension of a cyclic group by another cyclic group.

Life cycle of African trypanosomiasis parasites

Whilst feeding, an infected tsetse fly injects parasites in the form of **metacyclic trypomas-tigotes** into the skin tissue of the human host. The parasites multiply in the vicinity of the bite and then pass into the bloodstream via the lymphatic system. Once in the bloodstream they transform into long slender trypomastigotes and replicate by binary fission. They are transported to other sites in the body, such as the heart and other organs, where they replicate in the tissue fluid. Later in the disease they invade the central nervous system, and it is the tissue damage in the brain that leads to lethargy and confusion (the sleeping sickness) and eventual death.

A feeding tsetse fly becomes infected with bloodstream trypomastigotes which transform into procyclic trypomastigotes in the fly's midgut; these multiply by binary fission. The trypomastigotes are the flagellated form and are often referred to as the **trypanosomes**. When they leave the gut they transform into epimastigotes that migrate to the tsetse fly's salivary glands, where they multiply and transform into the metacyclic trypomastigotes that will infect the next human host and perpetuate the life cycle. During development in the salivary glands, metacyclic trypomastigotes initiate the expression of metacyclic variant surface glycoproteins (VSG). Differential activation of VSG genes in the bloodstream occurs to evade waves of antibodies, although it appears that the metacyclic stage aids the generation of population diversity. Humans are the main mammalian host for *T. brucei gambiense*, whereas *T. brucei rhodesiense* mainly infects cattle and wild game animals and humans are less common, incidental hosts.

Clinical features of African trypanosomiasis

A bite from a tsetse fly is extremely painful and causes a small indurated (hardened) lesion that can persist for several days. The marked inflammatory reaction (a chancre) resulting from parasite multiplication at the injection site can last for up to three weeks. Fever occurs when the parasites enter the bloodstream and can be accompanied by sweating, shivering, and an increased pulse rate. Early stages of the disease are associated with **lymphadenopathy** and anaemia, haemorrhages and **petechiae** may occur. The anaemia occurs primarily as a result of removal of immune-complex coated red cells by phagocytosis. The bleeding tendency arises from thrombocytopenia, vascular injury, and coagulopathy. In the later stages—when parasites invade the brain—mental dullness, apathy, excessive sleeping, and incontinence can occur; although despite the common name of the disorder, drowsiness is not always present.

lymphadenopathy
Swollen/enlarged lymph nodes.

petechiae
Red, pinpoint-sized haemorrhages of small capillaries in the skin or mucous membranes.

American trypanosomiasis (Chagas disease)

American trypanosomiasis occurs in Mexico, Central America, much of South America, and occasionally in the Southern USA. The infective organism, *T. cruzi*, is transmitted by nocturnal triatomine bugs such as the Assassin bug (*Triatoma infestans*). Infection has also been described via blood transfusion, organ transplantation, contaminated food, the placenta, and even breast milk.

BOX 7.10 *Affectionate bugs*

The group of triatomine bugs that spread Chagas disease are known as kissing bugs because of their predilection for feeding on people's faces.

Life cycle of *T. cruzi*

The bugs tend to feed around the edges of the mouth and eyes of the host and deposit meta-cyclic trypomastigotes on the skin surface through defaecation. The trypomastigotes enter the skin either by directly penetrating the conjunctiva or membranes of the nose and mouth or from being rubbed into the skin by scratching of the bite site by the human host. Once inside cells, such as those in the subdermal layer or phagocytic cells, the parasites develop into **amastigotes**, multiply by binary fission, and develop into trypomastigotes that then enter the bloodstream. The trypomastigotes do not replicate in the bloodstream and migrate to tissues such as heart and skeletal muscle, nerves, and smooth muscle of the gut. Once inside the cells the trypomastigotes differentiate into amastigotes which multiply to form pseudocysts containing up to 500 amastigotes. The amastigotes differentiate into more trypomastigotes, which rupture the cells, and burst into the bloodstream to travel and infect other cells in a cycle of cell infection, replication, and release, or are ingested by a feeding bug.

Inside the bug, trypomastigotes transform into **epimastigotes** and multiply in the mid-gut and differentiate into metacyclic trypomastigotes in the hind-gut where they can be transferred to the skin surface of a human host upon defaecation.

Clinical features of American trypanosomiasis

The disease begins with an acute phase immediately after infection that can last a few weeks or a few months. It is usually asymptomatic, although there is a swelling at the site of parasite entry, a chagoma, which may be accompanied by fever, anorexia, lymphadenopathy, mild hepatospleno-megaly (enlarged liver and spleen), and myocarditis (inflammation of heart muscle). Inflammation of conjunctiva is termed Romaña's sign and is a recognized marker of Chagas disease.

In most patients the acute phase resolves into an asymptomatic chronic phase that can last for years, or even decades, before a symptomatic chronic phase evolves. The most serious manifestation is heart disease in the form of arrhythmias and heart enlargement, which occurs in about 30% of patients. A smaller number develop gut abnormalities, such as loss of peristalsis and enlargement of the oesophagus and colon.

Laboratory detection of trypanosomiasis

The trypanosomes in the circulating blood phase can be detected by examining a sample of fresh anticoagulated whole blood, or the buffy coat, under a microscope for motile parasites, a so-called wet preparation. Giemsa-stained thick and thin films can be examined to directly visualize the parasites, and where necessary, identify the species. *T. cruzi* can be confused with *T. rangeli* which is not known to be pathogenic in humans, and *T. brucei gambiense* and *T. brucei rhodesiense* are morphologically indistinguishable.

kinetoplast
Mitochondrial DNA.

You can see in Figure 7.11 that on stained blood films trypanosomes appear with an undulating membrane, central nucleus, anterior flagellum, and posterior **kinetoplast.** They are between 14 and 33 μm in length. *T. cruzi* trypanosomes often adopt a characteristic C-shape.

The QBC method used for the detection of malarial parasites is also used for trypanosome detection and is the method of choice for African trypanosomiasis. In situations where there is a low parasitaemia, *xenodiagnosis* can be performed by allowing an uninfected vector bug to feed on patient's blood and then examining the bug's gut contents for the presence of parasites. PCR can be used for detection and species identification.

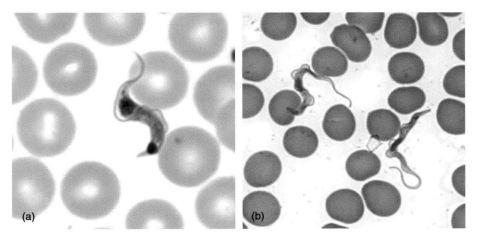

FIGURE 7.11
Trypanosomes (Giemsa-stained thin films; ×500 magnification). (a) *T. cruzi*, (b) *T. brucei*.

SELF-CHECK 7.8

How are trypanosomes detected in the laboratory?

7.5 **Leishmaniasis**

Flagellated protozoa of the genus *Leishmania* that are transmitted by night feeding female sandflies (*Phlebotomus* species) cause visceral and cutaneous leishmania in humans. Only the visceral form, also known as **kala-azar**, has protozoal life cycle stages associated with haemopoietic tissues—two species of parasite, *L. donovani* and *L. infantum*, are causative. More than 90% of cases of visceral leishmaniasis occur in India, Bangladesh, Nepal, Sudan, and Brazil. It is the most severe form of leishmaniasis and can be fatal if left untreated.

Life cycle of *L. donovani* and *L. infantum*

The infective stage of the life cycle, metacyclic **promastigotes**, are injected into the human host bloodstream by a feeding sandfly. Promastigotes actively invade neutrophils which are then phagocytosed by macrophages, whereupon the promastigotes invade the macrophages. Once inside the macrophage the promastigotes transform into amastigotes and replicate by simple division inside the **phagolysosome** of the macrophage—the very organelle designed to destroy foreign bodies. Promastigotes express surface lipophosphoglycan to resist destruction in the hostile lysosomal environment at the point where they infect the macrophage. Amastigotes do not express lipophosphoglycan and survive in the phagolysosome because their metabolism has evolved to be optimal in an acidic environment. Sheer numbers of amastigotes produced by replication cause the macrophage to rupture and release parasites to invade further macrophages and other organs or to be ingested by feeding sandflies. Once inside the sandfly's stomach the amastigotes transform into flagellated promastigotes that reproduce asexually before migrating to the sandfly's proboscis to be passed on at the next meal.

phagolysosome
Membrane-enclosed vesicle formed from the fusion of a lysosome (organelle containing digestive enzymes) and a phagosome (vacuole formed around foreign body inside a phagocytic cell).

Clinical features of visceral leishmaniasis

The clinical picture varies depending on the genotype of the infective organism and the host's immune response. Many infected individuals remain asymptomatic because they are able to preferentially activate T-lymphocytes; these produce gamma-interferon that is protective against progression to severe disease. Those whose disease does progress preferentially activate T-lymphocytes that produce interleukin-4, which promotes an antibody response but a lesser cellular protective response.

The incubation period typically lasts between 2 and 6 months, after which the onset of fever can be sudden. The acute phase can be accompanied by diarrhoea, joint pain, anorexia, and bleeding gums which are followed by progressive muscle wastage, fever, anaemia, and hepatosplenomegaly. Some patients have lymphadenopathy. Death is often caused not by the parasite itself but **opportunistic infections** such as pneumonia, tuberculosis, and dysentery because of a weakened immune system. In immunocompromised patients, such as those with human immunodeficiency virus (HIV) infection, visceral leishmaniasis behaves like an opportunistic infection.

Development of a normochromic, normocytic anaemia is common, with haemoglobin levels as low as 70 g/L. Splenomegaly can give rise to anaemia, leucopenia, and thrombocytopenia, and liver dysfunction can affect blood coagulation due to the reduced production of coagulation factors.

Some patients who recover can develop a secondary form of the disease called post kala-azar dermal leishmaniasis (PKDL), which can occur up to 20 years later. It is more commonly associated with *L. donovani* infection. PKDL manifests as small, hypopigmented lesions on the face which gradually enlarge and then spread over the body. The lesions can coalesce to form swollen, disfiguring plaques that resemble leprosy. Blindess may follow if they spread to the eyes.

opportunistic infection
An infection caused by organisms that do not normally cause disease in the presence of a competent immune system.

Laboratory detection of visceral leishmaniasis

The most common method for detecting *L. donovani* and *L. infantum* parasites is by light microscopy of a bone marrow aspirate. The parasites can also be demonstrated in splenic aspirate, lymph nodes, liver biopsy, and peripheral blood buffy coat.

Romanowsky staining reveals the amastigotes as round or oval organisms about 2–3 µm in length with pale blue cytoplasm and a large red nucleus. The cytoplasm exhibits a deep-red or violet, rod-shaped kinetoplast close to the nucleus. The amastigotes are contained within monocytes and macrophages, which you can see in Figure 7.12.

Rapid immunochromatography assays are available to detect parasite antigens, and PCR techniques are available to detect and speciate the parasites. Serological testing for antibodies is available and widely used in the field, but not all patients who are infected will develop the clinical disease and require treatment. Antibodies can remain after a patient is cured so these tests cannot confirm cure or indicate re-infection because the tests do not detect the parasites themselves. Immunocompromised patients will not generate antibodies and therefore will be negative in an antibody detection test even if they are infected.

SELF-CHECK 7.9

How is visceral leishmaniasis detected in the laboratory?

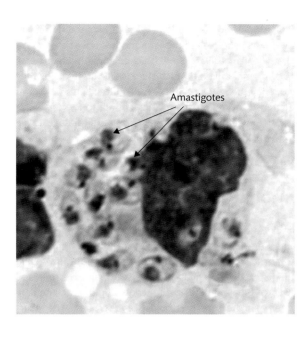

Amastigotes

FIGURE 7.12
Monocytes containing
***Leishmania* amastigotes**
(Giemsa-stained skin scraping;
×500 magnification).

7.6 **Filariasis**

Filarial worms are nematodes (roundworms), and eight species are known to infect humans: *Wuchereria bancrofti, Brugia malayi, B. timori, Loa loa, Mansonella perstans,* and *M. ozzardi,* which have blood-inhabiting larvae; and *M. streptocerca* and *Onchocerca volvulus* that do not. Of the peripheral blood-detectable organisms, only *W. bancrofti, B. malayi, B. timori,* and *L. loa* are associated with significant symptomatic disease in humans. *Dirofilaria* species cause incomplete infection as they are unable to mature into adults in a human host.

W. bancrofti, B. malayi, and *B. timori* are transmitted to humans by mosquitoes of the genera *Culex, Anopheles, Mansonia,* and *Aedes.* Vectors for *L. loa* are mainly the Deerfly (or Mangofly) species of *Chrysops silacea* and *C. dimidiata.*

Life cycle of *W. bancrofti,* *B. malayi,* **and** *B. timori*

The life cycles of *W. bancrofti, B. malayi,* and *B. timori* are virtually identical except for transmittance by different species of vector mosquitoes. An infected mosquito introduces third-stage filarial larvae (microfilariae) into the host bloodstream when it takes a blood meal. The microfilariae moult twice and migrate to the lymphatic vessels and lymph nodes, particularly in the arms, legs, scrotum, and breast. Here they mature into adult worms, mate, and produce more microfilariae. Mature female *W. bancrofti* are between 80 and 100 mm in length, those of the *Brugia* species being about half that length. Adult male worms are about half the size of females. An adult female can release 50 000 active, immature microfilariae into the peripheral blood each day. The microfilariae of *W. bancrofti* are about 250 μm in length, whilst those of *Brugia* species are about 200 μm in length. The presence of the adult worms in the lymphatic system causes the vessels to dilate, resulting in the lymph fluid travelling more slowly. Microfilariae appear in the peripheral blood within 6–12 months after the adult worms are established in the lymphatics, a situation termed microfilaraemia.

Microfilariae circulate in the peripheral blood and can show periodicity depending on the feeding habits of vectors in the region. Many vectors feed at night and it is advisable to take blood samples for diagnostic purposes when microfilariae will be circulating in larger numbers. A feeding mosquito ingests circulating microfilariae which shed their outer coat as they penetrate the gut wall of the mosquito. They then migrate to the mosquito's flight muscles in the thorax and enter cells where they transform to first-stage larvae, moult to form second-stage larvae, and then elongate to form the infective third-stage larvae. The third-stage larvae leave the flight muscles, pass through the haemocele (blood space in arthropods), and enter the mouth parts to be transmitted at the next blood meal.

Clinical features of lymphatic filariasis

tropical pulmonary eosinophilia
Nocturnal cough, wheezing, fever, and eosinophilia arising from marked sensitivity to microfilariae in the lungs.

W. bancrofti, *B. malayi*, and *B. timori* cause lymphatic filariasis in humans. The presence of the worms in the lymphatic system and the resultant tissue damage lead to swelling, scarring, bacterial infections, and a lung condition called **tropical pulmonary eosinophilia**. There are recurrent bouts of fever and patients experience heat, redness, and pain over infected lymphatic vessels. The reduced function of the lymphatic system causes fluid to accumulate and cause swellings (termed lymphoedema) in the arms, legs, breasts, and scrotum . The recurrent infections and inflammation can lead to hardening and thickening of the skin, which is termed elephantiasis because the swollen limbs with thick hard skin resemble those of elephants. Elephantiasis can lead to severe disfigurement, decreased mobility, and long-term disability. Additional features of *W. bancrofti* infection are fluid accumulation in the scrotum, a hydrocele, and chyluria, which is turbid urine containing emulsified fat or pus.

Life cycle of *L. loa*

During a blood meal an infected fly introduces third-stage larvae onto the skin surface of the human host. The larvae then enter the skin through the bite wound and mature into adults in the subcutaneous tissues, which takes about one year. Adult female worms are 40–70 mm long and males around 30 mm. The adults mate and produce microfilariae of a similar size to those of *W. bancrofti*. The *Chrysops* flies are diurnal feeders so the microfilariae are present in the peripheral blood during the day, and are mainly found in the lungs when not circulating. A feeding fly ingests microfilariae which moult and migrate from the gut to thoracic muscles via the haemocele. The microfilariae develop into first, second, and third-stage larvae, the latter being the infective stage that migrates to the fly's proboscis to infect a host at the next meal.

Clinical features of Loa loa filariasis

Some patients can be asymptomatic, whilst severe infections can result in encephalitis (brain inflammation), cardiomyopathy (inflamed heart muscle), and kidney failure.

The main clinical sign is puffy, diffuse subcutaneous swellings occurring predominantly on the limbs or face termed **Calabar swellings**, so-called because they were first recorded in 1895 in the coastal Nigerian town of Calabar. The swellings are red, itchy, and painful and arise from immune/allergic responses to worms migrating through subcutaneous tissues, to their metabolic products, or to dead worms. *L. loa* are sometimes referred to as the African eyeworm because they can be seen migrating across the conjunctiva. This does not cause loss of vision but can be irritating and painful; it takes about 15 minutes for a worm to cross an eyeball. Adult worms can cause hydrocele formation in the scrotum.

Laboratory detection of filariasis

Microfilariae can be isolated from peripheral blood, urine, hydrocele fluid, or biopsies. Blood specimens should be obtained based on the periodicity of the microfilariae in peripheral blood. The best time for phlebotomy in nocturnal periodicity is between 10.00 p.m. and 4.00 a.m. Parasites can be concentrated in blood samples by either passing through a filter or using Knott's technique of formalin centrifugation. Thick and thin blood films can be stained with Giemsa or haematoxylin.

Features of the sheath, cephalic space, and the presence/arrangement of nuclei in the tail (caudal nuclei) enable species identification. Pathogenic microfilariae are sheathed and non-pathogenic species are not. Not all sheaths stain with Giemsa, but they can be visualized by staining with haematoxylin. The main features of Giemsa-stained microfilariae of different species are outlined in Table 7.4 and examples of microfilariae appearances are shown in Figure 7.13.

TABLE 7.4 **Morphological features of microfilariae in Giemsa-stained blood films.**

Species	Sheath	Cephalic space	Column of caudal nuclei
W. bancrofti	Stains faintly	Short	Does not extend to tip of the tail
B. malayi	Bright pink	Long	Extends to tail tip; two isolated terminal nuclei separated by a constriction
B. timori	Does not stain	Longer than B. malayi	Greater number of single-file nuclei towards the tail than B. malayi
L. loa	Does not stain	Short	Long column of single nuclei extending to tip of tail
M. perstans	No sheath	Short	Extends to tip of a blunt tail
M. ozzardi	No sheath	Short	Does not extend to tip of the tail

BOX 7.11 *A practical tip*

Microfilariae can concentrate in the tails of a wedge blood film and eosinophilia is often present. In view of the occurrence of asymptomatic filariasis, a biomedical scientist encountering an unexpected eosinophilia should consider that parasites may be present and check the tails and edges for the presence of microfilariae.

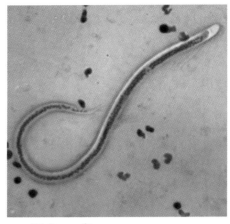

W. Bancrofti
(Thick film; x500 magnification)

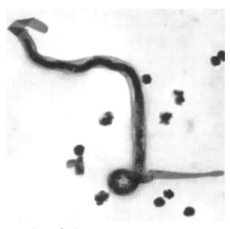

B. malayi
(Thick film; x500 magnification)

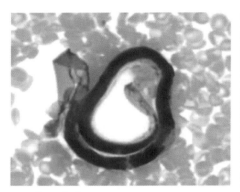

B. malayi
(Thin film; x500 magnification)

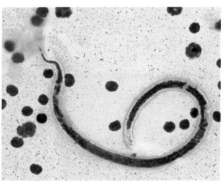

B. timori
(Thick film; x500 magnification)

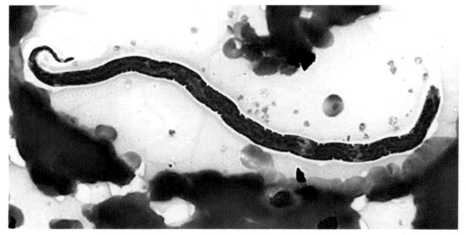

L. loa
(Thin film; x500 magnification)

FIGURE 7.13

Romanowsky stained microfilariae. Note the absence of red cells in the thick films and the presence of white cell nuclei.

Rapid immunochromatography assays are available to detect *W. bancrofti* antigens, and PCR techniques are available to distinguish between the two main causative organisms of lymphatic filariasis, *W. bancrofti* and *B. malayi*.

How are microfilariae differentiated in the laboratory?

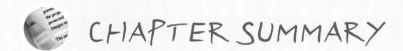 CHAPTER SUMMARY

- Human infective parasites with stages detectable in blood and bone marrow belong to the phyla Protozoa and Nematoda.

Malaria

- Malaria is a serious and sometimes fatal vector-borne infectious disease.

- The vectors for malaria are female *Anopheles* mosquitoes.

- The four main species of the protozoan genus *Plasmodium* that infect humans are: *P. falciparum*, *P. vivax*, *P. malariae*, and *P. ovale*.

- Once inside the human host the parasites enter hepatic, pulmonary, and red cell stages of the life cycle and reproduce asexually.

- The parasites undergo sexual reproduction in the mosquito.

- Synchronized release of parasites from red cells causes fever and haemolytic anaemia.

- *P. falciparum* infection is the most serious and potentially fatal.

- Some genetic disorders afford a degree of protection against malaria.

- The mainstay of laboratory detection and species differentiation of malaria is light microscopy.

- Supplementary diagnostic tools include rapid immunochromatography, quantitative buffy coat, PCR, and antibody assays.

Babesiosis

- Humans are incidental hosts to babesiosis parasites.

- The vectors are the Deer or Blacklegged tick (*Ixodes scapularis*) in the USA and the Sheep or Castor bean tick (*Ixodes ricinus*) in Europe.

- Babesiosis in Europe is mainly due to infection with *B. divergens*, and *B. microti* and *B. duncani* in the USA.

- Babesiosis is an intraerythrocytic, non-tropical, parasitic protozoan infection.

- *Babesia* parasites undergo unsynchronized release from red cells and cause a milder haemolytic anaemia than malaria. They do not re-infect vectors in human infection,

- The parasites are detected on thick and thin Giemsa-stained blood films. They have similarities to *P. falciparum* ring forms but Maltese Cross formations are diagnostic.

Trypanosomiasis

- There are two types of this parasitic protozoan disease—African and American trypanosomiasis, otherwise known as sleeping sickness and Chagas disease, respectively.

- In Africa, *T. brucei gambiense* and *T. brucei rhodesiense* are transmitted by the tsetse fly (*Glossina* species). In the Americas, *T. cruzi* is transmitted by nocturnal triatomine bugs.

- African trypanosomes travel in the bloodstream to organs such as the heart and replicate in the tissue fluid, and later invade the brain to cause the sleeping sickness.

- Triatomine bugs deposit parasites in their faeces onto the skin surface and the parasites enter the skin where they multiply and enter the bloodstream to travel to other tissues for further replication and ingestion by vectors.

- Trypanosomes are detected in blood samples by wet preparations and light microscopy. Quantitative buffy coat, xenodiagnosis, and PCR can also be used.

Leishmaniasis

- Protozoa of the genus *Leishmania* transmitted by female sandflies (*Phlebotomus* species) cause visceral and cutaneous leishmania in humans.

- Only the visceral form, also known as kala-azar, has life cycle stages associated with haemopoietic tissues and is due to infection by *L. donovani* or *L. infantum*.

- Parasites injected into the human host invade and divide in macrophages.

- The immune response of the host dictates the course of the disease.

- The parasites are detected by light microscopy of mainly bone marrow aspirates, but also splenic aspirate, lymph nodes, liver biopsy and peripheral blood buffy coat.

- Rapid immunochromatography assays, PCR techniques, and serological testing for antibodies can also be used.

Filariasis

- The nematode parasites *W. bancrofti*, *B. malayi*, and *B. timori* cause lymphatic filariasis and are transmitted to humans by mosquitoes of the genera *Culex*, *Anopheles*, *Mansonia*, and *Aedes*.

- Lymphatic filariasis is characterized by adult worms in the lymphatic system leading to swelling, scarring, bacterial infections, tropical pulmonary eosinophilia, and elephantiasis.

- The nematode parasite *L. loa* causes Loa loa filariasis and is transmitted to humans mainly by the Deerfly species of *C. silacea* and *C. dimidiata*.

- Adult *L. loa* live in subcutaneous tissues.

- Some individuals with Loa loa filariasis are asymptomatic whilst others develop the clinical disease, characterized by Calabar swellings.

- Adult filarial worms release microfilariae into the bloodstream to infect other tissues and to be ingested by feeding vectors.

- Microfilariae are detected microscopically from isolates of peripheral blood, urine, hydrocele fluid, or biopsies. Thick and thin blood films are stained with Giemsa or haematoxylin.

- Microfilariae are speciated based on features of the sheath, cephalic space, and presence/arrangement of nuclei in the tail (caudal nuclei).

- Rapid immunochromatography assays and PCR techniques are available to distinguish between *W. bancrofti* and *B. malayi*.

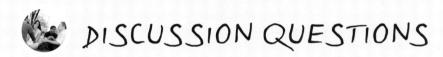

DISCUSSION QUESTIONS

7.1   Why are blood-borne parasites an evolutionary success?

7.2   Vector eradication can only ever be an unachievable social and medical ideal. Discuss.

7.3   Why does microscopy in the hands of an experienced scientist remain the mainstay of parasite detection and identification?

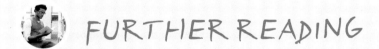

FURTHER READING

- **Hoffman SL, Abdalla SH, Pasvol G (ed.).** *Malaria: a Haematological Perspective*. Imperial College Press, London, 2004.

- http://www.malariasite.com

- **Bailey JW, Williams J, Bain BJ, Parker-Williams J, Chiodini P.** *Guideline: The Laboratory Diagnosis of Malaria*, 2005. British Society for Haematology website: http://www.bcshguidelines.com/pdf/Malaria2005.pdf

- **Bates I, Ekem I. Haematological aspects of tropical disease. In:** *Postgraduate Haematology*, 5th edn (ed. Hoffbrand AV, Catovsky D, Tuddenham EGD). Blackwell Publishing Ltd, Massachusetts–Oxford–Carlton, 2005.

Answers to self-check questions, case study questions, and discussion questions are provided in the book's Online Resource Centre, visit www.oxfordtextbooks.co.uk/orc/moore

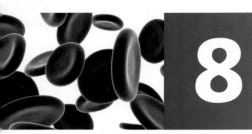

8

White blood cells in health and disease

Gavin Knight

The following chapter outlines the main types of white blood cell (WBC) encountered in the peripheral blood, their development, structure, and function.

The species of WBC that you will learn about in this chapter are neutrophils, lymphocytes, monocytes, eosinophils, basophils, and their precursors. Each of these species of WBC has a very particular function, and we can often suggest a differential diagnosis for a patient based on the way in which the WBCs are represented in the full blood count and their appearance using microscopy.

At the most basic level, WBCs are responsible for immunity through **phagocytic** means, through the production of antibodies which help in the destruction of foreign bodies, entering our system, or through cytotoxic mechanisms.

Broadly speaking, lymphocyte species called B cells and T cells are involved in adaptive immunity because they adapt to the specific antigens encountered, whereas other WBC species form part of our innate immune system, which treats all foreign antigens in the same way.

> **phagocytosis**
> The process of the ingestion and destruction of foreign and unwanted material, such as bacteria and effete red blood cells. Phagocytosis is performed by phagocytes principally neutrophils and monocyte macrophages.

Learning objectives

After studying this chapter you should be able to:

- Explain the functions of the different species of white blood cell.
- Describe the processes of maturation and differentiation of the different species of white blood cell.
- Describe Köhler illumination and explain how this method improves sample clarity when using microscopy.
- Draw the typical morphological characteristics of the different species of white blood cell and recognize the different species in a Romanowsky-stained blood film.
- Use the correct terminology to describe quantitative abnormalities in the WBC count.
- Describe some of the common causes of quantitative abnormalities in the WBC count.

8.1 Introduction

White blood cells (WBC), also known as leucocytes, are cellular components of the immune system. The concentration of white blood cells in the peripheral blood is usually maintained within tight limits, with a reference range of $4.0-10 \times 10^9$/L. The process of haemopoiesis was outlined in Chapter 3. Briefly, the pluripotent stem cell, under the influence of a number of growth factors and cytokines, undergoes the process of differentiation and maturation. Pluripotent stem cells can produce cells of erythroid, megakaryocytic, granulocytic, monocytic, and lymphoid lineages. However, this chapter is only concerned with the white cell components: granulocytes (neutrophils, eosinophils, and basophils), monocytes, and lymphocytes. The initial stages of white cell development occur in the bone marrow (BM), with maturation of all lineages—except a subset of lymphocytes called T lymphocytes—completing within the BM microenvironment. T lymphocytes require a stage of maturation within the thymus and migrate to this area of lymphoid tissue during development. With the exception of T lymphocytes, immature cells tend to remain within the bone marrow—which acts as a reservoir to subsidize the peripheral blood count if necessary. Because the myeloid precursors are held within the bone marrow, the bone marrow contains many more myeloid than erythroid cells where a ratio of between 2:1 and 12:1 in a normal adult bone marrow can be expected.

Cross reference

More detail regarding haemopoiesis can be found in Chapter 3.

8.2 Granulocytes

Granulocyte maturation

Granulocytes are WBCs that contain granules within their cytoplasm, and include neutrophils, eosinophils, and basophils. The process of granulocytic maturation involves a number of

BOX 8.1 Adult white blood cell count reference ranges

Total WBC count:	$4.0-10.0 \times 10^9$/L
Neutrophil:	$2.0-7.0 \times 10^9$/L
Lymphocyte:	$1.0-3.0 \times 10^9$/L
Monocyte:	$0.2-1.0 \times 10^9$/L
Eosinophil:	$0.02-0.5 \times 10^9$/L
Basophil:	$0.02-0.1 \times 10^9$/L

Some laboratories report their absolute cell counts as $\times 10^3$/μL and it is important to recognize the units used by your laboratory.

It is also important to recognise that reference ranges in your laboratory may be different, when interpreting result from patients in your laboratory, you must use your own local reference ranges.

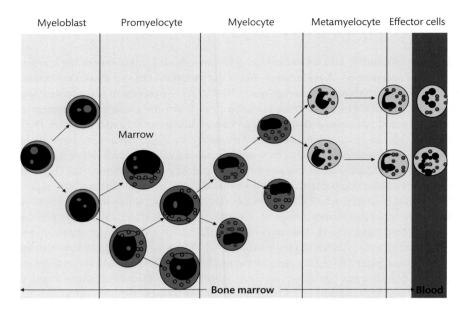

| Myeloblast | Promyelocyte | Myelocyte | Metamyelocyte | Effector cells |

Marrow

Bone marrow ——————————► Blood

FIGURE 8.1

Granulocyte maturation occurs within the bone marrow. Myeloblasts are shown on the far left. Cell division and maturation results in the production of larger promyelocytes. Promyelocytes demonstrate primary granules, but do not express species-specific characteristics. Promyelocyte division and maturation results in the myelocyte stage. Myelocytes contain species-specific granules and so morphologically can be identified as either neutrophil, eosinophil or basophil lineages. Myelocytes undergo further mitotic divisions before maturing into metamyelocytes. Metamyelocytes mature into effector cells without any further rounds of mitosis.

different stages, each relating to characteristic changes in cellular size, granularity, staining characteristics, and nuclear structure. The process of normal granulocyte differentiation and maturation occurs within the bone marrow, as shown in Figure 8.1. The earliest stage of concern in this chapter is called the **myeloblast** stage.

Myeloblasts

In a normal bone marrow up to 4% of cells are myeloblasts. Myeloblasts should not be apparent in the peripheral blood. These cells have a high **nucleocytoplasmic ratio**, i.e. the nucleus of the cell is almost as large as the cell itself, and a fine open lacy chromatin pattern is apparent, accompanied by prominent **nucleoli**. The cytoplasm of the cell stains a light shade of blue. The size of a myeloblast is 16 ± 4 μm.

The identification of myeloblasts in the bone marrow and peripheral blood is of great importance as increasing numbers can be suggestive of myeloid leukaemia. In the next chapters we will discuss leukaemias in greater detail and their association with an increased number of myeloblasts in the bone marrow and peripheral blood.

The next step in granulocytic development is the promyelocyte stage.

Promyelocytes

Promyelocytes are significantly larger than myeloblasts, measuring 20 ± 5 μm, although they demonstrate a lower nucleocytoplasmic ratio and occasional nucleoli. The cytoplasm has a deep blue coloration in comparison to the paler myeloblast, and contains primary granules. Primary granules

nucleolus (plural nucleoli)
An area of the nucleus composed of genes that encode ribosomal RNA, which is essential in the translation of transcribed proteins.

are retained in neutrophils, eosinophils, and basophils, and the function of these granules is identical in each of the cells outlined here. The nucleus of the promyelocyte is also slightly indented.

Promyelocytes should not be present in the peripheral blood. As we will see in the next chapter, an increase in the number of promyelocytes in the absence of other intermediate stages of maturation is associated with a subtype of acute myeloid leukaemia called acute promyelocytic leukaemia.

Cross reference
Chapter 9 gives more details on the development of acute leukaemia.

As promyelocytes mature, they become myelocytes.

Myelocytes

Myelocytes are smaller than promyelocytes, approximately 15 ± 5 μm in diameter, and they show evidence of chromatin clumping. Nucleoli are no longer visible. Secondary (or specific) granules are now present throughout the cytoplasm, enabling us to identify the granulocytic lineage to which these myelocytes belong. Secondary granules are so called because they are produced after the primary granules, and they possess a cell-specific function. Gradual changes in the structure of the myelocyte results in the metamyelocyte stage of maturation.

The myeloblast, promyelocyte, and myelocyte stages of maturation are all mitotic stages. At each of these stages, daughter cells are produced, so the larger the number of cells entering the cell cycle at the myeloblast stage, the greater the number of cells will become effector (mature) cells.

Metamyelocytes

Metamyelocytes contain distinctive primary and secondary granules. The nucleocytoplasmic ratio is much lower in metamyelocytes and the nucleus is kidney-shaped. As the metamyelocyte matures, the nucleus becomes increasingly curved, so that it almost resembles a horseshoe. Once the nucleus represents a horseshoe, these cells are no longer considered metamyelocytes, but are termed '**band forms**' or 'stab cells'.

band form (also called 'stab cells')
An immature granulocyte with a horseshoe-shaped nucleus.

Finally, the nucleus becomes segmented and the mature features of the **effector cell**—the neutrophil, eosinophil, or basophil—become apparent.

effector
A fully functional, mature cell.

SELF-CHECK 8.1

List the different stages of granulocyte maturation.

Neutrophils

In a healthy individual, early or intermediate stages of granulocyte maturation would not be expected within the peripheral blood, so only mature neutrophils, eosinophils, and basophils

BOX 8.2 *The dynamic morphology of granulocyte maturation*

An important concept to remember when examining the morphology of immature white blood cells is that the characteristic stages of development—myeloblast, promyelocyte, myelocyte, metamyelocyte, band form, and effector cell—are formed through a dynamic process. Each stage merges into another, so cells will often share features between different stages of maturation.

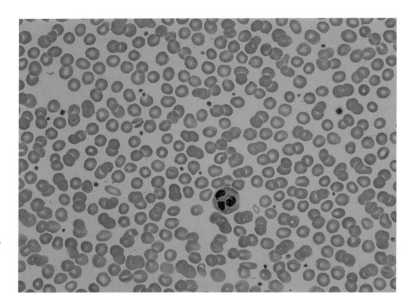

FIGURE 8.2

A mature neutrophil. Three nuclear lobes are joined by thin chromatin bridges, and cytoplasm shows azurophilic granules. Image courtesy of Jackie Warne, Haematology department, Queen Alexandra Hospital, Portsmouth.

should be found. Typical neutrophil morphology is shown in Figure 8.2. The reference range for neutrophils is $2-7 \times 10^9$/L. In reactive conditions such as inflammation or infection, less mature neutrophils may be found in the peripheral blood, with band forms becoming increasingly apparent as the reactive condition worsens.

A **leukaemoid reaction** may be found in the following: in very severe infections; as a response to certain cancers (carcinoma, melanoma, sarcomas, etc.); use of pharmaceuticals such as corticosteroids, minocycline, and myeloid growth factors; haemorrhage; haemolysis; and following alcoholic intoxication. A leucocyte count in excess of 50×10^9/L with all stages of myeloid maturation (including myeloblasts) being present defines a leukaemoid reaction. A leukaemoid reaction is very difficult to distinguish from chronic myeloid leukaemia and may be impossible to differentiate from chronic neutrophilic leukaemia. A leukaemoid reaction comprises polyclonal cells, whereas true leukaemia is composed of monoclonal cells. Providing the patient survives the inducing event, their leukaemoid reaction will resolve and blood counts will return to normal.

The process of **granulopoiesis** takes approximately 5–6 days to complete within the bone marrow.

SELF-CHECK 8.2

Define the term leukaemoid reaction.

As granulocytes mature, they are **sequestered** into the bone marrow storage compartment where they remain acting as a *reserve* to fight acute infection. As granulocytes are needed, they are released from this compartment into the peripheral blood where they will circulate for approximately 6–8 hours. Granulocytes are directed to the site of infection through the process of **chemotaxis**. Granulocytes can then adhere to the vascular endothelium prior to entering the tissues. This adherence to the vascular endothelium is called **margination** and is predominantly mediated by adhesion molecules such as L-selectin on leucocytes and E-selectin on endothelial cells. Marginating neutrophils can easily enter the tissues from their position on the vascular wall, where they can be involved in inflammation and phagocytosis.

Granulocytes, particularly neutrophils, can survive in the tissues for 2–3 days prior to cell death. The movement of granulocytes between the different compartments—bone marrow and reserve,

Cross references

Chronic myeloid leukaemia and chronic neutrophilic leukaemia are discussed in detail in Chapter 11.

Clonality is discussed in Chapter 9.

granulopoiesis

The growth, differentiation, and maturation of granulocytes.

sequester

To remove or separate.

chemotaxis

The process whereby chemical signals (for example, complement components C3a and C5a) and bacterial products (such as lipopolysaccharide) disseminate forming a concentration gradient for granulocytes to follow.

peripheral blood, and tissues—is a process of dynamic balance. As more granulocytes are required within a particular compartment, so more are released from reserves. The greater the pressure on the reserves, the greater the stimulus for proliferation within the bone marrow compartment.

In an acute setting, where tissue damage has occurred, neutrophils will be stimulated to enter the tissues from their marginating position. Rapidly, peripheral blood neutrophils will marginate to replace those entering the tissues, and will subsequently be replaced by the bone marrow reserve. Margination can happen very quickly, before the bone marrow can begin to synthesize a greater number of neutrophils. In this instance, a temporary reduction in the neutrophil count, called **neutropenia**, becomes apparent as all the neutrophils from the reserve have marginated in preparation for fighting the tissue infection. This neutropenia is short-lived, and as more neutrophils are synthesized, so they are released into the peripheral blood causing a rise in the neutrophil count. A neutrophil count in excess of the reference range is called a **neutrophilia**. These neutrophils will not have had time to mature within the bone marrow reserve, appearing in the peripheral blood as immature cells with large numbers of granules—they will be **left-shifted** and demonstrate **toxic granulation**, as shown in Figure 8.3.

Neutrophil lobes

A typical neutrophil has between three and five nuclear lobes connected to each other by thin strands of heterochromatin. A population of neutrophils showing an average of two nuclear lobes or fewer is considered **hyposegmented**. Conversely, a population of neutrophils where in excess of 3% of the total neutrophils show five nuclear lobes or more is considered **right-shifted** or **hypersegmented**.

Small regions of nuclear material protrude from the nucleus of neutrophils in females and some males. This excess nuclear material, called **drumsticks**, is consistent with an inactivated or **lyonized** X-chromosome.

left-shift

This describes an increase in the number of immature neutrophils within the peripheral blood.

toxic granulation

Occurs when neutrophils have been synthesized to fight an infection. The primary granules are more abundant in preparation for fighting infection and have a higher concentration of acid mucosubstances, which have prominent azurophilic-staining characteristics.

lyonization

Involves 'switching off' an X-chromosome in females through chromatin condensation. This chromatin condensation prevents the transcription and translation of genes contained within the additional X chromosome.

Cross reference

Hypersegmented neutrophils are introduced in the context of megaloblastic anaemias in Chapter 5.

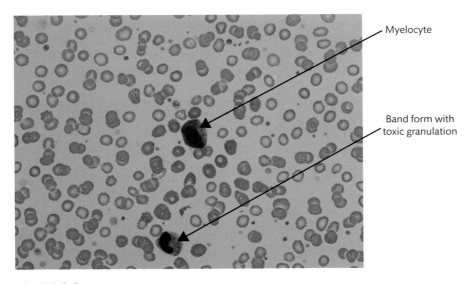

Myelocyte

Band form with toxic granulation

FIGURE 8.3

Left-shifted neutrophils. The cell at the bottom is a band form with toxic granulation and the large cell in the middle is a neutrophil myelocyte. Usually, myelocytes are not seen in the peripheral blood of a healthy individual; however, this patient is septic, with neutrophils and their precursors released in an attempt to combat the infection. Blood film also shows microcytic hypochromic red cells and rouleaux. Image courtesy of Jackie Warne, Haematology department, Queen Alexandra Hospital, Portsmouth.

It is important to make the distinction between left-shifted neutrophils and hyposegmented neutrophils. Left-shifted neutrophils are often a consequence of infection, inflammation, or pregnancy and denote an increased number of immature neutrophils or progenitors (myelocytes, metamyelocytes, and occasionally promyelocytes and myeloblasts) within the peripheral blood.

The **Pelger–Hüet anomaly** describes hyposegmented neutrophils with a singular or bilobed nucleus. The Pelger–Hüet anomaly may be inherited; most commonly, though, it will be seen as an acquired phenomenon, called the pseudo-Pelger–Hüet anomaly. In pseudo-Pelger–Hüet, the nucleus is usually bilobed, held together by a thin strand of chromatin, in what is referred to as the *pince-nez* configuration (named after circular spectacles with a pinching nose-bridge introduced in the 1840s). Pseudo-Pelger–Hüet neutrophils may also have a nucleus with a single lobe, often found in myelodysplastic syndrome.

Hypersegmented neutrophils may occur during infections, iron deficiency, and in **uraemic** patients. When a population of hypersegmented neutrophils is present, it is always important to consider whether the patient has any signs of vitamin B_{12} or folate deficiency. In patients with vitamin B_{12} or folate deficiency, megaloblastic anaemia develops. In these patients, DNA replication is often compromised and cell cycle arrest occurs within S-phase. Some of the neutrophils will be enlarged and contain twice as much DNA as normal. These enlarged neutrophils with increased DNA are called macropolycytes, as shown in Figure 8.4.

Neutrophil granulation

Primary and secondary granules are formed from the Golgi apparatus. Primary granules are synthesized at the promyelocyte stage of development and are found at the highest concentration within these cells. As the cell matures, and undergoes further cell divisions, the concentration of *primary* granules falls. During the myelocyte and metamyelocyte stages, in response to the myeloid transcription factor **C/EBPε**, synthesis of the antimicrobial containing *secondary* and *tertiary* granules occurs. C/EBPε-inducible antimicrobials may also be found in late primary granules, although formation of these primary granules ceases prior to the development of secondary and tertiary granules. Because the synthetic pathway of secondary granules is longer and occurs following the mitotic stages of development, secondary granules accumulate. More secondary granules are produced, providing the distinctive staining patterns used in the identification of different species of granulocytes and their precursors.

---

uraemia

The accumulation of urea within the blood.

C/EBPε

CCAAT enhancer binding protein is a factor important for the transcription of certain genes.

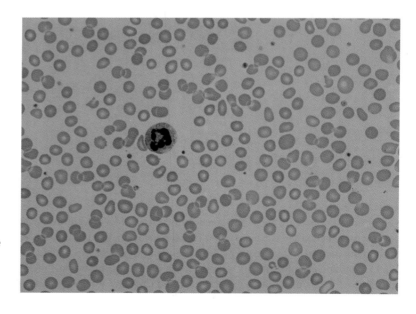

FIGURE 8.4

A macropolycyte in a patient with megaloblastic anaemia. The cell is much larger than a typical neutrophil, and contains excess DNA, which appears as a hypersegmented nucleus. Red cells should be macrocytic; however, in comparison to the macropolycyte, they appear small. Image courtesy of Jackie Warne, Haematology department, Queen Alexandra Hospital, Portsmouth.

Neutrophil granules contain approximately 300 different types of proteins, which are selectively distributed between the primary, secondary, and tertiary granules. These granules are released at different times, together orchestrating the neutrophil's multifaceted toxic response to foreign objects and inflammation.

Tertiary granules are **exocytosed** more readily than secondary granules, with gelatinase-containing granules exocytosed before gelatinase-negative granules. Finally, primary granules are exocytosed. The early release of gelatinase-containing granules is important as these facilitate the movement of the neutrophil through the vascular basement membrane prior to the release of bacteriostatic and bacteriocidal peptides.

exocytosis
Binding of cytoplasmic vesicles to the cell membrane leading to the release of the vesicle's contents into the extracellular environment.

SELF-CHECK 8.3

Outline the stages of granulocyte maturation in which the different types of granules are synthesized.

The identification of neutrophil granules is summarized in Figure 8.5.

A brief summary of some of the important peptides contained within the granules is provided below.

Primary granules

Myeloperoxidase (MPO) is a haem-containing enzyme important for the non-specific elimination of bacteria, viruses, and fungi. Hydrogen peroxide (H_2O_2) is generated by the membrane-bound NADPH oxidase following the reduction of oxygen to superoxide (O_2^-). Superoxide dismutates to H_2O_2 and is then utilized by MPO to form hypochlorous acid (HOCl), an important defence against a variety of microorganisms and viruses. MPO can also oxidize l-tyrosine to form tyrosyl radicals. Tyrosyl radicals have been shown to induce protein oxidation and lipid peroxidation, suggesting that host tissue damage can occur during acute inflammation.

Bacterial permeability-inducing factor (BPI) is a potent peptide with a binding specificity for lipopolysaccharide (LPS), and therefore exhibits specificity for Gram-negative bacteria, increasing bacterial membrane permeability and leading to cell death.

Lysozyme is an enzyme that can degrade the bacterial peptidoglycan cell wall by digesting the $\beta1 \rightarrow 4$ glycosidic bond between *N*-acetylglucosamine and *N*-acetylmuramic acid residues.

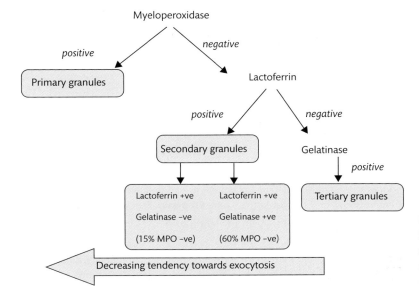

FIGURE 8.5
Differentiation between neutrophil granules based on myeloperoxidase, lactoferrin, and gelatinase components. Gelatinase may be found in approximately 60% of myeloperoxidase-negative granules.

Cross references

More detail of Gram-positive and Gram-negative bacteria can be found in the *Microbiology* text in this series.

Neutrophil elastase is discussed further in relation to the Kostmann syndrome later in this section.

Lysozyme is particularly effective at destroying Gram-positive bacteria, although it often requires cofactors such as lactoferrin, H_2O_2, or opsonins when directed against Gram-negative bacteria.

Sulphated mucopolysaccharides provide the azurophilic coloration of the primary granules.

Elastase is a highly destructive enzyme found within the primary granules. It has been shown to be particularly effective at degrading Gram-negative, but not Gram-positive, bacteria. The degradation of fungi and enterotoxins is also considered to be a vital role of elastase. Very high concentrations of elastase are found within primary granules, and are associated with significant tissue injury when released following degranulation.

Acid hydrolases include a wide range of different enzymes, including: acid phosphatase, β-galactosidase, β-glucuronidase, arylsulphatase, esterase, and mannosidase.

Secondary granules

Lactoferrin is an important enzyme which plays both bacteriostatic and bacteriocidal roles. A protein with a similar structure to transferrin, lactoferrin binds iron thereby preventing uptake by microorganisms. Lactoferrin may work in concert with lysozyme.

Lysozyme, as outlined in the 'Primary granules' section above.

Tertiary granules

Gelatinase is a matrix metalloproteinase capable of digesting denatured collagen, as well as intact collagen types IV and V. This digestive process enables neutrophils to migrate through the vessel basement membrane and enter the tissue fluid.

Secretory vesicles

Secretory vesicles are produced through the process of endocytosis during the final stages of neutrophil maturation in the bone marrow. They contain a variety of plasma proteins. Importantly, the membrane of the secretory vessel expresses a range of important adhesion proteins, alkaline phosphatase, and the complement regulator decay accelerating factor (DAF). Fusing of these secretory vesicles with the neutrophil membrane enables these proteins to be expressed on the cell surface, without the requirement for neutrophil degranulation.

In cases where toxic granulation is present, light microscopy may reveal the presence of **Döhle bodies**. Döhle bodies (Figure 8.6) are blue–grey in colour, appear as cytoplasmic inclusions, and are composed of remnants of endoplasmic reticular material.

Neutropenia

Neutropenia describes a reduction in the neutrophil count to below the lower end of the reference range. A neutrophil count of less than 0.5×10^9/L is considered serious as the risk of developing bacterial and fungal infections is high. At this neutrophil level, patients may be considered for isolation.

There are a number of causes of neutropenia, some more common than others. In the first instance, it is important to establish whether the patient has an isolated neutropenia, i.e. only their neutrophil count is low, or if the patient has **pancytopenia**. Pancytopenia is commonly associated with bone marrow failure and can be an indication or complication of malignancy.

pancytopenia

Describes a reduction in red cells, white cells, and platelets.

Isolated neutropenia can be drug-induced, immune in nature, or it can be a consequence of some viral or bacterial infections; particularly hepatitis virus HIV, and miliary tuberculosis. In addition, heredity may play an important role in some cases, with Kostmann's syndrome being the most common.

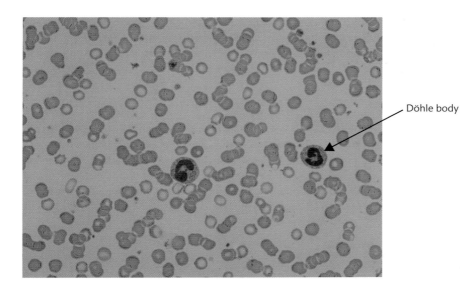

Döhle body

FIGURE 8.6

A female patient with sepsis. The neutrophil on the right shows a discrete blue patch in the upper right hand corner of the cytoplasm. This is a Döhle body. Of interest, the neutrophil in the centre has a drumstick protruding from the inner aspect of the nucleus. The red blood cells show significant rouleaux. Image courtesy of Jackie Warne, Haematology department, Queen Alexandra Hospital, Portsmouth.

BOX 8.3 *Neutropenia and ethnic variations*

A neutrophil count below the lower end of the reference range is considered neutropenia. This corresponds to a value below 2×10^9/L. However, it is important to consider ethnicity when interpreting low neutrophil counts, as Africans, Afro-caribbeans and those of Middle Eastern origin tend to have lower neutrophil counts; therefore the lower limit for such patients should be considered to be 1.5×10^9/L.

SELF-CHECK 8.4

Define neutropenia. Outline the medical risks for neutropenic patients.

Kostmann syndrome/severe combined neutropenia

This is a congenital neutropenia, commonly diagnosed within the first year of life following multiple severe bacterial infections or abscesses. Congenital neutropenia is associated with neutrophil counts typically below 0.2×10^9/L. Monocyte and eosinophil counts are often raised, leading to a white cell count within the reference range.

Kostmann syndrome is largely associated with mutations in the gene encoding neutrophil elastase (*ELA2*). Approximately 60% of all cases demonstrate *ELA2* mutations. These cases are either sporadic or are autosomal-dominant.

In autosomal-recessive neutropenia, as originally described by Kostmann, 30% of all patients demonstrate mutations in *HAX1*, the gene encoding HS-1 associated protein X (HAX). HAX plays an important role in regulating apoptosis. Deficiency of HAX1 predisposes these cells to apoptosis prior to their release from the bone marrow, and results in neutropenia.

Cases originally attributable to mutations in the granulocyte-colony stimulating factor (G-CSF) receptor have been shown to be somatic secondary mutations associated with Kostmann's syndrome, rather than causative.

There is a significant risk of patients with severe combined neutropenia developing myelodysplastic syndrome or acute myeloid leukaemia as part of the disease process. Both of these conditions are associated with significant morbidity and mortality and are discussed in detail in Chapter 11.

Cyclic neutropenia

This condition is characterized by oscillations in the neutrophil and monocyte counts. As the neutrophil count reaches its trough, often below the lower limit of the reference range, the monocyte count peaks, and vice versa. The oscillations are on a 21-day cycle. Bacterial infections are commonly encountered when the neutrophil count reaches its trough. G-CSF can be given to increase the neutrophil count during the trough period, thereby reducing the risk of infection. Mutations have also been identified in *ELA2*.

Autoimmune neutropenia

Autoimmune neutropenia can be divided into primary and secondary conditions. Primary autoimmune neutropenia is a very rare condition and will not be considered here.

Secondary autoimmune neutropenia is a common complication of drug therapy, malignancy, and can also be secondary to autoimmune diseases such as systemic lupus erythematosus (SLE).

Neutrophil destruction is likely to be due to the coating of neutrophils, called opsonization, with neutrophil-specific antibodies and complement components. These opsonized cells are then detected and removed by phagocytes in the spleen, liver, and bone marrow.

In secondary autoimmune neutropenia, prophylactic antibiotics are prescribed, and the patient may also be administered G-CSF to improve their neutrophil count. Ciclosporin A has been shown to improve the neutrophil count, although **splenectomy**—a reliable treatment for other autoimmune haematological disorders such as idiopathic thrombocytopenic purpura (ITP)—does not improve the neutropenia.

Neutrophil function

Neutrophils play the primary role in limiting the rate of microbial growth following infection. This antibacterial function is dependent upon both *oxidative mechanisms*, including the generation of hydrogen peroxide (H_2O), superoxide (O_2^-), hydroxyl radicals, nitric oxide, and *non-oxidative mechanisms* tending to be bacteriostatic. During infection, the process of inflammation is initiated. In the first instance, acute inflammation causes an increased permeability of blood vessels, initially mediated by histamine which is released by basophils, mast cells, and platelets.

Vasodilation

The increased vascular permeability initiated by histamine is important in mediating the efflux of neutrophils, monocytes, complement components, and antibodies from the circulation into the peripheral tissues. A second wave of vasodilation occurs in a histamine-independent manner, which is more prolonged and allows for a substantially increased migration of neutrophils from the peripheral blood into the area of infection.

The process of neutrophil migration from the blood to the tissues involves the neutrophil squeezing through the gap junctions between endothelial cells, a process called **diapedesis**, as shown in Figure 8.7. In order to successfully achieve an increased concentration of neutrophils within

splenectomy
The procedure of removing the spleen. The spleen is an important component of the reticuloendothelial system, playing a vital role in the removal of senescent red blood cells, bacteria, and virally infected cells. Splenectomy usually increases the lifespan of cells coated in immunoglobulin, and as such is a therapeutic option for individuals with autoimmune diseases of the haemopoietic system.

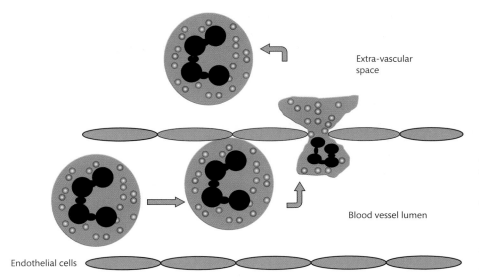

FIGURE 8.7
Diapedesis. Neutrophils adhere to the surface of the vascular endothelium, and migrate through the vascular wall via gap junctions between endothelial cells. Diapedesis enables neutrophils to access extra-vascular tissues to combat infection.

a particular area of the interstitial compartment, **chemotaxins** are required. Other mediators of vascular permeability include **kinins**, **prostaglandins**, **leukotrienes**, and the basic proteins found in neutrophil- and eosinophil-specific granules. Of note, in the latter stages of inflammation, neutrophils are replaced by other immune cells including macrophages and lymphocytes. Further detail of this process can be found in the *Immunology* text in this series.

Chemotaxis

Chemotaxis (Figure 8.8) is the process whereby cells move from one place to another when mediated by a chemical stimulus. Chemotaxis is a unidirectional process dependent upon one of five classes of compound:

- Products of bacteria
- Products of damaged tissue
- Complement factors C3a and C5a
- Neutrophil-derived products
- Plasma-derived chemicals

chemotaxins
Any group of small molecules that can induce chemotaxis.

kinins
A family of proteins that play an important role in inflammation, haemostasis, and pain.

prostaglandin
A lipid derived potent physiological mediator.

leukotrienes
A type of lipid related to prostacyclins involved in inflammation and allergic reactions.

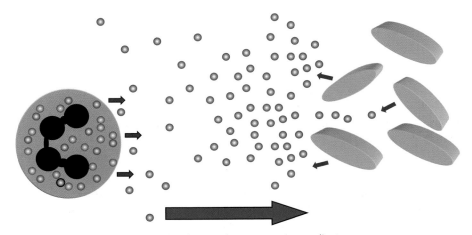

Increasing chemotaxin concentration gradient

FIGURE 8.8
Bacterial products are released (right) producing a concentration gradient. The highest concentration is at the source, becoming lower the greater the distance from the site of infection. Neutrophils can detect these concentration gradients and move towards the source in order to engage the infection.

Cross reference

More detail regarding the process of inflammation can be found in the *Immunology* text in this series.

lamellipodia

Lamellipodia are extensions of the cell cytoskeleton, and comprise actin projections which aid cell locomotion.

opsonins

Molecules coating the surface of cells which enhance the recognition and destruction of these coated cells by phagocytes.

FcγR

A receptor that recognizes a particular region (called the Fc region) on an IgG antibody.

Each of these compounds is released in a concentration gradient, with the highest concentration closest to the source, and with decreasing concentration the greater the distance from the origin. When neutrophils detect these chemotactic signals, they are able to move in straight lines against the concentration gradient by producing **lamellipodia**, the function of which is to help locomotion utilizing actin filaments. Repeated contraction and relaxation of these actin filaments is ATP-dependent.

SELF-CHECK 8.5

Describe the process of neutrophil migration from the peripheral blood to a site of infection.

The interaction between neutrophils and a bacterium

The interaction between neutrophils and bacteria is mediated by receptors on the surface of neutrophils that bind to **opsonins** coating the bacterium. The binding of specific antibodies (for example IgG) to the surface of the bacterium enables the neutrophil to interact with the bacterium via the **FcγR** receptor. Expressed on the neutrophil surface, FcγR signalling activates the neutrophil, leading to phagocytosis, degranulation, and **respiratory burst** activity.

Activation of phagocytosis involves the progressive manipulation of the neutrophil membrane, forming a vacuole which surrounds and internalizes the bacterium—called a **phagosome**. Fusion of neutrophil granules with the phagosome produces a phagolysosome, leading to the destruction of the ingested material, as shown in Figure 8.9.

During phagocytosis, the biochemical synthesis of bacteriotoxic compounds within the neutrophil is essential and these products must be directed to the phagosome in order to effectively kill the bacterium. Following phagocytosis, a huge increase in oxygen consumption occurs—called the respiratory burst—which allows the production of hydrogen peroxide and superoxide. Superoxide is generated through the increased availability of NADPH in response to a rising intracellular lactic acid concentration.

The phagocytic activity of neutrophils is clearly demonstrated in Figure 8.10, with this neutrophil engulfing cryoglobular material.

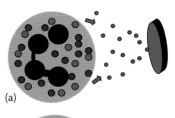
(a)

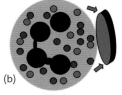
(b)

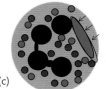
(c)

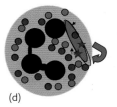
(d)

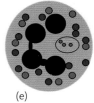
(e)

a. Chemotaxis

b. Binding to the bacterium

c. Engulfment & formation of a phagosome

d. Formation of the phagolysosome

e. Degradation of the bacterium

FIGURE 8.9

Formation of a phagolysosome. (a) Initially, neutrophils are attracted to a site of infection via a chemotactic concentration gradient. (b) Recognizing the bacterium as foreign, the neutrophil initiates phagocytosis. (c) Internalization of the bacterium within a membrane derived vacuole by the neutrophil produces a phagosome. (d) Fusion of lysosomes with the phagosome results in the formation of a phagolysosome and (e) Degradation of the bacterium.

Neutrophil   Intracellular cryoglobulin

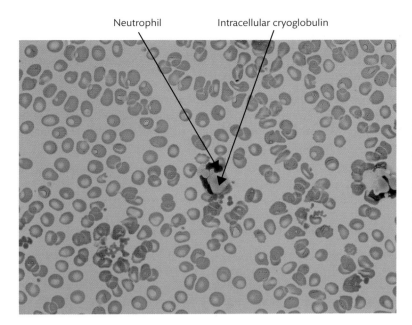

FIGURE 8.10
Neutrophils engulfing cryoglobulins. Cryoglobulin is a type of abnormal protein that precipitates at low temperatures and is usually found in patients with plasma cell related diseases. In this case, neutrophils have recognized cryoglobulins as abnormal and are utilizing their phagocytic properties in order to remove the cryoglobulin precipitates. In this case, the patient appears thrombocytopenic. Image courtesy of Jackie Warne, Haematology department, Queen Alexandra Hospital, Portsmouth.

Eosinophils

Eosinophils follow the same developmental pathway as neutrophils. However, their concentration in peripheral blood is much lower, with values expected to be within the region $0.02–0.5 \times 10^9$/L. From the myelocyte stage of maturation, eosinophil-specific granules start to form.

Eosinophils have a bilobed nucleus and large orange–red secondary granules which bind the stain eosin due to the high concentration of bactericidal arginine-rich basic proteins, including **major basic protein** (MBP), **eosinophil peroxidase**, and **eosinophil cationic protein** (ECP). Eosinophil-specific granules also contain **eosinophil-derived neurotoxin/eosinophil protein X** (EDN/EPX). These proteins are described in a little more detail in the following list:

MBP is known to disrupt the lipid bilayer of parasites and targets cells through interactions with anionic regions on these targets. This disruption results in an increase in membrane permeability and subsequent cell damage.

Eosinophil peroxidase is a haem-containing enzyme of the same family as myeloperoxidase. Eosinophil peroxidase is bactericidal and can form reactive singlet oxygen and hypobromous acid in the presence of H_2O_2 and bromide.

ECP also contains a large number of arginine residues and has ribonuclease (RNase) activity. Independent of its RNase function, ECP is known to be bactericidal and helminthotoxic (toxic to **helminths**) and can also induce degranulation of mast cells.

EDN/EPX are indistinguishable from one another and are actually believed to be the same protein. EDN/EPX is not restricted to eosinophils, but can also be found in basophils and monocytes. It has the same degree of bactericidal or helminthotoxic activity as ECP or MBP, although as the name suggests, EDN/EPX possesses neurotoxic activity.

helminth
A parasitic worm commonly found within the intestines.

SELF-CHECK 8.6

List the contents of eosinophilic secondary granules and provide, in note form, a one-sentence summary of the function of each.

Typical eosinophil morphology is shown in Figure 8.11.

Peripheral blood contains relatively few eosinophils in comparison to the bone marrow and tissues. Bone marrow holds significant reserves of eosinophils in the same manner as the neutrophils previously described.

Cross reference

T_{H2} cells are discussed in more detail in the T cell development section of this Chapter.

The development of eosinophils within the bone marrow is regulated by interleukin 3, interleukin 5 and GM-CSF. Interleukin 5, secreted by a subset of lymphocytes called CD4+T_{H2} cells, regulates eosinophils specifically and has been demonstrated to prolong their lifespan. This is an important feature, enabling eosinophils to fulfil their function in limiting helminth infections.

Eosinophils are known to be important mediators of allergic (hypersensitivity) reactions. In hypersensitivity reactions, eosinophils counteract the effects of basophils and mast cells. A number of compounds, including prostaglandins, inhibit the release of vasoactive amines from basophils and mast cells. Eosinophils also play a key role in the destruction of helminth parasite infections, including filariasis, hookworm, schistosomiasis, and trichinosis.

Charcot–Leyden crystal protein

A type of enzyme found within eosinophils and basophils that has the propensity to form crystals. Evidence of crystals in body fluids indicates allergy.

Individuals infected with the *Schistosoma* parasite, who have the disease schistosomiasis, demonstrate eosinophilia (meaning an increased number of eosinophils) in their peripheral blood. Following the opsonization of *Schistosoma* with IgG antibodies, eosinophils bind to the Fc fragment of the IgG using FcγR (receptors specific for the Fc fragment of IgG antibodies), inducing eosinophil degranulation and subsequent death of the helminth. Major basic protein, eosinophil peroxidase, eosinophil cationic protein, eosinophil-derived neurotoxin, and **Charcot–Leyden crystal protein** have all been shown to have a regulatory effect on helminth infections.

Eosinophilia describes an eosinophil count greater than 0.5×10^9/L—usually attributable to allergy or inflammation. However, in some situations an eosinophilia could be the consequence of Hodgkin lymphoma, chronic eosinophilic leukaemia, or idiopathic hypereosinophilic syndrome. In cases of prolonged eosinophilia, there is a significant risk of tissue damage following eosinophil degranulation. This tissue damage is characterized by tissue fibrosis and may ultimately lead to organ failure. In patients with prolonged eosinophilia, it is important to establish the cause and treat appropriately in an attempt to limit organ damage secondary to fibrosis. Figure 8.12 shows a blood film taken from a patient demonstrating eosinophilia.

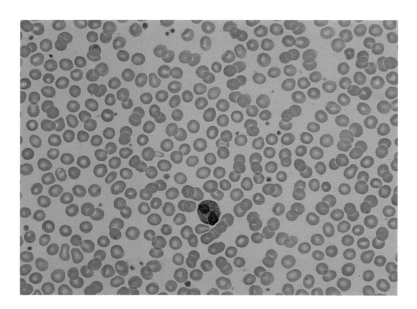

FIGURE 8.11

A typical eosinophil. The nucleus is bilobed, and there are distinctive orange (eosinophilic) granules within the cytoplasm. Image courtesy of Jackie Warne, Haematology department, Queen Alexandra Hospital, Portsmouth.

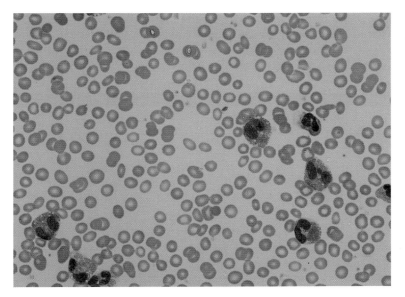

FIGURE 8.12
A patient with a severe allergy showing eosinophilia. Note the prominent orange granules within the cytoplasm of the eosinophils. Image courtesy of Jackie Warne, Haematology department, Queen Alexandra Hospital, Portsmouth.

Basophils

Basophils are the least common leucocyte in the peripheral blood with a concentration of $0.02–0.1 \times 10^9$/L. The nuclear structure of basophils is indented or comprises two nuclear lobes, and their cytoplasm is rich in purple–black granules, as shown in Figure 8.13. The granules are generally so large and numerous that they obscure the outline of the nucleus.

The basophil-specific granules contain acid mucopolysaccharides such as heparin, and large quantities of histamine. Degranulation of basophils results in the release of histamine and acute inflammation. As previously described, the release of histamine plays an important role in increasing vascular permeability.

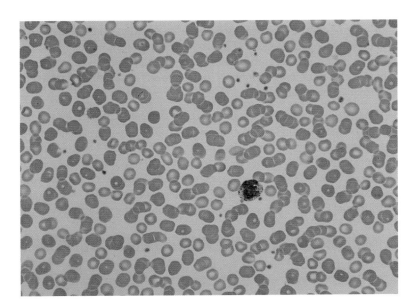

FIGURE 8.13
A normal basophil. Note the purple-black granules within the cytoplasm, and the indented shape of the nucleus. Image courtesy of Jackie Warne, Haematology department, Queen Alexandra Hospital, Portsmouth.

Cross reference
For further details about CML, please refer to the myeloproliferative neoplasms section in Chapter 11.

A basophil count of greater than 0.1×10^9/L is described as **basophilia**. A basophilia may be found in cases of acute hypersensitivity reactions, sometimes during viral infection, and may also be associated with haematological malignancies—in particular, chronic myeloid leukaemia (CML). Advancing CML is associated with progressive basophilia.

SELF-CHECK 8.7

Briefly describe the biological role of basophils.

8.3 Monocytes

Monocytes are found in the peripheral blood at a concentration of $0.2–1.0 \times 10^9$/L. The process of monocyte maturation is much simpler to follow than that of the granulocyte. Morphologically, monoblasts cannot readily be distinguished from the myeloblast, although as monoblasts mature they characteristically appear more like the monocytes we recognize in the peripheral blood.

SELF-CHECK 8.8

Outline the different stages of monocyte development.

A promonocyte is a large bone marrow derived cell with a large indented nucleus. Unlike pro-myelocytes, promonocytes tend not to demonstrate nucleoli and appear agranular using light microscopy. It takes approximately five days for the formation and release of a monocyte into the peripheral blood. Monopoiesis is outlined in Figure 8.14.

Monocytes have a large, highly indented, or C-shaped nucleus accompanied by greyish-blue cytoplasm and small numbers of azurophilic granules, the contents of which play an important role in the degradation of ingested particles. Typical monocyte morphology is demonstrated in Figure 8.15.

Monocytes are not effector cells, but rather a short (2–3 days) blood-borne stage in the development of tissue macrophages. In cases of infection, a monocytosis will often accompany a neutrophilia. The neutrophils act as the first line of defence against foreign pathogens, and monocytes are recruited to support neutrophils in the removal of pathogens and debris within the tissues to enable healing to occur.

Once monocytes enter the tissues, they mature to become macrophages, or histiocytes. Examples of macrophages include Küpffer cells of the kidney, lung alveolar macrophages and intraglomerular mesangial cells. Tissue macrophages continue synthesizing DNA and undergo mitosis. After several divisions, they can no longer undergo mitosis, and at this stage are considered to be mature macrophages. Mature macrophages may undergo the process of **endomitosis** until they produce *giant cells*, often found in areas of chronic inflammation. Unlike monocytes in the peripheral blood, macrophages may survive for months in the tissues.

endomitosis
A process involving the replication of a cell's nucleus in the absence of cytokinesis (cell division).

SELF-CHECK 8.9

Describe the process through which monocytes become giant cells.

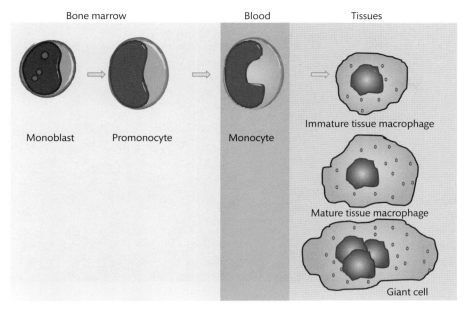

FIGURE 8.14

Monopoiesis. Monocytes begin the developmental process as monoblasts within the bone marrow. Mitosis and maturation result in the production of larger promonocytes. Promonocytes mature further into monocytes, which are typically found within the peripheral blood. Monocytes are an intermediate stage of maturation, and following exit from the blood vessel lumen into extravascular tissue, monocytes mature into tissue macrophages following a number of mitotic cycles.

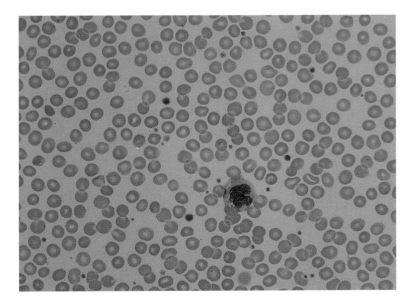

FIGURE 8.15

Peripheral blood monocyte. This monocyte has a characteristic c-shaped nucleus with pale blue cytoplasm. The cytoplasm in this monocyte contains vacuoles. Image courtesy of Jackie Warne, Haematology department, Queen Alexandra Hospital, Portsmouth.

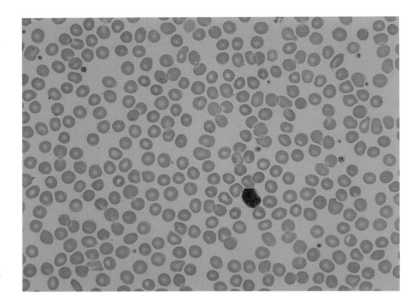

FIGURE 8.16

A single lymphocyte. The nucleus occupies the majority of the cell, with a thin, scanty rim of light blue cytoplasm to the periphery. Image courtesy of Jackie Warne, Haematology department, Queen Alexandra Hospital, Portsmouth.

8.4 Lymphocytes

Lymphocytes are mononuclear cells of variable size and are the second most abundant type of leucocyte found in the peripheral blood, accounting for 20–40% (1.0–3.0 × 10^9/L) of nucleated cells. Approximately 75% of circulating lymphocytes are T cells, although morphologically, differentiation between T cells and B cells cannot be accomplished reliably using Romanowsky-stained blood films. Between 10 and 15% of lymphocytes are B cells and the remaining 10–15% are **large granular lymphocytes (LGL)**.

Small lymphocytes have a round nucleus and a thin, often described as 'scanty', rim of cytoplasm with condensed chromatin. *Large lymphocytes* tend to have abundant cytoplasm with a more open, almost lacy, chromatin configuration. The cytoplasm of lymphocytes has a blue coloration when exposed to Romanowsky stain. Following activation, the cytoplasm becomes basophilic.

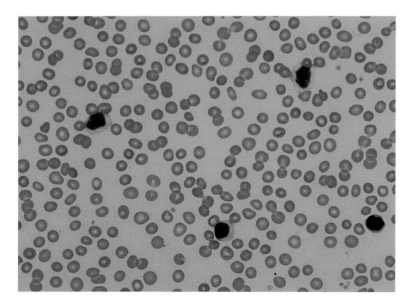

FIGURE 8.17

NK-cell leukaemia. Large numbers of circulating NK cells can be seen. Note the voluminous cytoplasm with the cytoplasmic granules when compared with the normal lymphocyte in 8.16. Image courtesy of Jackie Warne, Haematology department, Queen Alexandra Hospital, Portsmouth.

Typical lymphocyte morphology is shown in Figure 8.16.

Between 10 and 15% of lymphocytes are called large granular lymphocytes because they are larger than the average lymphocyte and include cytoplasmic azurophilic granules. The LGL population includes *natural-killer (NK) cells*, important in antibody-dependent, cell-mediated cytotoxicity, and also in the destruction of infected cells.

Figure 8.17 shows a photomicrograph of a blood film of a patient diagnosed with NK-cell leukaemia. Although the morphology is not quite representative of a normal NK cell, cytoplasmic granules are present within the cytoplasm of these lymphoid cells.

A raised peripheral blood lymphocyte count (called **lymphocytosis**) is often associated with viral infections, but may also been seen in bacterial infections and some haematological malignancies. Following activation, lymphocytes are described as '*reactive*' because, in the case of B cells, they begin to synthesize and secrete immunoglobulin, leading to the development of cytoplasmic basophilia. Antibody synthesis is the first step in the process leading to **plasma cell** formation—antibody secreting cells localized within the lymphoid tissues.

plasma cell
Antibody secreting terminal stage in B cell maturation following exposure to antigen.

BOX 8.4 *Describing white blood cell numerical abnormalities*

It is always important to use the correct terminology when describing quantitative abnormalities of white blood cells.

The prefix to the noun always denotes the species of white blood cell being described, whereas the suffix (emboldened below) denotes the quantitative abnormality.

So for an increased cell number, cell names ending in –phil become –philia, whereas cell names ending in –cyte become –cytosis:

Neutro**philia** = increased neutrophils

Eosino**philia** = increased eosinophils

Baso**philia** = increased basophils

Monocy**tosis** = increased monocytes

Lymphocy**tosis** = increased lymphocytes

Leucocy**tosis** = increased number of white cells

For a decrease in cell numbers, the suffix becomes –penia:

Neutro**penia** = decreased neutrophil count

Eosino**penia** = decreased eosinophil count

Baso**penia** = decreased basophil count

Monocyto**penia** = decreased monocyte count

Lympho**penia** = decreased lymphocyte count

Leuco**penia**—decreased white cell count

A reduced lymphocyte count (called lymphopenia) is a relatively common finding usually associated with acute disease such as trauma or infection, and may also be found in patients with immunosuppression. It is important to establish the cause of the lymphopenia, and to consider whether the patient is immunosuppressed.

Lymphocyte development

lymphopoiesis

The growth, differentiation, and maturation of lymphocytes within primary lymphoid organs.

Comprehensive coverage of **lymphopoiesis** is provided in the *Immunology* text in this series, although the development of lymphocytes will be addressed here in sufficient detail to provide a background for haematologists.

Lymphocytes provide the body with *adaptive immunity*. Adaptive immunity allows the body to develop a specific, tailored response to foreign antigens.

Cross reference

More detail regarding the process of lymphopoiesis can be found in the *Immunology* text in this series.

The process of lymphocyte development begins at the stem cell stage within the fetal liver and adult bone marrow. The haemopoietic stem cell differentiates into *common lymphocyte progenitors* (CLP). Exposure of CLP to a variety of lymphoid-specific cytokines selects for either a population of B cells (so-called because B cells were discovered in birds in the Bursa of Fabricius) or T cells. T cells are so-called because they require a stage of maturation within the thymus, whereas B cells develop within the bone marrow. Because the bone marrow and thymus are the initial sites for the development of B and T cells, they are called **primary lymphoid organs**.

Cross reference

More information on immunophenotyping can be found in Chapter 10 of this book.

B cell maturation

The first recognizable stage in the development of a B cell is the *progenitor (Pro)B cell*. The development of pro-B cells to **pre-B cells** requires interaction with bone marrow stromal cells. The pre-B cell shows evidence of immunoglobulin M (IgM) heavy-chain synthesis within the cytoplasm. Immunoglobulins are composed of two identical heavy chains and two identical light chains. As pre-B cells mature, light chains are synthesized and combine with the heavy chains, forming a complete surface-bound, **B-cell receptor (BCR)**. At this stage, the cell is called an **immature B cell**. Further changes to the B cell result in the surface expression of IgD. Co-expression of IgM and IgD surface receptors is found on **mature B cells** released from the bone marrow into the peripheral blood. These mature B cells are called **naïve B cells** (also unactivated or virgin B cells) because they have yet to encounter antigen. Stages of B-cell maturation can be determined by measuring the expression of different proteins on the cell surface by flow cytometry (immunophenotyping).

B-cell receptor (BCR)

The term BCR should be used with caution as it is context specific. In the context of immunology BCR represents the B-cell receptor, whereas in cytogenetics BCR represents breakpoint cluster regions.

SELF-CHECK 8.10

Describe the pattern of surface immunoglobulin expression throughout B-cell development.

B cell activation depends upon the interaction of a specific antigen and the structure and composition of that activating antigen. B-cell activation can be either:

- Thymus-dependent—requiring T cells to produce effector B cells; or
- Thymus-independent—not requiring T cells for the production of effector B cells.

The activation of B cells results in the development of highly proliferative behaviour, enabling the expansion of the activated B cell into a population of antibody synthesizing and secreting B cells.

variable region (or 'v region')

A region of an antibody that binds to an epitope on an antigen. All antibodies secreted by a particular plasma cell have the same variable region, although antibodies synthesized by different plasma cells have dissimilar variable regions.

As activated B cells proliferate, certain Ig-specific genes encoding the **variable region** of the BCR undergo point mutation—called **somatic hypermutation** (SHM) (see Box 8.5). The variable region of an Ig generates antigen-binding diversity within a specific class of antibody.

BOX 8.5 *Antibodies and somatic hypermutation*

An antibody contains two heavy chains and two light chains, each of which is composed of domains. The light chains (known as κ and λ based on their structure) contain a single constant domain (C_L) and a variable domain (V_L). Depending on the class of antibody produced, heavy chains contain three or four constant domains (C_H) and a single variable domain (V_H). Within the variable domains of the two chains, the **complementarity determining region** (CDR) is found. This CDR contains the antigen-combining site and provides the antibody or BCR with its specificity. Somatic hypermutation occurs within the CDRs following the interaction of a complementary antigen to a specific naive B cell. Somatic hypermutation increases the affinity of the CDR for the antigen, improving the effectiveness of the immune response.

Assessing V_H hypermutation plays an important role in establishing prognosis in certain B-cell malignancies. In B cell chronic lymphocytic leukaemia (B-CLL), malignant lymphocytes showing evidence of somatic hypermutation have been correlated with a good prognosis when compared with patients failing to show evidence of somatic hypermutation.

Complementarity determining region
The region of an antibody that complements the structure of its associated antigen.

Cross reference
For more information regarding CLL, see Chapter 12.

Somatic hypermutation occurs within a region of lymphoid tissue called the germinal centre. A germinal centre is illustrated in Figure 8.18. Cells undergoing somatic hypermutation are called **centroblasts**. Somatic hypermutation alters the amino acid sequence within the antigen-binding site of the variable region of an Ig in order to improve the specificity of the BCR for the stimulating antigen. In addition to somatic hypermutation, centroblasts undergo **class-switching recombination** (CSR), a process necessary for generating different types of immunoglobulin (particularly IgG and IgA). Combining CSR and SHM generates highly specific and reactive antibodies.

Following somatic hypermutation and CSR, **centrocytes** (as they are called at this stage), migrate to regions of secondary lymphoid organs where **follicular dendritic cells** (FDC) are concentrated. FDCs express antigen, and are one of a number of different types of **antigen-presenting cell** (APC). B cells expressing receptors with the highest affinity for the antigens presented on the FDC will be selected, expanding the population of B cells specific for that antigen. B cells expressing non-functional receptors or receptors with a weak affinity for the presented peptide will undergo apoptosis.

centroblasts
Highly proliferative cells found within the early germinal centre following antigenic stimulation.

class-switching recombination
The process of generating different types of immunoglobulin

centrocyte
A small non-dividing cell found within the germinal centre. The nucleus contains a cleft.

follicular dendritic cell
A cell with long branching processes found within lymphoid follicles. FDCs are important for enabling B-cell maturation.

antigen-presenting cell
Any cell that expresses MHC class II and can present antigenic material to elicit a T-cell response.

SELF-CHECK 8.11

Describe the process of somatic hypermutation and explain how this process alters the affinity of antibodies for their target antigens.

Following positive selection by FDCs, plasma cells are produced—secreting clones of antigen-specific antibodies. The lifespan of plasma cells is approximately 14 days, and in order for long-lived immunity to develop, a proportion of centrocytes must mature into **memory cells**. Memory cells provide a long-term record of previously encountered antigens, allowing a secondary immune response to occur following interaction with a previously recognized antigen.

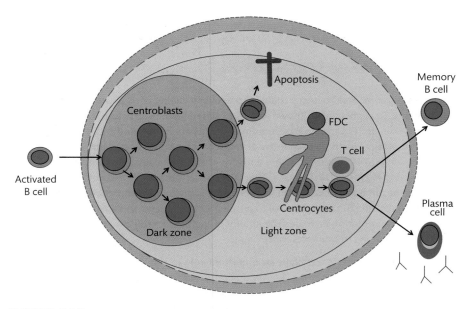

FIGURE 8.18

Structure of a germinal centre. Activated B cells enter the germinal centre from the T zone. Inside the germinal centre, the B cells become larger and, now called centroblasts, undergo repeated rounds of cell division and hypermutation in the variable region of an Ig within the dark zone. Following cell division, centrocytes enter the light zone where—if they encounter follicular dendritic cells—they survive, otherwise they are signalled for apoptosis.

A final encounter with antigen specific T cells is required before memory cells and plasma cells are produced.

BOX 8.6 *The germinal centre*

Germinal centres are found within lymphoid follicles. Following B-cell activation within an intrafollicular area, the B cell will enter a primary lymphoid follicle and begin to proliferate. Within three days a germinal centre forms and acts as a 'nursery' for the developing centroblasts. The germinal centre is composed of two distinctive anatomical sites: the *dark zone* and the *light zone*. Within the dark zone are actively proliferating centroblasts. As these centroblasts reduce their rate of proliferation, they migrate to the light zone. Within the light zone, non-proliferating centrocytes (as the developing centroblasts are called at this stage) interact with large numbers of follicular dendritic cells (FDC) and T_H cells (helper T cells, described in the next section). Centrocytes failing to appropriately interact with HLA-expressed antigenic peptides undergo apoptosis, ensuring only effective centrocytes remain. Finally the FDC-selected centrocytes mature into either antibody-secreting plasma cells or memory B cells.

T-cell development

T cells play a central role in the regulation of the immune system. Immature T cells leave the bone marrow or fetal liver and enter the peripheral blood. From here, immature T cells enter the thymus and are called **thymocytes**, where they will develop the surface expression of mature T-cell CD markers. On the thymocyte surface, specific molecules are expressed to enable T-cell function. T-cell receptors (TCR) are expressed on the T-cell surface following the selection of variable-genes encoding the TCR. T-cell receptors show diversity matched only by the BCR, with each T cell specific for a different antigen. The ability to select different variable region genes and combine these provides antigen-specific diversity, enabling an adaptive immune system to develop and function.

Accompanying the TCR is CD3, a protein essential for the transduction of signals into the cell following the binding of the TCR to its complementary antigen. In addition, CD4 and CD8 are co-expressed on the T-cell surface. These proteins interact with HLA (human leucocyte antigen) class II and HLA class I molecules, respectively.

Thymic selection then occurs, producing single positive CD4+ or single positive CD8+ thymocytes.

Not all T cells will develop into peripheral T cells (those found within the peripheral blood). The interaction of CD4+ and CD8+ thymocytes with each class of HLA molecules enables **self-peptides** to be presented to the thymocytes. In order to function correctly, thymocytes need to recognize and interact with HLA but should not recognize self-peptides—as in auto-immune diseases, where this process is dysregulated. Thymocytes failing to bind to HLA, or those binding to HLA too strongly—or avidly—are signalled for apoptosis. This process ensures that approximately 75% of thymocytes are lost during development, but those that survive are 'fit-for-purpose'.

self-peptides
These are short protein sequences presented to developing lymphocytes in order to inactivate self-reactive lymphocytes.

T-cell subtypes include helper T cells (T_H), cytotoxic T cells (T_C), suppressor T cells, and large granular lymphocytes (LGL), each having different functions. These functions are outlined below:

Helper T cells are subdivided into two types: T_H1 and T_H2. T_H1 cells promote the action of macrophages and another subtype of T cell called cytotoxic T cells (T_C). Interleukin 2 (IL-2) and gamma-interferon (IFN-γ) are secreted by T_H1 cells modulating cell-mediated immunity. B-cell activation and maturation is mediated by the T_H2 subsets through the secretion of IL-4 and IL-10.

Cytotoxic T cells express surface CD8 (abbreviated to CD8^+T_C), which interacts with HLA class I. HLA class I is expressed on most cells of the body, and therefore provides an excellent tissue non-specific way of presenting viral peptides to CD8^+T_C cells in order to induce cellular destruction. In contrast, HLA class II is expressed on cells of the immune system only.

The cytoplasm of T_C contains granules which are directed to the site of receptor binding following interaction between HLA class I-presented peptides, and CD8. Degranulation of T_C causes the release of perforins and serine proteases called granzymes, causing osmotic lysis and apoptosis of infected cells.

We have previously described the morphological appearance of LGLs. Of this LGL population, natural killer (NK) cells have an important function. NK cells express neither TCR nor BCR, but they are able to recognize antigens without being restricted in their function by antigen-specificity. Being cytotoxic T cells, NK cells have the ability to destroy infected cells through a process called *antibody-directed cellular cytotoxicity* (ADCC). Receptors to IgG antibodies, called FcγR—expressed on the NK cell surface—bind to antigen-bound IgG antibodies. Internal granular rearrangement within the NK cell focuses granules onto the area in which the antibody is bound, initiating degranulation and releasing perforins and granzymes.

SELF-CHECK 8.12

Outline the role of cytotoxic T cells (T_C) in controlling bacterial infections.

Interactions between B and T cells

B cells are particularly efficient antigen-presenting cells. The expression of antigenic peptides by HLA class II activates antigen-specific $CD4^+T_H$ cells. Binding to HLA class II-presented peptides enables $CD4^+T_H$ cells to secrete a range of cytokines which transform and activate B cells. Co-activation of the B cell through the interaction of CD40 and T cell expressed CD40L (L=ligand) is required to prevent B-cell apoptosis.

Now that lymphocytes and their subsets have been considered in some detail, we should examine some of the causes of numerical, morphological, and functional abnormalities of lymphocytes.

Infectious mononucleosis

Infectious mononucleosis (IM) is a benign **lymphoproliferative** disorder characterized by an *Epstein–Barr virus* (EBV)-mediated infection of B cells. EBV is a member of the human herpesvirus family that utilizes the CD21 receptor on the lymphocyte membrane to enter B cells. Infected B cells express viral antigens on their surface, initiating a rapid cytotoxic T-cell response and latterly—following B-cell activation—the production of EBV-specific antibodies.

EBV epidemiology

EBV infection occurs commonly in two defined age ranges: children aged 1–6 years, and individuals aged 14–20 years. EBV is spread through the saliva of infected individuals, and viral particles have also been identified in other bodily fluids. IM is commonly referred to as 'the kissing disease' because of the association between viral spread and this popular pastime amongst teenagers. Worldwide, approximately 80–90% of adults are **seropositive**, providing evidence of previous infection. Following an acute phase, EBV infection becomes latent, with the virus persisting in the patient for the remainder of their life. The immune system prevents the re-emergence of the virus, although when immunosuppression occurs re-emergence of the EBV infection can be detected.

Symptoms associated with infectious mononucleosis

Typically, symptomatic patients present with fever, malaise, and chills—which later develop into sore throat, **pharyngitis**, **exudative tonsillitis**, **palatal petechiae**, stiff neck, abdominal pain, and **lymphadenopathy**. In approximately 50% of cases, splenomegaly is apparent. Patients exhibiting splenomegaly should avoid strenuous activity due to the risk of splenic rupture—a severe and potentially life-threatening complication of IM. Approximately 50% of patients will be asymptomatic.

Differential diagnoses include cytomegalovirus (CMV), toxoplasmosis, streptococcal pharyngitis, and human immunodeficiency virus (HIV). These infections will be discussed in greater detail later in this section.

Laboratory investigations

The first step in the investigation of a patient with suspected IM is a full blood count, blood film, and heterophile antibody test. The full blood count will reveal a leucocytosis, often ranging from 12 to 25×10^9/L, predominantly composed of lymphocytes. Approximately 75% of lymphocytes are T cells. Lymphocytosis will usually occur after one week following the appearance of symptoms, peaking during the second or third week and lasting for up to eight weeks. Lymphocyte morphology is referred to as 'atypical' or 'reactive', and scalloping of the lymphocyte membrane around neighbouring red cells can be seen. Figure 8.19 shows a typical blood picture for a patient with IM as described above. The patient may also be neutropenic and thrombocytopenic.

Patients with IM develop **heterophile antibodies** called Paul–Bunnell antibodies. Heterophile antibodies do not react with human red cells, although they do cause agglutination of sheep, ox,

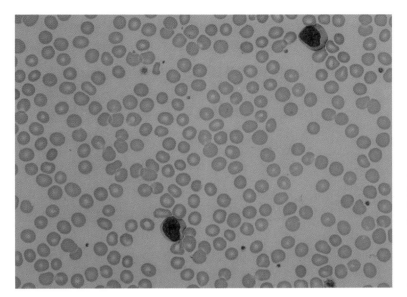

FIGURE 8.19

Blood film for a patient diagnosed with infectious mononucleosis. Two atypical lymphocytes are demonstrated, each with basophilic cytoplasm and one with membrane scalloping around juxtaposing red blood cells. Image courtesy of Sarah Bruty and Amelia Fitzpatrick, Haematology department, Southampton General Hospital.

and horse red blood cells. Other types of heterophile antibody, called **Forssman antibodies**, are not associated with IM, although they do occur in response to a range of infectious agents. Differentially, Forssman antibodies bind to guinea-pig kidney cells but not ox red cells, whereas IM heterophile antibodies react in the opposite fashion, binding to ox red cells but not guinea-pig red cells, see Table 8.1. The identification of non-Forssman heterophile antibodies provides a diagnosis of IM.

Testing for heterophile antibodies involves comparing the agglutination of horse red cells following mixing predetermined volumes of patient plasma with ground guinea-pig kidney cells and ox red cells. In patients with IM, stronger reactions are seen in the test containing guinea-pig kidney cells as Paul–Bunnell (PB) antibodies *are not* adsorbed by these cells. The ox cells *do* absorb PB antibodies, leaving fewer antibodies available to agglutinate the horse red cells. The opposite reaction occurs in the presence of Forssman antibodies.

A number of scientific reagent manufacturers have now developed tests for heterophile antibodies using latex agglutination techniques to differentiate between PB antibodies, Forssman antibodies, and others shown to react with multiple species. The specificity of latex agglutination tests means that differential absorption is no longer required to remove non-PB heterophile antibodies prior to testing, making latex agglutination tests much quicker and easier to use. Latex agglutination test results are shown in Figure 8.20.

It is important to recognize the limitations of the tests available. In patients infected with EBV under the age of four years, 50% fail to demonstrate PB antibodies. In older patients 71–91% of

Forssman antigen

A glycosphingolipid found on cell membranes in many different species. Antibodies directed against Forssman antigens are caused by a number of infectious agents, although they are not associated with infectious mononucleosis.

TABLE 8.1 The different patterns of antibody absorbance between heterophile antibodies.

Cell origin	Antibody reaction	
	Forssman	Paul–Bunnell
Ox cells	negative	positive
Guinea pig cells	positive	negative

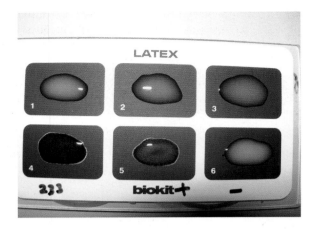

FIGURE 8.20

Results from a Biokit latex agglutination text. The two marked (+) and (−) are positive and negative controls. Note the patient next to the positive control (position 4). Clearly agglutination has occurred following the addition of patient plasma to the latex. This patient is diagnosed with infectious mononucleosis. All other patients on this slide are negative. Courtesy of Ann Figes, Haematology department, Royal Bournemouth Hospital.

patients exhibit PB antibodies. It is important to try to detect these antibodies at the appropriate stage in the infection to reduce the risk of obtaining a false-negative result. During the first week of infection, the false-negative rate could be as high as 25%, dropping to 5–10% in the second week. In the third week, false-negative results could still be as high as 5%.

Antibodies synthesized against the EBV-mediated antigens—*viral capsid antigen* (VCA) and *EBV nuclear antigen* (EBNA) are far more specific for diagnosing EBV infection, and are particularly useful in patients where there is a strong clinical indication of IM, but a negative PB antibody test. The acute phase of IM is associated with the presence of IgM antibodies called anti-VCA (VCA-IM), up to four months following infection. In the 3–12 months post infection, IgG anti-VCA (VCA-Ig) will be detectable and, once present, these IgG antibodies persist for life. Anti-EBNA will be present after the first 6–8 weeks and will also be present for life.

SELF-CHECK 8.13

Describe the findings you would expect from a patient referred to a haematology laboratory with suspected infectious mononucleosis.

Treating infectious mononucleosis

Patients diagnosed with IM are generally directed to rest and take analgesics such as paracetamol, aspirin, or ibuprofen to alleviate the symptoms. In approximately 30% of cases, IM is complicated with a concurrent β-haemolytic streptococcal infection. In these cases, the antibiotic amoxicillin may be prescribed, although there is a risk of skin rashes attributable to the formation of circulating immune complexes. These rashes resolve following withdrawal of the antibiotic.

Cytomegalovirus

CMV is a human β-herpesvirus transmitted through saliva, breast milk, sexual contact, placental transfer, and organ (including bone marrow) transplantation. Up to 70% of the population in industrialized nations is seropositive for CMV, although this figure is much higher in low socio-economic groups, homosexuals, and in developing countries. As with EBV, following the primary infection, CMV becomes latent, persisting lifelong and being controlled by the host's immune system. Dysregulation of the immune system can result in the re-emergence of CMV infection, with the largest reservoir of the virus comprising the myeloid compartment of the bone marrow.

immunocompetent

Describes a fully functioning immune system.

Immunocompetent, seronegative patients exposed to CMV generally exhibit many of the same symptoms as IM, outlined above. The majority of patients tend not to demonstrate pharyngitis, tonsillitis, or splenomegaly to the same extent, and in some cases describe the symptoms as 'flu-like'. In teenagers and older children there is no benefit in distinguishing these conditions. However, when encountered in pregnancy it is important to differentiate between the diagnosis of EBV, CMV, and toxoplasmosis, since CMV and toxoplasmosis can affect fetal development.

In pregnancy, CMV can cross the placenta, leading to congenital CMV. CMV is the most common congenital infection in the developed world, being identified in up to 6% of live births. In order to classify CMV as a congenital infection, it must be isolated within the first three weeks of life, otherwise CMV is considered the product of a postnatal infection.

Approximately 17% of patients with congenital CMV are asymptomatic, although those demonstrating clinical features may show hepatosplenomegaly, microcephaly (small head), jaundice, intrauterine growth restriction, thrombocytopenia, and petechiae. Some of these features may not be present at birth, but develop later in childhood.

Acquired CMV in **immunodeficiency** patients results in significant morbidity and mortality. Those at greatest risk are seronegative patients receiving an organ for transplantation from a seropositive donor. If the recipient is also seropositive, then reactivation of the virus can occur. Consideration must be given, especially for patients following stem cell transplantation, that blood is typed as CMV-negative to prevent infection by CMV.

immunodeficiency
Any inherited or acquired deficiency in the immune system.

Human immunodeficiency virus 1 (HIV-1)

The retrovirus HIV-1 is the causative agent of acquired immunodeficiency syndrome (AIDS). First reported in 1981 in the United States following a number of cases in which patients developed rare opportunistic infections or rare skin cancers, AIDS quickly spread throughout the developed and undeveloped world. Common complications include pneumocystis pneumonia (PCP) cased by *Pneumocystis jiroveci*, Kaposi sarcoma, and primary central nervous system lymphoma. In 2008, approximately 83 000 people were estimated to be living in the UK with HIV-1. With the introduction and improvement of antiretroviral drugs, the mortality rate from AIDS-related complications in the UK is approximately 500 people per annum.

HIV-1 can be transmitted from one individual to another through unprotected heterosexual or homosexual intercourse, from infected blood products, from intravenous drug abuse, or from an HIV-1 infected mother to her infant.

HIV-1 predominantly infects CD4+ T cells, and are called T-tropic strains, although CD4+ monocytes or macrophages can also be infected by M-tropic strains, through the binding of the CCR5 chemokine receptor. The lipid bilayer of the viral envelope expresses a transmembrane glycoprotein (gp41) associated with gp120. Gp120 binds to the CD4 ligand, and additional binding to the chemokine receptor CXCR4 enables the virus to enter host T cells. Once internalized, the viral RNA is reverse-transcribed to DNA, called a provirus, through the action of viral reverse transcriptase. The provirus is incorporated into the host's genome, with DNA replication enabling the synthesis of new virions. The expression of virions leads to the lysis of the infected T cell and the release of the virions into the patient's blood, enabling further infection of T cells.

Following infection by HIV-1, many patients are commonly asymptomatic. Those showing symptoms may present with fever, rash, and lymphadenopathy, all of which spontaneously resolve in a few weeks. Following a protracted chronic phase, the viral load—the number of copies of viral RNA in the patient's plasma—increases and the number of CD4+ T cells declines. Generally, AIDS is diagnosed when the patient's CD4+ count drops below 200 cells/mm^3, which often occurs at around 8 years post infection. Patients often succumb to opportunistic infection unless treated with one of the many effective antiretroviral agents designed to combat HIV-1.

Toxoplasmosis

Toxoplasma gondii is a protozoan parasite reportedly infecting approximately one-third of the world's population, and accounting for 1–2% of patients with suspected IM. Commonly, infection occurs following the ingestion of oocysts from cat faeces, contaminated and under-cooked meat, or water. Approximately 10–20% of infected individuals are symptomatic, and can be diagnosed with toxoplasmosis. Clinical features are similar to those found in IM, the most common of which is cervical lymphadenopathy.

Congenital toxoplasma infection can occur, but is only of risk to fetuses of seronegative mothers as *Toxoplasma gondii* does not cross the placenta in seropositive mothers. Clinical symptoms of congenital toxoplasma are variable, including neurological symptoms, encephalitis, anaemia, jaundice, rash, and petechiae.

Immunocompromised patients may be infected following a transplant from an infected individual; but, more commonly, infections are associated with the reactivation of a latent infection following the suppression of T lymphocytes. In immunocompromised patients, symptoms include pneumonitis, encephalitis, and myocarditis which, if left untreated, are associated with significant morbidity and mortality.

Plasma cells

Plasma cells are antibody-secreting cells found within the bone marrow and lymphoid organs. In a healthy individual, plasma cells would not be expected to be seen in the peripheral blood. However, occasionally during acute infections, and in some types of haematological malignancy (including plasma cell myeloma), plasma cells may be evident on a peripheral blood film.

Cross reference

Plasma cell neoplasms are discussed in greater detail in Chapter 12.

Plasma cells vary in size and shape, but typically contain an eccentric nucleus within deeply basophilic (blue) cytoplasm. The nucleus contains clumped chromatin and is surrounded by a prominent Golgi zone (a pale area) called a perinuclear halo. Figure 8.21 shows plasma cell morphology in a patient diagnosed with plasma cell leukaemia.

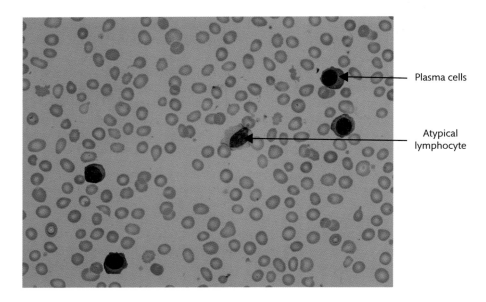

Plasma cells

Atypical lymphocyte

FIGURE 8.21

Plasma cells in the peripheral blood of a patient with plasma cell leukaemia. Four plasma cells are present, accompanied by an atypical lymphocyte in the centre. Note the presence of the deeply basophilic cytoplasm and perinuclear halo, characteristic features of plasma cells. Image courtesy of Jackie Warne, Haematology department. Queen Alexandra Hospital, Portsmouth.

8.5 **Light microscopy**

Light microscopy is an important aspect of laboratory haematology, enabling the morphology of blood cells to be evaluated and a manual differential count to be performed. Although the FBC can provide a broad range of information about a specimen, the appearance of red cells, white cells, and platelets can provide more information useful to clinicians when considering diagnosis.

Cross reference
More information on microscopy can be found in the **Biomedical Science Practice** volume of this series.

Microscope preparation

Keeping the light microscope in the best possible condition is essential to obtain the most information from a patient's blood film. The light microscope should be set up to ensure full and consistent illumination across the field of view—the area of the blood film seen through the eyepieces. The objective lens should be free from grease, and cleaned using an appropriate lens cloth. Dust should be removed from the light source. If in any doubt about how to clean your microscope, consult the manufacturer's instructions or your laboratory's standard operating procedure. The structure of a modern light microscope is provided in Figure 8.22.

The combination of a well-cared for microscope and a good quality blood film is necessary for diagnostic purposes.

Köhler illumination

The method used to achieve consistent illumination is called **Köhler illumination**. Used daily, Köhler illumination ensures optimal conditions for examining a specimen microscopically.

The first step in achieving Köhler illumination involves selecting the ×10 objective lens, placing a blood film on the stage and focusing the microscope. Next, the field diaphragm is reduced to enable visualization of a small point of light through the eyepiece. The x and y condenser

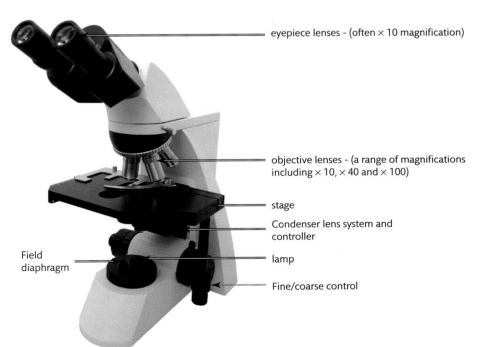

eyepiece lenses - (often × 10 magnification)

objective lenses - (a range of magnifications including × 10, × 40 and × 100)

stage

Condenser lens system and controller

Field diaphragm

lamp

Fine/coarse control

FIGURE 8.22

The basic structure of a modern light microscope. © Dragan Trifunovic/ istockphoto.com. True magnification involves multiplying the objective magnification by the eyepiece magnification: eg 40 × 100 = 400 × magnification.

adjustment screws are used to centre the small point of light within the field of view. At this point, the field diaphragm is centred under the condenser. Finally, the field diaphragm must be opened just sufficiently to ensure the entire field of view is illuminated. Consistent and reproducible illumination has now been achieved.

SELF-CHECK 8.14

List the steps involved in achieving Köhler illumination. Outline the benefits of setting a microscope up in this manner.

Specimen examination

A blood film should first be examined without the use of the microscope, i.e. macroscopically, to examine the coloration of the film, the thickness of the spread, and distribution of blood on the slide. Abnormal cellular aggregates are usually appreciable macroscopically. Once the requirements of macroscopic examination have been satisfied, microscopic examination can begin.

At low power, for example with a ×10 objective lens, assess the distribution of cells to identify any abnormal white cells, cell clumps, or fibrin strands present. Once the low power assessment has been completed, a ×40 or ×50 objective lens can be used to assess the detail of the cells. The ×40 objective is the standard lens to use, with air and oil lenses available. Remember, total magnification equals objective lens magnification multiplied by eyepiece lens magnification.

Each cell line should be examined, regardless of the reasoning for the request to examine the blood film. Often, having a striking abnormality under the microscope can distract the novice into examining only the most abnormal of cells; although, in practice, it is important to assess all cell lineages for number and appearance.

When examining white blood cells (as these are the focus of this chapter), the following should be assessed:

- The nuclear structure, including chromatin appearance and presence of nucleoli.
- The colour of the cytoplasm.
- The presence of granules within the cytoplasm, their colour, intensity, and whether or not granules are expected in that particular cell line.
- Abnormal maturation of the nucleus and the cytoplasm.
- Inclusion bodies or vacuolation and the associated lineage.
- The shape of the cell in comparison to what might be considered normal for each species of cell.
- The presence of any progenitor cells, intermediate stages of maturation, or cells otherwise abnormally localized to the peripheral blood.

By consistently following this pattern of investigation, no white blood cell abnormalities should be overlooked.

Manual differential count

For every automated FBC completed, a total white blood cell count will also be provided, along with a breakdown of the absolute numbers of the species of white blood cell and their relative percentages. The term 'white blood cell differential count' refers to the absolute numbers and percentages of the different species of WBC within the total white cell count. Depending upon the specification of the analyser, a three-population differential—assessing granulocytes, monocytes, and lymphocytes or neutrophils, lymphocytes and mixed

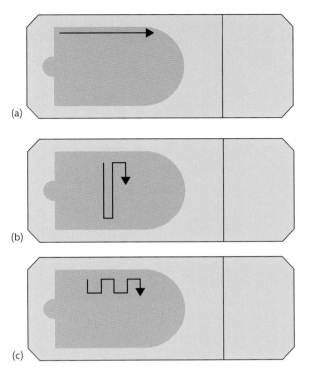

(a)

(b)

(c)

FIGURE 8.23

Diagrams of blood films showing tracking patterns employed in differential WBC: (a) tracking along the length of the film; (b) modified battlement method; and (c) battlement method; two fields are counted close to the edge parallel to the edge of the film, then four fields at right angles, then two fields parallel to the edge and so on. From Bain BJ. *Blood cells: a practical guide*, 4th edn. Oxford, Blackwell, 2006.

(monocytes, eosinophils and basophils) populations—might be used. However, a five-population differential is preferable—providing neutrophil, eosinophil, basophil, monocyte, and lymphocyte counts. Additionally, there are usually immature granulocyte parameters that can be measured.

Sometimes it is necessary for biomedical scientists to determine the differential count manually, especially when atypical white blood cells, such as WBC progenitors or **dysplastic** cells are present.

dysplastic
This refers to cells that have abnormal maturation characteristics.

A minimum of 100 white blood cells should be counted, with the identity of each species of white blood cell recorded on a cell counter. A well-prepared blood film, ideally using a sample less than 3 hours old, stained with a good quality Romanowsky stain should be used to ensure blood cell morphology is maintained. A ×400 magnification in conjunction with the *battlement method* should be used to obtain a good cross-section of the blood film. See Figure 8.23 for examples of the different methods employed to examine blood films.

The initial value obtained from the manual differential count is a percentage of each species of white blood cell. The absolute count, reported as $x \times 10^9$/L, for each species can be easily obtained using the percentages and the total white blood cell count obtained from the original FBC.

The various species of WBC have different migration patterns when spread on a glass slide. The better the quality of the blood film, the less pronounced the spreading characteristics of these white cells. Nevertheless, as a scientist it is important to obtain accurate and precise results and report these appropriately. Larger cells such as neutrophils and monocytes tend to spread to the periphery of the film (i.e. to the tip and the edges), whereas lymphocytes may be found at higher levels in the centre of the film. Because the battlement method (Figure 8.23(b)) is completed across the width of the slide, the edges and the middle of the film should be equally assessed, thereby reducing the risk of obtaining inaccurate results.

Some scientists recommend using a 'mini' battlement approach along the periphery of the slide, whilst others prefer working along the length of the slide from thick to thin in a region

METHOD Calculating the absolute cell counts from a manual differential

Now consider a patient who has a total WBC of 8.0×10^9/L, as determined by a standard haematology analyser. A biomedical scientist completes a 100-cell manual differential count obtaining the following data:

Neutrophils	72%
Lymphocytes	22%
Monocytes	3%
Eosinophils	2%
Basophils	1%
Total = 100%	

These data now need to be converted into absolute values, reported as $\times 10^9$/L.

The first step is to convert the percentages into decimal figures:

Neutrophils	0.72
Lymphocytes	0.22
Monocytes	0.03
Eosinophils	0.02
Basophils	0.01
Total = 1.00	

Now multiply the original total white cell count (in this case 8.0×10^9/L) by each of the decimals:

Neutrophils	$0.72 \times 8.0 = 5.76$
Lymphocytes	$0.22 \times 8.0 = 1.76$
Monocytes	$0.03 \times 8.0 = 0.24$
Eosinophils	$0.02 \times 8.0 = 0.16$
Basophils	$0.01 \times 8.0 = 0.08$
Total WBC = 8.0×10^9/L	

Remember to add each of your absolute counts together to ensure the final value equals the total white cell count originally obtained.

SELF-CHECK 8.15

A patient is shown to have an abnormal differential count using automated methods. Subsequent examination of the requested blood film demonstrates this differential count is incorrect. A manual differential cell count is completed providing the following percentages:

Neutrophils	64%
Lymphocytes	21%
Monocytes	12%
Eosinophils	3%
Basophils	0%

The total WBC is 16×10^9/L.

Based on the figures above:

1. Calculate the absolute count for each of the WBC species.
2. Indicate which of these species falls outside the reference range for the species absolute counts and whether they are high or low.
3. Using the correct white cell terminology describe which population(s) of cells is/are abnormal and how.

near the periphery of the film. Your training officer will have his/her own views. For the inexperienced morphologist, focusing on the monolayer and working across the width of the slide allows for full appreciation of the morphology without the risk of misinterpreting seemingly 'crushed' cells in the thick regions of the film.

BOX 8.7 *Practice identifying blood cells*

For educational purposes try obtaining some samples and corresponding FBC results from your laboratory. Produce your own films and compare your manual results with those obtained from the analyser. If you have any difficulties with cell identification, you can refer these to your training officer (or equivalent) for discussion and additional help.

CHAPTER SUMMARY

In this chapter we have:

- Determined the structure and of granulocytes morphological characteristics of each species of white blood cell.

- Outlined the granular contents of granulocytes and their impact on white cell function.

- Discussed some of the causes and consequences of abnormal white blood cell counts.

- Examined the methods of investigating suspected cases of infectious mononucleosis.

- Introduced the concept of Köhler illumination and the main considerations when setting up a light microscope.

- Outlined the methodology for completing a manual differential count and calculating the absolute values for each species of WBC.

DISCUSSION QUESTIONS

8.1 Consider the structure of the germinal centre. In combination with the information available in Chapter 12 and your further reading, critically discuss the relationship between the germinal centre and named lymphoid malignancies.

8.2 Compare and contrast the processes of monopoiesis and granulopoiesis.

8.3 Compare and contrast the effects of named bacterial and viral infections on the white blood cell count. Explain how the white cell differential and further haematological investigations can aid your diagnosis.

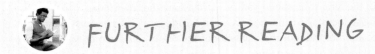

FURTHER READING

- Bain BJ. *Blood Cells: a Practical Guide*, 4th edn. Blackwell Publishing Ltd, Oxford, 2006.

- Hoffbrand AV, Moss PAH, Pettit JE (ed.). *Essential Haematology*, 5th edn. Blackwell Publishing Ltd, Oxford, 2006.

- Kindt TJ, Goldsby RA, Osborne BA. *Kuby Immunology* (6th edn). WH Freeman and Co., New York, 2007.

- Klein U, Dalla-Favera R. Germinal centres: role in B-cell physiology and malignancy. *Nature Reviews Inmunology* 2008: **8**; 22–3.

- Swerdlow SH, Campo E, Harris NL, Jaffe ES, Pileri SA, Stein H, Thiele J, Vardiman JW (ed.). *WHO Classification of Tumours of Haematopoietic and Lymphoid Tissues*. IARC, Lyon, 2008.

Answers to self-check questions, case study questions, and discussion questions are provided in the book's Online Resource Centre, visit www.oxfordtextbooks.co.uk/orc/moore

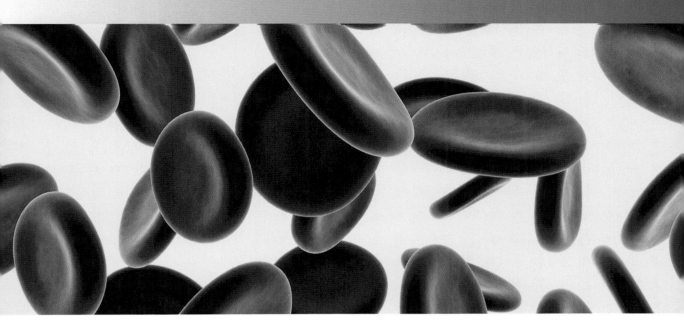

PART 3

Haematological Malignancies

An introduction to haematological malignancies

Gavin Knight

The study of cancers of the haemopoietic system is called **haemato-oncology**. The term 'haematological malignancy' is used to describe a range of cancerous conditions of the haemopoietic system and allows us to differentiate cancers of this system with cancers of other tissues. Haemato-oncology is a fascinating subject providing scientists with the opportunity to work at the cellular, genetic, or molecular level, enabling clinicians to piece together a wide variety of data for accurate diagnosis.

Throughout this chapter we will work through some of the cellular, molecular, and genetic mechanisms responsible for the development of these malignancies. Whilst it is invariably exciting to begin the investigation of a newly presenting haematological malignancy, it is essential to be mindful that every sample represents a patient and our actions should always be measured, respectful, and logical.

Learning objectives

After studying this chapter you should confidently be able to:

- Describe the main differences between the myeloid and lymphoid malignancies.

- Describe a number of conditions found in malignant haematology.

- Describe the role of the cell cycle in cell proliferation.

- Discuss the possible consequences of a dysregulated cell cycle.

- Critically discuss the role of the cancer stem cell in leukaemogenesis and lymphomagenesis.

- Describe the role of epigenetic processes as mechanisms of inducing malignant change.

- Explain the structure of chromosomes, and make appropriate use of chromosomal nomenclature.

- Discuss the role of different types of mutation in oncogenesis.

- Discuss the concept of clonality in relation to malignant haematology.

- Discuss the role of environmental factors in oncogenesis.

9.1 A background to haematological malignancies

haemopoiesis

This describes the process of producing the cellular constituents of the blood: red blood cells, white blood cells, and platelets.

self-renewal

A normal property of stem cells enabling the stem cell population to be regenerated without necessarily undergoing differentiation of daughter cells into specific cell lines.

oncogenic

The process of producing cancer.

dysregulation

Describes the abnormal function of one or more regulated processes.

maturational arrest

Occurs in malignant cells when they are unable to develop beyond a particular intermediate stage of maturation. This failure in development prevents the production of a population of effector cells.

apoptosis

The process of programmed cell death. One of the functions of apoptosis is to prevent acquired genetic mutations being passed on to daughter cells.

leukaemic phase

Describes the presence of malignant cells, derived from a lymphoma, having entered the peripheral blood from their associated lymphoid organ(s).

Cross reference

Chapter 3 deals with normal haemopoietic processes.

The haemopoietic system is responsible for the development of the effector cells we see in the peripheral blood: red blood cells, white blood cells (neutrophils, eosinophils, basophils, monocytes, and lymphocytes), and platelets through the process of **haemopoiesis**. The process of haemopoiesis begins with pluripotent stem cells, which have the capacity to develop into any one of the mature effector cells through their interaction with different growth factors and cytokines. Pluripotent stem cells also have the capacity for **self-renewal**, a process that ensures a sufficient supply of stem cells to enable the future production of mature effector cells.

If particular cancer-causing (**oncogenic**) genetic mutations are acquired by an individual stem cell, the process of stem cell maturation can become **dysregulated**. **Dysregulation** of haemopoiesis can result in:

- The failure to produce effector cells
- An accumulation of cells at a particular intermediate stage of maturation (**maturational arrest**)
- An increased cellular proliferation rate
- A failure of **apoptosis**

SELF-CHECK 9.1

Outline the effects of a dysregulation of haemopoiesis.

Not every haematological malignancy displays all of these features.

Capability of stem-cell self-renewal can be maintained in maturing populations of daughter cells. By inheriting the ability to self-renew, a population of cells with acquired genetic changes can rapidly accumulate and replace the normal haemopoietic components of the bone marrow. Cancer stem cells will be considered in greater depth later in this chapter.

Now that we have briefly considered some of the features of haematological malignancies, the range of these malignancies should be examined in a little more depth, starting with leukaemias and lymphomas before moving on to myelodysplastic syndromes, multiple myeloma and then myeloproliferative disorder.

Leukaemia and lymphoma

Leukaemia describes the presence of malignant haemopoietic cells within the peripheral blood or bone marrow. These malignant cells may be either *myeloid* (red blood cells, neutrophils, monocytes, eosinophils, basophils, platelets, or their precursors) or *lymphoid* (B-lineage, T-lineage lymphocytes, plasma cells, NK cells, or their precursors).

Lymphomas are *only* lymphoid in origin and are largely restricted to the lymphoid organs (spleen or lymph nodes), although we sometimes encounter patients with extranodal lymphomas (those originating outside the lymphoid organs). Often, lymphomas enter a **leukaemic**

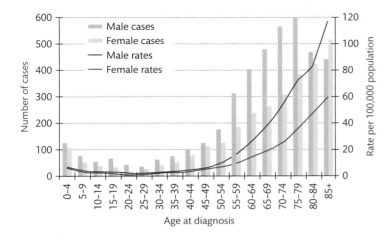

FIGURE 9.1

Cancer Research UK leukaemia data showing the incidence of leukaemia in 2006, stratified according to age and sex. Obtained with permission from Cancer Research UK: http://info.cancerresearchuk.org/cancerstats/types/leukaemia/incidence/index. Accessed 14/03/10.

Cross reference

Chapter 11 examines acute and chronic myeloid leukaemias.

blasts

A stage of differentiation of a blood cell as it passes from the stem cell stage to the mature cell stage that should only be found within the bone marrow in low numbers. Blasts may be further characterized by their lineage e.g. myeloblasts are of the myeloid lineage, lymphoblasts are of the lymphoid lineage.

Cross references

For more information on lymphoid malignancies please see Chapter 12.

For more information on myeloid malignancies please see Chapter 11.

phase, where malignant lymphoid cells, which were restricted to a particular lymphoid organ, overspill into the bone marrow and peripheral blood.

Leukaemias can be considered as either *acute* or *chronic*. Acute leukaemia is associated with an accumulation of immature cells called **blasts**—comprising at least 20% of the nucleated cells of the bone marrow with evidence of maturational arrest. Acute leukaemias are also clinically aggressive, leading to death relatively rapidly if untreated. Chronic leukaemias are less aggressive and have blasts below 20%. Maturational arrest does not occur in chronic leukaemias, although the cells often fail to undergo apoptosis, allowing the malignant cells to accumulate.

Cancer Research UK statistics for 2006 have been compiled to show the total number of male and female cases of leukaemia reported and their relative rates per 100 000 of the population. Figure 9.1 shows that males are more commonly affected throughout life. This data represents leukaemia in general, irrespective of acute or chronic, or any further subdivisions. The incidence is highest in the early years of life, declines through the twenties, and then increases rapidly in the latter half of the forties.

Lymphomas can be described as low grade or high grade. Low-grade lymphomas are associated with a lower cellular proliferation rate than high-grade ones, and low-grade lymphomas *tend* to progress slowly. Interestingly, low-grade lymphomas are more difficult to treat than high-grade lymphomas even though, if left untreated, high-grade lymphomas will cause death relatively quickly.

Additionally, we need to consider whether a particular case of lymphoma is a *Hodgkin lymphoma* (HL) or *non-Hodgkin lymphoma* (NHL). The name non-Hodgkin lymphoma describes a large group of solid lymphoid (lymphomatous) tumours which are very diverse in nature. This contrasts with Hodgkin lymphomas, which are relatively restricted in their pathology and are associated with a characteristic mutated B-lineage cell called the **Hodgkin and Reed–Sternberg cell**.

The presence of lymphoblasts in the bone marrow and peripheral blood indicates acute lymphoblastic leukaemia (ALL). In cases where there is clear evidence of primary lymphoblastic disease from a lymphoid organ or extranodal tissue, the term lymphoblastic lymphoma should be used.

Key Points

Becoming familiar with the terminology for leukaemias often takes some practice, and you will find some language variations between American and British textbooks. When discussing acute and chronic lymphoid leukaemias, it is important to use the correct suffix for the lineage in question. If you are discussing an acute leukaemia of lymphoid origin, the suffix –blastic must be used, and so the name would be acute lympho**blastic** leukaemia. In the chronic form you should use the suffix –cytic, so the disease would be termed chronic lympho**cytic** leukaemia. Large numbers of blast cells are evident in acute leukaemias as denoted by the name. In chronic leukaemias, the cells show maturation, and this is denoted by the suffix –cyte.

There are also variations in the myeloid lineage. Myeloid leukaemias may be described as myeloid, myelogenous, myeloblastic, or in America as non-lymphoblastic leukaemias. The best option here is to use myeloid as this can be used to describe either acute or chronic forms of the disease.

SELF-CHECK 9.2

List the four main types of leukaemia outlined so far.

SELF-CHECK 9.3

Outline the different grades used to describe the behaviour of lymphoma cells.

A comparison of the Cancer Research UK data for Hodgkin versus NHL from 2006 is particularly interesting. Examining Figure 9.2, it is apparent that Hodgkin lymphoma is much less frequently encountered than non-Hodgkin lymphoma (as demonstrated by Figure 9.3). It is important to ensure the axes for both graphs are read carefully before incorrectly interpreting these data. Hodgkin lymphoma is a disease primarily affecting the younger population, with the first incidence peak in the twenties and the second peak in the early sixties for men and again in the seventies for both sexes. Hodgkin lymphoma is generally

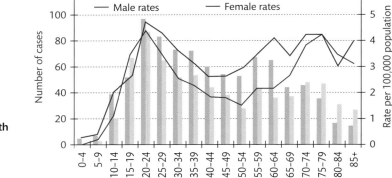

FIGURE 9.2

Cancer Research UK Hodgkin lymphoma data showing the incidence of leukaemia in 2006, stratified according to age and sex. Obtained with permission from Cancer Research UK: http://info.cancerresearchuk.org/cancerstats/types/hodgkinslymphoma/incidence/index. Accessed 14/03/10.

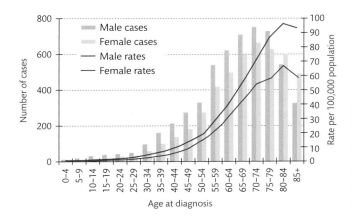

FIGURE 9.3

Cancer Research UK non-Hodgkin lymphoma data showing the incidence of leukaemia in 2006, stratified according to age and sex. Obtained with permission from Cancer Research UK: http://info.cancerresearchuk.org/cancerstats/types/nhl/incidence/index. Accessed 14/03/10.

more common in males than females, with the exception of the 15–19 age group, where the incidence is higher in females.

Non-Hodgkin lymphoma is a disease of increasing age. In infants, children, and teenagers, NHL is very unusual and the distribution between males and females is equal. Beyond the second decade, NHL is increasingly found in males more than females with a gradually increasing incidence until the mid fifties. Beyond the mid-fifties, there is a rapid increase in the incidence of NHL.

Myelodysplastic syndrome (MDS)

Myelodysplastic syndrome describes a range of heterogeneous blood diseases restricted to the myeloid lineage. In MDS, the predominant feature is an increased number of precursor cells within the bone marrow (bone marrow **hypercellularity**) and a concurrent reduction in the number of cells circulating in the peripheral blood (peripheral blood **cytopenia**). The premature death of immature haemopoietic cells within the bone marrow is called **ineffective haemopoiesis**. Clinically, when patients only exhibit signs of anaemia, MDS may be expressed as a low haemoglobin concentration with enlarged red cells (*macrocytic anaemia*). This anaemia will fail to respond to conventional treatments—vitamin B$_{12}$, folate, or iron—and is therefore called **refractory anaemia**. More severe symptoms, including recurrent infections, will be experienced if the patient has a severe reduction in the number of circulating mature white cells with a concurrent increase in the number of blast cells within the bone marrow and peripheral blood.

MDS used to be termed 'pre-leukaemia' because of the increased risk of transformation to an acute leukaemia in these patients. Pre-leukaemia is now a redundant term since most patients die of the complications of MDS before transformation to leukaemia can occur.

SELF-CHECK 9.4

Outline the common findings associated with myelodysplastic syndrome.

Multiple myeloma

Multiple myeloma (MM) is a malignancy of the lymphoid compartment and generally occurs in middle to old age. Examining the Cancer Research UK statistics for multiple myeloma (Figure 9.4),

hypercellularity

An increase in the number of cells within the bone marrow.

cytopenia

A reduction in one or more cell lines within the peripheral blood. If all cell lines (red cells, white cells, and platelets) are reduced, this is termed pancytopenia.

ineffective haemopoiesis

Describes an accumulation of immature cells within the bone marrow, the vast majority of which undergo apoptosis before maturing into effector cells.

Cross references

The importance of the micronutrients (iron, vitamin B$_{12}$, and folate) is explained in Chapter 5.

More detail can be found regarding the classification and pathogenesis of MDS in Chapter 11.

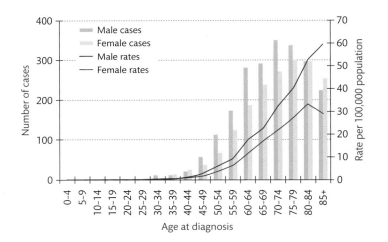

FIGURE 9.4

Cancer Research UK multiple myeloma data showing the incidence of leukaemia in 2006, stratified according to age and sex. Obtained with permission from Cancer Research UK: http://info.cancerresearchuk.org/cancerstats/types/multiplemyeloma/incidence/index. Accessed 14/03/10.

there is a subtle increase in incidence beyond the age of 30 years. There is a gradual increase from the mid forties, at which point the incidence rises markedly. Myeloma is more common in males than females.

Following stimulation by an antigen, the stimulated B cell will undergo a maturational process whereby either memory B cells (cells which enable a more rapid response to a repeat infection from the same organism), or antibody synthesizing and secreting plasma cells, are produced. MM is associated with the proliferation of malignant plasma cells. These malignant plasma cells accumulate in the bone marrow, causing myelosuppression and the activation of osteoclasts (phagocytic cells of the bone involved in bone remodelling). This increase in osteoclast activity causes a breakdown of bone, leading to spontaneous (pathological) fractures and punched-out lesions apparent on X-ray films. MM is characterized by the production of monoclonal antibodies, components of which may damage the kidney if present in the plasma at excessive concentrations.

Cross references

Multiple myeloma is discussed in further detail in Chapter 12.

Polycythaemia is included in Chapters 5 and 6, but as discussed in detail in Chapter 11.

Myelofibrosis and essential thrombocythaemia are discussed in further detail in Chapter 11.

SELF-CHECK 9.5

With which type of cell is multiple myeloma associated?

Myeloproliferative disorders

The collective term 'myeloproliferative disorder' refers to a range of haematological conditions affecting the myeloid lineage associated with an increased rate of proliferation. Three key disorders are contained under the umbrella of myeloproliferative disorder including:

- **Polycythaemia**—a monoclonal proliferation of red cell precursors and an accumulation of mature red cells causing an increased red cell mass.

- **Myelofibrosis**—proliferation of fibroblasts within the bone marrow resulting in a modification of the architecture of the bone marrow microenvironment and redistribution of haemopoietic precursors.

- **Essential thrombocythaemia**—inappropriate megakaryocyte proliferation causing a sustained increased platelet count.

In order to understand how haematological malignancies develop and exert a clinical effect, we need to examine some of the mechanisms through which a population of malignant cells can develop and expand.

In the next sections we will discuss the processes controlling cell maintenance, growth and proliferation in normal cells, and then examine how, when these processes malfunction, malignancy can develop.

9.2 Signal transduction

Signal transduction is the cellular process by which signals from the cell's environment regulate DNA transcription and translation, cell proliferation, and apoptosis. Figure 9.5 demonstrates an example of the signal transduction process. Notice how, in this case, an increase in the transcription and translation of target genes is induced as a consequence of intracellular signalling.

Signal transduction begins with an initiating factor, for example a growth factor (or ligand) binding to its receptor. This binding causes a conformational change, or dimerization, of receptors—leading to their activation through **phosphorylation**. Once a receptor has been activated, a biochemical cascade is initiated and activation of second messengers (also called signal transduction intermediates) directs the signal to its target. We refer to this process as an amplification cascade: it begins with what is essentially a very small stimulus, but results in an increasing number of additional intermediates becoming involved, causing a *cascade* through the *amplification* of the initial stimulus.

phosphorylation
The process of adding a phosphate group (PO₄) to an organic molecule.

Inhibition of the signal transduction cascade can cause the activation of transcription factors, or, conversely, may cause transcription factor repression. The consequence of this activation or inhibition of transcription factors is the control of gene transcription and translation. The products of these genes then play a specific role in controlling the cell cycle—for example, by inducing proliferation through the activation of the cell cycle.

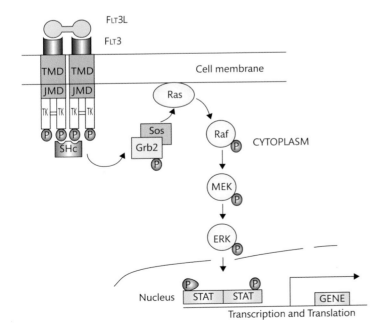

FIGURE 9.5

A signal transduction cascade initiated by the binding of the FLT3 ligand (FLT3L) to its receptor. Subsequent dimerization of the FLT3 receptor occurs leading to the phosphorylation (P) and activation of tyrosine kinase (TK) residues. Phosphorylation of TK induces downstream signalling events and the activation of STAT (Signal Transducer and Activator of Transcription) leading to the transcription and translation of FLT3L inducible genes. TMD = transmembrane domain, and JMD = juxtamembrane domain.

BOX 9.1 NFκB signalling

Dysregulation of signal transduction pathways is an important process in the development of haematological malignancies. The **Nuclear Factor κB (NFκB)** pathways relevant to haematology will be used for illustration below.

As you work through Chapter 12, you will encounter a number of haematological malignancies associated with the overactivity of NFκB pathways.

NFκB is a family of transcription factors containing DNA-binding, dimerization, nuclear translocation, and inhibitor binding domains. Usually located within the cytoplasm, and associated with inhibitors, NFκB is activated through two pathways—classical and alternate and is active in many signalling pathways. The *classical pathway* is activated by pro-inflammatory cytokines or the interaction of B-cell or T-cell receptors with their ligands, whereas the *alternate pathway* is activated by the TNF cytokine family. The multimeric complexes that result from the activation of these signal transduction pathways are structurally different, although once activated, these complexes can translocate from the cytoplasm to the cell nucleus, where they induce the transcription of a range of target genes.

NFκB signalling is essential for the development and maturation of B and T cells by suppressing apoptosis. Suppression of apoptosis is particularly important as B cells progress through the germinal centre following activation in an antigen-dependent manner to facilitate the development of highly specific memory B cells and plasma cells.

Constitutive activation of NFκB leads to the accumulation of cells through NFκB-initiated abnormal cell cycling and apoptotic failure; and is associated with a range of haematological malignancies including: follicular lymphoma; MALT lymphoma; activated B-cell type, diffuse, large B-cell lymphoma; anaplastic, large cell lymphoma; and in some EBV-related cases of Hodgkin lymphoma.

Now that the concept of signal transduction has been considered, we should examine one of the processes controlled by the signal transduction mechanism—the *cell cycle*.

SELF-CHECK 9.6

Outline the importance of signal transduction in regulating cell behaviour.

9.3 An introduction to the cell cycle

We have already established that both cellular proliferation and the failure of apoptosis have a role in the development of malignancies. Before moving on to consider specific details of oncogenesis, we should first consider how cells reproduce and try to understand some of the control mechanisms in place. Understanding the mechanisms controlling normal cellular reproduction can aid our understanding of how cells can become malignant when these control mechanisms malfunction.

The process of cellular reproduction comprises a series of phases which, when integrated, form a cycle—called the cell cycle. Figure 9.6 provides an outline of the main phases of the

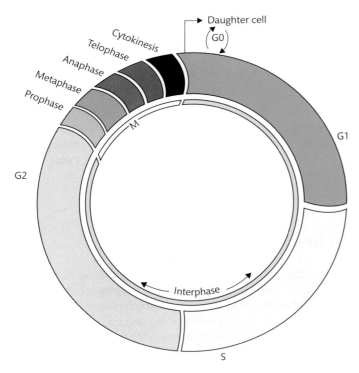

FIGURE 9.6

A brief outline of the main stages of the cell cycle. The cycle contains two gap phases (G1 and G2), a single synthesis phase (S), and mitosis (M). G1, S, and G2 phases constitute interphase, with the different phases of mitosis (prophase, metaphase, anaphase, telophase, and cytokinesis) leading to the production of two daughter cells. G0 represents an optional quiescent or 'resting' phase.

cell cycle. A single cycle usually produces two identical daughter cells from one 'parent' cell. Before the cycle is ready to produce daughter cells, sequential activation and termination of each phase of the cycle must be completed. The phases collectively producing the cell cycle include two gap phases abbreviated to G1 and G2, a synthesis phase (S), and mitosis (M). An additional phase, in which the cell 'rests' may follow mitosis, and is referred to as the quiescent stage (G0). These phases are organized into the following order to ensure the cell is fully prepared to reproduce:

$$G1 \rightarrow \quad S \rightarrow \quad G2 \rightarrow \quad M \,(G0)$$

During G1 phase, protein synthesis occurs, preparing the cell for the synthesis of DNA in S phase of the cell cycle. G1 is the longest phase of the cell cycle, completing in approximately 9 hours. Chromosomes are present as single **chromatids**.

S phase follows G1, and is involved in the synthesis of DNA. This synthesized DNA forms a duplication of all DNA within the cell. This process lasts approximately 5 hours, with mostly active (or early replicating) genes duplicating first, followed by largely inactive (or late replicating) genes.

G2 phase then follows, allowing the cell to make the final preparation for cell division.

G1, S, and G2 phases are collectively called interphase. Mitosis also includes a number of distinct phases: prophase, metaphase, anaphase, telophase, and finally cytokinesis. During mitosis, separation of duplicated chromosomes and division of the cytoplasm occurs, producing two distinct diploid cells.

> **chromatids**
> Subunits of chromosomes separated by a centromere. Chromatids become chromosomes following division of the centromere during mitosis.

SELF-CHECK 9.7

List the main phases of interphase and provide a brief description of each.

Cross reference
Metaphase will be discussed in relation to chromosomal structure and cytogenetic analysis in Chapter 10.

The cell cycle includes a number of regulators that induce or inhibit specific phases of the cycle. Between them, these regulators ensure that each phase begins and ends correctly, and that each phase takes an appropriate amount of time to complete.

Whilst the DNA is replicating, the replicating strand of DNA is checked for mutations. If mutations are detected, cell cycle regulators are activated and cell cycle arrest is induced.

Following cell cycle arrest, DNA repair enzymes will be activated; although, if repair is unsuccessful, apoptosis is induced. Inducing DNA repair or apoptosis prevents acquired DNA mutations from passing from one cellular generation to the next, thereby protecting the genome. Unrepaired mutations in the cell cycle machinery are associated with a wide variety of haematological malignancies.

Let's now explore the concept of the cell cycle in a little more detail.

An introduction to cell cycle control

To proliferate and become committed to the cell cycle, cells require particular signals to initiate mitosis. These signals are termed mitogenic and indirectly activate a family of cell cycle control proteins called **cyclin-dependent kinases** (CDKs). The concentration of CDKs remains constant throughout the cell cycle; however, their activity is regulated by another family of proteins called **cyclins**. One group of cyclin family members is called cyclin D (which actually comprises cyclins D1, D2, and D3), the transcription of which is induced through mitogenic signals (for example through Ras signalling). Particular cyclins will bind specifically with CDKs, and CDKs will not function unless they are bound to their appropriate cyclin partner. Table 9.1 shows the main CDK binding partner for each of the cyclins. Just as cyclin–CDK interactions push the cell cycle forward, control mechanisms are in place to inhibit these cyclin–CDK complexes, ensuring that each phase of the cell cycle completes at the appropriate time.

cyclin-dependent kinases
A group of enzymes, requiring cyclins, involved in the transfer of phosphate groups from donars to acceptors to enable the progression of the cell cycle.

mitogen
Any chemical or substance capable of inducing mitosis.

Initiation of the cell cycle

Prior to the initiation of a new cell cycle, the cycle is maintained in an inactive state—achieved through the actions of two families of cyclin kinase inhibitor (CKI):

- Inhibitors of CDK4 (INK)
- CDK inhibitory proteins (cip/kip)

These inhibitors form the CKI–CDK–cyclin complex. Binding of a **mitogen** (a growth factor, for example) to its binding site or receptor results in modification to this CKI–CDK–cyclin complex, allowing an interaction between a subgroup of cyclins—the D type cyclins—and their

TABLE 9.1 Key cyclins, their binding partners and typical expression within the cell cycle.

Cyclin	CDK-binding partner(s)	Typical expression in the cell cycle
Cyclin-D (-D1, -D2, -D3)	CDK4 or CDK6	Mid G1
Cyclin-E	CDK2	Late G1
Cyclin A	CDK2	S phase
Cyclin B	CDK1	Late G2/M

corresponding CDKs. The remodelling of this complex ensures that initiation of the cell cycle occurs in response to external requirements.

The cyclin D–CDK4 and the cyclin D–CDK6 complexes then interact with an important regulatory protein called retinoblastoma (pRb). Figure 9.7 outlines the process through which pRb is modified to allow cell cycle progression to occur. When the cell cycle is arrested, for example in the absence of cyclin D–CDK4, pRb binds to a **transcription factor** called E2F-1. By binding with E2F-1, pRb acts as a docking station, preventing E2F-1 from associating with its binding site in the promoter region of target genes. E2F-1 should only be released when appropriate signals are received by pRb. Because E2F-1 cannot bind to its binding site, E2F-1 sensitive genes are repressed, and so transcription of these genes cannot occur. Increasing intracellular concentrations of cyclin D–CDK4 and cyclin D–CDK6, in response to mitogenic activation, add phosphate groups to pRb, in a process called phosphorylation. This phosphorylation reduces the binding capacity of pRb for E2F-1, releasing E2F-1 transcription factors, and activating E2F-1 dependent genes. The release of E2F-1 promotes transcription of a range of genes, including the gene encoding cyclin E. Another protein bound to pRb is an enzyme called **histone deacetylase** (HDAC). The localization of HDAC to pRb and the promoter region of target genes causes modification of the chromatin structure within this region, thus inhibiting genes within the area.

> **transcription factor**
> A protein which plays a regulatory role in the transcription of particular genes.
>
> **histone deacetylase**
> A class of enzyme that removes acetyl groups from histones, thereby inhibiting DNA transcription.

SELF-CHECK 9.8

Describe the role of the retinoblastoma protein pRb.

Activation of cyclin E–CDK2 occurs in late G1 phase, just prior to cells entering S-phase, and induces factors necessary for S-phase progression.

> **Cross reference**
> HDAC and other epigenetic modifiers are discussed in greater detail later in this chapter.

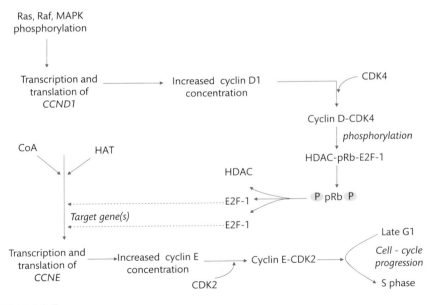

FIGURE 9.7

The induction of cyclin D via the mitogenic activation of Ras, Raf, or MAPK. Transcription of the cyclin D1 gene (*CCND1*) is induced, allowing translation of cyclin D1, thereby increasing its intracellular concentration. Cyclin D1 associates with CDK4 producing the Cyclin D-CDK4 complex. This complex phosphorylates pRb, releasing elongation factor 2-1 (E2F-1) and histone deacetylase (HDAC). Histone acetyltransferase (HAT) and coactivators (CoA) replace HDAC, and in the presence of E2F-1 allow the transcription and translation of *CCNE*. Cyclin E will then form a complex with CDK2, allowing cell cycle progression from late G1 to S phase.

Cell cycle progression

Cyclins A, B, B2, and B3 are mitotic cyclins and are involved in the progression of the cell cycle through S and G2 phases, although they are actually destroyed during mitosis itself. Cyclin A–CDK2 concentrations peak in early G2 following initial expression in late G1. Cyclin A–CDK2 is an essential component of the S phase as DNA replication is dependent upon its activity. In addition, cyclin A–CDK2 has been shown to play an inhibitory role in G1/S phase transition.

Cell cycle completion

Transition between G2 and M phases is largely controlled by cyclin B and CDK1 (also called cell division cycle 2). Cyclin B–CDK1 is initially expressed in early G2 phase, with a peak in concentration at the G2/M transition. Mitosis can only complete once cyclin B–CDK1 has been degraded. Once mitosis has completed, the cell cycle of the daughter cells may then begin.

Mitosis involves the condensation of duplicated sister chromatids across the equator of the cell. These sister chromatids are separated through the formation of a spindle complex and the associated microtubule network. Each chromatid, now called a chromosome, is localized to the opposite poles of the cell, allowing two genetically balanced daughter cells to be produced. This forms the basis of inheritance and, in the case of haematological malignancies, allows for abnormal genes to be passed on to subsequent generations and the production of a population of malignant cells.

TABLE 9.2 Common cell cycle control abnormalities in haematological malignancies.

Cell cycle component	Mechanism	Malignancy	Comments
RB1 (pRb)	Various	ALL	No prognostic implication
	Deletion	HL	Occurs in approximately 16% of cases
	Deletion	AML	Occurs in up to 55% of cases
	Mutation	CML	A product, rather than a cause of disease progression
CCND1 (cyclin D1)	Dysregulated	MCL	t(11;14)(q13;q32) *CCND1-IGH*
		Myeloma	As MCL (above)
		MGUS	As MCL (above)
CCND2 (cyclin D2)	Upregulation	CML	A downstream effector of BCR-ABL1
CCND3 (cyclin D3)	Upregulation	Myeloma	t(6;14)(p21;q32) *CCND3-IGH*
CCNE (cyclin E)	Upregulation	AML	Approx 25% of cases, but depends on subtype
	Upregulation	CLL	No data

Key: ALL, acute lymphoblastic leukaemia; AML, acute myeloid leukaemia; CLL, chronic lymphocytic leukaemia; CML, chronic myeloid leukaemia; HL, Hodgkin lymphoma; MCL, mantle cell lymphoma; MGUS monoclonal gammopathy of undetermined significance.

Dysregulation of the cell cycle through alterations in cell cycle machinery has been reported in a number of cases of haematological malignancy, and some of these are explored in Chapters 11 and 12. An outline of some of the most common abnormalities in haematological malignancies is provided in Table 9.2

Cancer stem cells

Stem cells are immunophenotypically CD34-positive (CD34+) precursor cells with the potential to differentiate and mature into many different types of effector cell, whilst undergoing the process of self-renewal. Cancer stem cells tend to be interspersed with more mature cancer cells, which lack the ability for self-renewal. Determination of the self-renewal characteristics of these cells is demonstrated through transplantation into immunodeficient mice. Cancer cells with the ability to populate the mouse with tumour cells are considered stem cells, whilst the more mature cancer cells fail to induce cancer.

Haemopoietic stem cells are rare, occurring in approximately 1 in 10 000 nucleated bone marrow cells. These stem cells can produce any of the myeloid or lymphoid lineages constituting the haemopoietic system whilst maintaining the stem cell pool. Stem cell division is either symmetric, producing two identical daughter cells (the typical model of mitosis) or asymmetric, producing dissimilar daughter cells—as demonstrated by Figure 9.8. These apparently disparate properties are important in maintaining bone marrow viability and can be achieved through the process of asymmetric cell division. Following mitosis, rather than two identical daughter cells being produced, one daughter cell will differentiate and mature to form an effector cell, whilst the other will maintain the stem cell phenotype, allowing the stem cell pool to be preserved. The selection pressure on the daughter cells should be sufficient to ensure that, depending on the body's physiological requirements, symmetric or asymmetric cell division will predominate. For example, following **myeloablative therapy** and stem cell transplantation, the transplanted stem cells may undergo symmetric division in the first instance to repopulate the bone marrow with stem cells. Following repopulation, asymmetric division will occur, producing a range of effector cells whilst conserving the stem cell pool.

Cancer stem cells have been associated with myeloid and acute lymphoid malignancies, although there is less evidence linking them with mature lymphoid malignancies. With myeloid malignancies it is difficult to ascertain whether stem cells acquire a malignant phenotype whilst retaining their self-renewal characteristics, or partially differentiated cells undergo genetic mutation reactivating the stem cell property of self-renewal.

In lymphoid malignancies, mature lymphoid cells have the potential to become self-renewing, highly proliferative cells following stimulation by antigen as they enter the germinal centre. In fact, the potential for self-renewal is maintained until the memory B-cell stage. Activation of this proliferative programme could lead to the expansion of malignant

myeloablative therapy
The process whereby the bone marrow is destroyed by high doses of chemotherapeutic agents in preparation for stem cell transplantation. Stem cell transplantation provides a potential cure for patients receiving this therapy.

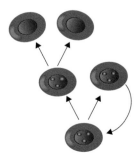

FIGURE 9.8
Stem cell kinetics. Stem cells have the capacity for differentiation or self-renewal depending upon physiological requirements. Here we can see one daughter cell undergoing maturation, whilst the other retains stem-cell characteristics.

BOX 9.2 *Stem cell immunophenotype*

Stem cells express a specific surface immunophenotype that enables identification and quantification using flow cytometry. The most important of the markers is CD34, and enumeration of this marker is useful in ensuring that sufficient stem cells have been harvested prior to myeloablative therapy and stem cell transplantation.

The common haemopoietic stem cell phenotype is: CD34+, CD38-, CD117+. Lineage-specific markers are typically absent (Lin-).

The three common markers that should be assessed to characterize stem cells are considered in more detail below:

CD34: A heavily glycosylated, monomeric, cell-adhesion molecule rich in O-linked carbohydrates and sialic acid. Approximately 42% of bone marrow blasts express CD34.

CD38: CD38 is a transmembrane, type-II glycoprotein expressed on early B and T lymphocytes, activated T lymphocytes, NK cells, and plasma cells.

CD117: Also known as c-Kit, CD117 is a transmembrane glycoprotein and receptor tyrosine kinase, the ligand of which is stem cell factor. CD117 is expressed on approximately 4% of normal marrow precursors, with the exception of lymphoid-lineage cells.

---

lymphocytes in the absence of 'true' cancer stem cells, and appears to be the explanation for why cancer stem cells are not found in lymphoid malignancies with a mature phenotype. By assessing variable heavy-chain hypermutation in malignant B cells, it is possible to establish the stage of maturation in which oncogenesis has occurred. Cells showing evidence of somatic hypermutation are derived from germinal centre or post-germinal centre cells, whilst those failing to show somatic hypermutation are usually derived from pre-germinal centre cells.

Oncogenesis through the accumulation of mutations at the post-germinal centre stage is thought to result in multiple myeloma and Hodgkin lymphoma.

Enumeration of cancer stem cells demonstrates the vast differences in the number of stem cells found in different types of cancer. In acute myeloid leukaemia, the abundance of CD34+CD38- cancer stem cells has been reported to be as low as 0.02-1%, whereas solid tumours are associated with much larger numbers of cancer stem cells. One explanation for the low numbers of cancer stem cells present in haemopoietic malignancies could be the large numbers of cytogenetic translocations associated with these malignancies inducing stem cell-like behaviour in the absence of CD34 expression.

Cross reference

More detail regarding germinal centres can be found in Chapter 8.

9.4 **Chromosomes and nomenclature**

Chromosomes are passed from one generation of a cell to the next. The DNA–histone composite found within chromosomes is called **chromatin**, and is composed of an assembly of nucleosomes. Figure 9.9 demonstrates the composition of the nucleosomes

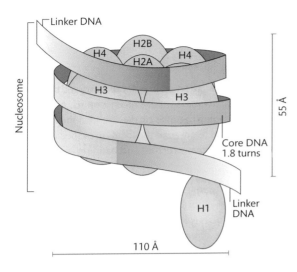

FIGURE 9.9

The structure of a nucleosome. Chromatin is formed by the assembly of nucleosome subunits. Nucleosomes contain eight histones, each wrapped in double-stranded DNA. Each nucleosome attaches to the next by linker DNA, stabilized by histone H1. Reprinted by permission from Macmillan Publishers Ltd: Georgopoulos, K., Haematopoietic cell-fate decisions, chromatin regulation and ikaros. *Nature Reviews Immunology* 2002: 2:162–174.

and their interaction with one another. Double-stranded DNA forms a nucleosome when wrapped around a histone octamer. Four histone proteins (H2A, H2B, H3, and H4) are duplicated to form the octamer. Each nucleosome contains 147 base pairs of DNA, with small segments of linker DNA attaching one nucleosome to the next. A single molecule of histone H1 may bind with the linker DNA and the nucleosome causing stabilization of this structure.

SELF-CHECK 9.9

Describe the components of a nucleosome.

The structure of chromatin varies in different stages of the cell cycle, with chromosomes in metaphase being composed of densely packed chromatin (not involved in the transcription process). It is only during metaphase that chromosomes are visible using light microscopy.

Whilst chromosomes can vary in size, shape, and DNA content, they all have a very similar structure. By understanding the normal structure of chromosomes, we can begin to appreciate the significance of chromosomal changes in haematological malignancies.

Chromosomal structure

Chromosomes have three key easily identifiable structural elements, as illustrated in Figure 9.10 The most prominent of these is the **centromere** which joins the two identical (sister) chromatids, produced after DNA replication. It is required for the formation of the kinetochore, where the fibres that pull each of the chromatids to opposite sides (poles) of the cell during anaphase attach, allowing the accurate passage of DNA from one generation to the next.

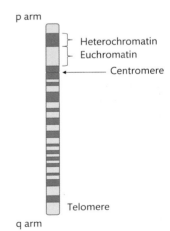

FIGURE 9.10

The basic structure of a chromosome, including an example of G-banding pattern.

Either side of the centromere are the two arms. The shorter of the two arms is called the **p-arm**. The p-arm is so called because it is 'petite'. The larger of the two arms is called the **q-arm**, so designated because it is next to p in the alphabet. The tip of each chromosome arm has a special DNA structure and is called the telomere.

banding pattern
A method of identifying chromosomes based upon their appearance following staining.

Now we have established the macro structure of the chromosome, let us consider the micro structure. By applying a variety of different stains to metaphase chromosomes, a **banding pattern** is generated. A brief summary of these banding patterns can be found in the following Method box. The cytogenetic bands can then be used to describe the location of specific genes. Refer to Fig. 9.10 for further clarification of chromosomal structure and banding patterns.

Each of the landmark bands is numbered from the centromere, in the direction of the chromosome tip, the telomere. To add further specificity, in less-condensed chromosomes bands may divide into sub-bands. Later in this book we will discuss a particular type of leukaemia called acute promyelocytic leukaemia (APL). The locus (plural loci) for one of the genes associated with APL, *RARA*, is 17q12. 17q12 is a specific direction to a particular place within the genome. The locus designation 17q12 tells us that *RARA* can be found on chromosome 17, on the long arm (q), band 12. A normal genome consists of 46 chromosomes and these banding pattern techniques allow the identification of very specific locations on chromosomes, and explain complex chromosomal information in a simple, effective manner.

Cross reference
Acute promyelocytic leukaemia is discussed in detail in Chapter 11.

The most important thing to remember about chromosomal nomenclature is that it is universal. All cytogeneticists report and discuss their results according to the International System for human Cytogenetic Nomenclature (ISCN). This means that communication regarding patients and scientific research can cross geographical borders, and regardless of the country, the terminology is standardized.

METHOD *Generating banding patterns in cytogenetic investigations*

- A variety of different methods can be used to produce banding patterns on chromosomes of interest. It is important when considering these techniques to remember that metaphase chromosomes are required. Using these techniques, cells are encouraged to progress through the cell cycle, and are then treated with a spindle inhibitor such as colchicine in order to arrest cell division in metaphase. The number of bands produced depends on the level of condensation of the chromatin; shorter chromosomes show fewer bands but retain the main 'landmark' bands.

- The most widely reported of the stains is Giemsa, which provides a *G-banding* pattern. The dark areas are composed of heterochromatin whilst light areas are composed of euchromatin. If you refer to Figure 9.10 you will notice the distribution of heterochromatin and euchromatin. Note that Giemsa stain is also one of the key stains used to assign blood cell morphology because of its robust and reproducible staining characteristics.

- *Q-banding* uses a fluorescent stain, such as quinacrine, to produce a distinct banding pattern. However, this pattern is not visible to the naked eye, and requires fluorescent microscopy to identify the appropriate banding patterns.

- *C-banding* involves the treatment of metaphase chromosomes with an acid and then a base prior to a final staining procedure using Giemsa. C-banding stains the centromere.

- *R-banding*, or reverse banding, provides a banding pattern opposite to that achieved by G-banding. Giemsa stain is still used with this technique, although in contrast to G-banding, the chromosomes are initially heated, modifying the uptake of this stain by the chromatin. The dark areas are composed of euchromatin, whilst light areas are heterochromatin.

Chromosomes in pathology

Many of the genes involved in leukaemias and lymphomas have been identified following recurring chromosomal rearrangements causing changes in the banding pattern. However, each chromosome band contains many genes and there are now much more sensitive techniques available to establish gene location, such as fluorescence *in situ* hybridization (FISH). FISH is a molecular cytogenetic technique, which can be used on interphase or metaphase chromosomes, and is discussed in greater detail in Chapter 10.

SELF-CHECK 9.10

How does G-banding help with the reporting of a particular gene locus?

The next sections examine different types of mutation at the genetic and chromosomal level in order to demonstrate how these aberrations can result in haematological malignancies.

Cross reference
Cytogenetic analysis is further considered in Chapter 10.

9.5 An introduction to genetic mutation

Variations in the sequence of a particular gene between individuals are commonplace, provide us with our genetic diversity, and are called **polymorphisms**. The different forms of a specific gene giving rise to polymorphisms are called **alleles**; the alleles for a given gene are found at the same locus, irrespective of their sequence. If an individual has inherited two different copies of an allele at a particular locus, they are called **heterozygous**, and if two identical alleles are inherited at any given locus, they are considered **homozygous** for that particular gene.

Key Points

The name of a gene should always be written in capital letters and italicized in order to differentiate between the gene and its product.

Example: The gene encoding retinoblastoma is referred to as *RB1*, whereas its protein product is abbreviated to pRb.

Non-germline mutations—those that are acquired and found only in somatic cells—occur throughout our lives and are, for the large part, detected by our DNA repair enzymes during the cell cycle. These mutations are either repaired, or the cell harbouring the mutation undergoes apoptosis. As we age, the likelihood of acquiring genetic mutations increases, and acquired mutations are commonly associated with malignancy. There are two particular families of genes that, when mutated, are associated with the development of cancer. These families of genes are:

- **Proto-oncogenes**—encode proteins that are often responsible for cell growth, proliferation, and survival. Mutations within proto-oncogenes may result in a protein product with a gain-of-function. Once mutated, proto-oncogenes are called *oncogenes*.

- **Tumour suppressor genes**—play an important role in controlling the cell cycle and preventing tumour development. An example of a tumour suppressor gene is *RB1*, which encodes pRb. In Section 9.3 we considered the role of pRb in the inactivation of the transcription factor E2F-1, thereby inhibiting the cell cycle—a characteristic role of a tumour suppressor. Tumour suppressor genes (TSG) are also called *anti-oncogene*s. Mutations within these genes often result in a loss-of-function. The result of this loss-of-function is analogous to removing the brakes from the cell cycle.

Section 9.4 considered the role of chromosomes in the packaging of genetic material. The respective roles of proto-oncogenes and tumour suppressor genes have been outlined above, and we will examine the ways in which the function of these genes can be altered or lost. Firstly, we will now consider the possible types of mutation affecting our genes at the nucleotide level, and will then consider major structural alterations of chromosomes. As demonstrated in Chapters 11 and 12, these mutations have an important role in the development (pathogenesis) of haematological malignancies.

Cross reference

For specific examples of types of chromosomal abnormalities in leukaemias and lymphomas, refer to Chapter 11 and 12.

SELF-CHECK 9.11

Briefly, compare and contrast tumour suppressor and proto-oncogenes.

Types of mutation

The sequence of nucleotides in a gene determines the sequence of amino acids in the polypeptide encoded. In turn, the sequence of amino acids in the polypeptide determines the structure and function of the polypeptide itself. Consequently, a mutation in a nucleotide sequence has a direct impact upon the polypeptide it encodes; it is so specific that a change in just one nucleotide is sufficient to render its polypeptide product dysfunctional.

The process of polypeptide synthesis (translation) requires a gene to first be transcribed into messenger RNA (mRNA). A sequence of three nucleotides in mRNA forms a *codon*, with each codon indirectly encoding a particular amino acid (or a signal denoting the beginning or end of transcription). Sequential codons form a so-called 'reading frame', the sequence of codons which is 'read' to determine the sequence of amino acids in the polypeptide product. Figure 9.11 demonstrates this complementary binding of the anti-codon to the codon, the production of sequence-specific polypeptides, and the consequences of the different types of mutation (as outlined below).

The alteration of a single nucleotide in a gene sequence is called a **point mutation**. A **missense mutation** encodes a different amino acid following a single nucleotide exchange, altering the original codon. By contrast, a **nonsense mutation** generates a codon not encoding an amino acid at all. Nonsense mutations prevent further transcription beyond the mutation and are therefore referred to as stop codons.

Missense mutations may be clinically silent (have no pathological affect) or may alter the structure–function relationship of the protein product. An alteration in the size or charge of the amino acid may change the conformational structure of the protein when folded into its tertiary structure, thereby altering its activity. A nonsense mutation fails to encode an amino acid and invariably results in shortened (or truncated) mRNA. If the sequence downstream from this nonsense mutation encodes a functional domain, this domain will not be transcribed and so the protein product loses its function.

The deletion or addition of a nucleotide (or nucleotide sequence) is likely to disrupt the reading frame, causing the synthesis of a structurally and/or functionally abnormal protein.

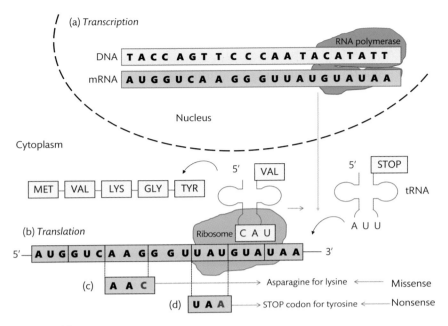

FIGURE 9.11

A simplified outline of transcription and translation. (a) mRNA is transcribed from the DNA template in the 3' to 5' direction by RNA polymerase (green). mRNA (purple) leaves the nucleus to interact with ribosomes in the cytoplasm (b). Following binding to the AUG start codon, tRNA anti-codons bind, in a complementary fashion, to the remaining codons in the mRNA sequence allowing the addition of specific amino acids to the polypeptide chain. Each amino acid binds to the next by a peptide bond. This transcription process is mediated by the ribosome (yellow). Nucleotide substitutions can alter the amino acid composition of the polypeptide. (c) A missense mutation—the nucleotide exchange of cytosine for guanine—changes the codon specificity from lysine to asparagine. (d) Exchanging the nucleotides uracil for adenine, in this instance, represents a nonsense mutation. A stop codon is formed in place of tyrosine, producing a shortened (truncated) polypeptide.

Let's look at some illustrative examples:

In the following example, the sentence is constructed of a number of three-letter words or syllables, each representing a codon. Each of these codons will encode an amino acid, providing we can understand each word included in the sentence. The first sentence (a) makes sense, is explanatory, and should be considered normal (wild type) DNA. In (b) we see the substitution of one of the letters (nucleotides) for another. Whilst the essence and structure of the sentence is preserved, the meaning has changed slightly. We can still encode an amino acid from the codon HAT (because we can still make sense of the word), but this will not necessarily be the *intended* amino acid. This is an illustration of a missense mutation. In (c) a nucleotide has been inserted into the sentence. We have tried to maintain the structure of the sentence by keeping to three-letter words. However, we can no longer understand the sentence as we now have a **frameshift mutation**. Translation will occur to the point at which the codon no longer makes sense (in this case ALT). As ALT does not make transcriptional sense, a premature stop codon is formed, and transcription ceases, resulting in a shortened protein product. This example illustrates the addition of nucleotides to a sequence, although it could also be reversed (d) to illustrate the loss of nucleotides.

(a)   THE CAT ATE ALL HIS DIN NER

(b)   THE HAT ATE ALL HIS DIN NER

(c)   THE CAT ATE ALT LHI SDI NNE R

(d)   THE CAT ATA LLH ISD INN ER

In addition, duplications of genes can occur, potentially resulting in an overexpression of the gene product. If a proto-oncogene is overexpressed in this way, the cell harbouring this duplication may have a growth or survival advantage, especially if the duplicated gene encodes a cyclin or an anti-apoptotic protein.

This section has so far considered the translation of polypeptides from mRNA following acquired DNA mutations, and the mechanisms through which the polypeptide product may be dysfunctional. The next section examines acquired alterations within the chromosomal constitution of a cell, and how these alterations can affect polypeptide synthesis.

SELF-CHECK 9.12

List each of the main types of DNA mutation and provide a brief description.

Quantitative and qualitative chromosomal abnormalities

Chromosomal abnormalities can be either quantitative (numerical) or qualitative (structural), many of which can have a profound effect on the host cell. In the following section we will consider the way in which numerical chromosomal abnormalities are reported, before examining some of the structural abnormalities found in malignancies. The most common of qualitative chromosomal abnormalities in haematological malignancies are translocations, although deletions and inversions are also frequently seen. There are also a range of other chromosomal abnormalities; for more information on these, a specialized cytogenetics textbook should be consulted.

Let us now consider the chromosomal complement of normal and malignant cells, by considering how a patient's karyotype is established.

Karyotype

Quantitative and qualitative chromosomal abnormalities can be identified quite easily through karyotypic studies. The **karyotype** is a description of the chromosomal complement of a cell—if abnormal, then the number of cells in which the abnormality was found should be written inside square brackets. In order to assess an individual's karyotype, chromosomes (autosomes and sex chromosomes) are harvested from cells of a particular tissue, stained, and during analysis are placed in decreasing order of size, location of the centromere, and chromosomal staining characteristics (also called the banding pattern). This arrangement of chromosomes is called a karyogram.

From a karyogram, alterations in the number of chromosomes should be readily apparent. **Ploidy** is the term used to describe the number of homologous chromosomes within a cell. Normal somatic cells are **diploid**: they contain *two pairs* of each autosome plus two sex chromosomes. A normal somatic cell contains 46 chromosomes and is described as **euploid**.

If the chromosomal complement is abnormal, having one or more chromosomes missing or gained in an otherwise chromosomally normal (euploid) cell, this is described as **aneuploidy**.

Examples of aneuploidy include monosomies and trisomies. The loss of a single chromosome results in a **monosomy** for that particular chromosome. The abbreviation for the loss of a chromosome is the minus sign (–). The karyotype for a female demonstrating a loss of chromosome 7 would read 45,XX,–7. The gain of a particular chromosome is called a **trisomy**, which is abbreviated to a plus sign (+). For a male patient with a trisomy 12, the karyotype would be reported as 47,XY,+12. For more comprehensive information regarding ploidy, please refer to Table 9.3.

Aneuploidy is frequently associated with haematological malignancies, and can be used to indicate the prognosis for a patient. For example, patients with an acute myeloid leukaemia (AML) with the loss of a chromosome 5 or 7 (–5 or –7) are considered to have a poor prognosis.

Examples of karyograms for two patients diagnosed with chronic lymphocytic leukaemia are shown in Figures 9.12 and 9.13.

The condition in which cells contain multiple sets of homologous chromosomes, also seen in some haematological malignancies, is called **polyploidy**.

Let us now examine some of the structural (qualitative) chromosomal abnormalities associated with haematological malignancies.

Translocations

Translocations in their simplest form comprise the exchange of genetic material between chromosomes. Look at Figure 9.14 which shows the mechanics of chromosomal translocation.

In most situations, the exchange of chromosomal material results in both chromosomes acquiring new genetic material. We call this exchange a reciprocal translocation. This exchange can have a number of effects on the genes within the translocated region.

TABLE 9.3 Nomenclature for describing cellular chromosomal content.

Ploidy	Number of chromosomes	Comments
Near haploid	23–29	As would normally be found in a germ cell (n = 23)
Low hypodiploid	30–39	
High hypodiploid	40–45	
Diploid	46	Normal chromosomal constitution for a somatic cell
Pseudo-diploid	46	Normal total chromosomal number, but composition is abnormal
Low hyperdiploid	47–50	
High hyperdiploid	51–65	
Hypo/hypertriploid	69 ± (66–80)	Approximately three times the haploid (n = 23) number
Near tetraploid	92 +/– 11 (81–103)	Approximately four times the haploid number of chromosomes

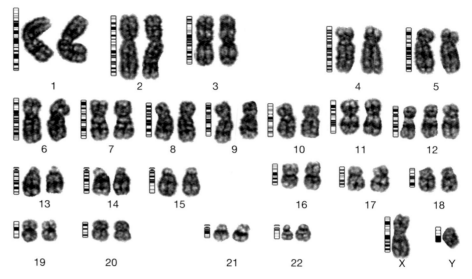

FIGURE 9.12

Karyogram for a male patient with chronic lymphocytic leukaemia. Chromosomes are aligned according to decreasing size and are matched into pairs according to banding pattern. This patient has an additional copy of chromosome 12 (trisomy 12) and deletion of the long arm of chromosome 13 (del13q). Image courtesy of Anne Gardiner, Cytogenetics department, Royal Bournemouth Hospital.

FIGURE 9.13

Karyogram for a female patient diagnosed with chronic lymphocytic leukaemia. This patient has additional copies of chromosome 3 (trisomy 3) and chromosome 18 (trisomy 18) plus t(7;11) (q21;p13). Image courtesy of Anne Gardiner, Cytogenetics department, Royal Bournemouth Hospital.

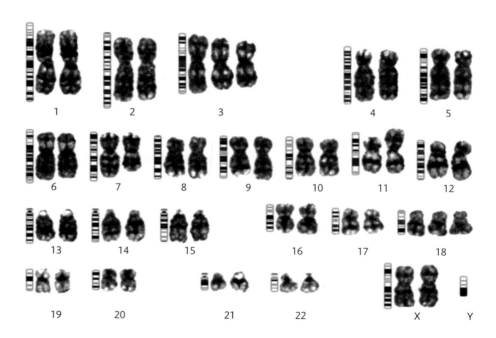

Firstly, the translocation may be clinically silent—it has no effect on the host cell. Secondly, translocations can result in the *overexpression of a gene*. This is usually due to the translocated gene becoming separated from its original promoter (the control region of a gene which regulates transcription), and being controlled by a stronger promoter located upstream of the

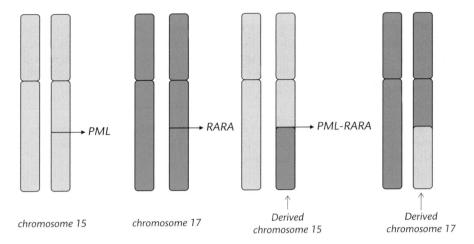

FIGURE 9.14

Translocation involving chromosomes 15 and 17 – t(15;17)(q22;q12). Two copies of each chromosome should be present in each diploid cell, but only one of each chromosome is involved in the translocation process. The *PML* gene is located on chromosome 15 (15q22) and *RARA* is located on chromosome 17 (17q12). The derived chromosome 15 harbours *PML-RARA* and is associated with acute promyelocytic leukaemia.

translocation site. The stronger promoter has an enhanced ability to induce transcription and translation. Thirdly, translocations can result in an *under-expression of a gene or its activity*. This can be due to a number of reasons including:

- Translocation leading to transcriptional control by a weaker promoter or loss of the promoter region.
- The **breakpoint** occurring within a specific gene, leading to a shortened (truncated) protein product.

Furthermore, due to the formation of a fusion (or chimeric) gene where two regions of different genes are brought together by a translocation, the *protein product may acquire a novel function*. When transcribed, the mRNA will comprise retained sequences from both genes, and the translation process will form a product called the **fusion protein** or **chimeric protein**. In many cases, some of the functional domains of both original proteins may be retained, but fused within a single molecule. In the majority of cases, the fusion protein will be unable to complete its wild-type function, or this function may be altered in some way.

breakpoint

An area of a chromosome, usually within a gene, where a region of chromosomal material is lost or exchanged with another chromosome.

Cross reference

Examples of fusion proteins can be found in Chapters 11 and 12.

Key Points

In order to describe a translocation, a lower case 't' is used followed by two pairs of brackets.

Within the first pair of brackets, the numbers of the chromosomes involved in the translocation are presented in numerical order. Each chromosome is separated by a semicolon e.g. t(9;22).

Within the second set of brackets breakpoints are included in an order that allows us to relate the chromosomes to their particular breakpoints. Again, each breakpoint is separated by a semicolon.

> **EXAMPLE: A specific translocation between chromosomes 9 and 22 found in chronic myeloid leukaemia, would be abbreviated as follows: t(9;22)(q34;q11). From this abbreviation we can determine that the breakpoints are 9q34 and 22q11. The description of each part of a karyotype is separated by a comma, so the karyotype for a male with this translocation would be 46,XY,t(9:22)(q34;q11).**

Whilst translocations can have a variety of effects on the behaviour of a cell, providing we know the function of the polypeptide transcribed from a particular locus, deletions have a more predictable effect and will be considered next.

Deletions

Another common cytogenetic feature found in haematological malignancies is the **deletion**. Deletions, as the name suggests, involve the loss of chromosomal material, including any genes found within that deleted region. A deletion may involve an entire chromosome, or part of a chromosome, either of which may have an overall effect on cell function. For example, if a key gene responsible for the regulation of the cell cycle (such as a tumour suppressor gene) is located within this deleted region, cell cycle control may be lost. Using appropriate chromosomal nomenclature, deletion is abbreviated as 'del'.

There are several types of deletion. Consider the structure of a chromosome in relation to Figure 9.15. A deletion occurring *within* a chromosome is called an **interstitial deletion**. Such deletions have two breakpoints, and result from the chromosome being wrongly repaired by the cell's DNA repair machinery. However, if there is only one breakpoint, and the rest of the chromosome arm is missing we have a **terminal deletion**. Small deletions found within a chromosome (often submicroscopic) are called **microdeletions**.

Inversions

Subtle changes in the banding pattern within a chromosome may indicate an inversion. Inversions also need two chromosome breaks and are the result of the portion of chromosome being rotated before being rejoined, causing the 5′ region to face in a 3′ direction and vice versa. Figure 9.16 demonstrates the mechanics of chromosomal inversions. Two types

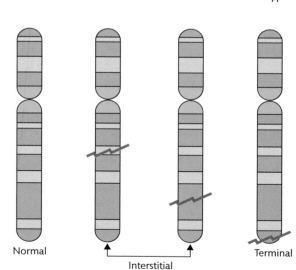

FIGURE 9.15

Chromosomal deletions. Zig-zagged lines represent chromosomal breakpoints. Left: normal chromosomal structure with the p and q arms separated by the centromere. Middle: examples of interstitial deletions. Right: a terminal deletion causes the loss of chromosomal material from the tip.

Normal   Interstitial   Terminal

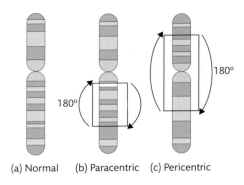

(a) Normal   (b) Paracentric   (c) Pericentric

FIGURE 9.16

Chromosomal inversions. (a) A normal chromosome is presented for comparison of the G-banding patterns. A paracentric inversion (b) is restricted to a single arm (in this case the q-arm) and shows a reversal of the banding pattern within the boxed region as a consequence of the 'rotation' of this chromosomal material. The pericentric inversion (c) involves both the p- and the q- arms and describes the rotation of chromosomal material around the centromere. The pericentric inversion also reverses the banding pattern.

of inversion can occur: a **paracentric inversion** and a **pericentric inversion.** A paracentric inversion is one in which a region restricted to one arm (p or q) is rotated through 180°. A **pericentric inversion** involves part of both arms of the chromosome so also includes the centromere and, unlike a paracentric inversion, may change the location of the centromere. An example of a pericentric inversion is inv(16)(p13;q22) and this is found in a particular sub-type of acute myeloid leukaemia.

So far, we have considered how gene expression can be altered through the process of mutation and the gene sequence and chromosomal complement of a cell altered. We have discussed that DNA mutations, if undetected by the cell's DNA repair machinery, can be passed on to daughter cells, causing an accumulation of cells, derived from the mutated progenitor. Epigenetic processes also allow constant modification of gene expression. Epigenetic processes are discussed in the next section.

Table 9.4 provides a comprehensive summary of the important translocations and inversions included within this book.

Cross reference

Inv(16)(p13;q22) is discussed in further detail in Chapter 11.

TABLE 9.4 The range of important cytogenetic translocations and inversions considered in this textbook.

Chromosomal abnormality	Product	Associated pathology
t(8;21)(q22;q22)	RUNX1-RUNXT1	AML with maturation
inv(16)(p13.1;q22)	CBFB-MYH11	Acute myelomonocytic leukaemia
t(16;16)(p13.1;q22)	CBFB-MYH11	Acute myelomonocytic leukaemia
t(15;17)(q22;q12)	PML-RARA	Acute promyelocytic leukaemia
t(11;17)(q23;q21)	PLZF-RARA	Acute promyelocytic leukaemia
t(11;17)(q13;q21)	NuMA-RARA	Acute promyelocytic leukaemia
t(5;17)(q35;q21)	NPM-RARA	Acute promyelocytic leukaemia
t(9;11)(p22;q23)	MLLT3-MLL	AML
t(6;9)(p23;q34)	DEK-NuP214	AML with maturation; acute myelomonocytic leukaemia
inv(3)(q21;q26.2)	RPN1-EVI1	AML; B-lymphoblastic leukaemia/lymphoma

(Continued)

TABLE 9.4 (Continued)

Chromosomal abnormality	Product	Associated pathology
t(1;22)(p13;q13)	RBM15-MKL1	Acute megakaryoblastic leukaemia
t(v;11q23)	v-MLL	AML; B-lymphoblastic leukaemia/lymphoma
t(9;22)(q34;q11)	BCR-ABL1	Chronic myeloid leukaemia; B-lymphoblastic leukaemia/lymphoma
t(12;21)(p13;q22)	TEL-AML1	B-lymphoblastic leukaemia/lymphoma
t(5;14)(p31;q32)	IL3-IGH	B-lymphoblastic leukaemia/lymphoma
t(1;19)(q23;p13.3)	E2A-PBX1	B-lymphoblastic leukaemia/lymphoma
t(14;18)(q32;q21)	IGH-BCL2	Follicular lymphoma; MALT lymphoma
t(11;14)(q13;q32)	CCND1-IGH	Myeloma; MGUS; mantle cell lymphoma
t(4;14)(p16.3;q32)	MMSET-IGH	Myeloma
t(14;16)(q32;q23)	IGH-CMAF	Myeloma
t(6;14)(p21;q32)	CCND3-IGH	Myeloma
t(14;20)(q32;q11)	IGH-MAFB	Myeloma
t(11;18)(q21;q21)	API2-MALT1	MALT lymphoma
t(1;14)(p22;q32)	BCL10-IGH	MALT lymphoma
t(2;17)(p23;q32)	CLTC-ALK	ALK positive large B-cell lymphoma
t(8;22)(q24;q11)	MYC-IGK	Burkitt lymphoma
t(2;8)(p12;q24)	MYC-IGL	Burkitt lymphoma
t(8;14)(q24;q32)	MYC-IGH	Burkitt lymphoma
t(2;5)(p23;q35)	ALK-NPM	Anaplastic large cell lymphoma ALK positive
t(1;2)(q21;p23)	TPM3-ALK	Anaplastic large cell lymphoma ALK positive

SELF-CHECK 9.13

A male patient's malignant cells are shown, using a variety of cytogenetic techniques, to have the following abnormalities in twenty cells examined:

47 chromosomes.

Deletion of chromosome 8.

Addition of chromosome 7.

Addition of chromosome 12.

Translocation of chromosome 15 long arm—band 22, and chromosome 17 long arm—band 12.

Write this patient's karyotype in abbreviated form.

9.6 **Epigenetics**

Epigenetics explores how gene expression can be altered whilst maintaining wild-type DNA sequences. Epigenetic processes are entirely normal, although, when they occur inappropriately, can predispose to malignancy. An excellent definition of epigenetic processes was proposed by Adrian Bird of the Institute of Cell Biology in Edinburgh as *'... the structural adaptation of chromosomal regions so as to register, signal or perpetuate altered activity states ...'*. Epigenetic processes can involve region-specific DNA sequences, or post-translational modification of histone proteins. **Hypermethylation** (the addition of methyl (CH_3) groups), a process whereby genes may be 'switched off' to repress DNA transcription, is an important epigenetic event. Epigenetic processes also describe the removal of methyl groups resulting in **hypomethylation**. **Acetylation** will be considered here as an important regulator of transcription.

A range of other epigenetic processes may also be utilized in transcriptional regulation, including phosphorylation—the addition of phosphate groups (PO_4^{3-}) to target proteins; and histone ubiquitination—the addition of the protein ubiquitin, to histone molecules H2A and H2B. These processes are beyond the scope of this book.

We will now examine hypermethylation, hypomethylation, and acetylation in turn.

Hypermethylation

A family of enzymes called **DNA methyltransferases** (DNMTs) attach methyl groups to **CpG islands** throughout the genome, as illustrated in Figure 9.17. DNA methyltransferases are found to be overexpressed in many haematological malignancies.

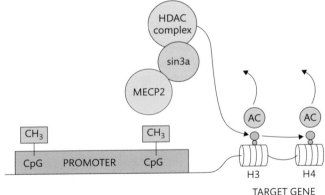

FIGURE 9.17
Epigenetic processes. Methylation of cytosine within CpG islands allows the assembly of an inhibitory complex involving HDAC and sin3A. This inhibitory complex causes chromatin remodelling by deacetylating histone H3 and H4 lysine residues. Transcriptional activators that normally bind to acetylated lysine fail to localize to this region, causing transcriptional repression.
CpG = CpG island within the promoter region;
MECP2 = Methyl-CpG-binding protein 2;
HDAC = Histone deacetylase;
AC = Acetylation.

CpG islands are regions of DNA rich in cytosine and guanine nucleotide repeats, found within the promoter regions of approximately 40% of all mammalian genes. The transcriptionally repressive process of hypermethylation is thought to be mediated by the binding of specific proteins containing a methyl-binding domain (MBD) to methylated CpG islands. The localization of MBD containing repressors and co-repressors inhibits DNA transcriptional machinery, preventing the production of mRNA. One of the key repressive enzymes to be localized in this fashion is HDAC. As such, hypermethylation enables the repression of specific genes.

In the context of haematological malignancies, hypermethylation of tumour suppressor genes results in their inactivation. Such inactivation of tumour suppressor genes can potentially cause the subsequent accumulation of mutations within the genome of the cell, attributable to a reduction in the intracellular concentration of tumour suppressor proteins.

The pattern of methylation is passed to subsequent generations of daughter cells, silencing tumour suppressor genes in a progenitor cell, which in turn will cause silencing of the tumour suppressor in all subsequent generations of cells. This heritable silencing of tumour suppressors increases the probability of further mutations accruing within this lineage, predisposing these cells to malignant transformation.

The following mechanisms outline the process of silencing tumour suppressor genes through hypermethylation:

- *Biallelic methylation* of a particular tumour suppressor gene means that both copies of that gene are silenced, rendering the host cell deficient in a particular tumour suppressor protein.

- *Monoallelic hypermethylation with simultaneous mutation of the accompanying tumour suppressor allele.* In this scenario, a single copy of the tumour suppressor gene is silenced by methylation, but the alternative allele has been mutated in some way, inhibiting the function of the tumour suppressor protein. This situation also causes the host cell to become deficient in a particular tumour suppressor protein.

Hypermethylation has the same effect as a tumour suppressor deletion or mutation: loss-of-function. Pro-apoptotic genes, cell cycle regulators, and DNA repair genes are examples of other families of genes that may be silenced through epigenetic processes.

Now that the role of hypermethylation in gene silencing has been considered, we should examine the role of hypomethylation on gene transcription.

Hypomethylation

Whilst the importance of hypermethylation can be seen in the repression of specific genes, another epigenetic mechanism may result in an overexpression of certain genes and their products. This mechanism is called hypomethylation. Hypomethylation, or demethylation, is the opposite of hypermethylation and is a process through which the methyl groups attached to DNA are removed. This demethylation results in gene activation as methyl-binding proteins can no longer localize within the promoter region of target genes. The failure of this localization subsequently inhibits binding to a range of transcriptional repressors and co-repressors which inhibit DNA transcription and translation. Often in haematological malignancies, widespread hypomethylation occurs (called global hypomethylation), the result of which is the activation of a number of oncogenes including cyclins and anti-apoptotic genes—allowing transcription and translation to occur. Overexpression of oncogenes can play an important role in oncogenesis.

Acetylation

Acetylation involves the addition of acetyl-Coenzyme A (CoA) -derived acetyl groups ($-COCH_3$) to histone lysine residues in the presence of the enzyme histone acetyltransferase (HAT). Acetylated lysines, usually associated with histones H3 and H4, are unevenly distributed throughout chromatin, although are associated with the 'open' chromatin structure **euchromatin.** The term euchromatin describes regions of chromatin possessing active genes. These regions are therefore subject to DNA transcription. Euchromatin is also associated with hypomethylated CpG islands, ensuring transcriptional repressors fail to localize in this region. In contrast, **heterochromatin**, the 'closed' or 'clumped' chromatin, retains hypoacetylated histones and is associated with hypermethylated CpG islands, both of which repress transcription and translation.

In hypermethylated regions, the localization of large inhibitory protein complexes prevents transcription and translation through a variety of mechanisms (refer to Figure 9.17). Localization of HDAC removes acetyl groups from H3- and H4-associated lysine residues. Co-localization of sin3a (bridging HDAC to specific transcription factors) and mi-2 (involved in the nucleosome remodelling and histone deacetylation complex (NuRD)) enables chromatin remodelling and the inhibition of transcription.

The removal of acetyl groups from lysine is believed to inhibit transcription and translation in two ways:

- The positive charge of the histone-associated lysine residues is regained following neutralization by the acetyl groups. This positive charge induces chromatin clumping, preventing access of the DNA transcriptional machinery to target genes.

- Acetylated lysines associated with H3 and H4 act as binding sites for proteins containing a **bromodomain**. These bromodomain-containing proteins are largely considered to be involved in the regulation of transcription and translation. Removal of the bromodomain binding site causes gene repression.

Here we have considered some of the genetic and epigenetic mechanisms responsible for altering cell behaviour and ultimately increasing the probability of oncogenesis. However, to put these concepts into the context of clonal disorders, the next section provides a definition of clonality, and the ways in which we can establish whether a population of cells is a malignant clone. The next section will conclude with discussing the acquisition of additional mutations which can cause an alteration in the behaviour of the clonal subpopulation. With this in mind, let's have a look at clonality.

> **bromodomains**
> Originally identified in the Drosophilia protein brahma. A bromodomain comprises a sequence of 110 amino acids derived from a four-helix bundle. When the helices interact, they produce a hydrophobic binding pocket with a conserved amino acid sequence that recognizes acetyl lysine.

SELF-CHECK 9.14

Briefly discuss the roles of hypomethylation, hypermethylation, and acetylation in the control of transcription and translation.

9.7 Clonality

Unrepaired mutations occurring within a single stem cell or haemopoietic progenitor will be passed on to all subsequent generations of cells derived from that mutated cell, as shown in Figure 9.18. As these daughter cells share the same genetic or molecular features, although they are distinct from the wild-type population of cells, this population of

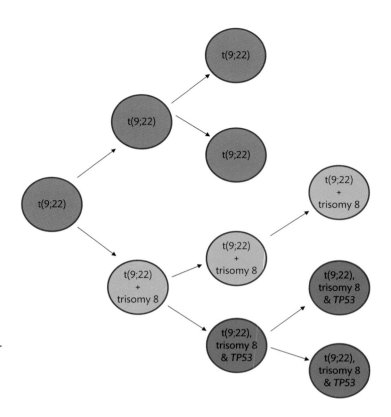

FIGURE 9.18

A clonal population of cells. All cells in this figure are derived from a single mutated stem cell harbouring t(9;22), typically found in CML. Daughter cells also acquire additional mutations, forming subclones (represented by the different colours). These subclones accumulate mutations, altering their behaviour in a process called clonal progression. In this example, trisomy 8 is acquired in a cell already harbouring t(9;22). One of the daughter cells of this subclone acquires a *TP53* mutation, resulting in the loss of a valuable tumour suppressor—forming another subclone with a greater survival advantage and likely resistance to therapy.

mutated cells is called a clone. Haematological malignancies are clonal disorders and, as such, the malignant cells all share the same basic genetic or molecular abnormalities. The remainder of this section describes some of the ways that are used to determine the clonality of a particular group of cells.

Cytogenetic analysis

Cytogenetically, a population of cells can be called a clone if a minimum of two cells share an additional chromosome, or a minimum of three cells share the same deletion in the absence of any other abnormal cytogenetic features. Two or more cells need to show the same translocation to constitute a clone.

Philadelphia chromosome

This denotes the derived chromosome 22 der(22q−) not to be confused with t(9;22). The translocation process is abbreviated to t(9;22).

light chain restriction

An overexpression of either kappa or lambda light chains. This overexpression of a single type of light chain would be the product of a monoclonal population of B cells.

A good example of a clonal disorder is chronic myeloid leukaemia (CML). Following the extraction of a bone marrow aspirate for cytogenetic analysis, the cultured cells will be investigated for a specific chromosomal abnormality called the **Philadelphia chromosome**. This chromosome is known as der(22q−) as it is derived (der) from a reciprocal translocation, although there is a net loss of chromosomal material from the long arm of chromosome 22 (22q−). Specifically, the translocation t(9;22)(q34;q11) producing der(22q−) will be investigated and should be found in all the malignant cells within the myeloid lineage. Morphologically, CML appears as an accumulation of mature and maturing granulocytes. There are generally all stages of maturation of neutrophils present, with an increase in basophils and eosinophils also occurring, especially as the disease progresses. Platelet defects will also be apparent. Even though CML appears morphologically heterogeneous, this condition is clonal because all malignant cells possess the Philadelphia chromosome.

Immunophenotyping

Using immunophenotyping, it can be rather difficult to establish whether a population of cells is clonal. When a B-lineage malignancy is suspected, we can investigate membrane-bound immunoglobulins specifically to assess kappa (κ) or lambda (λ) **light-chain restriction**. A single B cell will express a single type of light chain, either kappa or lambda, but never both. Figure 9.19a shows a monoclonal population of B lymphocytes, with kappa light-chain restriction. We would expect approximately 65% of cells to express kappa light chains, with the remainder expressing lambda. Generally speaking, kappa or lambda light chains found in excess of those ranges are described as light-chain restricted and therefore clonal. Ratios within the reference range suggest a polyclonal population of B cells have produced these light chains, which is a normal response to infection.

If aberrant markers are expressed on a range of malignant cells, for example the T-cell antigen CD7 expressed on myeloid cells as shown in Figure 9.20, this is also an indication of a clonal population. However, selective loss or gain of antigen expression often makes the immuno-phenotyping of aberrant markers an unreliable process.

Cross references

Cytogenetic analysis is discussed in greater detail in Chapter 10.

See the *Microbiology* text in this series for more information on immune response to infection.

A more in-depth outline of CML can be found in Chapter 11.

More detail regarding the process of immunophenotyping and an explanation of CD markers can be found in Chapter 10.

Morphology

It is important to recognize that the cells constituting a clonal population do not necessarily look the same (homogeneous morphology)—and in malignancies such as CML, they appear heterogeneous. Investigations such as cytogenetic analysis, or polymerase chain reaction (PCR) should be completed to determine clonality.

DNA mutations and their products

Genetic mutations play an important role in oncogenesis, often resulting in a structurally and functionally abnormal protein product. Using DNA analysis techniques such as polymerase

Cross references

Some of the methods used to indentify DNA mutations and their products are outlined in Chapter 10.

Myeloproliferative diseases are discussed in greater detail in Chapter 11.

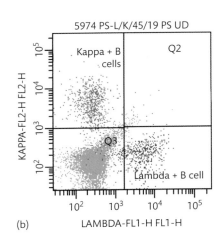

FIGURE 9.19

Flow cytometric evaluation of light chain status. (a) Patient shows only kappa light chains (red), quadrant 1 (Q1). The patient has a clonal population of B cells which are kappa light chain restricted. (b) A polyclonal B-lymphocyte population in which both kappa and lambda light chains are detected. Cells in Q2 and Q3 are considered negative for kappa and lambda. Images courtesy of Adnan Mani, Department of Immunology, Southampton General Hospital.

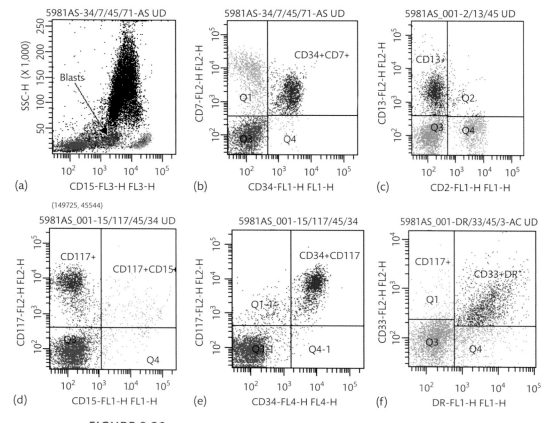

FIGURE 9.20

Aberrant expression of CD7 in acute myeloid leukaemia (AML). CD7 is a T-cell marker, but may be found abnormally expressed on cells of a myeloid lineage in AML. (a) Shows the general distribution of cells within the sample, the target population is shown in red. (b) Cells co-express CD34 and CD7. (c) Cells show bright expression of CD13 (a marker of granulocytes and monocytes), but do not express CD2 (a marker of T-cells). (d) Blast population (red) expresses CD117, the stem cell factor receptor, but not CD15 (another marker of granulocytes). (e) Confirms that cells co-express CD34 and CD117. (f) Cells co-express CD33 (a marker of monocytes and myeloid progenitor) and HLA-DR. The blast phenotype is: CD34+, CD117+, CD13+, CD33+, HLA-DR+, CD7+ and CD2-, CD15-. Images courtesy of Adnan Mani, Department of Immunology, Southampton General Hospital.

Cross reference

JAK2 mutations are discussed in greater detail in Chapters 6 and 11.

chain reaction, mutated proteins or genes can be identified in a population of cells. If the cell population shares an identical mutation, these cells are clonal. An example of a mutated protein is the JAK2 receptor, derived from the valine to phenylalanine substitution at position 617 (V617F) associated with a number myeloproliferative diseases including polycythaemia vera.

Clonal progression

Clonal progression, sometimes called clonal evolution, refers to the acquisition of mutations within a pre-existing clone of cells, as shown in Figure 9.18. As the cells with the additional mutation proliferate, they form a sub-clone. Depending upon the function of the mutated gene or genes, the behaviour of the malignant population will change, and in many cases will become more aggressive. Markers of aggressiveness include the spread of malignant cells to other sites (metastasis), or resistance to previously effective therapy. For example, mutation of the tumour suppressor gene *TP53* is associated with a poor prognosis because radiotherapy and many chemotherapeutic agents activate the p53 protein through the DNA damage they induce. This mutation renders these *TP53* mutated cells resistant to many forms of traditional anti-cancer therapy. With wild-type p53, following chemotherapy or radiotherapy, p53 would be activated, and as a consequence, the apoptotic machinery would be initiated, causing death of the malignant cells.

We have now considered all the important changes that can occur within a cell to cause malignant transformation, but how many of these mechanisms need to occur before a cell will transform? Section 9.8 considers this in relation to the oncogenic mechanisms discussed thus far.

SELF-CHECK 9.15

Provide, using your own words, a definition of a clone.

9.8 **Mechanisms of oncogenesis**

This chapter considers the development of haemopoietic tumours. The development of leukaemia is called **leukaemogenesis**, and the same process resulting in lymphoma is called **lymphomagenesis**. The process through which myeloid develops is called **myelomagenesis**.

The development of cancer is a consequence of the loss of a cellular control mechanism, possibly causing an increase in the proliferation rate, or the loss of apoptotic control. Ultimately, the result is an inherent genomic instability within the tumour cells, predisposing the malignant clone to further genetic alteration and clonal progression.

Clonal progression usually heralds an evolution in the behaviour of the tumour cells and can cause resistance to commonly used therapeutic agents. However, the cause of the change from a normal to a malignant cell is unlikely to be the response to a single mutational event. Rather, oncogenesis is due to a multi-step process causing a gradual reduction in cellular control. As we have previously discussed, alterations in proto-oncogenes are likely to cause gain-of-function mutations, and mutations in tumour suppressor genes cause a loss of cellular control. Mutations in both tumour suppressor genes and proto-oncogenes are common in haematological malignancies, but will a single mutation in a single gene cause cancer? Undoubtedly, the answer to this question is 'no'.

Take, for example, a mutation in a tumour suppressor gene. Tumour suppressors have a number of functions, but the endpoint of their action is to ensure that the cell cycle completes appropriately, without the incorporation of any mutations within the replicated DNA sequence. Mutating a tumour suppressor gene on its own will not cause cancer. Instead, alterations in tumour suppressor genes (TSG) will increase the likelihood of *additional* mutations occurring in other areas of the genome, and will then go unchecked because of the initial mutation. For example, the loss of a tumour suppressor may be the first mutation within a cell. If this TSG mutation is followed by a mutation in either the same cell or in that cell's progeny by an activating (or gain-of-function) mutation within a proto-oncogene, uncontrolled proliferation will occur. Once uncontrolled proliferation occurs, additional mutations are likely, leading to clonal progression.

This multi-step process of oncogenesis was proposed by Ernest Knudson in 1971 and is called *Knudson's hypothesis*. This hypothesis states that a minimum of two steps (or two-hits) are required within a single cell to cause cancer, and this has been repeatedly demonstrated in a wide range of tumours.

The acquisition of somatic mutations is a proven way of developing genetically unstable cells leading to a haematological malignancy. However, this model largely describes oncogenesis in an ageing population, where the accumulation of somatic mutations occurs over time. Clearly this process does not explain all types of haematological malignancy. Undoubtedly, there is a heritable component to many haematological malignancies, and the next section examines some of those conditions leading to an increased risk of developing malignancy but also abide by Knudson's hypothesis.

SELF-CHECK 9.16

Using appropriate examples, explain Knudson's hypothesis.

9.9 Inheritance and leukaemia

A wide range of heritable conditions can predispose individuals to haematological malignancies. A number of these heritable conditions can result in childhood leukaemias. Some of these conditions may be associated with the inheritance of a single inactivating mutation within a tumour suppressor gene, leaving the individual open to further mutations in accordance with Knudson's multi-hit hypothesis. Others, such as Down syndrome, Fanconi syndrome, and Diamond–Blackfan anaemia are associated with alternative mechanisms of oncogenesis, including failure of DNA repair and immunodeficiency. Table 9.5 demonstrates the range of familial conditions associated with a predisposition to haematological malignancies. This section briefly introduces a selection of inherited factors.

Trisomy 21

Trisomy 21, commonly called Down syndrome, is associated with an increased risk of leukaemia. The highest risk is associated with patients below four years of age, with the risk progressively decreasing beyond this age. Children with trisomy 21 commonly undergo a brief period in which the production of their myeloid cells within the bone marrow becomes grossly abnormal (**transient abnormal myelopoiesis**—TAM). When examined in the laboratory, TAM is virtually indistinguishable from acute myeloid leukaemia. The key differentiating feature is that TAM spontaneously remits within two to three months. Approximately 25% of patients with TAM will later go on to develop acute megakaryoblastic leukaemia (cancer of the platelet precursors)—a particularly rare subgroup of AML. Individuals who have a mosaic genotype for trisomy 21, i.e. a mixture of cells with either two or three copies of chromosome 21, are also at risk of TAM. In these mosaic cases, only the trisomic cells are implicated in TAM, indicating that the additional copy of chromosome 21 is essential for this haematological syndrome to manifest itself. Currently, the reason for the association between trisomy 21 and leukaemogenesis is unknown.

Cross reference

Trisomy 21 is discussed in the context of a myeloid proliferation related to Down syndrome in Chapter 11.

Fanconi syndrome

Fanconi syndrome or Fanconi anaemia (FA) is associated with progressive bone marrow failure and reduced peripheral blood cell counts of all three lineages (pancytopenia): red cells,

TABLE 9.5   Hereditary diseases associated with the development of haematological malignancies. Adapted from Segal GB, Lichtman MA. Familial (inherited) leukaemia, lymphoma, and myeloma: an overview. *Blood cells, molecules and diseases.* 2004; 32: 246-261.

Syndrome	Inheritance pattern	Malignancy
DNA repair		
Ataxia telangiectasia	Recessive	BCL, TCL, T-ALL, T-PLL
Bloom	Recessive	ALL, AML lymphoma
Fanconi	Recessive	AML
Nijmegen breakage	Recessive	Lymphoma, leukaemia
Rothmund–Thomson	Recessive	AML
Seckel	Recessive	AML
Werner	Recessive	AML
Conditions leading to secondary mutations		
Amegakaryocytic thrombocytopenia	X-linked	AMML
Diamond–Blackfan	Dominant and recessive	AML
Familial platelet disorder	Dominant	AML
Kostmann	Dominant and recessive	AML, AMoL
Schwachman–Diamond	Recessive	ALL, AML, AMML, AMoL, EL, JMML
Tumour suppressor Li–Fraumeni	Dominant	ALL, Hodgkin, Burkitt, CML B-CLL
Neurofibromatosis	Dominant	AML, JMML
Immunodeficiency Common variable immunodeficiency	Dominant and recessive	BCL
Severe combined immunodeficiency disease	Recessive	BCL
Wiskott–Aldrich	X-linked	ALL, Hodgkin lymphoma
X-linked lymphoproliferative syndrome	X-linked	EBV-linked BCL

Key: ALL, acute lymphoblastic leukaemia; AML, acute myeloid leukaemia; AMML , acute myelomonocytic leukaemia; AMoL, acute monocytic leukaemia; BCL, B-cell lymphoma; B-CLL, B-cell chronic lymphocytic leukaemia; CML, chronic myeloid leukaemia; EBV, Epstein–Barr virus; EL, erythroleukaemia; JMML, juvenile myelomonocytic leukaemia; T-ALL, T-acute lymphoblastic leukaemia; TCL, T-cell lymphoma; T-PLL, T-prolymphocytic leukaemia.

white cells, and platelets. The risk of developing AML is 15 000-fold higher in FA patients in comparison to the normal population. Inherited in an autosomal-recessive fashion (i.e. the patient must have two copies of the mutated gene in order for the disease to manifest itself), the precise biology of the disease is unknown, although it is recognized that patients with FA are more susceptible to DNA cross-linking and therefore are more likely to undergo DNA mutation. To date, eight key genes have been associated with the development of FA: *FANCA–FANCG*. *FANCD* has been subdivided into *FANCD1* and *FANCD2*. Of these *FANC* genes, *FANCA*, *C* and *G* are most commonly mutated. 60–70% of patients show mutations within *FANCA*. Groups *C* and *G* account for approximately 20% of mutations. Although the mechanisms are poorly understood, *FANC* proteins have been shown to be involved in DNA repair and cell checkpoint control. Failure of this mechanism is thought to allow the accumulation of genetic mutations.

Cross reference

Fanconi anaemia and Diamond–Blackfan anaemia were introduced in Chapter 5.

Diamond–Blackfan anaemia

Diamond–Blackfan anaemia (DBA) is a particularly interesting congenital disease as it is the first condition to be associated with the mutation of a ribosomal protein, RPS19. The mechanisms responsible for DBA-associated pathologies are incompletely understood. The gene encoding RPS19 is located at locus 19q13, and mutations within this gene are found in 25% of patients. Alternative gene loci have also been implicated in DBA pathogenesis. DBA is associated with an increased risk of AML, and although clinically and biologically heterogeneous, usually presents within the first year of life with a failure of red cell production (erythropoiesis), an anaemia associated with enlarged red cells (a macrocytic anaemia), and a significant reduction in the number of developing red cells within the bone marrow (erythroid aplasia).

So far, some of the heritable factors causing a predisposition to oncogenesis have been considered. Now we should examine some of the environmental factors demonstrated to play a role in oncogenesis, and in particular the development of haematological malignancies.

9.10 Environmental causes of haematological malignancies

So far, we have examined some of the molecular and cytogenetic causes of cancer. Later chapters will demonstrate the consequences of the mutations already introduced, and how their very real impact on cell proliferation and survival can ultimately cause malignant transformation. Sometimes mutations will occur through a very traceable series of events, such as the inheritance of a dysfunctional tumour suppressor gene. In other situations, the cause may not be so straightforward, and we need to look into alternative hypotheses to explain the causes of these tumours.

It is important to be aware of environmental factors. Whilst it is very easy to view ourselves as discrete autonomous units, in fact we are the opposite, although we may not be conscious of it. Our bodies are constantly adjusting and adapting to environmental stimuli. The vast majority of these environmental factors are totally harmless, although in some situations, these may be oncogenic. In this section we will look at some of the environmental factors associated with haematological malignancies.

Ionizing radiation

It is well established that individuals surviving the detonation of atomic bombs in 1945 in Nagasaki and Hiroshima had an increased risk of developing haematological malignancies. The first type of malignancy to manifest itself following irradiation from an atomic bomb detonation is leukaemia. Individuals can also be exposed to ionizing radiation through treatment for solid tumours, occupational exposure in medical radiology or as a radiation scientist (such as those working in nuclear processing plants). It is believed that Marie Curie and her daughter, Irene, both died from leukaemia following their work with radiation. Health risks are substantially lower as a consequence of recent changes in working practices within these environments, as occupational exposure has been reduced.

The most common types of leukaemia associated with atomic bomb detonations are acute leukaemias and chronic myeloid leukaemia. The Life Span study for atomic bomb survivors has provided the majority of the information used to shape our understanding of these malignancies following exposure to radiation. Recent work completed in Nagasaki suggests that two other haematological conditions may follow atomic bomb exposure: myelodysplastic syndrome (MDS) and monoclonal gammopathy of undetermined significance (MGUS)—a clonal disorder of plasma cells, identified by an excess production of a single type of immunoglobulin in the absence of any clinical symptoms—two conditions usually affecting the elderly. The group, investigating in excess of 50 000 atomic bomb survivors, suggests an increased incidence of these conditions in survivors. The closer the survivor to detonation, the greater the risk of developing haematological malignancies in later life. It seems likely that irradiated stem cells predispose individuals to haematological malignancies later in life.

Non-ionizing radiation

There is a great deal of public concern and media attention directed towards the issue of non-ionizing radiation in the form of extremely low-frequency electromagnetic fields (ELF-EMF) associated with overhead power cables. The particular concern is that these low-frequency fields can induce DNA damage, especially in children, causing childhood leukaemia. In 2005 Draper *et al.* published a paper examining 29 081 children with cancer, including 9700 with leukaemia. Draper noted an increased risk of leukaemia (although not other childhood cancers) associated with children living within 200 metres of a high-voltage power line compared with those living at distances greater than 600 metres from the source. However, the group concede that these results may be due to chance or secondary to a mechanism other than ELF-EMF. To date, there is no convincing evidence of a genuinely increased risk of childhood leukaemia due to ELF-EMF.

Cross references

For more information on myelodysplastic syndromes, refer to Chapter 11.

Late effects of therapy in leukaemogenesis are discussed in detail in Chapter 11.

Late effects of therapy

Many patients treated with radiotherapy (ionizing radiation) and chemotherapy eg for solid organ tumours may subsequently develop haematological malignancies, most commonly leukaemias. These leukaemias are called **'secondary' leukaemias** because they arise as a consequence of exposure to a known **mutagen**. By contrast, spontaneously occurring malignancies are called **de-novo leukaemias** as they have no traceable cause. These will be further discussed in Chapters 11 and 12.

mutagen
A chemical substance known to induce DNA mutations.

Chemotherapeutic agents, for example alkylating agents or topoisomerase II inhibitors, work by inducing DNA damage in cells with a high proliferation rate, resulting in cell death through the activation of apoptotic pathways. However, because these therapeutic agents are so toxic, they tend to have innocent bystander effects where non-malignant cells (such as haemopoietic progenitor cells) accrue mutations and become precancerous. Patients developing secondary acute myeloid leukaemia following radiotherapy and chemotherapy commonly have a preceding myelodysplastic syndrome which later transforms into AML.

At the forefront of concern for these so-called 'late effects' cancers are patients treated for childhood leukaemia. The most common type of childhood leukaemia is common acute lymphoblastic leukaemia (c-ALL) which accounts for 26% of all childhood cancers in the United Kingdom, and is associated with a 5-year survival rate of 80%. These patients tend to have an increased risk of late-effect cancers because of their survival potential due to their young age. That is, their young age increases the likelihood that they will survive ALL—however, if they do survive, they then have a greater chance of developing a late-effect cancer when they get older.

Infectious agents

There are a number of infectious agents, viral and bacterial, associated with haematological malignancies. This section outlines a number of the more common types and their association with malignant transformation.

Epstein–Barr virus (EBV)

EBV is a member of the human herpesvirus family and is the cause of infectious mononucleosis (glandular fever). EBV was the first virus to be associated with human cancer, having been derived from the tissue of patients with Burkitt's lymphoma. In some individuals, EBV is associated with a number of haematological malignancies, although this does not necessarily mean that anyone exposed to EBV (or, indeed, has suffered from glandular fever) is destined to develop cancer.

Cross reference

Germinal centres are discussed in greater detail in Chapter 8.

EBV can infect a wide range of cells including B and T lymphocytes. When naïve B cells are infected, some will migrate to germinal centres—found within lymph nodes and important in the process of B-cell maturation—where they will develop into plasma cells or memory B cells. These memory B cells contain residual viral DNA, and cause the patient to become a carrier of EBV DNA. Over time, carrier status can result in malignant transformation and the onset of B-cell lymphoma particularly in patients with ineffective immune systems. Although not an exhaustive list, these lymphomas include Hodgkin lymphoma and primary central nervous system lymphoma. EBV-positive tumours are more commonly found in immunocompromised than immunocompetent patients.

Human T-lymphotrophic virus-1 (HTLV-1)

HTLV-1 can be isolated from most cases of adult T-cell leukaemia (ATL) and is commonly found in Africa, the Caribbean, and Japan. The mechanism of transformation is particularly complex, and is thought to involve the inactivation of tumour suppressor genes, the activation of cell cycle regulators, and the up-regulation of anti-apoptotic proteins. The end result is a clone of T cells with an increased proliferation rate and an inability to undergo apoptosis. This cellular behaviour increases the probability of mutations and can result in malignant transformation. Of those patients infected with HTLV-1, up to 3% may develop ATL.

Human herpesvirus-8 (HHV8)

This is a member of a group of viruses that includes herpes simplex 1 and 2, cytomegalovirus (CMV), and EBV. Herpesviruses persist for the life of the host and affect between 60 and 90% of adults.

Human herpesviruses comprise linear, double-stranded DNA within a protein capsid. Initially infecting epithelial cells, following primary infection the virus enters a latent period within the periaxonal sheath of a variety of nerves. Reactivation of the virus involves migration along sensory neurones to the mucocutaneous interface, a process that enables the virus to avoid immune recognition.

HHV8 is recognized as an important cause of Kaposi sarcoma in HIV patients, and can also infect CD19+ B cells, leading to the development of B-cell lymphomas associated with immunosuppression.

Helicobacter pylori

Gastric *Helicobacter pylori* infections are associated with the development of gastritis, peptic ulceration, and the development of gastric carcinoma. Infection by *Helicobacter pylori* is also strongly associated with the development of a marginal zone B-cell lymphoma of mucosa-associated lymphoid tissue (MALT) type. MALT lymphoma is a form of marginal zone lymphoma, which comprises transformed B lymphocytes. MALT lymphoma accounts for approximately 8% of all non-Hodgkin lymphomas. Evidence suggests that the mechanism of lymphomagenesis is due to chronic inflammation caused by infection, as supported by the fact that, in low-grade cases, eradication of *Helicobacter pylori* results in a resolution of the MALT lymphoma. One study revealed that in uncomplicated, low-grade cases, 79% of patients were cured by eradicating the *H. pylori* infection. However, patients with tumours extending beyond the mucosa and submucosa (i.e. those with invasive properties) have a less favourable outcome when treated with antibiotics and require traditional cytotoxic therapy.

Benzene

Many polycyclic and aromatic hydrocarbons are carcinogenic. Benzene is a well-established leukaemogen, having been associated with leukaemia since as early as 1928. In order to become toxic, benzene must first be metabolized in the liver primarily by cytochrome P4502E1 (CYP2E1). The outcome of this process is to generate phenol which is then further metabolized to catechol, hydroquinone, and 1,2,4-benzentriol. 1,4-benzoquinone is subsequently generated by the degradation of catechol (in which bone marrow peroxidases have been implicated). These metabolic derivatives are thought to bind to various intracellular proteins and enzymes such as topoisomerase II to influence DNA indirectly. It is this impact on DNA which is believed to have a leukaemogenic effect.

The association between benzene and leukaemia is strong, although inconsistent between subtypes. AML has the strongest association, as repeatedly demonstrated, whereas chronic lymphocytic leukaemia (CLL) has a far weaker association. The correlation with ALL and CML is ambiguous and requires further, more comprehensive, investigation. Individuals associated with exposure to high levels of benzene include those employed in the petrochemical, shoe, rubber, and paint industries.

Cross references

HHV8 is discussed in relation to large B-cell, lymphoma-associated Castleman disease and primary effusion lymphoma in Chapter 12.

Marginal zone lymphomas are discussed in greater detail in Chapter 12.

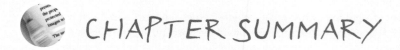

CHAPTER SUMMARY

In this chapter we have:

- Established the role of the cell cycle in the development of daughter cells.

- Examined the definitions and main subgroups of haematological malignancy.

- Examined the mechanisms involved in oncogenesis.

- Discussed the role of the cancer stem cell in leukaemogenesis and lymphomagenesis.

- Established that a population of identical cells, all derived from the same mutated parent, constitutes a clone.

- Outlined the process of clonal progression.

- Identified the link between loss-of-function mutations in tumour suppressor genes and gain-of-function mutations in proto-oncogenes established in the context of Knudson's multi-hit hypothesis.

- Discussed cytogenetic terminology and introduced chromosome structure in relation to haematological malignancies.

- Outlined a range of mutations at the genetic level and linked these to abnormalities in the polypeptide product potentially leading to a malignant phenotype.

- Examined the role of epigenetic processes as genetic modifiers, and linked these processes to the alteration of the expression level of a range of different proteins.

- Examined some of the heritable and environmental causes of cancer and established links between these causes and genetic mutation.

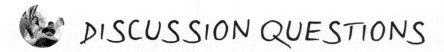

DISCUSSION QUESTIONS

9.1 Using appropriate examples, critically discuss the effect of chromosomal abnormalities on cell cycle control and the subsequent development of haematological malignancies.

9.2 Abnormal DNA methylation patterns influence tumour suppressor function in haematological malignancies. Discuss this statement.

9.3 Critically discuss the roles of infectious agents in lymphomagenesis.

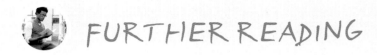

FURTHER READING

- Chen J, Odenike O, Rowley JD. *Leukaemogenesis: more than mutant genes*. *Nature Reviews Cancer* 2010:**10**;23–36.

- Degos L, Linch DC, Löwenberg B (ed.). *Textbook of Malignant Haematology* (2nd edn). Taylor & Francis, Oxon, 2005.

- Hoffbrand AV, Catovsky D, Tuddenham EGD (ed.). *Postgraduate Haematology* (5th edn). Blackwell Publishing Ltd, Massachusetts–Oxford–Carlton, 2005.

- Keutgens A, Roberit, Viatour P, Chariot A. *Deregulated NF-kB activity in haematological malignancies*. *Biochem. Pharmacol.* 2006:**72**;1069–80.

- Segal EB, Lichtman MA. *Familial (inherited) leukaemia, lymphoma and myeloma: an overview*. *Blood cells, Molecules and Diseases* 2004:**32**;246–61.

Answers to self-check questions, case study questions, and discussion questions are provided in the book's Online Resource Centre, visit www.oxfordtextbooks.co.uk/orc/moore

10

The laboratory investigation of haematological malignancies

Gavin Knight

As a biomedical scientist, it is often exciting to be involved in the investigation of a new haematological malignancy. Getting 'hands on' in the examination of blood films and other laboratory-generated data in these cases can be particularly rewarding. However, it is essential that we remain mindful of the fact that every sample represents a patient who is likely to be unwell, emotional, or intimidated by the process of investigation. In every instance we must remember that these patients are human beings and it is our duty to treat the sample with respect, regardless of the scientific principles to be learnt from the case. Many of these patients will continue to be treated at the hospital in which they present, and over time we can observe changes in their results as a consequence of the treatment regimens they are prescribed. The investigations we complete and the results generated have an important bearing on the patient's management. It is often regarded that working in a laboratory distances you from a patient. However, this is not the case. Instead you are part of a multidisciplinary healthcare team and your actions as a biomedical scientist can have a profound impact on patient care.

This chapter outlines some of the diagnostic procedures followed when a patient presents to a medical professional with symptoms that are suggestive of haematological malignancy and therefore require laboratory investigation. The particular investigative methods outlined here are pertinent to biomedical scientists and other laboratory personnel, but exclude non-laboratory diagnostic techniques and investigations, such as radiological and surgical exploration.

The chapter begins by discussing some of the most common presenting symptoms associated with malignancies, putting them into a biological and physiological context. We then examine the range of laboratory tests often required for a definitive diagnosis. Whilst the focus of this chapter is on haematology, we also discuss a range of molecular biological and cytogenetic investigations essential for the diagnosis and classification of haematological malignancies. Biochemical and microbiological investigations have been omitted in the interests of focus, but can be explored in the companion titles, *Clinical Biochemistry* and *Medical Microbiology*.

Learning objectives

After studying this chapter you should be able to:

- Discuss the common symptoms experienced by patients presenting with a haematological malignancy and explain the physiological cause of these symptoms.
- Describe the investigative process in establishing the diagnosis of a specific haematological malignancy.
- Describe the common findings from the initial full blood count and blood film analysis associated with malignant haematological conditions.
- Compare and contrast a bone marrow trephine with a bone marrow aspirate and outline the different stains that can be used to provide diagnostic information.
- Describe some of the typical cytogenetic abnormalities associated with a range of haematological malignancies, and outline some of the techniques available for their identification.
- Discuss the role of named molecular techniques in the investigation of haematological malignancies.

10.1 **Patient presentation**

Before we begin examining the laboratory procedures for diagnosing and monitoring haematological malignancies, it is important to consider some of the symptoms exhibited by patients when they present to the medical team. The range of these symptoms is particularly broad, and any combination can be present in any one patient. It is also important to realize that these symptoms can be explained using normal physiological principles. These principles will be discussed in the context of the symptoms outlined below.

The symptoms associated with malignant disease include:

- Pallor
- Lethargy
- Pharyngitis
- Recurrent infections
- Easy bruising
- Pyrexia
- Night sweats
- Bone pain
- Flu-like symptoms
- Lymphadenopathy
- Splenomegaly
- Hepatomegaly
- Asymptomatic

Let us now consider each of these in turn.

Pallor (a pale coloration to the skin) and **lethargy** are often attributable to anaemia with an associated reduction in oxygen delivery to the tissues. This reduction in oxygen delivery is a

lethargy
Tiredness or fatigue.

normocytic normochromic anaemia

A particular form of anaemia associated with red cells of a normal size and coloration. Although there can be a number of causes, in the context of a malignancy the most likely causes are anaemia of chronic disease or myelosuppression.

Cross reference

Normocytic normochromic anaemias were first introduced in Chapters 5 and 6.

ecchymoses

Bruises caused by the leakage of blood from blood vessels.

cellularity

The proportion of cells within the bone marrow.

punched-out lesions

Caused by the catabolic effects of osteoclast activating factors on bony structures.

Cross reference

Myeloma is discussed in more detail in Chapters 9 and 12.

consequence of a reduced haemoglobin concentration, or a reduction in the number of circulating red cells. A **normocytic normochromic anaemia**, where the red cells appear of normal size and normal coloration (haemoglobinization), is most frequently encountered with a malignancy.

Pharyngitis and recurrent infections are the consequence of a dysfunctional immune system. As we shall see later on in this chapter, although the white blood cell (WBC) count may be raised, this should not be used to imply that the white cells are functional. This raised WBC count (*leucocytosis*) may be due to circulating leukaemic cells. There is a common misconception by students that a raised WBC as part of a haematological malignancy is a consequence of the body fighting infection. In fact, the raised WBC is usually due to either circulating malignant cells, or non-malignant cells displaced by clonal cells within the bone marrow.

Easy bruising is caused by two main effects:

1. A reduced platelet count (thrombocytopenia)
2. Dysfunctional platelets

A combination of the two may also be apparent. In either case, platelets are unable to form a primary platelet plug, which is essential to prevent leakage of blood from blood vessels. In a patient with a normal platelet count, day-to-day bumps and scrapes go unnoticed, but for patients with thrombocytopenia or dysfunctional platelets, easy bruising occurs. Easy bruising may take the form of **ecchymoses** or *petechiae*.

Each of the symptoms outlined above is associated with a condition called **myelosuppression**— the failure of the myeloid component of the bone marrow to produce red cells, white cells, and platelets as a consequence of either a therapeutic agent or a malignant clone. Myelosuppression was initially believed to be the consequence of malignant stem cells competing with normal stem cells for their microenvironment. Although this is partly true, it has been demonstrated that malignant blasts actually secrete cytokines which suppress the proliferation of normal blasts. The consequence of this suppression is that mature effector cells will not be produced, causing a reduction in all myeloid cell lines (pancytopenia).

Pyrexia (a rise in the body's core temperature) and *night sweats* are often symptoms associated with malignant B lymphocytes and their precursors in response to the synthesis and secretion of cytokines. In particular, interleukin (IL) -1, tumour necrosis factor-α (TNFα), and IL-6 are associated with fever and weight loss. During an infection, the normal physiological response is for white cells to increase in number and secrete a range of cytokines to:

- Potentiate the white cell colony
- Stimulate the hypothalamus to increase the body's temperature
- Stimulate the proliferation of haemopoietic stem cells
- Stimulate the proliferation of B cells and promote switching between different types of antibody (isotype-switching)

Increases in white cell numbers will cause an increase in the concentration of circulating cytokines and `potentiate their physiological role. However, the white cell count is unlikely to rise as a consequence of elevated cytokine levels because the cytokines produced by the malignant blasts have a myelosuppressive effect on the normal blasts of the bone marrow.

Bone pain can have a number of causes. An increase in the bone marrow **cellularity**, as a consequence of large numbers of malignant cells, can compress the nerves running through the bone, causing pain. Secondly, in myeloma, malignant plasma cells synthesize and secrete osteoclast activating factors, promoting the degradation of bone. The result of bone degradation is the gradual loss of bone density and, when examined on X-ray, **punched-out lesions** throughout the skeleton become apparent.

In lymphoma, the spleen or a lymph node may be the primary site of the malignancy. These sites tend to become enlarged and can be felt (palpated) during a clinical examination. *Lymphadenopathy* (one or more enlarged lymph nodes) is often painless. The nodes feel rubbery, and can become quite large in a short space of time. *Splenomegaly* (an increase in the size of the spleen) is often found in splenic lymphoma, although this is not always the case. Splenomegaly is associated with a wide range of illnesses and haematological malignancies. In cases of splenomegaly, the left side of the abdomen can become severely distended and puts pressure on the other visceral organs. Thrombocytopenia (a reduction in a patient's platelet count) may be apparent because platelets accumulate in the enlarged spleen and may result in easy bruising. There may be a concurrent increase in the size of the liver, **hepatomegaly**, due to reduced blood flow through the enlarged spleen and pooling of blood in the liver. A combination of hepatomegaly and splenomegaly is called **hepatosplenomegaly**.

Finally, it is important to note that some patients may be *asymptomatic*, although a haematological malignancy may be identified and diagnosed through a routine full blood count investigation. The FBC could be requested as part of routine monitoring for an unrelated condition, for example diabetes.

When a patient presents to a doctor with any of these symptoms, the doctor will take a thorough medical history and perform a clinical examination. If an obvious cause is not apparent, then more information is needed before a diagnosis can be made, so blood tests are requested. Although a range of blood tests may be requested for the first-line investigation of these symptoms, this chapter will focus on those most pertinent to haematology. The first investigation we will consider is the full blood count.

Cross reference

The full blood count was first described in Chapters 2 and 4.

SELF-CHECK 10.1

Outline the main presenting symptoms associated with a haematological malignancy.

10.2 The full blood count

The full blood count (FBC) is a broad measure of the red cells and their contents, white cells and platelets. The FBC provides us with an enormous amount of **quantitative** data, although it has limited value as it does not provide **qualitative** data, and as such is unable to demonstrate how those cells are functioning. The FBC is also non-diagnostic in the large majority of cases. The FBC fails to give a reason for particular indices being outside their reference range. Therefore, in response to an abnormal FBC, the results should be considered in the context of the patient's clinical details and further investigations requested.

Although the FBC can provide important information about haematological malignancies, the presence of a malignancy will not always cause abnormal FBC results. In localized malignancies such as occurs in some lymphomas, it is possible that the patient may have a normal FBC. Normal FBC results may also be found in the early stages of malignancies before the bone marrow has been compromised.

quantitative
Types of data that deal with numerical values; for example, the number of platelets in one litre of blood.

qualitative
Non-numerical data; for example, the ability of a platelet to function correctly.

co-morbidities
Two or more co-existing diseases.

Key FBC findings

You may expect to see changes in the following FBC parameters in some patients with haematological malignancies. It is important to note that every patient is different, and some may have **co-morbidities** (from more than one disease process) which may alter the blood profile.

Cross reference

More information on lymphomas can be found in Chapters 9 and 12.

Cross reference

More detail on polycythaemia vera can be found in Chapter 11.

Red cell count

The red cell count may be either reduced or increased. A *reduced* RBC count could be a consequence of myelosuppression or may be attributable to bleeding, especially in patients with thrombocytopenia or abnormal haemostasis. As mentioned earlier in this chapter, a normocytic normochromic anaemia is commonly associated with malignancy, and whilst the red cells will look normal, they may be reduced in number within the peripheral blood. By contrast, the RBC may be *increased* in polycythaemia vera where a clonal proliferation of red cell precursors increases the number of circulating red cells.

Mean cell volume (MCV) and haemoglobin (Hb)

Whilst a normocytic normochromic anaemia is usually associated with haematological malignancies, a macrocytosis (raised MCV) may be apparent in some patients. A macrocytosis is commonly found in patients receiving cytotoxic therapy, or those with myelodysplastic syndrome as a consequence of **cell cycle arrest**. In conjunction with the raised MCV, the haemoglobin concentration is often normal or slightly low.

In diseases such as polycythaemia, an iron deficiency may develop because of the increased production of red cells and the use of venesection to reduce the haematocrit. This will eventually lead to a microcytosis (low MCV), reduced haemoglobin concentration, and a gradual reduction in the red cell count.

Raised mean corpuscular haemoglobin concentration (MCHC)

The MCHC is calculated from the average haemoglobin concentration of each of the red cells counted. In patients with autoimmune haemolytic anaemia (AIHA), a condition often associated with B-cell malignancies, red cells lose their biconcave disc shape and become spherical (called spherocytes). Part of the red cell membrane is removed by macrophages in response to membrane-bound autoantibodies, whilst the volume of the cell stays the same. This reduction in cell size accompanied by a maintained cell volume causes the MCHC to increase.

cell cycle arrest

Occurs when the G1–S–G2–M transitions become disrupted. Arrest usually occurs in late G1 or S phases as a consequence of the activation of tumour suppressor proteins in an attempt to initiate DNA repair. Alternatively, it can be seen during S phase where synthesis of DNA is disrupted.

White blood cell count

The white cell count represents the number of both mature and immature white cells. In the case of a haematological malignancy, an increased white blood cell (WBC) count may be the result of malignant cells circulating in the peripheral blood, or attributable to normal cells being displaced by the malignant clone. When examining malignant cells, the raised WBC count may represent an increased proliferation rate, a failure of apoptosis, or both.

A reduced WBC count may also be found, particularly as a consequence of myelosuppression. In myelofibrosis, an increased or decreased WBC count may be seen, depending upon whether the fibrotic marrow has displaced immature cells to the peripheral blood, or suppressed leucocyte development.

An important practice point to remember is that even though the WBC count may be within the reference range, this does not necessarily mean these white cells are normal and indeed, the relative proportions of the different speices of WBCs may be markedly abnormal.

Cross reference

More information about clonality can be found in Chapter 9.

Abnormal differential

The differential count examines the range of species of white blood cell: neutrophils, lymphocytes, monocytes, eosinophils, basophils, and their precursors. Each of these should be found within a defined reference range, as determined by testing a representative group of the local population. An abnormal differential is commonly found in haematological malignancies, broadly representing the events occurring within the bone marrow. In lymphoid malignancies, a **reversed ratio** may be found. Normally, the neutrophil count is higher than the lymphocyte count, but in lymphoid malignancies the reverse is often found. A reversed ratio may also occur in viral infections and in children up to the age of seven years, so it is important not to jump to diagnostic conclusions, but consider all findings logically and perform further investigations as necessary.

Platelets

In haematological malignancies, thrombocytopenia is the most commonly identified platelet abnormality, and can be attributable to myelosuppression. However, in splenomegaly, thrombocytopenia can also be evident due to pooling of platelets within the spleen. A raised platelet count (thrombocytosis) may be associated with myeloproliferative conditions such as polycythaemia vera, and in a mandatory finding in **essential thrombocythaemia** (for which there are specific diagnostic criteria). Thrombocytosis may be a reactive phenomenon mediated by inflammatory cytokines.

Whilst this section focuses on findings associated with haematological malignancies, these can also be associated with benign conditions. A raised WBC count may be found in people with bacterial infections, although it may be decreased following a viral infection. Platelets may be decreased following a haemorrhage, and increased during an inflammatory illness. AIHA may not always be associated with malignancy, it can be a complication of another autoimmune disease or infection, and the MCHC may be increased following treatment with certain types of drugs, or following a transfusion reaction. In some types of haematological malignancy, the FBC may be normal.

In cases where abnormal FBC results have been generated or a specific request has been made by a doctor, the next step is to examine a peripheral blood film. The blood film can give us important information regarding the appearance (**morphology**) of the cells, and some of the features apparent on the film may be of diagnostic use. The blood film can also help confirm the legitimacy of the FBC results.

SELF-CHECK 10.2

List examples of data provided by a full blood count analysis.

10.3 Blood film

A blood film should always be examined when a patient has a suspected haematological malignancy. Clinical laboratories have their own guidelines to determine the point at which a blood film examination is indicated.

The indices provided by the FBC should be representative of the cells seen when using a microscope, although in some cases the FBC findings may be inaccurate. For example, **dysplastic** changes in white cells alter their morphology and physical properties to the point that the analyser cannot determine their species. In these instances, the blood film is an important mechanism for identifying the true nature of the FBC results. Some of the limitations of using a FBC alone are outlined below.

- The FBC may suggest that a patient's platelet count is low, but it is considered good practice to examine a blood film to check for **platelet clumps** and fibrin **strands**, either of which would artificially reduce a patient's platelet count *in-vitro*. Where there is an unexpectedly low platelet count, the sample should be checked for a clot before the blood film is made.

- A patient's MCV may be within the reference range. However, when examining a blood film, two distinct populations of red cells, small and large (**dimorphic**), can be distinguished.

reversed ratio
A lymphocyte count that is higher than the neutrophil count.

essential thrombocythaemia
A clonal proliferation of megakaryocytes leading to an increased platelet count.

Cross reference
More information regarding essential thrombocythaemia can be found in Chapter 11.

dysplasia
The abnormal development or maturation of cells, tissues, or organs.

platelet clumps
Aggregates of platelets within a FBC, demonstrable on a blood film. Often artefactual, facilitated by the presence of EDTA in blood tubes.

dimorphic
Two distinct populations of red cells in the same FBC sample.

When each population of red cells has their volume averaged, the mean sits within the reference range. An indication of this may come from a raised red cell distribution width (RDW). *Note*: The RDW is often measured as part of an automated FBC, but is not always reported.

- The technological methods used to determine the identity of white blood cells is unreliable when there are signs of dysplasia, or when large numbers of immature cells are present. This could result in misclassification of a particular species of WBC.

The peripheral blood film also allows examination of the structural features of the cells, and identification of any inclusion bodies present. We can obtain many diagnostic hints to aid in the classification process by examining: the cytoplasmic granular contents of granulocytes; the size and haemoglobinization of red cells; the size and number of platelets; the nuclear configuration (nucleoli and chromatin structure) of white cells; and the presence of immature forms.

Blood film examination

Romanowsky stain should be used to obtain the most information from the blood film. According to the *International Committee for Standards in Haematology* (ICSH) Romanowsky stain should be composed of Azure B (an acidic stain) and Eosin Y (a basic stain). These stains bind to basic and acidic intracellular or extracellular components of blood, respectively.

By using Romanowsky stain we would expect to see cell nuclei staining purple, with nucleoli staining a much lighter blue. The cytoplasm of the cell differs according to the function of the cell or its stage of maturation, and therefore its chemical composition. Table 10.1 demonstrates the typical cytoplasmic staining of the different haemopoietic cells following Romanowsky staining.

TABLE 10.1 Typical Romanowsky staining characteristics of erythroid, myeloid, and lymphoid cells.

Lineage	Cell	Cytoplasm	Granulation
Erythroid	Early erythroblast	Dark blue	
	Late erythroblast	Light blue	
	Reticulocyte	Bluish tinge	
	Red blood cell	Dark pink	
Myeloid	Myeloblast	Pale blue	None
	Promyelocyte	Blue	Azurophilic
	Myelocyte	Pink	Lineage specific granules (see mature cells)
	Metamyelocyte	Pink	Lineage specific granules
	Neutrophil	Pink/orange	Purple
	Eosinophil	Pink	Red/orange
	Basophil	Blue	Purple/black
	Monocyte	Grey/blue	
Lymphoid	Lymphocyte	Blue	
	Plasma cell	Dark blue	

Ideally, when examining the blood film for the first time, a low-power lens should be used so that the distribution of cells can be ascertained. Any cellular clumps or fibrin strands should be easily recognizable at low power.

Once the low-power examination is complete, a higher powered lens (×40 magnification) should be used. This more detailed examination should enable the appreciation of cell structure and identification of key cell lines. Any immature cells otherwise retained within the bone marrow should be easily recognizable. In cases of malignancy a differential count of 200 white blood cells should be completed to determine the proportions of the different cells and their precursors. Precursor cells found within the peripheral blood would be counted on an *ad hoc* basis, but as part of the differential count. The term **leucoerythroblastic blood picture** is used to describe a blood film containing immature white cells and immature red cells.

The cytoplasmic contents of granulocytes and the nuclear lobes of polymorphs should be readily appreciable. Examination of the shape, size, structure and chromatin distribution of the nucleus, and identification of nucleoli in lymphocytes is of utmost importance. Should blasts be present, evidence of **Auer rods** should be sought to assist with malignancy classification. Figure 10.1 describes typical morphological characteristics associated with blast cells.

Identification of Auer rods confirms a malignancy to be of myeloid origin, although the absence of Auer rods does not suggest a lymphoblastic malignancy. Only 50% of myeloid malignancies exhibit Auer rods within the cytoplasm of blast cells.

Experience in blood film examination is essential in order to obtain the greatest amount of information from the patient sample. Often, alterations in blood cell morphology can make the identification of individual cells, particularly white blood cells, very difficult. Experience of examining blood films is crucial when identifying features of a particular cell's lineage. The difficulty in identifying cells could lead to the incorrect diagnosis being made, or important diagnostic features being overlooked. Whenever the opportunity arises, this should always be taken to gain valuable experience in blood film examination.

leucoerythroblastic blood picture
A blood film showing nucleated red cells and immature white cells.

Auer rods
Eosinophilic primary granules are abnormally assembled in rod-like structures and are a marker of myeloid malignancies.

Cross reference
See Chapter 8 for the morphology of white blood cells.

SELF-CHECK 10.3

What is the significance of identifying Auer rods in a population of blasts?

Whilst a blood film is important for the examination of peripheral blood cells, a bone marrow sample is a key diagnostic tool. The bone marrow is the site of haemopoiesis and is informative of the pathological process taking place.

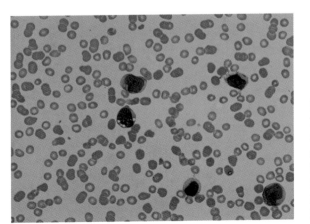

FIGURE 10.1

Typical blast cell morphology. This peripheral blood film shows examples of myeloblasts. The blast in the top right contains an Auer rod next to the cell membrane. The presence of Auer rods is conclusive evidence of the myeloid lineage of these cells. The high nucleocytoplasmic ratio and the presence of nucleoli are both characteristics of blast cells. Image courtesy of Jackie Warne, Haematology Laboratory, Queen Alexandra Hospital, Portsmouth.

10.4 **Bone marrow assessment**

Bone marrow samples

Whilst blood film examination can give us a great deal of information about a patient's disease and can aid in a diagnosis, we need to assess the patient's bone marrow to fully appreciate the nature of their disease. With the exception of T-lymphocyte production, the process of haemopoiesis occurs within the bone marrow. It is therefore important to examine the bone marrow to obtain as much information as possible about the patient's pathology.

In cases involving a suspected haematological malignancy of a lymph node (or group of lymph nodes), samples from the lymph node(s) should be used for primary diagnostic purposes. However, the bone marrow should also be assessed to allow the evaluation of the haemopoietic tissue as this will give us an indication of the presence of malignant cell infiltrates; the architecture of the bone marrow; the distribution and proportions of cells; the presence of abnormal inclusions within the cells; and the overall cellularity.

The following samples can be used to assess the patient's bone marrow:

- Aspirate
- Trephine
- Trephine imprint/roll

The sternum, around the area of the second intercostal space, or the iliac crests are the most commonly chosen sites for bone marrow aspiration. A combination of aspirate and trephine dictates the use of either the anterior or posterior iliac crests, utilizing the same skin incision for both procedures, whereas a lone bone marrow trephine *must* be perfomed on the iliac crest because of the risk of puncturing the thoracic cavity.

Each of these samples will be considered below.

Routine bone marrow assessment involves the collection of a bone marrow aspirate and, often, a trephine biopsy. It is essential if the aspirate gives a '**dry tap**' or is **haemodiluted** that a trephine is obtained for diagnostic purposes.

dry tap

An unsuccessful bone marrow aspirate which yields either no bone marrow material, or insufficient amounts for analysis. A dry tap could be caused by poor technique, but is more likely to be due to bone marrow fibrosis or hypercellularity.

haemodilute

When aspirated contents of the bone marrow are excessively diluted with peripheral blood.

Bone marrow aspirate

Samples collected from a bone marrow aspiration can be used for morphological examination, Perls' staining (to assess iron stores), immunophenotyping, and cytogenetic and molecular genetic testing. An image of a well-produced bone marrow aspirate slide is shown in Figure 10.2. All of these investigations are important in order to provide as much information on the patient's condition as possible. Differential cell counts can be performed easily on a well-stained bone marrow (BM) aspirate as the cellular morphology is well preserved. A minimum of 500 cells should be counted for the BM differential, with the trails of bone marrow behind the fragments being the best position to find cells originating from the bone marrow. A bone marrow fragment at the tip of an aspirate slide is shown in Figure 10.3. Outside this localized area, the differential may start to include cells from peripheral blood contaminating the bone marrow from the aspiration, and may therefore be inaccurate. Table 10.2 shows the reference ranges for a bone marrow differential count for an individual aged between 21 and 56 years of age.

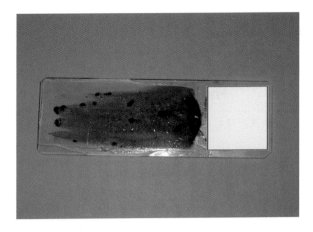

FIGURE 10.2

Bone marrow aspirate. A macroscopic view showing the distribution of the marrow on the slide. The densely stained region on the right is the origin. Tails are to the left. Bony particles can be seen at the tips of the tails. Image courtesy of Dr Robert Corser, Haematology Dept, Queen Alexandra Hospital, Portsmouth.

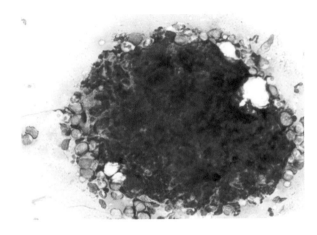

FIGURE 10.3

High magnification of bony particle. Large numbers of cells are contained within the fragment, and these can be used to estimate bone marrow cellularity. Image courtesy of Dr Robert Corser, Haematology Dept, Queen Alexandra Hospital, Portsmouth.

METHOD *Bone marrow aspirate*

Bone marrow aspiration begins with the rupture of the sinusoidal membrane. The fine needle enters the bone marrow and liquid marrow is withdrawn using a syringe. The liquid nature of the bone marrow is a consequence of peripheral blood leaking into the bone marrow from damaged blood vessels.

Once aspirated, the fluid can be smeared onto a slide, dried, fixed, and stained using Romanowsky stain.

Excess aspirate can be aliquoted into EDTA anticoagulant and used to make additional films, but EDTA can alter cellular morphology and cause the loss of subtle diagnostic clues. The films are prepared for interpretation in the haematology laboratory, and the turnaround time can be as little as an hour. EDTA anticoagulated bone marrow can be forwarded on for immunophenotyping analysis if necessary.

TABLE 10.2 Reference ranges for haemopoietic constituents in bone-marrow-derived samples, for patients between 21 and 56 years of age.

Cell	Mean value (%)	Range (%)	Comments
Myeloblasts	1.4	0–3	WHO classification of acute leukaemia ≥20%
Promyelocytes	7.8	3.2–12.4	'Blast-equivalents' in leukaemia diagnosis
Myelocytes	7.6	3.7–10	Mitosis does not occur beyond this stage
Metamyelocytes	4.1	2.3–5.9	
Band forms	–	–	
Neutrophils	34.2	23.4–45	
Eosinophils	2.2	0.3–4.2	
Basophils	0.1	0–0.4	
Monocytes	1.3	0–2.6	
Erythroblasts	25.9	13.6–38.2	Myeloblast equivalent in erythroleukaemia
Lymphocytes	13.1	6–20	
Plasma cells	0.6	0–1.2	Increased in myeloma and other plasma cell diseases
Myeloid : erythroid ratio	2:4	1.3–4.6	This is a ratio and as such is not reported in percentage terms

Bone marrow aspirates should be examined using low power, intermediate, and then high power. At low power, an assessment of the bone marrow cellularity should be made along with the identification of abnormal cells within the marrow. Megakaryocytes and macrophages should also be examined for abnormalities. At high power, the maturational stages of myeloid and erythroid lines should be appreciated and a differential count completed. The myeloid to erythroid ratio should be calculated and areas of necrosis determined. Finally, iron stores should be assessed using Perls' stain.

An initial (baseline) bone marrow aspirate is a useful tool as it can be used diagnostically, but it also allows clinicians to compare subsequent bone marrow aspirates to the original following treatment. The baseline marrow therefore allows us to assess whether a particular disease is progressing or improving following treatment.

Bone marrow trephine

In comparison with the bone marrow aspirate, the trephine is a core biopsy of marrow in which the architecture is maintained, see Figures 10.4 and 10.5. Bone marrow trephines do not need to be performed in all cases, although, once obtained, the sample should be fixed and prepared prior to staining with a minimum of haematoxylin & eosin (H&E) and a reticulin stain. Romanowsky stain can also be used, and a high-quality Giemsa stain can provide much

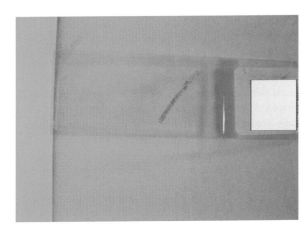

FIGURE 10.4

Bone marrow trephine. This is a core biopsy in which the bone marrow architecture has been maintained. Image courtesy of Dr Robert Corser, Haematology Dept, Queen Alexandra Hospital, Portsmouth.

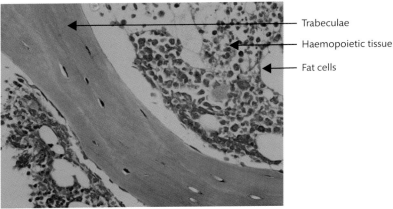

— Trabeculae

— Haemopoietic tissue

— Fat cells

FIGURE 10.5

Microscopic evaluation of the bone marrow structure can be assessed using a bone marrow trephine. The bone marrow architecture is maintained, allowing cell to cell interactions and distribution to be assessed. Image courtesy of Dr Robert Corser, Haematology Dept, Queen Alexandra Hospital, Portsmouth.

BOX 10.1 Bone marrow trephine

A bone marrow trephine is the removal of a core of bone marrow tissue, measuring a minimum of 16 mm, from the iliac crest. The trephine biopsy maintains the architecture of the bone marrow and allows the relationship between different cell types within the bone marrow to be assessed; for example, immature erythrocytes with macrophages, or the localization of immature myeloid cells within the marrow.

Once collected, the biopsy is placed in formalin and labelled appropriately with the patient's details. To summarize the process of preparation, the sample is transported to the histopathology laboratory for processing where it undergoes a process of decalcification to remove bony particles contained within the tissue. The tissue is then ready for embedding prior to cutting sections for staining. Once stained, the proportions of different cell species and their interrelationship can be assessed.

more information than an H&E stain, including the identification of cell lineage and the detection of fibrosis (supplemented using a reticulin stain).

In contrast to the aspirate, the trephine is prepared by the histopathology laboratory primarily because of the requirement for specialized techniques and equipment. The turnaround time for the trephine biopsy is approximately two days. A trephine biopsy is essential for patients with suspected myeloproliferative disorders, particularly when a bone marrow aspirate has provided a dry tap, as is often the case in myelofibrosis. In lymphoid malignancies with suspected bone marrow involvement, a trephine biopsy is important for providing information regarding the distribution of cells infiltrating the marrow. This may help dictate when therapy is initiated, and is also an important baseline for comparison with post-treatment trephines.

Trephine imprint or the trephine roll

The trephine imprint is often indicated in the absence of a bone marrow aspirate. Following biopsy, the trephine is rolled over the surface of a glass slide, depositing bone marrow material, see Figure 10.6. The trephine biopsy is then placed in fixative ready for transportation to the histopathology laboratory. The trephine roll, however, can be processed by the haematology laboratory in the same manner as the bone marrow aspirate. The trephine roll can then be used to complete a differential count prior to the receipt of the processed trephine biopsy. The turnaround time can be as little as an hour.

Haematological malignancies often disrupt the normal distribution of cellular elements within the bone marrow. Granulocytes and their precursors differentiate and mature next to bony trabeculae, and appear to diffuse away from the trabeculae—towards the centre of the bone where many of the marrow sinusoids (blood vessels) are located—as they mature. Erythroblasts form discrete colonies with other red cell precursors and, along with megakaryocytes, are often found in small islands associated with sinusoids. Lymphocyte aggregates are commonly found, although are not associated with paratrabecular areas.

The dissociation between normal developmental patterns and those seen in cases of bone marrow involvement with a range of malignancies often accounts for the presence of immature haemopoietic cells within the peripheral blood.

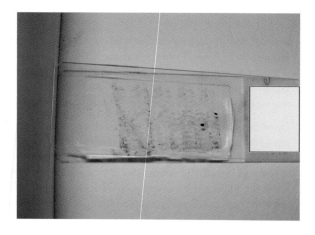

FIGURE 10.6

A trephine imprint. When a bone marrow aspirate cannot be taken, a trephine is indicated. It is often useful to obtain an imprint of the trephine surface prior to histological processing of the trephine so the morphology of the cells can be fully appreciated. Image courtesy of Dr Robert Corser, Haematology Dept, Queen Alexandra Hospital, Portsmouth.

> ## Key Points
>
> When examining bone marrow trephines it is important to consider the normal distribution pattern of haemopoietic elements. In the case of normal lymphoid aggregates, they are absent from paratrabecular regions. However, as we will discuss in Chapter 12, when bone marrow involvement occurs in follicular lymphoma, paratrabecular infiltration is commonly found.

SELF-CHECK 10.4

Compare and contrast the bone marrow aspirate and the trephine.

When examining a bone marrow slide, one of the important features to assess is the cellularity. This gives an indication of the integrity of the bone marrow and its capability for haemopoiesis.

Bone marrow cellularity

Examination of a patient's bone marrow can provide an indication of cellularity—the percentage of cells within the area of the marrow being examined. The trephine is particularly good for being able to assess cellularity, although bone fragments contained within the tails of an aspirate can also provide a good indication of the bone marrow cellularity when a trephine is unavailable.

Bone marrow comprises yellow and red components. Yellow marrow is composed of adipose tissue, whereas red marrow is haemopoietic tissue. When the haemopoietic activity of the marrow reduces, replacement of red marrow with yellow marrow occurs; reciprocally, an increase in haemopoietic activity replaces yellow marrow with haemopoietic tissue.

It is absolutely essential when assessing bone marrow to consider the age of the patient. Bone marrow in normal individuals progressively becomes less cellular with age. Up to 3 months of age, 100% cellularity can be expected. From 3 months to 10 years, this gradually reduces to approximately 80%. At 30 years, the marrow will comprise approximately 50% cells, and at 70 years, this decreases to approximately 30%. Generally, for an adult, bone marrow is considered **normocellular** within the range of 40–70%.

A percentage of cells within the bone marrow greater than 70% is termed **hypercellular**, whereas a reduction in the percentage of cells within the marrow to less than 40% is termed **hypocellular**.

Let us now consider the process of bone marrow infiltration.

normocellular
The percentage of haemopoietic cells to bone marrow falls within the expected range based on a patient's age.

hypercellular
Denotes an increase in the size of the haemopoietic compartment of the bone marrow, or an increase in the number of cells within the marrow. These cells do not have to be haemopoietic in origin, but can be metastatic.

hypocellular
A reduction in the size of the haemopoietic component of the marrow and an increase in the size of the yellow marrow (fatty marrow) compartment.

SELF-CHECK 10.5

What is the generally accepted reference range for bone marrow cellularity?

SELF-CHECK 10.6

What is the name given to an increased or reduced cellularity, and what are the respective percentage cut off points of each?

Patterns of infiltration

The term bone marrow infiltration refers to a process whereby malignant cells originating from outside the bone marrow become deposited within the bone marrow environment. It is important to determine patterns of infiltration, particularly in patients with suspected or confirmed lymphoproliferative conditions but also in metastatic diseases such as breast or prostate cancers, where there is evidence of bone marrow involvement due to the effects these malignant cells have on haemopoiesis. By determining the pattern of infiltration through the examination of a bone marrow trephine, we can obtain important information to assist diagnosis and the formulation of a prognosis. Four main types of infiltrative pattern occur:

- Paratrabecular
- Interstitial
- Nodular
- Diffuse

trabeculae

Bony processes which extend from the outer bony tables into the marrow cavity.

Paratrabecular infiltration: malignant cells accumulate along the periphery of the **trabeculae**, displacing myeloid precursors and fatty tissue. Figure 10.7 shows typical paratrabecular patterns of infiltration. Paratrabecular infiltration is commonly found in patients with bone marrow involvement in a particular type of lymphoproliferative disease called follicular lymphoma.

Interstitial infiltration involves the accumulation of malignant cells between the tissues of bone marrow, i.e. between the haemopoietic elements. Fat spaces remain intact, as shown in Figure 10.8.

Cross references

More detail about follicular lymphoma can be found in Chapter 12.

Chapter 11 discusses the French–American–British (FAB) classification of myeloid leukaemias.

Chapter 12 discusses the French–American–British (FAB) classification of lymphoid leukaemias.

Nodular infiltrates are small, rounded accumulations of tumour cells within the bone marrow, as shown in Figure 10.9. These can occur in any location within the marrow and have a limited effect on haemopoiesis.

Diffuse bone marrow infiltration occurs throughout the bone marrow. The architecture and cellular interactions of normal haemopoietic elements are disrupted by the sheets of malignant cells accumulating within the marrow environment, as shown in Figure 10.10.

Here, the methods for assessing the morphology of haemopoietic cells, both in the peripheral blood and the bone marrow, have been established. The different types of

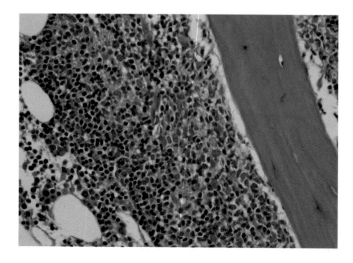

FIGURE 10.7

Paratrabecular infiltration of the bone marrow by lymphoid cells. The trabeculae (solid mauve structure on the right), run the length of the microscopic field. The swathe of cells running adjacent to the trabeculae are malignant lymphoid cells. From a patient with follicular lymphoma. Reprinted from St J Thomas J. The diagnosis is of lymphoid infiltrates in the bone marrow trephine. *Current Diagnostic Pathology* 2004:**10**:236–45, with permission from Elsevier.

bone marrow sample and patterns of infiltration within these samples have also been considered. We now need to examine the different methodologies available for identifying cell lineages.

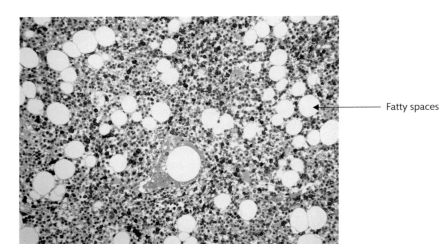

Fatty spaces

FIGURE 10.8
Interstitial infiltration. Here the bone marrow structure is intact, with few, widely interspersed, clumps of malignant lymphocytes. The fatty spaces and haemopoietic tissue are all intact. Kindly provided by Professor SA Pileri.

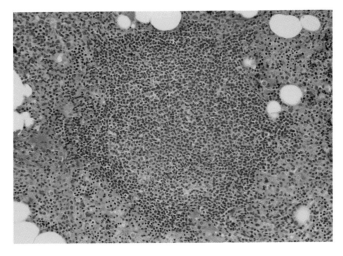

FIGURE 10.9
Nodular infiltration. All haemopoietic elements are maintained, except for discrete areas where malignant lymphoid cells accumulate. Fatty spaces are intact. Reprinted from St J Thomas J. The diagnosis is of lymphoid infiltrates in the bone marrow trephine. *Current Diagnostic Pathology* 2004:**10**:236–45, with permission from Elsevier.

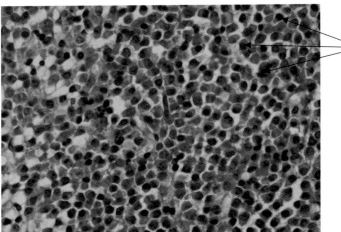

Malignant lymphocytes

FIGURE 10.10
Diffuse bone marrow infiltration. All normal haemopoietic tissue is replaced by malignant lymphoid cells. Haemopoiesis will be compromised. Reprinted from St J Thomas J. The diagnosis is of lymphoid infiltrates in the bone marrow trephine. *Current Diagnostic Pathology* 2004:**10**:236–45, with permission from Elsevier.

SELF-CHECK 10.7

Define bone marrow infiltration.

10.5 Cytochemistry

Cytochemistry is used to confirm the presence or absence of particular markers within cells. This can assist in the identification of cell lineage. For example, particular enzymes, such as myeloperoxidase, may be present in myeloid cells but absent from lymphoid cells. Being able to confirm the presence or absence of these enzymes helps us to establish cell lineage and to classify haematological malignancies appropriately.

Although a wide range of different cytochemical stains are available, this section will focus on a small selection including:

- Myeloperoxidase (MPO)
- Sudan black B (SBB)
- Alpha-naphthyl acetate esterase (ANAE)
- Chloroacetate esterase (CAE)
- Periodic acid–Schiff (PAS)
- Acid phosphatase (AP)

These cytochemical stains are summarized in Table 10.3.

This section does not focus on the chemistry of these reactions, but rather the endpoint required for interpretation. Please refer to Figures 10.11(a–e) in accordance with each of the sections below.

Cytochemistry utilizes microscopic techniques to assess the characteristics of cells following exposure to a range of cytochemical stains. By far the most significant of these is Romanowsky stain, and this should be the platform upon which the diagnosis of a particular haematological malignancy is based. However, other cytochemical stains can prove useful in characterizing cells otherwise difficult to categorize microscopically using Romanowsky stain alone.

Except where Auer rods are present, using Romanowsky stain to differentiate between myeloblasts and lymphoblasts is very difficult and is subject to error. Without utilizing alternative techniques, there is a risk of miscategorization of the cell, and possible misclassification of the malignancy. Differentiation between monoblasts, erythroblasts, and megakaryoblasts also requires the application of alternative techniques, since these cells are morphologically similar, although they differ in their cytoplasmic contents. This cytoplasmic variation can be exploited by using cytochemical stains to produce different colours, which can be interpreted and quantified. However, the use of cytochemistry is also limited, and distinguishing between undifferentiated blasts and megakaryoblasts cannot be achieved using cytochemistry alone. The inability to differentiate between these blasts was one of the important considerations with the implementation of immunophenotyping in the diagnosis of haematological malignancies.

Now we should examine the main cytochemical stains in greater detail.

Cross references

Section 10.3 gave details of blood film examination.

See Chapter 11 for the French-American-British (FAB) classification of myeloid leukaemias.

See Chapter 12 for the French-American-British (FAB) classification of lymphoid leukaemias.

TABLE 10.3 Cytochemical staining characteristics of haemopoietic progenitors and mature cells.

Stain	Lineage	Colour	Cell/maturational stage	Reaction	Comments
MPO	Myeloid	Brown	Early myeloblast	–ve	*Negative in:*
			Late myeloblast	–/+ve	ALL, AMKL &
			Promyelocytes	++ve	undifferentiated leukaemia
			Myelocytes	++ve	
			Metamyelocytes	+ve	
			Neutrophils	+ve	
			Eosinophils	+ve	
			Basophils	+ve	
			Monocytes	+/–ve	
SBB	Myeloid	Black	*as above*		
ANAE	Myeloid	Red/brown	Monoblasts	+ve	
			Granulocytes	+ve	
CAE	Myeloid	Bright blue	Myeloblasts	–ve	
			Granulocytes	+ve	Increases with maturation
PAS	Myeloid/ lymphoid	Pink/red	Erythroblasts	–ve	
			Maturing/mature RBCs	–ve	
			Immature granulocytes	–ve	Leukaemic erythroblasts +ve
			Mature granulocytes	+ve	Eosinophil/basophil granules –ve
			Monocytes	+/–ve	
			Megakaryocytes	++ve	
			Platelets	++ve	
AP	All cells	Red granules	T-cells	++ve	Good for distinguishing B/T cells
			B-cells	+ve	
			Granulocytes	++ve	Leukaemic monocytes ++ve
			Megakaryocytes	++ve	
			Plasma cells	++ve	

Key: All, acute lymphoblastic leukaemia; AMKL, acute megakaryoblastic leukaemia; –ve, negative; +ve, positive; –/+, occasionally positive; +/–, occasionally negative; ++ve, strongly positive.

Myeloperoxidase

Myeloperoxidase is a member of the peroxidase family of enzymes and is found primarily within the azurophilic granules of granulocytes (neutrophils, eosinophils and basophils), but *may* also be found within monocytes. A positive reaction utilizing the chromogen 3,3'diaminobenzidine (DAB) provides a brown granular inclusion within the cytoplasm. Early myeloblasts are negative for MPO, but as they mature, they become MPO-positive. Strong reactions with DAB are seen in promyelocytes and myelocytes. Cells of monocytic lineage will also stain with DAB. A negative reaction does not distinguish between undifferentiated leukaemia, acute lymphoblastic leukaemia, or acute megakaryoblastic leukaemia.

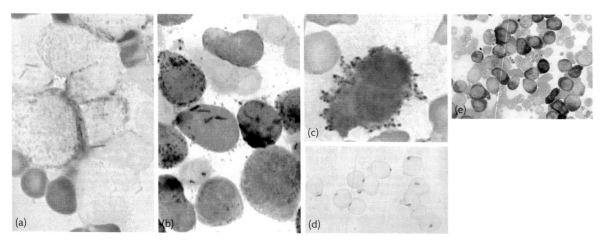

FIGURE 10.11

(a) Myeloperoxidase staining of myeloblasts. Cytoplasm shows diffuse staining of granules and Auer rods are apparent. (b) Myeloblasts stained with Sudan black B. (c) Periodic acid–Schiff stains this dysplastic micromegakaryocytes demonstrates pink cytoplasm and granules. (d) Acid phosphatase providing distinct red staining in lymphoblasts in a case of T-cell acute lymphoblastic leukaemia. (e) Combined esterase α-naphthyl acetate esterase (ANAE) and chloroacetate esterase (CAE). ANAE provides a dark brown coloration to leukaemic monocytes, whereas CAE stains granulocytes bright blue. Reproduced by permission from Lewis et al., 2001, Dacie & Lewis Practical Haematology 9th edn. © Elsevier.

Sudan black B

Sudan black B provides comparable information to myeloperoxidase and can therefore be used to identify granulocytes and *some* monocytes. SBB is a lipophilic stain which binds to the lipid membrane surrounding granules in granulocytes and some monocytes. A positive reaction causes a black and granular inclusion within the cytoplasm.

α-Naphthyl acetate esterase and chloroacetate esterase

Both of these enzymes are part of the esterase group and can be used singly, or in combination with one another. ANAE is useful in the identification of normal and leukaemic monoblasts. ANAE is also useful to identify, through a red/brown coloration, granulocytes in myelodysplastic syndromes and in leukaemia. CAE is useful for identifying granulocytic maturation, as positivity (demonstrated by a bright-blue coloration) increases with maturation. Myeloblasts are generally negative for CAE.

Periodic acid–Schiff

PAS reacts with the 1,2-glycol groups found in carbohydrates, predominantly in glycogen, to produce a pink to bright-red reaction. Normal erythroid cells and their precursors are negative when exposed to PAS, although erythroblasts in erythroleukaemia are generally positive. Cells of all other lineages are likely to show a reaction. Immature granulocytes are negative, although become increasingly positive throughout the maturation process. Cytoplasmic PAS reactions are seen in eosinophils, whilst eosinophil granules are negative. Basophils are often positive, although basophil granules do not stain with PAS. Monocytes may or may not be positive, with variable reactions from fine to coarse granulation. Megakaryocytes are strongly positive, as are platelets, and normal lymphocytes may show granular positivity.

Leukaemic lymphoblasts may be strongly positive, and malignant plasma cells may show variable staining results.

Acid phosphatase

The acid phosphatase reaction produces red granules or a diffuse pattern in all haemopoietic cells. The degree of the reaction is particularly important when discriminating between B and T cells, with the T cells showing the strongest reaction. Acid phosphatase has historically been of value in identifying T-cell leukaemias because of the strong reactive pattern when compared to the B-cell lineage. Acid phosphatase is also of value in identifying AML with monocytic involvement where strong cytochemical reactions are apparent.

SELF-CHECK 10.8

Provide a brief outline of the reaction patterns and colours associated with the myeloperoxidase, Sudan black B, and Periodic acid–Schiff stains.

As we have determined, cytochemistry is important for identifying cell lineage in haematological malignancies. However, cytochemistry has been largely superseded by the introduction and use of immunophenotyping as the main method for the identification of haemopoietic lineages.

Now that we have considered some of the commonly used cytochemical stains and their application in the differentiation of haemopoietic cell lineages, the methodology of immunophenotyping and its value in the diagnosis of haematological malignancies will be examined.

10.6 Immunophenotyping

Although immunophenotyping has a wide range of applications, we will briefly examine the role of immunophenotyping and its application to haematological malignancies. Either peripheral blood or a bone marrow aspirate preserved in EDTA anticoagulant can be used for immunophenotyping analysis.

In 2006, recommendations were made by an international group of expert haematologists in Bethesda, USA, to address the use of immunophenotyping in the diagnosis and monitoring of haematological malignancies. These recommendations largely complement the 'WHO classification of tumours of haematopoietic and lymphoid tissues', and also aim to reduce redundancy in the investigative process by using evidence-based practice to reduce the number of unnecessary requests for immunophenotyping.

Figure 10.12 summarizes the Bethesda group's recommendations for the appropriate use of immunophenotyping in the context of haematological malignancies. Sections in blue bubbles are considered appropriate requests for immunophenotyping whilst those highlighted in yellow are not considered to be valid reasons for immunophenotyping requests.

Cross reference

The WHO classification of tumours of haematopoietic and lymphoid tissues is discussed in detail in Chapters 11 and 12.

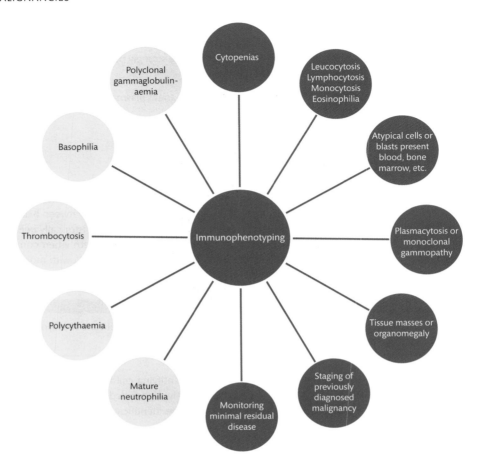

FIGURE 10.12

A summary of the Bethesda group's recommendations for the applications of immunophenotyping, where malignancy is in question. All cases highlighted in blue would form an appropriate basis for immunophenotypic investigation. Isolated scenarios in yellow do not require immunophenotypic investigation.

monoclonal antibodies (mAbs)

These are manufactured to recognize a particular epitope on a specific antigen. Although mAbs produced by different manufacturers may have the same name, they may recognize a different epitope on the specified antigen.

cluster of differentiation (CD) antigen

The standardized notation used to describe a range of molecules associated with the differentiation and maturation of cells. CD markers can be measured using epitope-specific monoclonal antibodies.

The process of immunophenotyping involves the use of **monoclonal antibodies (mAbs)** directed against intracellular or extracellular **cluster of differentiation** (CD) antigens, of which 350 are currently recognized. Monoclonal antibodies directed against specific CD antigens are called *anti*-CD, followed by the respective number of the CD antigen, for example anti-CD19. CD antigens are expressed on all cells; some CD antigens may be expressed across all lineages, and others are much more specific, being expressed on a single lineage, or at a particular stage of maturation. If you look at Figure 10.13 you will see an illustration of mAbs binding to two different types of CD marker, allowing immunological identification of the cell.

Panels of mAbs directed against different CD antigens provide a very powerful tool for identifying cells accurately, regardless of the cell's morphological features.

In order for the antibodies to bind intracellular antigens, fixation procedures (to prevent cell lysis) and permeablization procedures (to allow the monoclonal antibody to enter the cell) are necessary.

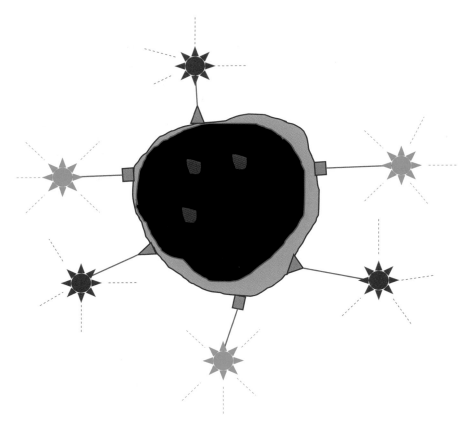

FIGURE 10.13

An illustration of two discrete fluorochrome conjugated monoclonal antibodies of differing specificity (as suggested by the different shaped surface antigens) binding to the surface of a malignant blast. An analyser with multiple channels would be able to detect the fluorescene from these different fluorochromes simultaneously, providing evidence of antigenic co-expression.

Monoclonal antibodies are joined to **fluorochromes**, molecules which emit light at a particular wavelength when excited by a laser. The light emitted from each fluorochrome can be measured using a detector, and is used to identify whether or not a particular CD marker is expressed by a specific population of cells. We can measure a number of fluorochromes simultaneously by using a flow cytometer with multi-channel capabilities. In order to do this, mAbs joined to fluorochromes emitting light at different wavelengths must be selected. We can use the data generated to assess whether or not a particular set of antigens are co-expressed on particular cells, which can help the identification of the cell.

A wide range of fluorochromes have been manufactured; some of the most common are listed in Table 10.4 with their relative excitation and emission wavelengths.

The data generated using immunophenotyping can help to establish whether a particular condition is malignant or reactive by distinguishing between a monoclonal or polyclonal cell population. If the cells are malignant, we can use immunophenotyping to ascertain whether they are myeloid or lymphoid, undifferentiated, or express markers of both myeloid and lymphoid lineages. Immunophenotyping is also important to allow us to define the stage of

fluorochrome

A chemical which, when excited by light of a particular wavelength, will emit light of a different but predictable wavelength, measurable using a photodetector.

> ### BOX 10.2 *Monoclonal antibodies*
>
> The technique to produce monoclonal antibodies was devised by Milstein and Köhler and reported in 1975. Monoclonal antibody production involves fusing normal-immunoglobulin (Ig) -producing cells, stimulated to produce Ig following sensitization with an appropriate antigen, with myeloma cells. Normal Ig synthesizing cells do not survive in culture conditions for long, and myeloma cells do not reliably produce Ig, although they survive continuously under culture conditions. This technique produces 'hybridomas' that continually produce antibodies directed to the epitopes expressed by the sensitizing antigen. These hybridomas can be separated by producing single-cell colonies which will expand to form a clonal population, and the specificity of the antibody can be determined. These colonies can be cultured to constantly produce reagent monoclonal antibodies. For any given epitope, the corresponding monoclonal antibodies will all have the same structure, specificity, and binding strength (avidity), meaning that these monoclonal antibodies can be used reproducibly for diagnostic and research purposes.
>
> The seminal findings, in which the synthesis of anti-sheep red blood cell antibodies were generated, were reported in Köhler and Milstein, 1975 (see the Reference list at the end of this book).

Cross reference

See Chapter 9—Introduction to haematological malignancies; Section 9.7: Clonality.

maturational arrest within the malignant cell population. In a lymphoid population, immunophenotyping can establish whether the cells are of B or T lineage, or express markers of both.

SELF-CHECK 10.9

What sort of information can be provided through the use of immunophenotyping?

There is no single CD marker that signals malignancy. CD markers are expressed on normal cells, often in a lineage-restricted manner. Aberrant expression of CD markers, or a coexpression of markers, can suggest an abnormality; the range of markers as a whole needs to be assessed to

TABLE 10.4 Approximate maximum excitation and emission wavelengths for commonly used fluorochromes in immunophenotyping.

Fluorochrome	Excitation max (nm)	Emission max (nm)
Allophycocyanin (APC)	650	660
Fluorescein isothiocyanate (FITC)	490	520
Peridinin chlorophyll protein (PerCP)	488	578
Phycoerythrin (PE)	564	576
Rhodamine	550	573
Texas Red	596	615

establish a diagnosis. For example, as shown in Figure 10.14, in B-cell CLL the typical markers are CD 5+ve, CD19+ve, CD23+ve, FMC7–ve. Using this combination of CD markers, B-CLL can be confidently diagnosed, even though, individually, each of these is a normal CD marker.

Cross reference

CLL is discussed in detail in Chapter 12.

Limitations of immunophenotyping

The immunophenotyping technique has its limitations. In malignancies involving mature cells, such as CML, the expression of CD antigens is consistent with mature myeloid cells and therefore immunophenotyping is of no benefit in the diagnosis of this condition. However, there is value in using immunophenotyping to establish the lineage of blasts in people with CML in blast crisis. Although approximately 70% of cases of CML in blast crisis become acute myeloid leukaemias, specific subtypes—for example, erythroleukaemia or lymphoblastic leukaemias—may develop and are subject to different types of therapy and prognoses. At the time of writing this chapter, there is limited benefit in the use of immunophenotyping for the diagnosis or classification of myelodysplasia (MDS), although again, immunophenotyping can be useful for classifying leukaemia in cases where MDS has transformed. Research is focusing on immunphenotyping for potential markers of MDS.

Whilst immunophenotyping is a very powerful tool, and it is relatively simple to perform the preparatory work and sample processing, analysis of the results may be rather more difficult. The ability to analyse results correctly and formulate a diagnosis requires a great deal of training and experience. New flow cytometers are expensive pieces of equipment to purchase, and monoclonal antibodies conjugated to fluorochromes (primary mAbs) can also be costly.

Cross reference

The pathogenesis of CML and its disease course are discussed in Chapter 11.

Cross references

See Chapter 11—Introduction to classification systems: Myeloid neoplasms.

See Chapter 12—Introduction to classification systems: Lymphoid neoplasms.

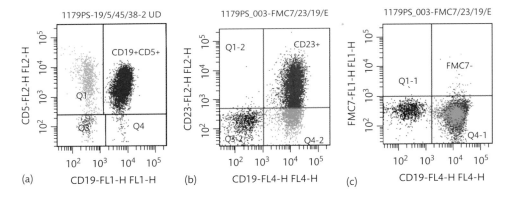

FIGURE 10.14

The typical B- chronic lymphocytic leukaemia (CLL) phenotype. Each scattergram is divided into quadrants—with the quadrant on the bottom left in this case, blue—are always antigen negative (a) cells are tested against anti-CD5 (y-axis) and anti-CD19 (x-axis). There is a population of cells that is CD5 positive and CD19 negative (Q1) which correlates with a T-cell population; CD19 positive and CD5 negative cells are shown in Q4. The population of cells highlighted red are the malignant B cells and are CD5 positive and C19 positive (Q2). (b) CD19 positive cells have been selected and, again in quadrant (Q2) show co-expression of CD23. (c), CD19 positive cells rarely co-express FMC7, as shown by the small number of cells within Q2 in this scattergram. The results show CD5+ve, CD19+ve, CD23+ve, FMC7–ve. Immunophenotyping data courtesy of Adnan Mani, Department of Immunology, Southampton General Hospital.

Now that some of the general considerations of immunophenotyping have been examined, we should now concentrate on how some of the technical considerations affect the way immunophenotyping is used in practice.

Technical considerations for immunophenotyping

The British Committee for Standards in Haematology (BCSH) has set out guidelines for the use of immunophenotyping for the laboratory investigation of haematological malignancies of myeloid and lymphoid origin. Revised guidelines were set out in 2002, but the BCSH has yet to update these guidelines based on current best practice. As such, this section will broadly mirror the recommendations of the 2002 BCSH guidelines.

The process of immunophenotyping begins by selecting a panel of monoclonal antibodies against which the patient cells are tested. The selection of antibodies largely depends upon the malignancy suspected, as indicated by morphology using Romanowsky and, in some cases, cytochemical stains. For a suspected acute leukaemia a first-line panel should be used initially, followed by a second-line panel, if indicated. First- and second-line panels are used for the investigation of acute leukaemias and chronic lymphoproliferative disorders, although the monoclonal antibodies in these panels are different.

In a suspected case of *acute leukaemia*, the first-line panel helps us identify:

- Myeloid or lymphoid lineages to enable a diagnosis of AML or ALL
- B- or T-lineage cells in ALL
- Mixed phenotypic leucaemias
- Stage of maturation in a non-lineage restricted manner, for example, by expression of CD34 or HLA-Dr

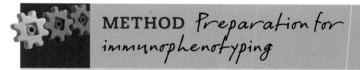

METHOD *Preparation for immunophenotyping*

- Using peripheral blood as an example—once the panel of choice has been selected, the red cells are lysed, and the remaining cells washed to remove red cell stroma.

- The sample is thoroughly mixed and known volumes of blood are aliquoted into separate labelled tubes. These are then incubated with the range of monoclonal antibodies from the selected panel.

- Following incubation, the contents of each tube are washed to remove excess antibody which would otherwise interfere with the results (for example, by providing a false-positive result).

- The sample is now ready for analysis.

- Information regarding the number of tubes to be tested and the specificity of the monoclonal antibodies contained within each tube should be inputted into the analyser software prior to analysis.

- The analyser will provide a prompt when the analysis of each tube is complete and the next tube can begin.

- The amount of time taken for measuring fluorescence depends upon the number of cells (events) counted.

- Once complete, the data can be analysed.

And the second-line panel should then be used selectively to provide the following important information:

- If B- or T-lineage ALL: determination of the appropriate subtype
- If a myeloid leukaemia: unusual variants including erythroid and megakaryocytic lineages

However, in a *chronic lymphoproliferative disease*, the first-line panel should be used to determine a diagnosis of a B- or T-cell disorder. A second-line panel should be applied to identify particular subgroups of lymphoproliferative disease based on the results of the first-line panel.

The first stage of analysis is to identify the population of cells to be analysed. Analysis is achieved using two particular measurements: **forward scatter** (FSC) and **side scatter** (SSC). These are plotted on a scatter graph. Forward scatter represents the size of each of the cells in the sample and is measured based on the amount of light (generated by a laser) diffracted by the cell membrane. FSC is plotted on the x-axis. Side scatter, plotted on the y-axis, is detected at 90° to the path of the light from the source and represents the internal complexity of each cell. The data representing cell size and internal complexity can then be used to identify the cell species according to the structural properties of that cell. For example, neutrophils are relatively large, with a high SSC due to their internal complexity (highly granular with a multi-lobulated nucleus).

Cross references

See Chapter 11—Introduction to classification systems: Myeloid neoplasms.

See Chapter 12—Introduction to classification systems: Lymphoid neoplasms.

SELF-CHECK 10.10

What is the difference between forward scatter (FSC) and side scatter (SSC)? How does this enable us to identify different populations of cells?

Analysis begins with the assessment of anti-CD45, a pan white cell marker, used to exclude any remaining red cell debris or platelets from the analysis; see Figure 10.15. Anti-CD45 is substituted for the FSC measurement on the x-axis. Blast expression of CD45 is significantly lower than that of normal lymphocytes and monocytes, allowing separation of these three mononuclear populations, as shown in Figure 10.16. The use of forward scatter and side scatter alone may allow an overlap between the blast population and the lymphocyte and monocyte populations because of the similar light scattering characteristics of this heterogeneous population of blasts.

Once the appropriate cell population has been selected, a gate can be applied. **Gating** is a very powerful technique for identifying and subsequently classifying a range of haematological malignancies according to the combined antigenic expression on a particular population of cells. Gating can be performed on the FSC/SSC plot, where a population of cells is selected

gating
The process of selecting a particular population of cells on which to base further immunophenotyping analysis.

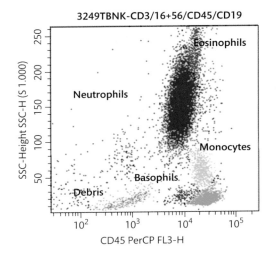

3249TBNK-CD3/16+56/CD45/CD19

FIGURE 10.15

CD45 can be used in place of forward scatter against side scatter to enable leucocytes to be identified according to CD expression and cellular internal complexity. Neutrophils are coloured red, eosinophils purple, monocytes turquoise and basophils dark blue. The green population are lymphocytes. Immunophenotyping data courtesy of Adnan Mani, Department of Immunology, Southampton General Hospital.

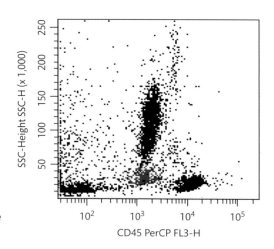

FIGURE 10.16

CD45 expression to identify a population of blasts. Due to the size and internal complexity of blasts, they tend to overlap the distributional patterns of lymphocytes and monocytes when forward scatter and side scatter are used alone. When CD45 is used in place of forward scatter, the blast population (coloured red) becomes a discrete entity due to the poor expression of CD45 on the blast surface.

based on size and internal complexity, although there is a risk that this population will be contaminated by cells of another lineage, as previously highlighted in the context of blasts. Using CD45 provides an excellent way of selecting a pure population of cells because the cell populations are clearly separated.

Once a reaction has been determined between the mAb and the target antigen, to call these cells 'antigen-positive' we need to establish whether or not the cells actually express the antigen at a sufficient density. If no fluorescence is measured, this clearly indicates the cells do not express a particular antigen, although weak fluorescence also needs to be considered.

Based on comprehensive scientific research, antigen-positive is considered for acute leukaemia when a minimum of 20% of cells express a particular antigen, compared with 30% for lymphoproliferative disorders. For example, if we examined B-CLL cells for CD38-expression, and established that 25% of cells expressed CD38, we would consider the B-CLL population CD38-negative. If 30% of the CLL cells expressed CD38, this population would be termed CD38-positive. The use of this arbitrary cut-off point underlines the intrinsic potential for inaccuracy of the techniques.

Having established the pattern of antigen expression on the gated population, we can compare these data with pre-established criteria for different types of malignancy to ascertain the correct diagnosis. For example, we know that if a population of cells are shown to have the following phenotype: CD13+, CD33+, CD117+, CD34– and HLA-DR–, as shown in Figure 10.17 this is characteristic of acute promyelocytic leukaemia.

The identification of lineage is of vital importance in being able to establish the correct diagnosis for a patient with a haematological malignancy. For example, if a population of cells express CD13, CD33, and CD34, we can be confident that these cells are of the myeloid lineage, and because of the expression of CD34, a stem cell marker, these cells are myeloblasts. Lack of CD34 expression implies these cells are beyond the 'blast' stage of maturation.

Cross reference

Zap 70 is discussed in greater detail in Chapter 12.

Certain antigens, such as CD38 and Zap-70 in B-CLL, act as prognostic markers, which are of importance when deciding upon therapeutic intervention, communication between healthcare professionals, and keeping the patient informed of their disease. Immunophenotypic analysis is an important tool in diagnosis and prognostication, although additional diagnostic and prognostic information can be elucidated using cytogenetic analysis.

Cytogenetic testing is a specialized procedure, unavailable in the majority of hospital pathology departments. Specialist referral centres are often used to provide this service, and it is

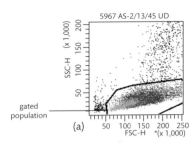

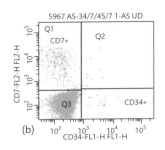

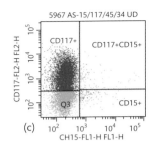

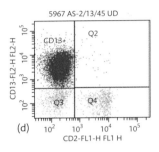

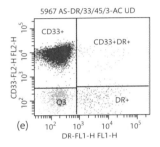

FIGURE 10.17

Acute promyelocytic leukaemia (APL). (a) Cells of interest are gated. All immunophenotypic data is analysed in relation to this gated population. As we can see by these different colours, this is not a homogeneous population of cells, although we are interested in the large red population of cells in this analysis. Quadrant 3 (Q3) is negative throughout a–e. (b) There is a population of CD34 negative, CD7 positive cells (Q1), although these are normal T cells contaminating the malignant cell population. The majority of the other cells are CD7 negative and CD34 negative (Q3). CD34 is a stem cell marker. (c) There is a clear population of CD117 (also called c-kit) positive cells (Q1), which are CD15 negative. (d) The malignant cells express CD13 (Q1), but not CD2 (Q2). CD2 is a pan T-cell marker and is co-expressed with CD7. (e) The population of interest (red), Q1, expresses CD33, but does not express HLA-DR. The red population has the immunophenotype: CD13+ve, CD33+ve, CD34−ve, HLA-DR−ve CD7−ve, CD117+ve, typical of acute promyelocytic leukaemia. Immunophenotyping data courtesy of Adnan Mani, Department of Immunology, Southampton General Hospital.

important to have an awareness of the procedures in place and the data obtainable using these techniques as they are of increasing importance in the field of haemato-oncology.

SELF-CHECK 10.11

What is the purpose of gating?

10.7 Cytogenetic analysis

The term cytogenetics is a fusion of cytology (the study of cells) and genetics, the study of genes. Cytogenetics is the process of studying genetic material at the cellular level and is important in assessing heritable, congenital, and acquired genetic diseases. A considerable amount of scientific and clinical research shows that assessing the cytogenetic profile of patients with haematological malignancies is vital for:

- Diagnosing particular haematological malignancies
- Selecting appropriate therapies (in specific cases)
- Assessing a patient's prognosis
- Identifying clonal progression

The tissue required to complete a cytogenetic analysis depends upon the histological origin of the malignancy and the location of abundant tumour cells. If, for example, we have a patient with a suspected malignancy *localized* in a lymph node, cytogenetic analysis of that lymph node should be performed. Performing a cytogenetic analysis of the bone marrow in this case would not be of value, even if a bone marrow sample has been received.

A bone marrow aspirate usually provides good-quality cells for culture and hence the assessment of patients with acute and chronic leukaemias and for patients with bone marrow infiltration (Section 10.4). Whether bone marrow or peripheral blood is to be used for the analysis, the sample should be collected into preservative-free, lithium–heparin tubes.

SELF-CHECK 10.12

What is the purpose of performing cytogenetic investigations on patients with a suspected haematological malignancy?

---

karyotype

The chromosomal complement for a cell, or population of cells.

The requirements and procedures for cytogenetic analysis tend to vary between centres, but the patient's **karyotype** will probably be established to identify any numerical chromosomal abnormalities. Comparative genomic hybridization (CGH) can be used to rapidly screen cells for copy number abnormalities whereas G-banding and FISH are most commonly used to establish any numerical or structural chromosomal abnormalities associated with malignant cells.

Although an important and commonly used technique, G-banding does have its limitations. It can be impossible to identify microdeletions (submicroscopic deletions of chromosomal material) or some types of translocation, especially when the banding pattern of the chromosomes has not been disrupted. Translocations unidentifiable using standard microscopic techniques are called **cryptic translocations**. In cases involving cryptic translocations, more powerful techniques may be used. A good example of a cryptic translocation is t(12;21)(p13;q22), found in childhood ALL, where the regions of chromosome exchange have an identical banding pattern to the normal chromosomes 12 and 21, and so cannot be detected using G-banding and light microscopy. Molecular cytogenetic techniques provide more reliable data to establish the cytogenetic profile of patients with haematological malignancies.

cryptic translocation

This occurs when the original morphology and banding pattern of a chromosome is maintained following translocation. This means the translocation may go undetected.

Comparative genomic hybridization (CGH) is a relatively fast screening technique used to identify changes in chromosome copy number, as outlined in Figure 10.18. Once CGH analysis is completed and changes in copy number are established, more specific techniques—such as FISH or DNA sequencing—are used to identify the precise chromosomal defect.

CGH does not require cell culturing prior to analysis. Tumour DNA is extracted, conjugated with a green fluorescent probe, and mixed with normal DNA which is conjugated to a red fluorescent probe. The green and red labelled DNA is then hybridized to pre-prepared human metaphase chromosomes, and the ratio of green to red fluorescence measured. A ratio of

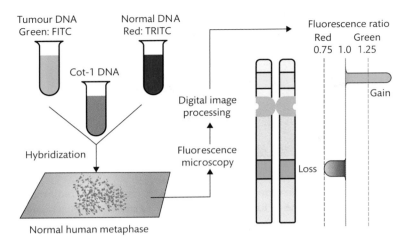

FIGURE 10.18

Comparative genomic hybridization. Tumour DNA is labelled green and normal DNA labelled red. These are mixed in a 1:1 ratio and hybridized to metaphase chromosomes. The ratio of green to red fluorescence is measured. Values >1 are suggestive of chromosomal gains whilst <1 suggest losses. Adapted by permission from BMJ Publishing Group Limited. Weiss MM, et al. Comparative genomic hybridisation. *Molecular Pathology* 1999:**52**;243–51.

greater than one demonstrates chromosomal gain, whereas a ratio of less than one indicates a loss of chromosomal material.

Fluorescence in-situ *hybridization* (FISH) uses fluorescent probes to bind in a complementary fashion to the particular chromosomal segments to be investigated. FISH can enable very accurate, rapid analysis for particular qualitative chromosomal abnormalities, and has

BOX 10.3 *Cytogenetic techniques*

Using peripheral blood as an example, the technique requires approximately 5–10 ml of lithium heparin-anticoagulated whole blood.

- Cultures containing ~1 × 10⁶ WBC/ml culture medium (typically RPMI) are set up under sterile conditions, and incubated at 37 °C. Depending upon the target cells, a mitogen may be added to stimulate cell division.

- To harvest the cells from the culture, either colchicine or other spindle inhibitors are added to induce cell cycle arrest in metaphase.

- When it is thought that an appropriate number of cells have accumulated in metaphase, a hypotonic solution is added to burst the red cells and swell the cultured cells.

- The cells are then fixed and dropped gently onto microscope slides. The chromosomes spread to produce metaphases, which are then stained and analysed microscopically. At least 30 cells arrested in metaphase should be examined for cytogenetic abnormalities.

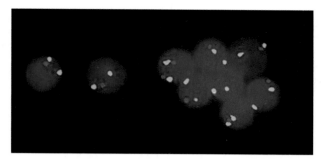

FIGURE 10.19

Fluorescence *in situ* hybridization, using a probe for *ATM* locus 11q23 (red), and one for the centromere of chromosome 11 for this CLL patient. There should be equal numbers of red and green fluorescent spots within each cell. There are fewer red spots, indicating the loss of *ATM* in the majority of these interphase cells. Courtesy of Anne Gardiner, Cytogenetics laboratory, Royal Bournemouth Hospital.

complex karyotype

Describes the situation where more than three acquired cytogenetic abnormalities are found within a population of tumour cells.

the advantage that either metaphase chromosomes or interphase nuclei can be used as the target. FISH is an important technique for assessing individuals with cryptic translocations and those with **complex karyotypes**. By using one or more probes labelled with different fluorochromes it is possible to examine different chromosomal segments, which allows us to identify deletions, additions, and translocations relatively easily, as shown in Figures 10.19 and 10.20. However, unlike G-banding it is not a 'global technique' examining the whole genome, it only provides an answer to the specific question asked by the use of particular probes.

The cytogenetic assessment of patients with suspected and confirmed haematological malignancies is essential in order to conform to the World Health Organization's (WHO) classification of haematological and lymphoid neoplasms.

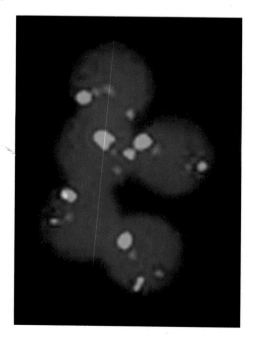

FIGURE 10.20

Fluorescence *in situ* hybridization for the same patient as 10.19, but with two different probes. A probe for the *TP53*, locus, 17p13 (red), and the centromeric probe (green) shows equal numbers of green and red fluorescent spots. There is no evidence of *TP53* loss in this patient. Courtesy of Anne Gardiner, Cytogenetics laboratory, Royal Bournemouth Hospital.

Consider the different conditions in the following list of cytogenetic markers associated with different types of haematological malignancy. This is by no means an exhaustive list, although it demonstrates some of the important cytogenetic findings in a range of different malignant conditions. In some cases, these abnormalities have been linked with prognosis. Pre-treatment cytogenetic data is one of the most important prognostic factors for patients with AML and ALL.

Cytogenetic abnormalities in malignant conditions

AML

Cytogenetic abnormalities can help direct the medical professional to a diagnosis, especially in certain cases where a particular cytogenetic event is closely associated with a specific disease. For example, t(15;17)(q22;q12) is diagnostic for acute promyelocytic leukaemia, and for this particular translocation, targeted therapy in the form of **all-*trans* retinoic acid (ATRA)** is available. Identification of t(15;17) is associated with a good prognosis and survival prospects because of the success of ATRA in treating these patients.

Other cytogenetic abnormalities in AML associated with a good prognosis include t(8;21)(q22;q22), inv(16)(q13;q22), and t(16;16). Intermediate prognostic markers include a trisomy 8, trisomy 21, and the majority of fusion partners associated with the breakpoint 11q23. Poor prognostic markers in AML include t(6;9)(p23;q34), inv(3)(q21;q26) del(5q) and del(7q).

ALL

For ALL, good prognostic markers include **hyperdiploidy** (more than 47 chromosomes), but particularly the presence of 51–65 chromosomes (high hyperdiploidy) and t(1;19)(q23;p13). By contrast, poor prognostic markers include t(9;22)(q34;q11) and t(4;11)(q21;q23).

MDS

In MDS, patients with either a 5q– or 7q– are associated with better survival prospects (a good prognosis) than those with either a trisomy 8 (associated with an intermediate prognosis) or those with the loss of the entire chromosome 5 or 7 (a poor prognostic marker). Because of the good prognosis associated with 5q–, the WHO has established a new subcategory for the classification of MDS—MDS with associated del(5q) or 5q– syndrome.

---

all trans retinoic acid (ATRA)

A vitamin A derivative which interacts with the PML–RARα fusion protein in acute promyelocytic leukaemia and, at pharmacological concentrations, can induce differentiation of cell cycle arrested promyelocytes, allow their maturation, and the induction of apoptosis.

hyperdiploidy

Human cells containing in excess of 47 chromosomes.

BOX 10.4 Cytogenetics and clonality

Identifying a monoclonal population of cells by immunophenotyping suggests that these cells are malignant, whereas a polyclonal population of cells is likely to be normal or reactive. If cytogenetic analysis shows a chromosomal addition or structural abnormality, excluding a loss, *two cells must share that abnormality* to be considered clonal. If the loss of a chromosome is detected using cytogenetic analysis, *a minimum of three cells must share this abnormality* in order for a clonal disorder to be confirmed.

microRNAs

Small fragments of RNA, 20–23 nucleotides in length, which bind in a complementary fashion to mRNA to inhibit translation.

Cross references

See Chapter 9–Introduction to haematological malignancies–for more information on karyotypes.

For more information on CML, please see Chapter 11.

imatinib mesylate

A signal transduction inhibitor which can be used to target the ATP binding pocket conserved on the Abl transcript of BCR-Abl. Inhibition of BCR-Abl inhibits the phosphorylation of downstream effector molecules, reinstating apoptosis and overriding the other dominant effects of BCR-Abl. Imatinib can also inhibit c-Kit and the platelet-derived growth factor receptor (PDGFR).

Cross references

See Chapter 12–Introduction to classification systems: Lymphoid neoplasms.

Thrombophilia is considered in greater detail in Chapter 15.

CLL

When del13q14 is the only chromosome abnormality detected in CLL it is associated with a good prognosis, as is a normal karyotype. Del13q14 is not associated with the loss of the tumour suppressor gene *RB1*, but rather with the loss of two members of a **microRNA** (miRNA) family of genes found telomeric to *RB1*. In particular *miR-15a* and *miR-16-1* are deleted which downregulates the anti-apoptotic protein BCL2. Loss of miR-15a and miR-16-1 allows overexpression of BCL2, protecting the cell from apoptosis.

Trisomy 12 may be associated with either a good or poor prognosis, whereas 11q23 abnormalities (loss of *ATM*; Figure 10.19) and 17p deletion (loss of *TP53*) are associated with a poor prognosis. Deletion of either of these genes and mutation of the remaining allele reduces the patient's response to DNA-damaging drugs often used in the treatment of CLL, so alternative therapies should be used.

CML

Identification of the Philadelphia chromosome der(22) or the translocation t(9;22)(q34;q11) is important to enable the appropriate therapeutic selection for patients with CML. This translocation results in the production of a BCR–Abl fusion protein with increased tyrosine kinase activity, causing the signal transduction intermediates interacting with this tyrosine kinase to be 'switched on'. This will lead to an increased transcription and translation of the genes activated by this signal transduction cascade, causing CML. Patients with this translocation have a better prognosis than those with atypical CML in which t(9;22) is absent. Individuals with t(9;22) can be treated with the signal transduction inhibitor, **imatinib mesylate**, which prevents activation of the downstream signal transduction intermediates, reversing the molecular effects of BCR–Abl. The introduction of signal transduction inhibitors is an exciting move towards targetting malignant diseases according to gene expression and cytogenetic data.

Non-Hodgkin lymphoma (NHL)

NHL is a broad term used to describe a range of different subtypes of lymphoma that are epidemiologically, clinically, and biologically distinct from Hodgkin lymphoma. Particular cytogenetic abnormalities are associated with particular subtypes and aid in their diagnosis. Cytogenetic analysis can be performed on malignant lymphocytes obtained from peripheral blood, bone marrow or cells aspirated from a lymph node.

In follicular lymphoma t(14;18)(q32;q21) is found in more than 90% of cases, or less commonly t(2;18)(p11.2;q21) and t(18;22)(q21;q11.2). Overexpression of BCL-2 is due to the translocation of this gene to the immunoglobulin heavy-chain gene locus (*IGH*), or the κ or λ light-chain loci on chromosomes 2 and 22, respectively, although t(2;18) and t(18;22) are rarely seen. Overexpression of BCL-2 prevents apoptosis in cells where this is expressed.

In 80% of cases of Burkitt lymphoma, t(8;14)(q24;q32) causes the translocation of *MYC* to the *IGH* locus. This leads to overexpression of the transcription factor c-Myc and subsequent B-cell proliferation.

In Mantle cell lymphoma, t(11;14) (q13;q32) is found in over 70% of cases and induces overexpression of *BCL-1/* cyclin D1 through the translocation of this gene with the *IGH* locus. Overexpression of cyclin D1 pushes the cell cycle from G1 to S phase, driving proliferation in these cells. Rarely in cases without a t(11;14) other cyclins associated with different translocations have been found to be overexpressed.

In certain situations, the tests outlined so far are insufficient for us to be able to obtain the appropriate diagnostic and prognostic information for a particular disease. In these cases further information can be obtained using molecular techniques.

10.8 **Molecular techniques**

The use of molecular techniques has improved diagnosis, the selection of therapeutic agents, and provides important prognostic information for a range of haematological malignancies. The polymerase chain reaction (PCR) and variants, DNA sequencing technologies, and gene expression profiling all provide important information to help treat and monitor disease. Of course, not all molecular techniques are available in every laboratory, but there are referral centres and centres of excellence providing these services, allowing us to utilize their expertise in this field. These techniques are also used for research into a wide variety of pathologies, not just haematological malignancies, although a greater understanding of the pathogenesis of haematological malignancies is due largely to the development and availability of these techniques.

Some of the methods used to provide diagnostically and prognostically useful information to haematologists are outlined below. PCR is a basic technique, the product of which can be used for a wide range of important molecular techniques. PCR can be utilized for the investigation of *TP53* polymorphisms in malignancies to the identification of individuals with Factor V Leiden mutations in the investigation of thrombophilia.

Polymerase chain reaction

This technique is extremely important in amplifying particular segments of DNA and can be used to identify specific mutations within the sequence being studied. Once a region of DNA has been selected, providing the sequence of the ends is known, the process of amplification can begin.

The PCR technique involves the use of a single-stranded DNA template, oligonucleotide primers and deoxynucleotides (to excess), and a DNA polymerase to generate multiple copies of a target sequence. A series of cycles of heating (to 95°C) to separate the complementary DNA strands, and cooling (to 50°C) to anneal the oligonucleotide primers, is used. The addition of deoxynucleotides in the presence of the heat-tolerant DNA polymerase, *Thermus aquaticus* (*Taq*), results in the extension of the oligonucleotide primers and the formation of a complementary strand to the template DNA during the extension phase at 72°C. The cycle can be repeated many times, each time generating successively greater copy numbers of the target sequence for analysis.

If a particular region of DNA is of interest within a tumour, this tissue can be compared to non-tumour cells (wild-type cells) from the same patient. For example, if tumour cells from a patient with B-cell CLL were being examined, DNA could be extracted from neutrophils for comparison. Neutrophil DNA would be considered wild-type, and any differences between the two could be considered to be due to the disease process.

The next step could involve the addition of a **restriction enzyme**, which recognizes specific nucleotide sequences. If a particular sequence is present, the DNA will be cut at that point producing two fragments. Using electrophoresis, we can visualize the products of the PCR and the effects of the restriction enzyme. By ascertaining whether the DNA has been cut, compared to a **wild-type region of DNA**, we can infer the presence of particular point mutations within this region.

Although PCR is an excellent technique to facilitate further investigation into the molecular biology of particular malignancies, the following techniques have played a pivotal role in our understanding of the biology of malignant disease. DNA sequencing technology allows us to examine the nucleotide sequence of entire genes. Knowing the sequence of a particular gene can assist in the selection of restriction enzymes for screening tests or can aid our understanding of the nature of gene mutations in both health and disease.

restriction enzymes
These enzymes recognize specific nucleotide sequences and can cut DNA wherever the sequence occurs. This selective cutting allows fragments to be formed which can be indicative of mutations within a specified sequence through the loss or gain of these restriction sites.

wild-type DNA
Denotes germline DNA. Mutations found within tumour cells when compared to wild-type DNA are considered to be acquired.

DNA sequencing technology

The use of DNA sequencing technology has dramatically improved our understanding of a range of lymphoid malignancies, particularly B-cell chronic lymphocytic leukaemia (CLL). The importance of DNA sequencing technologies will be illustrated using the example of somatic hypermutation. Elucidating the DNA sequence for the immunoglobulin heavy-chain hypervariable region (IgVH) determines whether the B cell has undergone somatic hypermutation. Somatic hypermutation is usually defined as less than 98% homology with the germline DNA sequence.

Somatic hypermutation is an entirely normal process within B cells, and follows an encounter with an antigen. These somatic mutations cause an increased strength of antigen binding and enhance the specificity for that antigen by the antibody. If somatic hypermutation has occurred, the B cell has passed through a lymph node-derived germinal centre. If the DNA sequence demonstrates an unmutated IgVH region, this suggests that the B cells have not passed through the germinal centre.

Cross reference

Germinal centres were introduced in Chapter 8.

Correlating IgVH mutational status with clinical outcome indicates that patients demonstrating hypermutated IgVH have a significantly better prognosis than those with unmutated IgVH genes. Patients with unmutated IgVH are likely to have a more aggressive disease, require treatment earlier, and have a reduced survival rate.

DNA sequencing is an important, but expensive and technically demanding, technique only available to a relatively small number of laboratories. Surrogate markers (such as Zap-70 in the case of B-CLL, measured using immunophenotyping) can be used as a more accessible marker of IgVH mutational status without the cost implications of sequencing.

The molecular biological methods mentioned so far are available, albeit indirectly, to a large number of laboratories within the UK. The final technique in this chapter—the use of gene expression studies, or the gene microarray—is only available as a research tool at present, although it has provided an abundance of information to help us understand the mechanics of malignancy. In Chapters 11 and 12 we discuss classification systems, and the techniques available to accurately and reproducibly categorize diseases according to a framework of guidelines as outlined by the World Health Organization. These classification guidelines are likely to expand over the next few years to incorporate data from gene expression studies, as this technology becomes more readily available and more pathobiological information is uncovered.

Gene expression studies

The use of gene expression studies, or the DNA microarray, is increasing within the scientific community, although it is still largely a research rather than a diagnostic tool. Although the principle behind the technique is fairly simple, practically, the technique can be rather difficult to employ. The data generated is indicative of the expression level of a particular gene or set of genes within a disease. By using the term expression level, we are focusing on the amount of mRNA produced when compared to controls. Expression can be normal, low, or high.

The DNA sequence of a number of target genes is obtained and incorporated into an array in the form of probes. These probes are arranged in a carefully recorded order, and inputted onto an analytical database. Separately, patient samples are processed to yield mRNA. This mRNA is then converted to complementary DNA (cDNA) (using reverse transcriptase) to which a fluorochrome is attached. This fluorochrome-labelled cDNA is added to, and incubated with, the DNA probes. Any complementary sequences shared between the DNA probe and the cDNA will result in the binding (annealing) of the complementary sequences. After washing off the excess cDNA, the microarray can be analysed, with the intensity of fluorescence being measured photometrically. The intensity of fluorescence will be proportional to the concentration of labelled cDNA binding to its complementary probe: if the cDNA is present in high quantities (mirroring the high levels of the original mRNA), the fluorochrome will generate an intense signal. By contrast, low levels of cDNA will generate a weak signal.

Gene expression studies provided the first indication that Zap-70 expression may be linked with the prognosis of patients diagnosed with B-cell CLL.

The results of gene expression studies can be influenced by a range of factors, although this book focuses on some of the key pathological influences. Epigenetic processes, such as the hypermethylation of genes, or the hypoacetylation of histones, will result in gene repression and downregulation since mRNA will be synthesized either at a reduced rate, or will fail to be synthesized. Reduced or absent mRNA decreases the fluorescence generated from this technique and can be interpreted as underexpression of a gene. The hypermethylation of *CDKN2A* and *CDKN2B* causes the loss of expression of the INK cell cycle regulators p16 and p15, respectively. The loss of p16- and p15-mediated cell cycle control ensures dysregulation of the cyclin D–CDK4/6 complex, and the hyperphosphorylation of pRb. *CDKN2A and CDKN2B* silencing through methylation or deletion occurs in approximately 60% of cases of non-Hodgkin lymphoma, and results in dysregulation of the cell cycle.

In mantle cell lymphoma, t(11;14)(q13;q32) is associated with an upregulation of cyclin D1 as a consequence of its translocation to the immunoglobulin heavy-chain locus. The use of the strong promoter in this region causes an increase in the transcription of cyclin D1. Therefore, using gene expression studies and an appropriate probe for cyclin D1 mRNA, overexpression would be demonstrated.

The results from gene expression studies can be consolidated by many other molecular techniques, including PCR and electrophoresis, in order to investigate the cause of abnormal mRNA expression.

Cross references

See Chapter 9—Introduction to haematological malignancies; Section 9.3—Introduction to the cell cycle, and Section 9.6—Epigenetics.

Lymphomas are discussed in greater detail in Chapter 12.

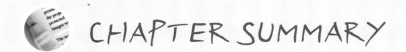

CHAPTER SUMMARY

In this chapter we have:

- Examined the laboratory work involved in the investigation, diagnosis, and monitoring of patients with suspected haematological malignances.

- Outlined commonly associated symptoms and discussed their causes in relation to the underlying molecular and biochemical mechanisms of haematological malignancies.

- Discussed a variety of laboratory techniques used in diagnosis and monitoring, and have focused on those closely allied with haematology; including cytogenetics, immunophenotyping, and molecular biology.

- Discussed the range of samples that can be used for the investigation of haematological malignancies, including peripheral blood, bone marrow aspirates, trephines, and lymph node biopsies.

DISCUSSION QUESTIONS

10.1   Compare and contrast the value of cytochemical and immunophenotypic methods in the investigation and diagnosis of haematological malignancies.

10.2   Compare and contrast the bone marrow aspirate and bone marrow trephine. Explain which sample is appropriate for the assessment of lymphocyte infiltration of haemopoietic tissue.

10.3   'G-banded chromosomes are sufficient to identify all important cytogenetic abnormalities in haematological malignancies.' Critically discuss this statement.

 FURTHER READING

●   Bain BJ. **The bone marrow aspirate in healthy subjects**. *British Journal of Haematology* 1996:**94**;206–9.

●   Bain BJ, Clark D, Lampert IA, Wilkins BS. *Bone Marrow Pathology*. Blackwell Publishing, Oxford, 2001.

●   Lewis SM, Bain BJ, Bates I (ed). *Dacie and Lewis Practical Haematology*, 9th edn. Churchill Livingstone, London, 2001.

●   Weiss MM, Hermsen MAJA, Meijer GA, van Grieken NCT, Baak JPA, Kuipers EJ, van Diest PJ. **Comparative genomic hybridisation**. *Molecular Pathology* 1999:**52**;243–51.

Answers to self-check questions, case study questions, and discussion questions are provided in the book's Online Resource Centre, visit www.oxfordtextbooks.co.uk/orc/moore

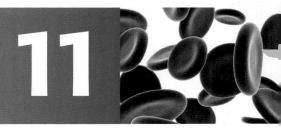

An introduction to classification systems: myeloid neoplasms

Gavin Knight

The discovery of leukaemia is generally attributable to Hughes Bennett and Rudolph Virchow independently in 1845. The first description of leukaemia was actually published in 1844 by the French physician Alfred Donné in his text '*Cours de microscopie complémentaire des études médicales, Anatomie microscopique et physiologie des fluides de l'Economie*'. In more than a century and a half since this initial discovery, we now recognize a wide range of different types of haematological malignancy, not just leukaemia.

Chapter 9 examined the basic theories of haemato-oncology and established that leukaemia can be subdivided into acute and chronic forms. In this chapter, we examine a range of haematological malignancies, including leukaemias, and explain how we can subdivide these into myeloid or lymphoid lineages and then further subdivide them according to various cellular, molecular, genetic, and clinical features. This chapter focuses on myeloid-related neoplasms, whereas Chapter 12 examines those of lymphoid origin.

By providing an appropriate classification system, clinicians can use specific criteria to consistently recognize particular disease entities, distinguish similar and dissimilar malignancies, and provide appropriate treatment to improve the patient's prognosis. If haematologists have the appropriate scientific and clinical information, therapy can be prescribed on a more appropriate basis and, in the long-term, reduce morbidity and mortality.

The next two chapters consider the importance of classification and examine some of the more recent developments in classification systems. Laboratory techniques are used to provide the data necessary to accurately classify malignant haematological diseases, as outlined in Chapter 10.

Learning objectives

After studying this chapter you should confidently be able to:

■ Describe the importance of classification systems and understand the basis of their development.

■ Describe the main differences between the World Health Organization (WHO) and French–American–British (FAB) systems in the classification of acute myeloid leukaemia.

■ Critically discuss the types of haematological malignancy recognized by the FAB and WHO systems.

■ Describe the common translocations identified in haematological malignancies and, where appropriate, their role in classification.

■ Discuss the classification of myelodysplastic syndromes.

11.1 **Why is classification important?**

As we established at the beginning of this chapter, we have knowledge of a wide range of different types of haematological malignancy. Each malignant disease varies with its origin, clinical behaviour, morphology, cytogenetic profile/, and molecular makeup. In addition, the way a disease responds to therapeutic agents varies between different types of cancer and, based on our knowledge of the molecular basis of cancer, some therapies are more appropriate for treating a particular disease when compared to others. The best way of ensuring that a patient is prescribed the appropriate medication is to obtain a correct diagnosis and to ensure that, as scientists and clinicians, we have a universal language to describe the disease. The terminology assigned to a particular disease in the UK has to be standardized to have the same meaning throughout the world. This can be achieved via a clear framework allowing us to pigeonhole specific diseases.

From a research perspective, it is important that scientists are able to confidently both investigate and report internationally recognized diseases. Having a standardized diagnostic framework can ensure that research can be reported and interpreted globally. An appropriate classification system is important because it allows the subdivision of patients with different prognoses, ultimately helping to direct future research and therapeutic options.

Ultimately, classification systems need to be dynamic. We need to be able to change different aspects of these systems as technology and scientific understanding develops. As we will see, the French–American–British (FAB) system outlined below used morphology and cytochemical stains as the basis of classification, although this was eventually superseded by a system that utilizes molecular and cytogenetic approaches. At present, the WHO system does not recognize results from gene-expression analysis, although in the future, this may be an important consideration for classification.

Let's now consider the main classification systems frequently encountered in your studies and in the clinical haematology laboratory.

11.2 **The main classification systems**

The FAB system has provided the cornerstone of classification of leukaemias and myelodysplastic syndromes since 1976. FAB uses cellular morphology and the arbitrary value of 30% blasts to differentiate between acute leukaemias and other myeloproliferative conditions.

Patients are diagnosed with acute leukaemia when their blast count exceeds 30%. In these patients, more aggressive therapy is indicated than those with <30% blasts. The FAB diagnostic criteria required to classify a patient with acute leukaemia are listed below. As you will see later on in the chapter, (b) and (c) below relate to specific disease entities.

(a) At least 30% of all nucleated blood cells in the bone marrow must be blasts.

(b) 50% or more of the total nucleated cells should be erythroblasts, with 30% or more of the non-erythroid cells also being blast cells (this allows for the diagnosis of erythroleukaemia).

(c) Morphological features of acute promyelocytic leukaemia are present, irrespective of the blast count (this allows for the diagnosis of acute promyelocytic leukaemia).

As diagnostic techniques have improved and the limitations of FAB are increasingly recognized, immunophenotyping and cytogenetic techniques have been incorporated into this classification system in order to improve both the sensitivity and specificity of diagnosis. Morphology should still be used for the initial diagnosis, whilst immunophenotyping and cytogenetic data should be used to increase our confidence in classification and to improve reproducibility between users. In 2001, the World Health Organization (WHO) published a revised system for the classification of a range of neoplasms, not just restricted to those of haemopoietic origin. Of key importance to this system is the new 20% **blast threshold** for the classification of acute myeloid leukaemias. Clinical research has demonstrated that there is a significant improvement in the survival of patients who fall into this 20–30% blast margin when given the opportunity to be treated with more aggressive chemotherapeutic agents.

blast threshold
The minimum percentage of blasts required to diagnose a leukaemia as acute. WHO currently specifies 20% blasts to make this diagnosis.

The FAB system

The FAB classification system is largely based on morphology, and should only be used to make a diagnosis in untreated patients with a normocellular or hypercellular marrow. Many chemotherapeutic agents can affect the morphology of cells, as can the choice of anticoagulant and the age of the sample, making a classification system based on morphology unreliable. Morphological examination of blood and bone marrow slides is essential and must be supported by a 200 white cell differential count of peripheral blood and a 500 white cell differential count of bone marrow before a diagnosis can be made.

Cross reference
For more details on myelodysplastic syndromes see Section 11.3.

The FAB system divides acute leukaemias into myeloid and lymphoid categories, based on the cellular characteristics evident through the use of Romanowsky and cytochemical stains; the myeloid category is subdivided as M0 through to M7, and the lymphoid L1 to L3. The blood film should be stained to a high quality using Romanowsky stain, with additional cytochemical stains used to establish cell lineage and origin as necessary. Using Romanowsky stain alone, it is often difficult to differentiate between lymphoblasts, myeloblasts, monoblasts, erythroblasts, and megakaryoblasts—and so more specific cytochemical investigation or immunophenotyping is required. Table 11.1 outlines the subtypes of acute myeloid leukaemias. The table demonstrates that for each of the conditions listed a myeloid abbreviation (M0–M7), and a name are provided. This name describes the stage of maturational arrest present or the predominant cell found in each particular disease. For acute lymphoblastic leukaemias, this is not the case. Lymphoblastic leukaemias are described according to differences in nuclear size and cytoplasmic features. Using immunophenotyping, it is possible to classify lymphoblasts according their stage of maturation, but this is only of value when considering the L3 subtype. More detail can be found on the classification of acute lymphoblastic leukaemia in Chapter 12.

Cross reference
See Chapter 12 for a classification of precursor lymphoid neoplasms.

BOX 11.1 *FAB classification*

The FAB classification was published in 1976 after seven haematologists from France, America, and Britain examined the blood cell morphology of 200 cases of leukaemia. The proposals outlined paved the way for the morphological classification of acute leukaemias and, later, myelodysplastic syndromes.

Acute myeloid leukaemia

We should now examine the disorders the FAB group recognizes as acute myeloid leukaemias. Seven categories are recognized by the FAB group as distinct myeloid leukaemias, although the therapeutic choice is broadly similar for all types of AML, with the exception of acute promyelocytic leukaemia. The following pathologies are summarized in Table 11.1 for easy reference.

TABLE 11.1 **The FAB classification of acute myeloid leukaemia. On the left we have the abbreviated form, with the full name expansion following. A description of the morphological findings is included, as well as cytochemical reactions as this forms the basis of the FAB system. Cytogenetic features have been included for interest where appropriate.**

Sub group	Name	Morphological findings	Cytogenetics	Cytochemistry
M0	Undifferentiated	MPO/SBB positive in <3% blasts—further investigation required by immunophenotype. No Auer rods.		<3% pos for SBB, MPO, CAE
M1	Without maturation	≥90% blasts with ≥3% MPO/SBB positive ≤10% monocytes/granulocytes		>3% pos for SBB, MPO, CAE
M2	With maturation	≥30% blasts (but up to 89%). Granulocytes ≥10%; monocytes ≤20%	t (8;21); t (6;9)	MPO/SBB/CAE pos
M3	Acute promyelocytic	Significant numbers of promyelocytes. <30% myeloblasts	t (15;17)	MPO/SBB/CAE/AP pos
M4	Myelomonocytic	≥30% blasts; ≥20% granulocytes and monoblasts*	inv(16)/t(16;16)**	CAE/ANAE***
M5a	Monoblastic	≥80% monocytic component (with ≥80% monoblasts) of non-erythroid cells		ANAE pos, MPO SBB neg
M5b	Monocytic	≥80% monocytic component (with <80% monoblasts) of non-erythroid cells		ANAE pos, MPO SBB neg
M6	Erythroleukaemia	Blasts ≥30% non-erythroid cells; erythroblasts ≥50% all nucleated bone-marrow cells		ANAE/PAS/AP and Perls' pos
M7	Megakaryoblastic	No Auer rods		MPO/SBB/CAE neg Based on immunophenotyping

Key: ANAE = alpha naphthyl acetate esterase; AP = acid phosphatase; CAE = chloroacetate esterase; MPO = myeloperoxidase; PAS = Periodic acid–Schiff; SBB = Sudan black B.

*Plus additional evidence of monocytes in PB (>5 × 10⁹/l)/± BM consistent with M2
**M4 subtype with increased eosinophils (M4Eo)
***Useful for differentiation between lineages

Acute myeloid leukaemia, undifferentiated (M0)

The least mature AML is classified as M0. There is no morphological evidence of maturation or differentiation, with large numbers of blasts of uncertain lineage apparent. Due to their lack of differentiation, less than 3% of blasts in M0 are positive for the cytochemical stains Sudan black B (SBB), myeloperoxidase (MPO), and chloroacetate esterase (CAE). There is usually no evidence of Auer rods in cases of M0.

Cross reference

Chapter 10 contains greater detail regarding the use and specificity of cytochemical stains.

Acute myeloid leukaemia without maturation (M1)

As we progress to M1, we start to see evidence of differentiation into the myeloid lineage. There is a variable nucleocytoplasmic ratio, with some cells larger than others. There is also evidence of nucleoli. We will start to see cytoplasmic granules and we may occasionally see Auer rods. In excess of 3% of blasts will express MPO, SBB, and CAE, and can be called 'MPO/SBB/CAE-positive'. Maturing granulocytes and monocytes should be apparent, but each of the two populations will comprise less than 10% of the non-erythroid compartment.

Acute myeloid leukaemia with maturation (M2)

M2 demonstrates further evidence of differentiation, and these cells are clearly of myeloid origin. Of the bone marrow non-erythroid cells, blasts and promyelocytes dominate. Blasts comprise 30–89%, but maturing forms of the other lineages are increased. In excess of 10% of non-erythroid cells should be maturing granulocytes (unlike in the bone marrow findings of M1), and less than 20% should be maturing monocytes. Cytochemical reactions are usually positive for MPO, SBB, and CAE. Auer rods may be present.

Acute promyelocytic leukaemia (and variant) (M3)

M3 is a particularly interesting form of AML. A maturational arrest evident at the pro-myelocyte stage occurs, resulting in acute promyelocytic leukaemia (APL). Large numbers of promyelocytes accumulate, with a corresponding reduction in mature granulocytes. In the case of M3, the threshold of 30% blasts is not usually exceeded, but morphology forms the basis of the diagnosis of AML, as outlined in Section 11.2. In actual fact, for the purposes of classification, the FAB group consider promyelocytes to be 'blast equivalents'. The promyelocytes contain large numbers of coarse purple/red granules which may make the nucleus difficult to see on the peripheral blood film. When apparent, particularly in the trephine, the nucleus appears bilobed. Auer rods are frequently found, with cells containing bundles of Auer rods called **faggot cells**.

A variant of M3 (M3v) has been recognized exhibiting different morphological features. Promyelocytes are either microgranular or hypogranular in this subtype, and the white cell count at presentation tends to be higher. Cases with a higher white cell count are associated with a poorer prognosis. The standard myeloid cytochemical stains MPO, SBB, and CAE are positive, and acid phosphatase also gives a strong reaction.

faggot cells

Immature granulocytes that contain bundles of Auer rods. These are commonly seen in acute promyelocytic leukaemia.

Acute myelomonocytic leukaemia (M4)

In M4, acute myelomonocytic leukaemia, myeloblasts constitute 30% or more of the total cell count, and there is also monocytic and granulocytic maturation in excess of 20% of all non-erythroid cells. In excess of 20% monoblasts should be present in the bone marrow in addition to the 30% or more of myeloblasts, with $>5 \times 10^9$/L monocytes or their precursors in the peripheral blood. Cytochemistry can also be used to identify the relevant lineages accurately. In particular, CAE can be used for granulocyte identification and α-naphthyl acetate esterase (ANAE) for the monocytic lineage to enable appropriate differentiation of the lineages. Auer rods may be apparent.

Acute monoblastic/monocytic leukaemia (M5)

M5 is subdivided into M5a and M5b, depending on the monoblast composition of the bone marrow. M5a is associated with >80% monoblasts and M5b <80% monoblasts within the bone marrow. Non-specific esterases, such as ANAE, can be used to identify the monocytic lineage. Myeloid markers MPO and SBB are negative, but dysplastic features are often present on a Romanowsky-stained film. Auer rods may be found within the cytoplasm.

Erythroleukaemia (M6)

The last two stages of the FAB classification further differentiate and specialize, with M6 representing erythroleukaemia. Erythroblasts comprise 50% or more of all nucleated bone marrow cells and myeloblasts constitute >30% of non-erythroid cells as outlined in Section 9.2. Cells usually provide positive reactions for ANAE, Periodic acid–Schiff (PAS), acid phosphatase, and Perls' stain. Auer rods may be present in the malignant cells.

Acute megakaryoblastic leukaemia (M7)

M7, acute megakaryoblastic leukaemia, is apparent through increased numbers of megakaryoblasts, some of which show cytoplasmic blebbing—the process under which platelets are produced. Cytochemical techniques can be used, although they are of limited value. MPO, SBB, and CAE fail to demonstrate reactions in this lineage, and Auer rods are not evident. Nowadays, immunophenotyping is most frequently used to distinguish between M0 and M7, as these both share similar morphology and cytochemical reactions.

SELF-CHECK 11.1

Outline the main types of acute leukaemia identified by the FAB system.

Now that the FAB classification has been considered, let's have a look at the way classification has been improved by the World Health Organization system.

The World Health Organization classification system

The WHO system for the classification of haematological malignancies revolutionized the way in which these malignancies are reported. Evidence-based practice is the cornerstone of this system, which initially uses morphological assessment for classification purposes, but then utilizes immunophenotype and cytogenetic data to further subgroup patients into their respective disease groups. Using the WHO system, the biology behind the disease (pathobiology) is also considered, with a parallel between the malignant cell and normal cell counterpart being drawn where appropriate. In addition, therapy-related malignancies (i.e. those leukaemias secondary to previous chemo- or radiotherapeutic procedures), and those considered to be a progression of myelodysplasia, are classified as particular disease entities. This clarification is important as these secondary conditions often have a less favourable prognosis when compared with primary (*de novo*) malignancies.

Seven main *myeloid subgroups* have been established by the WHO system and include:

1. Acute myeloid leukaemia and related precursor neoplasms.

2. Myeloproliferative neoplasms

3. Myeloid and lymphoid neoplasms with eosinophilia and abnormalities of *PDGFRA*, *PDGFRB*, or *FGFR1*

4. Myelodysplastic/myeloproliferative neoplasms

5. Myelodysplastic syndromes

6. Acute leukaemias of ambiguous lineage

7. Histiocytic and dendritic cell neoplasms

And five *lymphoid subgroups*:

1. Precursor lymphoid neoplasms

2. Mature B-cell neoplasms

3. Mature T-cell and NK-cell neoplasms

4. Hodgkin lymphoma

5. Post-transplant lymphoproliferative disorders

The lymphoid neoplasms will be considered in the next chapter.

SELF-CHECK 11.2

What are the main myeloid diseases categorized by the WHO system?

Since we have already examined the FAB requirements for the classification of an AML, we should look at the ways in which we can provide a diagnosis of AML, according to the WHO system.

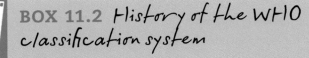

BOX 11.2 *History of the WHO classification system*

The World Health Organization classification system of haematological malignancies represents the collaboration between the European Association for Haematopathology and the Society for Haematopathology. Prior to publication, a Clinical Advisory Committee was developed with over 40 international panel members to ensure the system was valid. The first WHO version, published in 2001, based on the revised European and American classification of lymphoid neoplasms (REAL), now applies to all haematological malignancies.

In 2008, the fourth WHO version was published, although it still contains a number of provisional disease entities requiring more research before becoming committed to the definitive document.

Acute myeloid leukaemia and related precursor neoplasms

The WHO classifies AML based on an excess of 20% myeloblasts in the peripheral blood or bone marrow *or* the presence of the following cytogenetic abnormalities irrespective of the blast percentage:

- t(8;21)(q22;q22)
- inv(16)(p13.1;q22)
- t(16;16)(p13.1;q22)
- t(15;17)(q22;q12)

In addition, the following recurrent cytogenetic features are also considered important in the WHO classification, but require a blast count of 20% or higher to be classified as acute leukaemia:

- t(9;11)(p22;q23)
- t(6;9)(p23;q34)
- inv(3)(q21;q26.2)
- t(3;3)(q21;q26.2)
- t(1;22)(p13;q13)

Individuals harbouring these mutations usually have very specific morphological features highly suggestive of the mutations listed above, although a definitive diagnosis should not be made without access to the appropriate cytogenetic data. In addition, AML with the mutated nucleophosmin gene (*NPM1*) and CCAAT enhancer binding protein α-gene(*CEBPA*) have been included as provisional disease entities as these mutations have an impact on the disease course. However, further research and evidence is needed before these mutations are permanently included in this classification.

The WHO group recognizes seven distinctly different subcategories of AML:

- Acute myeloid leukaemia with recurrent genetic abnormalities
- Acute myeloid leukaemia with myelodysplasia-related changes
- Therapy-related myeloid neoplasms
- Acute myeloid leukaemia not otherwise specified (NOS)
- Myeloid sarcoma
- Myeloid proliferations related to Down syndrome
- Blastic plasmacytoid dendritic cell neoplasm

Acute myeloid leukaemia with recurrent genetic abnormalities is based on the presence of one of nine recurrent genetic abnormalities identified as providing a predictable clinical outcome for these patients. Additional mutations involving *NPM1* and *CEBPA* will not be considered further in this book as they are included as 'provisional entities' in the WHO classification and their importance has yet to be fully elucidated.

If features of multilineage dysplasia are present in the blood or bone marrow findings of a patient with AML, the disease will be classified as *AML with myelodysplasia-related changes*. AML with myelodysplasia-related changes predominantly recognizes secondary myeloid leukaemias following a myelodysplastic course or cases showing an MDS-related karyotype.

Also recognized and classified are acute myeloid leukaemias, myelodysplastic syndromes, and myeloproliferative disorders secondary to previous exposure to chemotherapeutic agents or ionizing radiation in a clinical setting. *Therapy-related neoplasms* tend to have characteristic patterns of presentation and prognosis.

In the fourth edition of the WHO classification, the category *acute myeloid leukaemia not otherwise specified* has been modified to reflect our updated knowledge of diseases previously considered in this group. Myeloid sarcoma has been removed from this group and been awarded a discrete category. Future amendments to this category are likely to occur as the nature of evidence-based practice furthers our level of understanding of these diseases at the genetic or molecular levels.

Myeloid proliferations related to Down syndrome is another important new category that relates particularly to the processes of transient abnormal myelopoiesis and Down syndrome-related acute megakaryoblastic leukaemia. Both these conditions are associated with mutations in the *GATA1* transcription factor, and should therefore be treated separately to non-Down syndrome-related myeloid diseases.

Another newly classified condition reported by WHO is *blastic plasmacytoid dendritic cell neoplasm*. Although a rare disease with ambiguous origins, WHO have included this as an acute myeloid leukaemia.

Reading below you will see that the main categories within the AML section of the WHO guidelines are outlined. Where appropriate, the molecular basis of the disease is introduced.

AML with recurrent genetic abnormalities

This particular subgroup includes four main genetic abnormalities identified through clinical research as having either a good or poor prognosis. The classification of AML with recurrent genetic abnormalities should only be applied to *de novo* malignancies, even if the mutations described below are encountered in cases of secondary leukaemia. The use of standard cytogenetic tests, as outlined in Chapter 10, is usually sufficient to identify these abnormalities.

The identification of recurrent cytogenetic abnormalities should always be considered in the first instance in order to successfully classify acute myeloid leukaemias.

AML with t(8;21)(q22;q22) – RUNX1–RUNX1T1 (formerly AML1–ETO)

The translocation t(8;21)(q22;q22) involves the fusion of *RUNX1* (formerly known as *AML1*), found on the long arm of chromosome 21 with the functional co-repressor *RUNX1T1*, formerly known as *ETO* (*eight twenty-one*) on chromosome 8.

Figure 11.1 depicts chromosomes 16 and 21, and the location of the genes *CBFB* and *RUNX1*, respectively. Working through Figure 11.1 you can see that in a normal situation, the protein product RUNX1 (CBFα), acts as a molecular bridge allowing the binding of core binding factor-β (CBFβ) to the CBF binding site. This, in the presence of other transcription factors which are localized to the CBFα/CBFβ complex, allows for the active transcription of target genes.

In Figure 11.2, the N-terminal region of CBFα is fused with the majority of the RUNX1T1 protein forming a chimeric (fusion) protein, preventing the formation of a stable DNA binding complex involving CBFβ. Instead, functional repressors become involved with RUNX1–RUNX1T1, inhibiting transcription and translation of target genes and causing a failure of cell maturation and differentiation.

The RUNX1–RUNX1T1 chimeric protein is insufficient to be independently leukaemogenic, but requires a secondary event to promote leukaemogenesis—as predicted by Knudson's hypothesis.

Cross reference
Knudson's hypothesis is outlined in Chapter 9.

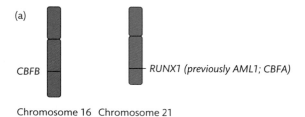

FIGURE 11.1

(a) The locus for the CBFα gene (*RUNX1*) is situated on chromosome 21q22, and CBFβ (*CBFB*) is located on chromosome 16q22. (b) The binding of CBFα to the CBF binding site permits the subsequent binding of CBFβ. This complex enables histone acetyltransferase (HAT) and co-activators (CoA) to bind, allowing histone modification and transcription and translation of CBF inducible genes.

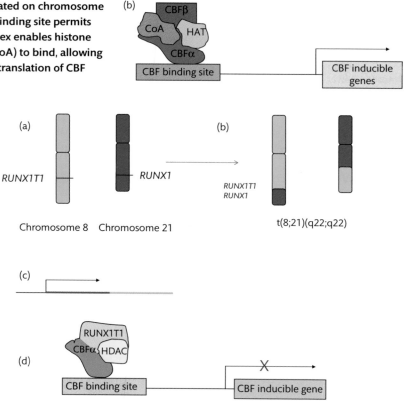

FIGURE 11.2

Repression of the CBF complex through the fusion of RUNX1 (encoding CBFα) with the transcriptional repressor RUNX1T1. Translocation of *RUNX1* found on chromosome 21 (21q22) and *RUNX1T1* on chromosome 8 (8q22) (a and b) produce a fusion gene (c) which is transcribed and translated into the chimeric protein RUNX1–RUNX1T1. RUNX1–RUNX1T1 binds to the CBF binding site (d), but instead of enabling transcription and translation of target genes through the binding of CBFβ and transcriptional activators, transcriptional repressors are recruited, inhibiting maturation and differentiation of cells containing this translocation.

AML with inv(16) (p13.1;q22) or t(16;16)(p13;q22): CBFB–MYH11

The pericentric inversion inv(16) and translocation, t(16;16), are both involved with the disruption of the *CBFB* gene, and the consequent function of CBFβ protein product is disrupted. If you look at Figure 11.3, you will see that, through this inversion or translocation process, *CBFB* is fused with the gene encoding the smooth muscle myosin heavy chain (SMMHC)–*MYH11*.

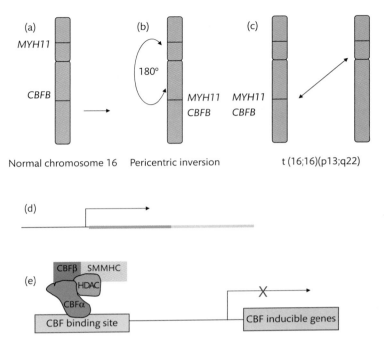

FIGURE 11.3

Disruption of the CBF pathway. The normal chromosome 16 (a) contains the gene encoding CBFβ (16q22) and the gene encoding the smooth muscle myosin heavy-chain gene (*MHY11*) (16p13). Through pericentric inversion (b), rotation of chromosomal material involving the centromere, or translocation (c), results in *CBFB* and *MYH11* becoming fused. (d) Transcription and translation of the fusion protein follows. (e) *CBFβ*–SMMHC is able to recruit potent transcriptional corepressors (HDAC (histone deacetylase) and other co-repressors) to the CBF complex, inhibiting maturation and differentiation of cells containing this chimeric protein.

The chimeric protein product, CBFβ–SMMHC, recruits a range of transcriptional repressors and histone deacetylases to the CBF binding site. The consequence of recruiting these repressors is that the transcription and translation of target genes is prevented. A number of studies have demonstrated that inv(16) or t(16;16) alone are insufficient to be leukaemogenic, although they can contribute to a malignant phenotype in the presence of a second mutation.

AML with t(15;17)(q22;q12)–PML–RARA

Translocation t(15;17)(q22;q12) is present in approximately 98% of patients diagnosed with acute promyelocytic leukaemia (APL). The t(15;17)(q22;q12) is associated with the translocation of the promyelocytic leukaemia gene (*PML*), so-called because it was first identified in patients with this disease, with the retinoic acid receptor α- (*RARA*) gene. If you refer to Figure 11.4 you will see that in a normal situation, retinoic acid, when bound to its receptor (RARα/RXR), induces the dissociation of transcriptional repressors, and the binding of transcriptional activators. In Figure 11.5 we can see that t(15;17)(q22;q12) produces the chimeric protein PML-RARα. PML-RARα interacts with a variety of co-repressors, including histone deacetylase (HDAC), inhibiting the retinoic acid-responsive genes necessary for granulocytic maturation beyond the promyelocyte stage. It has also been suggested that the methylating enzymes Dnmt1 and Dnmt3a are recruited by PML-RARα, causing transcriptional repression through promoter methylation.

The range of retinoic acid responsive genes involved in the pathogenesis of APL has yet to be elucidated, although recent evidence suggests that the transcription factor PU.1, necessary

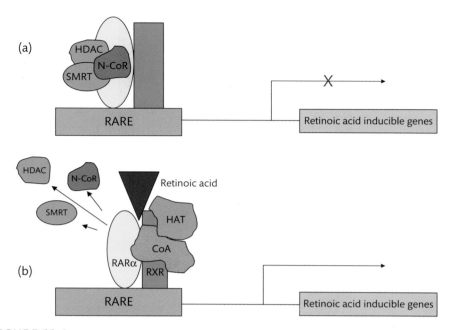

FIGURE 11.4

The action of the wild-type retinoic acid receptor. The retinoic acid receptor-α (RARα) forms a heterodimer with the retinoid X receptor (RXR) in the presence of the retinoic acid response element (RARE) binding site. This heterodimer, when unbound to retinoic acid, binds a range of functional co-repressors including histone deacetylase (HDAC), SMRT, and N-CoR (a). Chromatin is remodelled, preventing transcription. When retinoic acid binds to its receptor (b), the repressors dissociate from the receptor complex and allow the binding of the transcriptional activators histone acetyltransferase (HAT) and other coactivators (CoA), allowing histone modification. Binding of functional activators permits transcription and translation of target genes and the maturation of promyelocytes to neutrophils.

for granulocytic differentiation, can be indirectly inhibited by PML–RARα. Inhibition of PU.1 blocks differentiation, leading to an accumulation of myeloid precursors. Treatment with all-*trans* retinoic acid (ATRA) and combinations of chemotherapy including ATRA restores granulopoiesis by removing the block of differentiation and maturation, and allows the production of mature neutrophils to continue.

In addition to t(15;17), a number of other translocations involving *RARA* have also been identified. The most common of these include:

- t(11;17)(q23;q21) fusing the promyelocytic leukaemia zinc finger (*PLZF*) gene to *RARA*
- t(11;17)(q13;q21), fusing nuclear matrix associated (*NuMA*) to *RARA*
- t(5;17) in which nucleophosmin (*NPM*) is fused to *RARA*

There is also evidence of der(17)which fuses stat5b with RARα. Differences in these molecular mechanisms alter the sensitivity of these cells to ATRA. Cells containing *PML*, *NPM*, and *NuMA* fusions are sensitive to ATRA therapy, whilst those with *PLZF* and *stat5b* fusions are insensitive. In the original version of the WHO classification published in 2001, the *RARA* variants above were also considered as AML with recurrent cytogenetic abnormalities and were included with t(15;17). However, because these variants provide different clinicopathological diseases, they have since been removed from this classification.

If you consider all cases of AML, approximately 30% will harbour t(8;21)(q22;q22), inv(16) (p13;q22), t(16;16)(p13;q22), or t(15;17)(q22;q12).

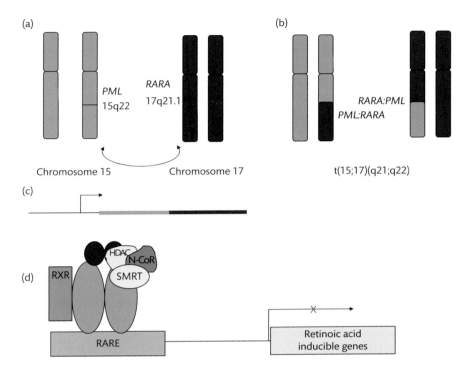

FIGURE 11.5

The inhibitory complex generated by t(15;17) in acute promyelocytic leukaemia (APL). A balanced and reciprocal translocation occurs between the long arms of chromosomes 15 and 17 (a) involving the genes *PML* and *RARA*, generating the fusion genes *PML:RARA* (b). Transcription of this fusion gene (c) ensures that components of both *PML* and *RARA* are retained and incorporated into the chimeric protein PML–RARα. PML–RARα retains important functional domains including the retinoic acid response element (RARE) binding domain, the RXR (retinoid X receptor) binding domain in RARα, and the PML homodimerization domain. (d) PML binds transcriptional repressors, HDAC, N-CoR and SMRT, with high affinity, and these become localized to the RARE via PML–RARα binding. Chromatin modification via the co-repressors prevents transcription and translation of target genes, in this case resulting in a maturational arrest at the promyelocyte stage of development.

AML with t(9;11)(p22;q23)–MLLT3–MLL

The cytogenetic abnormalities t(8;21), inv(16), and t(16;16) are very specific. Here, two genes are involved, and fusion of the two produces a chimeric protein with an altered structure–function relationship.

The original WHO classification for AML with recurrent genetic abnormalities included any primary AML with 11q23 abnormalities. 11q23 abnormalities are a much more heterogeneous group of mutations than the others within this classification, with the only constant being that 11q23 is involved. There are over 50 different partners which have been documented to combine with the mixed-lineage leukaemia gene (*MLL*), although the most common found in AML is MLLT3 in t(9;11), present in approximately one-third of cases.

The latest (2008) update of the WHO classification specifies t(9;11) as a recurrent genetic abnormality, but excludes all other mutations from this *MLL* category.

AML with t(6;9)(6p23;9q34)–DEK–NUP214

The translocation resulting in the formation of the *DEK–NUP214* (previously known as *DEK–CAN*) fusion gene is associated with a poor prognosis. A rare condition, accounting for between 0.5 and 4% of all cases of AML, t(6;9) is associated with an aggressive malignancy refractory to common chemotherapeutic agents, with a survival time of less than 12 months.

Originally classified as either acute myeloid leukaemia with maturation (M2) or, less frequently, as acute myelomonocytic leukaemia (M4), using the FAB system, AML with t(6;9) should only be classified as such following comprehensive cytogenetic analysis—even though the genotype is considered predictable by the discrete morphological characteristics usually demonstrated. Peripheral cell counts demonstrate pancytopenia, whilst bone marrow investigations reveal a hypercellular marrow with an absolute basophilia and signs of unilineage or multilineage dysplasia.

> **internal tandem duplications (ITD)**
> These arise from the duplication of sequences from within a gene. In relation to FLT3, ITD of the juxtamembrane region of the gene results in constitutive activation of FLT3.

Internal tandem duplications of *fms*-related tyrosine kinase (FLT3–ITD) are found in approximately 70% of patients harbouring t(6;9), with the combination of the two associated with a higher white cell count, blast percentage, and worse prognosis.

AML with inv(3)(q21;q26.2) or t(3;3)(q21;q26.2)–RPN1–EVI1

The paracentric inversion inv (3)(q21;26.2) or t(3;3)(q21;q26.2) results in the fusion of *RPN1* with *EVI1*, forming a fusion gene. *EVI1* encodes a nuclear DNA-binding protein, which, when dysregulated through fusion with another protein causes the inappropriate expression of EVI1. Following fusion, the stronger *RPN1* promotor region controls the transcription of *EVI1*, resulting in the overexpression of EVI1 and an increased proliferative potential in blast cells harbouring this fusion product.

Morphologically, this subgroup of AML demonstrates significant platelet abnormalities including, in some cases, thrombocythaemia and giant hypogranular platelets, with a background of anaemia. Neutrophil dysplasia including hypogranulation and the Pelger–Huet anomaly are also common features.

Patients with this chromosomal abnormality have a poor prognosis.

AML (megakaryoblastic) with t(1;22)(p13;q13)–RBM15–MKL1

An uncommon cytogenetic abnormality, t(1;22), is associated with infant and childhood acute megakaryoblastic leukaemia, accounting for approximately 10% of all childhood AMLs.

The gene *RBM15*, also called *OTT* following its identification as a fusion partner in the translocation One Twenty Two, encodes the RNA-binding motif protein 15 found in high concentrations in haemopoietic progenitors. Wild-type RBM15 is thought to be involved in the inhibition of differentiation and, in addition, inhibits proliferation. When dysregulated through the fusion with MKL1, also called megakaryoblastic leukaemia-1 (*MAL*, *BSAC*, or *MRTF-A*), RBM15 maintains megakaryoblasts in an immature state.

Experimentally, the knock-down of *RBM15* is associated with an increased number of marrow megakaryocytes; and, accompanied with the inhibitory apoptotic inhibitor MKL, is a likely candidate in the pathogenesis of acute megakaryoblastic leukaemia harbouring t(1;22)(p13;q13).

Morphologically, patients with t(1;22) have increased numbers of megakaryoblasts, some of which are small, and demonstrate cytoplasmic blebbing. Marrow fibrosis is a common feature as with all pathologies demonstrating megakaryoblast/megakaryocyte accumulation.

Once recurrent cytogenetic abnormalities have been considered, we should identify the presence of dysplasia. Approximately 30% of cases will have been classified with recurrent cytogenetic abnormalities, but an appropriate designation needs to be found for the remainder of cases with AML.

SELF-CHECK 11.3

List the genetic abnormalities considered of diagnostic value in classifying acute myeloid leukaemia.

SELF-CHECK 11.4

Briefly, explain the function of t(15;17)(q22;q12) in leukaemogenesis.

Acute myeloid leukaemia with myelodysplasia-related changes

This subgroup of the AML classification can, unlike the recurrent genetic abnormalities subgroup, occur in *de novo* or secondary leukaemias.

A patient may be diagnosed with acute myeloid leukaemia with myelodysplasia-related changes (AML–MRC) in the following circumstances:

1. AML arising from a previous MDS or MDS/myeloproliferative disorder
2. AML with a specific *MDS-related* cytogenetic abnormality
3. AML with multilineage dysplasia

In the case of AML with multilineage dysplasia, two or more of the myeloid lineages must exhibit signs of dysplasia in ≥50% of the cells in the affected cell lines in order to fulfil the term multilineage, and the blast count must exceed the 20% threshold to be considered an acute leukaemia. If the 20% threshold is not exceeded, the patient is likely to be diagnosed with one of the following:

- Refractory cytopenia with multilineage dysplasia (RCMD)
- Refractory anaemia with excess blasts (RAEB)
- Chronic myelomonocytic leukaemia (CMML)
- Atypical chronic myeloid leukaemia (aCML)

These conditions are addressed later in this chapter.

Examples of dysplasia might include:

- Megakaryocytes with a reduced number of nuclear lobes (hypolobulated megakaryocytes) or those with widely dispersed lobes
- Abnormally small megakaryocytes (micromegakaryocytes)
- Hypolobulated neutrophils
- Hypogranular neutrophils
- Multinucleated erythroblasts
- **Dyskaryorrhexis**

Dyskaryorrhexis
Abnormal bursting of the cell nucleus

AML with multilineage dysplasia is associated with an unfavourable prognosis; patients may be resistant to standard therapies, and survival rates are low.

SELF-CHECK 11.5

Describe some of the dysplastic features you may expect to see in the blood or bone marrow of a patient with an acute leukaemia or myelodysplastic syndrome with multilineage dysplasia.

We have now considered whether the patient has a recurrent genetic abnormality, or if they show signs of myelodysplasia-related changes. Evidence of either of these allows us to apply the appropriate classification, as highlighted above. However, if neither recurrent genetic abnormalities nor myelodysplasia-related changes are present, we should consider *therapy-related myeloid neoplasms*.

Therapy-related myeloid neoplasms

This classification requires the patient to have been previously treated with, or exposed to:

- Alkylating agents
- Ionizing radiation
- Topoisomerase II inhibitors

By definition, the disorders included in this group are attributable to previous medical interventions and are therefore considered **iatrogenic**. The patient's medical records should contain information related to their exposure to any of the agents considered to predispose to haematological malignancies, although access to this information can often be difficult, especially if the patient is from overseas or has moved around the country. Therefore, a thorough medical history should be taken to establish whether exposure to any of these agents has occurred and, if so, when the patient was exposed.

Haematological malignancies that fall within this category include therapy related (t-) acute myeloid leukaemia (t-AML), myelodysplastic syndrome (t-MDS), and myelodysplastic/myeloproliferative neoplasms (t-MDS/MPN). Most patients present with dysplastic features and, in the case of alkylating agents or ionizing radiation, abnormalities of chromosome 5 or 7.

In the 2001 version of the WHO guidelines, the different types of therapy associated with secondary malignancies was outlined in particular detail. However, in the 2008 version, the classification has been simplified on the premise that a combination of these therapies is usually indicated in patient treatment and, therefore, separation of malignancies based upon exposure to one particular therapeutic agent is largely academic. However, for educational purposes, each of the classes of therapy associated with therapy-related myeloid neoplasms are outlined below.

Alkylating agents

Alkylating agents are a group of compounds with electrophilic properties which add alkyl groups to biologically important molecules (a reaction called **alkylation**). Of particular interest is the mechanism by which alkylating agents interact with DNA. The result of this interaction may be a failure of mitosis, preventing cell division. Inhibition of cell division is of particular importance when treating malignancies, as preventing cell proliferation and inducing apoptosis can reduce a patient's **tumour burden**.

The mode of action is dependent upon the properties of the alkylating agent. Some alkylating agents are monofunctional, where a single strand of DNA is alkylated, whereas bifunctional agents can cause cross-linking between two strands of DNA. Examples of alkylating agents include cyclophosphamide, melphalan, Chlorambucil, and nitrosoureas. Figure 11.6 demonstrates the action of alkylating agents.

Ionizing radiation

Leukaemias are associated with this particular form of radiation. **Ionizing radiation** is known to cause a range of different cancers, and the dose of radiation has been well established. Exposure to ionizing radiation even at doses as low as <0.2 **Grays** has been associated with

iatrogenic

A term used to describe a disease or condition caused by medical intervention.

alkylation

The transfer of an alkyl group (C_nH_{2n+1}) from one molecule to another.

tumour burden

The size of an individual's tumour or the number of tumour cells involved in a particular malignant case.

ionizing radiation

Radiation in the form of either high-energy waves or particles which, when interacting with atoms, can remove electrons, thus producing a charge (ion).

Gray

The unit of measurement for the absorbed dose of radiation (i.e. the amount deposited in the mass of a particular material). One Gray = one joule per kilogram.

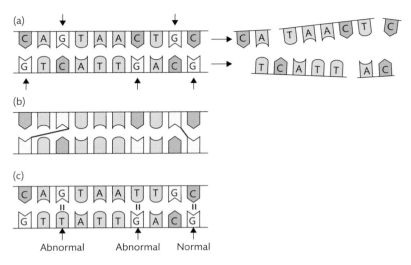

FIGURE 11.6

Mechanisms of DNA disruption through alkylating agent activity. Alkylating agents bind to guanine (G) and cause modification as outlined in a, b and c. (a) Alkylated guanine (represented by yellow icons) is cleaved by repair enzymes, causing DNA fragmentation. (b) Cross-linking guanine bases between DNA strands (as shown) or within strands prevents DNA strand separation, inhibiting DNA transcription. (c) Aberrant binding of guanine to thymine (T) instead of cytosine (C) results in the incorporation of point mutations into the DNA template.

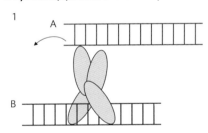

Topoisomerase II binds to DNA segment B (blue).

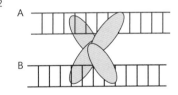

In addition, Topoisomerase II now binds to supercoiled DNA segment A (red).

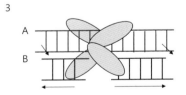

Topoisomerase II cleaves DNA strand B and begins to move supercoiled strand A towards strand B.

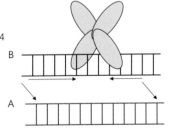

DNA strand A passes through strand B, reducing the mechanical stress caused by supercoiling. Topoisomerase re-ligates strand B.

FIGURE 11.7

(1) Topoisomerase II binds to double-stranded (ds) DNA (B). (2) Whilst bound to B, topoisomerase II binds to a second dsDNA which is considered supercoiled. In order to reduce the tension in the DNA coil, helix A needs to pass through helix B. (3) In order to mediate this DNA transfer process, strand B needs to be cleaved. Reversible cleavage is achieved by topoisomerase II, enabling strand A to pass through prior to re-ligation (4).

leukaemogenesis. Exposure to ionizing radiation can be through medical treatment, occupation, or in some cases, environment.

Both alkylating agents and ionizing radiation have a latent period of five to ten years prior to the development of therapy-related myeloid neoplasms.

Topoisomerase II inhibitors

Topoisomerase II (Topo II) is an enzyme intrinsically involved in the cell cycle through its ability to make cuts in double-stranded (ds) DNA. These cuts not only enable transcription, replication, and recombination to occur, but they also allow for supercoiled DNA to relax by allowing the passage of one segment of dsDNA through another. Figure 11.7 demonstrates the process of Topo II-mediated DNA cleavage and transport. The transit of DNA molecules through one another is permitted by the induction of a transient cleavage complex involving a strand of DNA, which is rejoined (re-ligated) following the passage of the second DNA molecule.

Administration of Topo II inhibitors (also known as Topo II poisons) is associated with large numbers of DNA breaks, although the precise mechanism depends upon the particular type of drug used. In the case of *etoposide* and *teniposide*, Topo II is prevented from rejoining (re-ligating) the dsDNA breaks it initiates, causing the formation of multiple permanent DNA breaks. Ultimately, cell cycle arrest and apoptosis is induced. Other examples of Topo II inhibitors include doxorubicin and daunorubicin.

The way in which the malignancy presents is largely influenced by the therapy to which the patient was previously exposed. Patients treated with alkylating agents or radiotherapy present as an acute leukaemia or MDS, whereas patients treated with Topo II inhibitors present purely with a leukaemia. Leukaemias and myelodysplastic syndromes caused by exposure to alkylating agents or ionizing radiation commonly occur within 5–10 years from exposure compared with topoisomerase II inhibitor exposure, which usually develops within 12 months post exposure.

Leukaemias associated with alkylating agents or ionizing radiation have a poor prognosis compared to those caused by topoisomerase II inhibitors. In addition, patients who have been exposed to Topo II inhibitors are much more likely to possess 11q23 translocations because of the functional activity of the Topo II enzyme in causing dsDNA breaks.

SELF-CHECK 11.6

Compare and contrast the causes of secondary leukaemia associated with different therapies.

For the majority of other cases not fitting into the categories already discussed, the current classification system provides an area in which to deposit these cases: *acute myeloid leukaemia not otherwise specified*.

Acute myeloid leukaemia not otherwise specified

This section largely covers the AMLs that cannot be classified according to the WHO subgroups previously described. No consistent cytogenetic features can be used for diagnosis, and so morphology, cytochemistry and immunophenotyping must be used. There are stringent criteria that must be considered and met in order to provide an appropriate classification for leukaemias in this subgroup. Look back at the different types of acute myeloid leukaemia outlined by the FAB group in Table 11.1 and you will notice the similarity with this subgroup, as shown in Table 11.2. Some new disease entities have been recognized and included, but will not be considered in any detail in this book.

TABLE 11.2 Acute myeloid leukaemia not otherwise specified. The approximate frequencies of these conditions have been outlined, but in some cases it is difficult to obtain a precise figure as these vary between reports. For convenience, these, where appropriate, have been cross referenced to the FAB system.

Subtype	Frequency (%) cases of AML	Cross reference to FAB type
AML with minimal differentiation		M0
AML without maturation	10%	M1
AML with maturation	30–45%	M2
Acute myelomonocytic leukaemia	15–25%	M4
Acute monoblastic and monocytic leukaemia*	5–8%	M5a
Acute monocytic leukaemia*	3–6%	M5b
Acute eythroid leukaemia:		
erythroid/myeloid	approx 5%	M6
pure erythroid leukaemia		
Acute megakaryoblastic leukaemia	3–5%	M7
Acute basophilic leukaemia	<1%	
Acute panmyelosis with myelofibrosis	v rare ? data	

*In the WHO classification, acute monocytic leukaemia is combined to form acute monoblastic and monocytic leukaemia.

Myeloid sarcoma

Myeloid sarcoma describes the accumulation of myeloblasts within one or more anatomical sites outside the bone marrow, causing destruction of the normal tissue within that region. Myeloid sarcoma is considered the diagnostic equivalent of AML, and can occur in conjunction with established AML or other myeloproliferative or myelodysplastic syndromes. Treatment is aggressive to maximize the chances of survival, and bone marrow transplantation is often indicated.

Myeloid proliferations related to Down syndrome

The incidence of Down syndrome (DS) is approximately 1 in every 700 births and is associated with a constitutional trisomy 21. Infants and children with Down syndrome have a predisposition to acute lymphoblastic leukaemia, with a 20-fold higher risk of developing the disease in comparison to the general population. These infants are also predisposed to acute myeloid leukaemia, and have a 500-fold increased risk of developing acute megakaryoblastic leukaemia (AMKL).

The development of DS-AMKL is known to be a multi-step process, although the precise genetic requirement in this disease has yet to be determined. There is a requirement for trisomy 21, although we do not know which genes present on chromosome 21 are important in the pathogenesis of DS-AMKL. A Down syndrome critical region (DSCR) has been identified as being important in determining the clinical phenotypes of patients with DS, and there are candidate genes present within this region that could be involved in leukaemogenesis.

Importantly, mutations within the haemopoietic transcription factor GATA1 have been identified, and are always present in cases of DS-AMKL. GATA1 mutations are not associated with

Cross reference

For further information on trisomy 21 and Down syndrome, please refer to Chapter 9.

non-DS AMKL. GATA1 is an essential transcription factor required for erythropoiesis and mega-karyopoiesis. The loss of GATA1 function results in the accumulation of abnormal megakaryocytes within the liver and bone marrow, and the failure of these megakaryocytes to produce platelets.

Mutation of *GATA1* is an *in-utero* event with these mutations clustering in exon 2 of *GATA1*. Point mutations, insertions, and deletions have all been documented and produce a premature stop codon. Transcription and translation of mutated *GATA1* produces a truncated transcription factor called GATA1s in which the transcriptional activation domain is absent.

Recently, *JAK3* mutations have been identified in a small group of patients with DS-AMKL, and are associated with increased STAT signalling and cellular proliferation.

The multi-step process of myeloid leukaemogenesis in DS is relatively well described. Between 4% and 10% of infants with trisomy 21 develop a transient leukaemia, also called *transient abnormal myelopoiesis* (TAM) and *transient myeloproliferative disease* (TMD). All these cases studied express GATA1s. In the vast majority of cases, this transient leukaemia resolves spontaneously within three months. In approximately 20% of patients, by the age of four years, AMKL develops following a myelodysplastic stage. This is probably due to residual cells harbouring the GATA1s mutation developing additional mutations and leading to a full leukaemic phenotype.

Clinical and laboratory findings include a raised white cell count with an increased number of megakaryoblasts. The patient may demonstrate thrombocythaemia or thrombocytopenia and show signs of hepatomegaly. Hepatomegaly is due to the retention of neonatal hepatic haemopoiesis and the accumulation of malignant megakaryoblasts within the liver. Abnormal cytokines released by the megakaryoblasts induce fibrotic changes within the liver.

Patients with DS have an increased sensitivity to cytarabine and anthracyclines. Low doses of cytarabine have been shown to cure up to 80% of patients with DS-AMKL.

Blastic plasmacytoid dendritic cell neoplasm

Plasmacytoid dendritic cells (pDC) are usually found in clusters within T-cell rich areas of lymphoid tissue and are important mediators of innate and adaptive immunity. Virus and bacterially derived products stimulate dendritic cells to synthesize large quantities of interferons following their interaction with receptors, such as toll-like receptors, expressed on the pDC surface.

The origin of these cells is unclear and further investigation is required to establish the definitive origin of these cells, although this malignancy itself is associated with an accumulation of plasmacytoid dendritic cell precursors. This malignancy is highly aggressive with a median survival of approximately 12 months. Prior to diagnosis, comprehensive immunophenotypic analysis should be completed to ensure the accurate classification of this disease.

Acute leukaemias of ambiguous lineage

These are a rare group of malignancies derived from a multipotential haemopoietic stem cell and show no lineage-specificity. The classification of these disorders has changed significantly since the introduction of the first WHO classification of haematological neoplasms in 2001. In the 2001 classification, two important leukaemias were included as outlined below:

Biphenotypic leukaemia

Prior to the original WHO classification, biphenotypic leukaemia was described as mixed-lineage or hybrid leukaemia—accounting for less than 5% of acute leukaemias. Biphenotypic leukaemia was identified when a single population of blast cells was shown to express both myeloid and lymphoid antigens, either cytoplasmically or on the cell membrane. Using the scoring system as recommended by the European Group for the Immunological classification of Leukaemias (EGIL), it became possible to differentiate between biphenotypic leukaemias and those with the aberrant expression of a marker from another lineage. However, because of inconsistencies in many cases a replacement for the EGIL scoring system is now being sought.

Bilineal leukaemia

Bilineal leukaemia, accounting for less than 1% of acute leukaemias, is characterized by two distinct populations of blast cells of different lineage. Commonly, blasts of myelomonocytic lineage occur in conjunction with T-lineage blasts.

These entities have now been reclassified to include six main diseases which can be separated into two categories:

1. Acute undifferentiated leukaemia
    a. Acute undifferentiated leukaemia
2. Mixed phenotype acute leukaemias
    a. Mixed phenotype acute leukaemia with t(9;22)(q34;q11.2); *BCR–ABL1*
    b. Mixed phenotype acute leukaemia with t(v;11q23); *MLL* rearranged
    c. Mixed phenotype acute leukaemia, B/myeloid, not otherwise specified
    d. Mixed phenotype acute leukaemia T/myeloid, not otherwise specified
    e. Mixed phenotype acute leukaemia, not otherwise specified—rare types

Acute undifferentiated leukaemia can be considered a separate disease entity as phenotypically there are no lineage-specific markers expressed either cytoplasmically or on the cell surface. Conversely, mixed phenotype leukaemias are an expansion of biphenotypic leukaemias from the 2001 WHO classification and show lineage-specific phenotypic antigens, although a combination of lineage-specific antigens will be expressed either within the cytoplasm or on the cell surface. For example, blasts with a B- or T-lineage phenotype accompanied by cytoplasmic myeloperoxidase or monoblastic markers would be sufficient to diagnose mixed phenotypic acute leukaemia.

Bilineal leukaemia is now incorporated into *mixed phenotype acute leukaemia T/myeloid, not otherwise specified*—there are no specific cytogenetic features although coexisting populations of blast cells are identifiable in the same patient.

The presence of *BCR–ABL1* is a poor prognostic indicator and is only of relevance to this classification category if an underlying CML can be excluded.

Patients demonstrating 11q23 rearrangement also have a poor prognosis. *MLL* can be considered to be a promiscuous gene as it has a number of fusion partners. In this classification, 'v' has been used in the abbreviation t(v;11q23) to demonstrate variable translocation partners rather than specifying each in turn.

11.3 **Myelodysplastic syndrome**

Myelodysplastic syndrome is diagnosed when one or more of the myeloid cell lines display signs of dysplasia. Generally, signs of dysplasia will be seen in 10% or more of cells within a particular lineage, when peripheral blood and bone marrow slides are examined. Myelodysplastic syndrome is a disease usually associated with a hypercellular bone marrow, but with the patient showing variably low peripheral blood counts. The patient's blast percentage may be normal or raised, but will not exceed the critical 20% value diagnostic for AML.

It is important when assessing patients' blood films for signs of dysplasia that optimal staining procedures are followed using a good quality Romanowsky stain. Samples should be less than two hours old to ensure cellular morphology is maintained. Samples older than two hours start to show EDTA changes, making the assessment of dysplastic features difficult. Table 11.3 provides an outline of the signs of dysplasia which may be indicative of MDS.

In addition to the role FAB has played in the diagnosis and classification of acute leukaemias, FAB has also played an important role in the classification of MDS. MDS has, for many years, been considered to be a precursor to acute leukaemia and some of the subtypes do over-lap with acute leukaemias. When we compare and contrast the FAB and WHO systems, MDS should be considered to be a disease entity in its own right, rather than a leukaemic precursor. FAB utilized morphological examination in order to develop five distinct subtypes (see Table 11.4) to this heterogeneous disease, but this classification system does not correlate with the clinical features demonstrated by these patients.

In some cases using the FAB system, significant heterogeneity within particular subtypes is evident, and this is one of the features addressed by the World Health Organization. The FAB and WHO classification systems for MDS are mutually exclusive. If you recall, the FAB system uses the arbitrary blast count of 30% as the blast threshold required to fulfil the classification of AML compared to 20% for the WHO system. The subgroup *refractory anaemia with excess blasts in transformation* (RAEB-t) was defined by the FAB group as 21–30% blasts within the bone marrow. This, according to the WHO system, can now be classified as *acute myeloid leukaemia with myelodysplasia-related changes*.

Chronic myelomonocytic leukaemia, the last of the five groups defined as MDS, is now classi-fied as a myelodysplastic/myeloproliferative disease according to the WHO system.

TABLE 11.3 Morphological changes associated with dysplasia.

Red blood cells
Ringed sideroblasts*
Vacuolization: red cell precursors should not contain cytoplasmic vacuoles
Nuclear budding
Multinuclearity: suggestive of dysregulated cell division
Nuclear lobulation: only one nucleus should be present
Internuclear bridging
Karyorrhexis: appears as though the nucleus is bursting
Changes associated with megaloblastic anaemia

Granulocytes
Alterations in cell size: may be very small or commonly very large
Nuclear hypolobulation: many neutrophils showing less than 3 nuclear lobes
Reduced granulation: agranular or hypogranular neutrophils**

Auer rods: abnormal fusion of lysosomes—in MDS suggests RAEB-2.

Megakaryocytes
Micromegakaryocytes: small megakaryocytes
Hypolobulated nucleus: one nucleus with no lobes
Multinucleation: a number of discrete nuclear lobes

*demonstrated using Perls' stain. >15% ringed sideroblasts is suggestive of refractory anaemia with ringed sideroblasts.
**Care must be taken to ensure that hypogranulation or agranular neutrophils are not artefactual due to poor staining technique.

Any case of MDS secondary to either the use of alkylating agents or radiotherapy should be considered as a therapy-related neoplasm and called t-MDS.

The International Prognostic Scoring System (IPSS) was developed in 1997 to correlate disease classification with patient prognosis. This system allows patient prognosis to be determined based on the risk of progression to acute myeloid leukaemia. The IPSS criteria for determining risk of AML progression is outlined below.

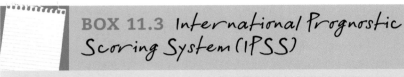

BOX 11.3 *International Prognostic Scoring System (IPSS)*

The International Prognostic Scoring System (IPSS) was developed to establish associations between patient blast count, cytogenetic features, levels of cytopenia, and patient prognosis. The IPSS score should be calculated at the point of diagnosis. For each feature (outlined below) a score between 0 and 2 is given. These scores are staged in increments of 0.5. The important thresholds include:

Blast percentages
<5%
5–10%
11–20%
21–30%* (now not considered as MDS, but AML with myelodysplasia-related changes)

Cytopenia
Haemoglobin <100g/L
Neutrophil count <1.8×10^9/L
Platelet count <100×10^9/L

Karyotype

Good:
Normal
–Y
del(5q)
del(20q)

Intermediate:
Other abnormalities

Poor:
Complex karyotype
Abnormalities of chromosome 7

Taken together, this information was incorporated into an easy-to-use table:

	Score				
Prognostic variable	0	0.5	1.0	1.5	2.0
BM blasts	<5	5–10	–	11–20	21–30
Karyotype	good	intermediate	poor		
Cytopenias	0/1	2/3			

These scores can then be associated with patient prognosis:

Low = 0
INT-1   = 0.5–1.0
INT-2   = 1.5–2.0
High   = >2.5

Based on risk category, low-risk patients had a median survival of 5.7 years; intermediate survival was subdivided into INT-1 and INT-2 with survival rates of 3.5 years and 1.2 years, respectively. High-risk patients were calculated as having a median survival of 0.4 years.

The WHO have recently released a prognostic scoring system (WPSS) using the WHO classification system. Initial external validation finds this a powerful prognostic algorithm, but a more comprehensive review is required.

Let's now consider the breakdown of the groups of MDS as considered important by the FAB group.

The FAB classification of MDS

Outlined below are the five groups of MDS as classified by the FAB group. This classification has now been modified and superseded by the WHO system. Table 11.4 provides a convenient quick reference guide for FAB classification.

TABLE 11.4   The peripheral blood and bone marrow features associated with myelodysplastic syndrome as outlined by the FAB group.

	Peripheral blood	Bone marrow
Refractory anaemia / refractory cytopenia	Anaemia	Blasts <5%
	Neutropenia or thrombocytopenia	Ringed sideroblasts ≤15% erythroblasts
	Blasts ≤1% and monocytes ≤1 × 10^9/L	
Refractory anaemia with ringed sideroblasts	Anaemia; neutropenia or thrombocytopenia	Blasts <5%
	Blasts ≤1% and monocytes ≤1 × 10^9/L	Ringed sideroblasts >15% erythroblasts
Refractory anaemia with excess blasts	Anaemia; >1% but <5% blasts; monocytes <1 × 10^9/L	Blasts ≥5% but ≤20%
Refractory anaemia with excess blasts in transformation	Blasts ≥5% (OR) Auer rods in PB/BM	Blasts >20% but <30%
Chronic myelomonocytic leukaemia	Blasts <5%; monocyte count >1 × 10^9/L	Up to 20% blasts ± promonocytes

The subgroups considered by FAB include:

- Refractory anaemia (RA)
- Refractory anaemia with ringed sideroblasts (RARS)
- Refractory anaemia with excess blasts (RAEB)
- Refractory anaemia with excess blasts in transformation (RAEB-t)
- Chronic myelomonocytic leukaemia (CMML)

Refractory anaemia

Refractory anaemia (RA) is categorized by <5% blasts within the bone marrow, and <1% within the peripheral blood. The bone marrow is usually hypercellular, whilst peripheral cell counts are low (cytopenia); this is as a consequence of **ineffective haemopoiesis**. RA usually includes patients with a low red cell count with dysplastic features unresponsive to vitamin B_{12}, folate, or iron therapy. Although the name of this category suggests that only red cells should be dysplastic, RA also includes a unilineage neutropenia and thrombocytopenia.

refractory
Does not respond to standard treatment.

Refractory anaemia with ringed sideroblasts

RARS fulfils the same criteria as RA outlined above, except that, when using Perls' stain, >15% of erythroblasts in the bone marrow have a partial or complete ring of siderotic material (contains iron) surrounding the nucleus. These siderotic rings are believed to contain ferric iron (Fe^{3+}) deposited in mitochondria surrounding the nucleus of erythroblasts. Fe^{3+} is not incorporated into haemoglobin effectively, and therefore accumulates within the mitochondria—since this is the site where iron is usually added to protoporphyrin IX by the enzyme ferrochelatase to produce haem.

Cross reference
Haemoglobin production is outlined in detail in Chapter 4.

Refractory anaemia with excess blasts

RAEB is characterized by dysplasia in all three lineages and peripheral blood cytopenias in at least two. The bone marrow comprises 5–20% blasts and <5% in the peripheral blood. RAEB provides a high risk of transformation to acute leukaemia since a number of genetic hits have occurred in order to make cells in RAEB genetically unstable, as demonstrated by the high blast count and the degree of dysplasia.

Refractory anaemia with excess blasts in transformation

The haematological features associated with RAEB-t are identical to those outlined for RAEB. However, peripheral blood blasts are >5% and bone marrow blasts are 21–30%. Auer rods are frequently found as inclusions within the blasts. According to the WHO classification, RAEB-t is now classified as an acute leukaemia since the blast count exceeds 20%.

Chronic myelomonocytic leukaemia

CMML is now considered a myelodysplastic/myeloproliferative disease because of the high white cell counts associated with the peripheral blood picture. CMML accounts for 20–25% of cases of MDS when considered as a member of this disease group. An increased monocyte count accompanied by <5% blasts in the peripheral blood, and up to 20% in the bone marrow, is characteristic of CMML. CMML is considered in greater detail within the myelodysplastic/myeloproliferative diseases section of this chapter (Section 11.4).

The World Health Organization classification of MDS

In 2001 the classification for MDS was revamped in order to group together cases of MDS displaying similar clinical, morphological, cytogenetic, and prognostic features. As part of this process some of the FAB groups have been separated in order to generate homogeneous groups of dysplastic disorders. In other cases, new categories have been introduced to respond to our enhanced understanding of MDS. In the 2008 version of the WHO classification, MDS was further modified to address recent clinical findings in this area. Although patients may initially be classified in one of the lower-risk subgroups, their disease may progress over time, eventually becoming an acute leukaemia with multilineage dysplasia.

The main types of MDS recognized by the WHO are:

- Refractory cytopenia with unilineage dysplasia
- Refractory anaemia with ringed sideroblasts
- Refractory cytopenia with multi-lineage dysplasia (RCMD)
- Refractory anaemia with excess blasts 1 (RAEB-1)
- Refractory anaemia with excess blasts 2 (RAEB-2)
- Myelodysplastic syndrome unclassified (MDS-U)
- MDS associated with isolated del(5q) (5q– syndrome)
- Childhood MDS (provisional entity)

Table 11.5 provides a convenient quick reference guide.

Refractory cytopenia with unilineage dysplasia

According to the WHO group, refractory cytopenia with multilineage dysplasia includes these main disease entities. RA is now used to describe dysplasia restricted to the erythroid lineage. The peripheral blood film shows signs of a macrocytic anaemia, and the bone marrow shows evidence of erythroid dysplasia. By amending the requirements for entry into this category, RA has become homogeneous, therefore it is now easier to monitor these patients and inform them of their likely prognosis.

Furthermore, two new groups have been added to this system: *refractory neutropenia* (RN) and *refractory thrombocytopenia* (RT). These groups also present with unilineage dysplasia with more than 10% of cells from these lineages demonstrating dysplasia. For the purposes of identifying dysplasia in megakaryocytes, the WHO recommends evaluating the morphology of a minimum of 30 megakaryocytes.

Refractory anaemia with ringed sideroblasts

This category is an extension of RA, outlined above. The same peripheral blood film abnormalities are expected, although the bone marrow shows >15% ringed sideroblasts when stained with Perls' stain.

TABLE 11.5 The WHO method for diagnosing myelodysplastic syndrome. Characteristic blood and bone marrow findings have been outlined.

WHO subgroup	Blood	Bone marrow
Refractory cytopenia with unilineage dysplasia	Anaemia or ≥10% dysplastic neutrophils or abnormal platelets	Erythroid dysplasia Restricted neutrophil dysplasia or restricted megakaryocytic dysplasia
Refractory anaemia with ringed sideroblasts	Anaemia	Erythroid dysplasia +>15% ringed sideroblasts
Refractory cytopenia with multilineage dysplasia	Bi/pancytopenia	Dysplastic features in >10% of 2+ cell lineages
Refractory anaemia with excess blasts-1	<5% blasts & cytopenias	Uni/multilineage dysplasia with 5–9% blasts
Refractory anaemia with excess blasts-2	5–19% blasts & cytopenias	Uni/multilineage dysplasia with 10–19% blasts or Auer rods
Myelodysplastic syndrome, unclassified	Cytopenias	
Myelodysplastic syndrome with isolated del(5q)	Anaemia with normal/increased platelets	Erythroid hypoplasia plus mono/binuclear megakaryocytes

Refractory cytopenia with multilineage dysplasia

This new group introduced by the WHO recognizes dysplastic features in >10% of cells in two or more cell lineages. The peripheral blood film shows cytopenias in two or more cell lineages.

In the 2001 version of the WHO guidelines, *refractory cytopenia with multilineage dysplasia and ringed sideroblasts* was considered as a discrete disease entity in cases of multilineage dysplasia with >15% ringed sideroblasts. In the updated version, this category has been removed and included as part of this generic multilineage grouping.

Refractory anaemia with excess blasts-1

The WHO has subdivided the RAEB category, as devised by the FAB group, into two—based on clinical observations of patients within the original RAEB group and correlating these findings with the blast count and the presence of Auer rods.

RAEB-1 includes patients with peripheral blood blasts <5%, and 5–9% bone marrow blasts. Dysplastic features may be seen in one or more cell lineages. Patients classified as RAEB-1 have a more favourable prognosis than those with a RAEB-2 classification. Patients diagnosed with RAEB-1 have a mean survival of 23.3 months compared to 16.1 months for RAEB-2.

Refractory anaemia with excess blasts-2

This group is an extension to RAEB-1, with 5–19% blasts in the peripheral blood, and 10–19% blasts in the bone marrow. If Auer rods are present, providing the blast count is <20%, patients are classified as RAEB-2, regardless of any other features. Interestingly, a number of authors have questioned the validity of including the presence of Auer rods in a poor prognostic group, as Auer rods have been shown to be an independent marker of a good prognosis. This may be addressed in the next WHO classification.

Patients classified as RAEB-2 have a worse prognosis than those classified as RAEB-1 (see RAEB-1 for clarification of survival data).

Myelodysplastic syndrome unclassifiable

The importance of MDS-U should not be underestimated just because it contains unclassifiable cases. Over the coming years, with further clinical research and the emergence of improved availability of new technologies, we should be better equipped to provide a more appropriate classification for these cases. In the 2001 WHO classification, this group contained cases of unilineage myeloid and megakaryocytic dysplasia previously added to the RA category by the FAB group. However, these were moved in the 2008 classification to be included in the group *refractory cytopenia with unilineage dysplasia*.

Cases should qualify for MDS-U when less than 10% of myeloid cells show signs of dysplasia in the presence of MDS specific cytogenetic abnormalities, a number of which have been outlined in the IPSS box earlier in this section.

MDS associated with isolated del(5q)

These patients are usually female and typically present with a normal or raised platelet count, a macrocytic anaemia and normal white cell count. The bone marrow morphology is specific for 5q– syndrome, with mononuclear or binuclear megakaryocytes and erythroid hypoplasia, allowing a prediction of the patient's cytogenetic profile. Cytogenetic evaluation is essential for these patients to confirm the 5q– status and to provide a definitive diagnosis. The 5q– syndrome is associated with a good prognosis. Recent evidence suggests that *RPS14*, which produces part of the 40S ribosome subunit, is deleted in these patients, causing **haploinsufficiency**. Loss of *RPS14* reduces protein production within the cell harbouring 5q–.

haploinsufficiency
Occurs when one of a pair of genes on homologous chromosomes is silenced through deletion or mutation. The intracellular concentration of the 'normal' gene product is insufficient to complete its intended biological role.

Childhood myelodysplastic syndrome

These are an extremely rare group of diseases which are largely attributable to heritable syndromes, the most notable of which is Down syndrome. Only primary myelodysplastic syndromes are considered in this category under the provisional classification of refractory cytopenia of childhood (RCC). It is important when investigating these patients to consider the broad differential diagnoses including infectious agents, vitamin deficiencies and inherited bone marrow failure syndromes.

RCC covers a range of myelodysplastic syndromes, the behaviour of which is different to MDS in adults. The majority of cases are associated with a hypocellular marrow, in contrast to the hypercellular marrows seen in adults. As the WHO considers RCC a provisional entity, no further discussion regarding this pathology will be made.

Now that the myelodysplastic syndromes have been considered, we should examine the myeloid diseases overlapping with myelodysplastic syndromes. Myelodysplastic/myeloproliferative diseases exhibit dysplastic features and a higher cell count since these cells have a larger proliferative component than purely myelodysplastic syndromes.

SELF-CHECK 11.7

Compare and contrast the WHO and FAB systems for the classification of myelodysplastic syndromes.

11.4 Myelodysplastic/ myeloproliferative diseases

This category was introduced by the WHO to include diseases demonstrating dysplastic features, plus a hypercellular bone marrow and increased peripheral cell counts. Included within this category are:

- Chronic myelomonocytic leukaemia (CMML)
- Atypical chronic myeloid leukaemia (aCML)
- Juvenile myelomonocytic leukaemia (JMML)
- Myelodysplastic/myeloproliferative disease, unclassifiable

We will now examine each of these conditions in a little more depth.

Chronic myelomonocytic leukaemia

CMML, initially classified as a myelodysplastic syndrome by the FAB group, is characterized by a hypercellular bone marrow and a normal or increasing white cell count. A sustained peripheral monocytosis ($>1 \times 10^9$/L) is apparent with no obvious reactive cause. Monocytes are precursors to tissue macrophages and usually increase in number during bacterial infections or following tissue damage to remove cell debris. Bacterial infection and tissue damage should be excluded prior to a diagnosis of CMML being made. Variable signs of dysplasia should be apparent in the myeloid series. Cytochemical stains, including ANAE, can be used to identify cells of a monocytic lineage, where cells will stain red/brown, whilst CAE can assist in differentiating dysplastic granulocytes staining bright blue. There should be no evidence of the Philadelphia chromosome, or the BCR–ABL1 transcript (otherwise suggestive of a diagnosis of chronic myeloid leukaemia).

CMML is subdivided into two groups based on the number of blood and bone marrow blasts (the term blast in this instance includes the promonocyte stage of maturation): CMML-1 comprises <10% bone marrow blasts with <5% peripheral blood blasts, and CMML-2 demonstrates 10–19% bone marrow blasts with 5–19% peripheral blood blasts. Clinical evidence suggests that patients with a higher blast count have a poorer prognosis and are at greater risk of transforming to AML.

Atypical chronic myeloid leukaemia, *BCR–ABL1* negative

Although the name of this disease suggests that it is a variant of chronic myeloid leukaemia, atypical CML (aCML) is caused by a separate pathological process. Atypical CML is not associated with the Philadelphia chromosome, and does not show evidence of BCR–ABL1 at the molecular level.

Within both the peripheral blood and bone marrow, aCML often shows evidence of multi-lineage dysplasia.

The prognosis for patients diagnosed with aCML is particularly poor, with a median survival of 14–25 months. The majority of patients succumb to complications of bone marrow failure, including overwhelming infections, complications of anaemia, or bleeding. Up to 20% of patients will transform to acute myeloid leukaemia.

Juvenile myelomonocytic leukaemia

This is a rare myelodysplastic/myeloproliferative condition associated with infants and young children, accounting for approximately 2% of all childhood leukaemias. Characterized by a proliferative neutrophil and monocytic compartment, juvenile myelomonocytic leukaemia (JMML) can be differentiated from CML through the absence of the Philadelphia chromosome and the lack of BCR–ABLl.

In the vast majority of cases, dysregulation of Ras leading to its hyperactivity can be identified. Some 35% of patients have gain-of-function mutations of *PTPN11* which encodes Shp2, a protein tyrosine phosphatase; 35% of patients have gain-of-function mutations in either *NRAS* or *KRAS*; and 15% of patients have mutations of *NF1*– necessary for the activation of GTPase, the negative regulator of Ras activation.

Current guidelines for the classification of JMML include a monocyte count in excess of 1×10^9/L. Blasts should not be in excess of 20% and there should be no evidence of *BCR–ABL1*. The total WBC may be more than 10×10^9/L and in some cases the patient's HbF percentage may be higher than expected for their age. Immature granulocytes may be present in the peripheral blood, and these may be hypersensitive to GM-CSF in cell culture or alternative techniques. Chromosomal abnormalities may be apparent, but at present this classification does not recognize *NF1*, *NRAS*, *KRAS*, or *PTPN11* gene mutations. The JMML working group have also suggested that clinical appreciation of splenomegaly in addition to an age limit of 13 years of age should be included in the diagnostic criteria.

Myelodysplastic/myeloproliferative disease, unclassifiable

Myelodysplastic/myeloproliferative disease, unclassifiable (MDS/MPD-U) should not be considered to be a subgroup where inadequately investigated cases are placed, but rather those conditions with a proliferative element showing dysplasia in one or more cell lines.

MDS/MPD-U may be misclassified in cases where patients have been administered chemotherapy, which would induce dysplastic change, or growth factors, which cause myeloproliferation. Care must be taken to exclude both scenarios prior to a diagnosis being made.

Cytogenetic features characteristic of specific disease entities, for example the Philadelphia chromosome and BCR–ABL1 fusion product, should be excluded, with patients classified according to the WHO criteria dictated by those cytogenetic abnormalities.

We should now change focus from those diseases with a myelodysplastic component to purely myeloproliferative neoplasms.

11.5 **Myeloproliferative neoplasms**

Myeloproliferative neoplasms have a blast count below 20% and are generally associated with an increased bone marrow cellularity. Typically, peripheral cell counts are raised—particularly in the early phases—but in later stages bone marrow fibrosis can occur. Fibrosis compromises haemopoiesis leading to peripheral blood cytopenias.

Of the conditions outlined below, polycythaemia vera (PV), essential thrombocythaemia (ET), and primary myelofibrosis (PMF) can morph into one another throughout their natural course. Criteria for the diagnosis of myelofibrosis secondary to polycythaemia vera and essential thrombocythaemia have been clearly outlined by the WHO.

One of the most important mechanisms of oncogenesis in PV, PMF and ET is the acquisition of a point mutation in the JAK2 tyrosine kinase. Found in approximately 90% of cases of PV, 50% of PMF patients and 30% of ET, the substitution of amino acids valine for phenylalanine at position 617 results in the constitutional activation of this tyrosine kinase and enhanced sensitivity to specific growth factors, including Epo, GM-CSF, Tpo, IL-3, and stem cell factor.

Key Points

JAK2 is a receptor-associated tyrosine kinase involved in the signalling from a number of cytokine receptors including EpoR. JAK2 also acts as a chaperone facilitating the trafficking of EpoR to the Golgi for post-translational modification prior to receptor expression on the cell surface.

Binding of cytokines to their JAK2-associated receptor induces the formation of either homo- or heteromeric receptors and the clustering of JAK2. Receptor-associated JAK2 kinases then phosphorylate one another (in a process called transphosphorylation), and tyrosine residues within the cytokine receptor undergo phosphorylation. STAT molecules associate with the receptor and are phosphorylated, leading to the activation of downstream signalling pathways. Of particular importance is the association between JAK2 and the STAT pathway. Subsequent dimerization of STAT and localization within the nucleus results in increased transcription and translation of STAT-inducible genes.

JAK2 is composed of seven JAK homology domains (JH1-7). JH1 comprises the tyrosine kinase domain and JH2 the pseudokinase or tyrosine kinase-like domain. The pseudokinase domain negatively regulates JH1 controlling phosphorylation and activation of JAK2. Wild-type V617, located within JH2, preserves the inactive conformation of a critical structure called the activation loop. V617F modifies the structure of JH2, preventing inhibition of JH1, allowing continuous signalling utilizing the newly positioned activation loop.

Polycythaemia vera

Polycythaemia vera (PV) is characterized by an increase in an individual's red cell mass >25% above the patient's mean predicted value. In half of patients, thrombocytosis is a feature and two-thirds of patients demonstrate neutrophilia. Surrogate markers, including patient haematocrit (discussed later in this section) and haemoglobin concentration have been adopted, although these should be interpreted in the context of the patient's clinical examination and medical history.

Cross reference

Polycythaemia vera is contrasted with erythrocytosis in Chapter 6.

METHOD *Calculating a patient's mean red cell mass*

In nuclear medicine, red cell mass is measured using sodium radiochromate (^{51}Cr) or sodium pertechnetate (^{99m}Tc) -labelled red cells as per the International Committee for Standardization in Haematology (ICSH) guidelines. The value obtained should be compared to the patient's predicted RCM, and is calculated as follows:

For males: [(1486 × surface area) – 825]ml

For females: [(1.06 × age) + (822 × surface area)]ml

PV is a clonal disorder, and so all defective cells will be the product of a mutated progenitor and nucleated cells will harbour any cytogenetic abnormalities present in that progenitor cell. The vast majority of patients harbour *JAK2 V617F* mutations. Other patients demonstrate variant mutations within JAK2, leading to constitutional activation of this receptor and increased tyrosine kinase signalling.

In the absence of clear molecular evidence of clonality, the difficulty with diagnosing PV is determining whether the erythrocytosis is the consequence of a clonal population of red cells, or another event raising the red cell count and haematocrit—secondary erythrocytosis.

To exclude secondary erythrocytosis, serum erythropoietin should be measured and is expected, in PV, to be low for the degree of erythrocytosis; pulse **oximetry** should be used to investigate for insufficient oxygen in the blood (hypoxaemia) and would be expected to fall within the reference range in PV; investigations such as high performance liquid chromatography (HPLC) or isoelectric focusing (IEF) to exclude high-affinity haemoglobins, should be completed; and renal pathology should be excluded, as reduced blood flow through the glomerulus may induce erythropoietin (Epo) production, and consequently, raise the red cell count. Additionally, in some cases of liver disease, Epo-like peptides may be synthesized, leading to an increased red cell count, so these should be investigated.

A major diagnostic criterion is the haematocrit. This threshold result is stratified according to *JAK2* mutation and is indicative of PV (as in Table 11.6).

The combination of a high haematocrit or raised red cell mass, plus evidence of *V617F*, provides the diagnosis of PV. In cases where *V617F* is absent, a raised haematocrit or raised RCM is necessary, plus the exclusion of any cause of secondary erythrocytosis or another acquired genetic abnormality within the haemopoietic cells (excluding BCR–ABL1). A combination of two or more of the following can also be used in the absence of an additional acquired genetic abnormality: prolonged thrombocytosis, neutrophilia, or low serum Epo concentration.

oximetry

A non-invasive method for determining the amount of oxygen within arterial blood.

TABLE 11.6 Stratification of haematocrit according to sex and *JAK2 (V617F)* mutational status.

	V617F positive	*V617F* negative
Males	>0.52	>0.48
Females	>0.60	>0.56

> **BOX 11.4** *PV guidelines*
>
> Comprehensive guidelines outlining the strategy employed in investigating and diagnosing PV are provided by the British Committee for Standards in Haematology (BCSH); reference details can be found in the Reference section at the end of this book.

Primary myelofibrosis

Primary idiopathic myelofibrosis (PMF) is a clonal disorder characterized by the proliferation of immature myeloid precursors. Mutation of the pluripotent stem cell precursor is believed to induce the proliferation of erythroblasts, megakaryoblasts, and their progeny. Megakaryoblasts are thought to play a key role in the development and potentiation of the myelofibrotic phenotype. Megakaryoblasts can stimulate fibroblast proliferation via basic fibroblast growth factor b (b-FGF) and transforming growth factor β (TGF-β) leading to the development of fibrosis.

In the early stages, PMF is characterized by a leucoerythroblastic blood picture featuring teardrop poikilocytes. An increased white cell count composed primarily of raised neutrophils, often with raised eosinophils and basophils, is a feature. Extramedullary haemopoiesis is commonly associated with PMF, and an associated hepatosplenomegaly is also frequently encountered. In keeping with the megakaryocytic component of this disease, a raised platelet count is often observed in the early stages. As the disease progresses, thrombocytopenia develops, and the white cell count drops as haemopoiesis becomes compromised by the increasing marrow fibrosis. In up to 10% of patients, PMF transforms to AML.

Essential thrombocythaemia

Essential thrombocythaemia (ET) is a clonal disorder of megakaryocytes, characterized by a persistently raised platelet count $>450 \times 10^9$/L in the absence of any reactive condition. Reactive conditions should be identified via thorough clinical examination or a raised ESR or CRP. Previously, ET was suggested with a platelet count $>600 \times 10^9$/L for a duration of two months or more, but the WHO have amended this based on some patients experiencing the complications of ET at platelet counts below 600×10^9/L. Other myeloproliferative disorders should also be excluded where practical, although in some patients ET may coexist with another disease entity.

Diagnosis relies on the exclusion of diseases which may cause a secondary thrombocytosis. Iron deficiency should be excluded as this is associated with a reactive increase in platelet count.

It is also important to exclude the presence of the Philadelphia chromosome and BCR–ABL1 to ensure CML is not missed.

Detailed investigations should be completed to ensure the patient has none of the morphological or cytogenetic features of any other myeloid neoplasm. The best diagnostic tool for this is bone marrow examination, allowing for the morphology of megakaryocytes and other haemopoietic progenitors to be fully appreciated.

Cross reference
Bone marrow assessment was outlined in Chapter 10.

Chronic myelogenous leukaemia, *BCR–ABL1* positive

Chronic myelogenous leukaemia (CML), also known as chronic myeloid leukaemia or chronic granulocytic leukaemia (CGL), is the most clinically researched haematological malignancy in history. CML was the first malignant disease to be associated with a particular chromosomal abnormality, the **Philadelphia chromosome**, and the first to have significant reported success with a molecular targeted therapy—imatinib mesylate.

In 1960, Nowell and Hungerford made the association between the typical morphological features we see in patients diagnosed with CML and a minute chromosome, the shortened chromosome 22. In 1973, the origin of this shortened chromosome 22 became clear, when Rowley identified t(9;22), the Philadelphia translocation. The precise breakpoints to this translocation have been identified as: t(9;22)(q34;q11).

CML is a clonal disorder of pluripotent stem cells causing proliferation of myeloid precursors, and their differentiation into mature effector cells. These effector cells are likely to be qualitatively abnormal, so they are functionally impeded. CML is not associated with maturational arrest, but there is a failure of apoptosis. In the case of CML, an increased proliferation rate accompanied by apoptotic failure results in an increased white cell count. In many cases the red cell count and platelet count are also increased.

The defining feature of CML is the Philadelphia (Ph) chromosome or the presence of the fusion product of t(9;22)(q34;q11), BCR–ABL1. Using cytogenetic analysis, 95% of patients demonstrate the Ph chromosome. A further 2.5% of patients have a masked (cryptic) translocation undetectable using conventional cytogenetic techniques, despite evidence of BCR–ABL1 using molecular techniques. The remaining 2.5% are considered to be Ph chromosome negative, with no evidence of the Ph chromosome and no molecular evidence of BCR–ABL1.

Atypical morphology in the absence of the Ph chromosome can be considered atypical CML, whereas those with typical morphology are called Ph-negative CML.

The key fusion gene found within the Philadelphia chromosome der(22), *BCR–ABL1*, is formed from the proto-oncogene *ABL1*, originally located on chromosome 9—encoding a non-receptor tyrosine kinase, and the *BCR* (breakpoint cluster region) gene. The actual physiological role of the BCR protein has yet to be effectively demonstrated. The Philadelphia translocation can produce protein products of three sizes: p190 (190 kDa), p210 (210 kDa), and p230 (230 kDa) depending upon the site of the breakpoint within the *BCR* gene—p210 is by far the most common of the three fusion products found in CML. Figure 11.8 shows a simplified version of the formation of the different sized fusion proteins.

The clinical course of CML can be subdivided into three distinct phases: chronic phase, accelerated phase, and blast crisis. Each of these phases has distinctive associated clinicopathological features, as previously considered and outlined by the WHO.

The majority of patients who present are in *chronic phase*, which may last between 2 and 7 years. Chronic phase is usually associated with a hypercellular bone marrow with peripheral leucocytosis, and is responsive to therapy. The majority of patients at presentation have

Philadelphia chromosome
This denotes the derived chromosome 22 der(22) not to be confused with t(9;22). The translocation process is abbreviated to t(9;22).

BCR located at 22q11

ABL1 located at position 9q34

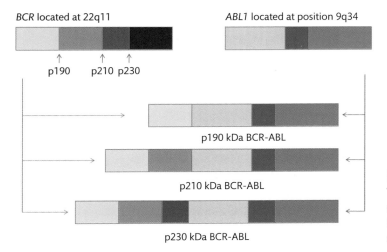

p190 p210 p230

p190 kDa BCR-ABL

p210 kDa BCR-ABL

p230 kDa BCR-ABL

FIGURE 11.8

The formation of BCR–ABL1 fusion proteins of differing size. *ABL1* remains intact, but different breakpoints within *BCR* can result in different-sized fusion genes and proteins.

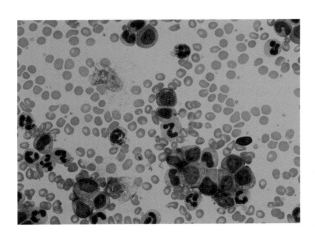

FIGURE 11.9

CML in chronic phase. Large numbers of myeloid cells are present within the peripheral blood. Varying degrees of maturation are present, although many are in the process of maturing. Image courtesy of Jackie Warne, Haematology department, Queen Alexandra Hospital, Portsmouth.

splenomegaly or hepatosplenomegaly, and this can be reduced in chronic phase using standard chemotherapeutic agents. Figure 11.9 shows a peripheral blood film from a patient in chronic phase. Note the large numbers of differentiated, maturing cells. There is no evidence of maturational arrest

As the disease progresses to *accelerated phase*, it becomes more difficult to treat. The blast count will rise, although remains less than 20%, and the basophil count will equal or exceed 20%. The leucocytosis will become difficult to control, and will be accompanied by either a persistent thrombocytopenia (<100 × 10⁹/L) or a thrombocytosis (in some cases >1000 × 10⁹/L). The presence of thrombocytopenia is part of the disease process, and is not secondary to **cytoreductive therapy**. Additional cytogenetic abnormalities may be found, suggesting disease progression.

Blast crisis describes the transformation to acute leukaemia. The blast count is 20% or higher, and immunophenotyping is often required to determine the lineage of the acute leukaemia. Figure 11.10 shows a case in which blast crisis has transformed to acute leukaemia.

cytoreductive therapy
A form of therapy effective at reducing high blood cell counts. An example of cytoreductive therapy is hydroxycarbamide.

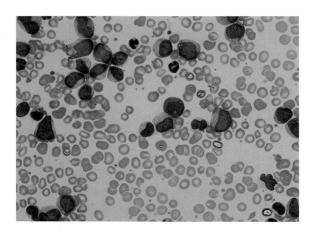

FIGURE 11.10

CML in blast crisis. Large numbers of blasts are apparent in the peripheral blood. Note the prominent nucleoli. Some mature neutrophils are apparent. Image courtesy of Jackie Warne, Haematology department, Queen Alexandra Hospital, Portsmouth.

Cross reference

CML was briefly introduced in Chapter 9.

SELF-CHECK 11.9

Give a brief account of the different phases of chronic myeloid leukaemia.

Chronic neutrophilic leukaemia

Chronic neutrophilic leukaemia (CNL) is an exceptionally rare myeloproliferative disorder associated with a neutrophil leucocytosis in the absence of infection, inflammation, or confounding myeloid malignancy.

CNL is a disorder classified through the process of exclusion, providing the peripheral blood leucocyte count is >25 × 10^9/L and composed of >80% neutrophils or band forms. Less than 10% of the peripheral blood leucocytes should be immature granulocytes. The bone marrow appears hypercellular, with increased granulopoiesis evident. There should be no evidence of any cytogenetic abnormalities characteristic of other myeloid diseases; for example, the Philadelphia chromosome should not be present, nor should be the BCR–ABL1 fusion product, which in itself is diagnostic for CML. Other myeloproliferative disorders and myelodysplastic syndromes should also be excluded. The majority of patients demonstrate hepatosplenomegaly.

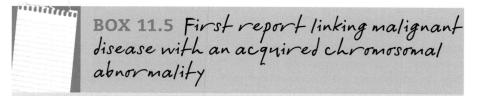

BOX 11.5 *First report linking malignant disease with an acquired chromosomal abnormality*

Nowell and Hungerford's original findings were the first linking a malignant disease to an acquired chromosomal abnormality. The minute chromosome reported, using microscopic examination of cells derived from seven patients diagnosed with chronic granulocytic leukaemia, was later identified as chromosome 22, and is now abbreviated to der(22): the Philadelphia chromosome. (See the Reference list at the end of this book for Nowell and Hungerford, 1960.)

Historically, a number of cases of CNL have been associated with multiple myeloma, and recent evidence suggests that the neutrophilia may be driven by malignant plasma cells in an inflammatory process, rather than being an independent clonal neutrophilic leukaemia.

Chronic eosinophilic leukaemia, not otherwise specified, and hypereosinophilic syndrome

A raised eosinophil count is a common feature of allergic reactions, parasitic infections, and malignancy to name but a few, and it is important to consider these when attempting to make a diagnosis of chronic eosinophilic leukaemia (CEL) or idiopathic hypereosinophilic syndrome (HES).

A significant overlap between CEL and HES exists and the WHO has made an attempt to allow differentiation between them. The defining feature common to both conditions is a raised eosinophil count >1.5 × 10^9/L for six months or more.

All reactive causes of an eosinophilia should be excluded, as should any malignant condition known to cause a raised eosinophil count, either directly (as part of the malignant clone), or indirectly (through chemical mediation). An abnormal T-cell population should also be excluded, which could promote a sustained eosinophilia through the activity of interleukin-5 (IL-5).

CEL is diagnosed when a clonal population of eosinophils is identified, or there is an increase in myeloblasts (below 20%) accompanied by a persistently raised eosinophil count. If the clonal nature of the eosinophils cannot be established, and the blast percentage is not raised, then a diagnosis of idiopathic HES is appropriate.

Mastocytosis

Mast cells are important effectors in both innate immunity and in IgE-associated immune responses. Increased numbers of mast cells showing clonal gene rearrangements and a propensity to accumulate in one or more organ systems, is called mastocytosis. The main categories of mastocytosis, named according to the organ system within which the clonal mast cells are identified and their behaviour, are listed below:

- Cutaneous mastocytosis
- Indolent systemic mastocytosis
- Systemic mastocytosis with associated clonal haematological non-mast cell lineage disease
- Aggressive systemic mastocytosis
- Mast cell leukaemia
- Mast cell sarcoma
- Extracutaneous mastocytoma

In addition there are a number of extremely rare subvariants to these mast cell diseases.

Commonly, a point mutation within the *c-KIT* gene is identified, leading to a substitution of valine for aspartic acid at position 816 (ASP816VAL or D816V) within the KIT receptor. The ligand for KIT is stem cell factor (SCF). D816V is an activating mutation causing enhanced and inappropriate signalling through KIT in a ligand-independent manner. Other KIT mutations have been documented, and these tend to be associated with the mastocytosis variants.

There are a range of mast cell disorders demonstrating mutations within platelet-derived growth factor receptor (PDGFRA) and PDGFRB, but these should be considered as distinct entities and classified as myeloid or lymphoid neoplasms with eosinophilia and abnormalities of PDGFRA, PDGFRB, or fibroblast growth factor receptor 1 (FGFR1) (outlined in the next section).

Depending upon the subtype of mastocytosis present, there are variable clinical and laboratory features, so bone marrow analysis is important to assess the number and distribution of mast cells. This can also assist in establishing prognosis. The spleen, liver, and lymph nodes are also commonly affected. If mast cells exceed 20% of nucleated cells within the bone marrow, mast cell leukaemia should be diagnosed. Mast cells are likely to feature in the peripheral blood where a diagnosis of mast cell leukaemia is suspected, with levels of 10% of the total WBC count not uncommon.

Chronic myeloproliferative disease, unclassifiable

As the name suggests, chronic myeloproliferative disease, unclassifiable (CMPD-U) should be used when we are unable to classify a thoroughly investigated CMPD as a specific disease entity.

The presence of the Philadelphia chromosome and the fusion product BCR–ABL1 should be excluded, otherwise the condition should be considered CML. It is important that CMPD-U is not used for inadequately investigated cases.

Myeloid and lymphoid neoplasms with eosinophilia and abnormalities of PDGFRA, PDGFRB, or FGFR1

The diseases contained within this category are diverse and uncommon. The main diseases are listed below.

- Myeloid and lymphoid neoplasms with platelet-derived growth factor receptor A gene (PDGFRA) rearrangement
- Myeloid neoplasms with platelet-derived growth factor receptor B gene (PDGFRB) rearrangement
- Myeloid and lymphoid neoplasms with fibroblast growth factor receptor-1 gene (FGFR1) abnormalities

The majority of cases demonstrate a degree of eosinophil involvement, with the eosinophil count generally over 1.5×10^9/L. The malignant progenitor cell is thought to be a stem cell capable of forming myeloid or lymphoid lineages, and this is reflected in the classification title for these diseases. This would explain why in some cases there is an overt lymphoblastic leukaemia accompanied by eosinophilia. Care must be taken with this diagnosis to ensure the eosinophilia is a consequence of genetic mutation rather than aberrant growth factor release from the malignant lymphoid cells.

Although three main disease entities are classified under this heading, many of those possessing PDGFRA or PDGFRB mutations comprise chronic eosinophilic leukaemia (CEL).

Patients demonstrating the cryptic *FIP1L1–PDGFRA* fusion del (4q12) or *PDGFRA* rearrangements, are included within the category 'Myeloid and lymphoid neoplasms with *PDGFRA* rearrangement'.

Patients generally possess mutations at the locus 5q31–33 involving the *PDGFRB* gene. Translocations are the common finding, unlike mutations involving 4q12, where cryptic deletion is commonly present. A number of these cases also produce CEL. Other cases may represent a variety of myeloproliferative diseases but these commonly demonstrate eosinophilia.

Abnormalities with the gene *FGFR1* are associated with translocations involving the 8p11–12 locus. These translocations give rise to a range of both myeloid and lymphoid diseases.

BOX 11.6 *Growth factors*

Platelet-derived growth factor receptor

The receptor for platelet-derived growth factor (PDGF) contains α- and β-subunits which dimerize following the binding of PDGF. PDGF has mitogenic activity, i.e. mitosis can be induced when it is bound to its receptor. The binding of PDGF to PDGFR initiates the dimerization of PDGFRα- and PDGFRβ-subunits and autophosphorylation of intracellular tyrosine kinase domains. This phosphorylation induces the activation of intracellular signalling. Mutations within PDGFRα or PDGFRβ can switch this tyrosine kinase on, leading to inappropriate signalling.

Fibroblast growth factor receptor-1

This receptor is involved in intracellular signalling, inducing proliferation, cell growth, and differentiation in response to the binding of fibroblast growth factor (FGF). The extracellular region is involved in ligand binding, whilst the intracellular region contains a tyrosine kinase domain, which, when activated, is important in initiating signal transduction pathways. The translocations involving *FGFR1* induce overactivity of the receptor causing dysregulation of cell growth and proliferation.

CHAPTER SUMMARY

In this chapter we have:

- Outlined the importance of appropriate classification systems.

- Compared and contrasted the French–American–British (FAB) and World Health Organization (WHO) classifications for myeloid malignancies.

- Examined the morphological, genetic, and molecular events commonly associated with different types of myeloid malignancy.

- Dismantled many of the subgroups adopted by the WHO system, and examined the diseases that comprise these groups in order to gain an understanding for the reasoning behind the classification process.

- Examined the arbitrary nature of the FAB system, and attempted to overcome this by using evidence-based practice to provide a framework for diagnostic and treatment strategies.

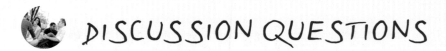

DISCUSSION QUESTIONS

11.1 In the light of the recent developments in molecularly targeted chemotherapeutics, critically discuss the value of classifying specific diseases according to the WHO category *AML with recurrent genetic abnormalities*.

11.2 Critically discuss the investigative steps required for the investigation of a patient in CML blast crisis.

11.3 Critically discuss the distinction between MDS and MDS/MPN.

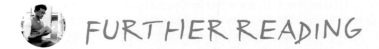

FURTHER READING

- Cotta CV, Bueso-Ramos CE. New insights into the pathobiology and treatment of chronic myelogenous leukaemia. *Annals of Diagnostic pathology* 2007: **11**; 68–78.

- Degos L, Linch DC, Löwenberg B (ed.). *Textbook of Malignant Haematology*, 2nd edn. Taylor & Francis, Oxon, 2005.

- Hoffbrand AV, Catovsky D, Tuddenham EGD (ed.). *Postgraduate Haematology*, 5th edn. Blackwell Publishing Ltd, Massachusetts–Oxford–Carlton, 2005.

- Malinge S, Izraeli S, Crispino JD. Insights into the manifestations, outcomes, and mechanisms of leukemogenesis in Down syndrome. *Blood* 2009: **113**; 2619–28.

- Nimer SD. Myelodysplastic syndromes. *Blood* 2009: **111**; 4841–51.

- Swerdlow SH, Campo E, Harris NL, Jaffe ES, Pileri SA, Stein H Thiele J, Vardiman JW (ed.). *WHO Classification of Tumours of Haematopoietic and Lymphoid Tissues*. IARC, Lyon, 2008.

- Vitoux D, Nasr R, de The H. Acute promyelocytic leukemia: new issues on Pathogenesis and treatment response. *Int. J. Biochem. Cell Biol.* 2007: **39**; 1063–70.

- Wang ZY, Chen Z. *Acute promyelocytic leukemia: from highly fatal to highly curable*. *Blood* 2008: **111**; 2505–15.

Answers to self-check questions, case study questions, and discussion questions are provided in the book's Online Resource Centre, visit www.oxfordtextbooks.co.uk/orc/moore

12

An introduction to classification systems: lymphoid neoplasms

Gavin Knight

In the previous chapter we examined the fundamental considerations of classification systems for the purposes of identifying and reporting haematological malignancies. The principles are the same for myeloid and lymphoid malignancies, although the range of diseases is remarkably diverse. As we will see in Section 12.1, the desire to classify lymphoid malignancies has involved complex and almost farcical events in history, the limitations of which were a consequence of technical difficulties and a lack of understanding of the process of lymphocyte development and maturation. Even in the twenty-first century, the classification of lymphoid diseases has proved problematic, but we are closer now than ever before in achieving a classification system that accurately reflects the clinicopathological processes of lymphomagenesis and lymphoid leukaemogenesis.

In this chapter we consider the process of classifying lymphoid diseases, of which ninety different disorders are recognized by the WHO. These are broadly subdivided into six different categories. This chapter cannot consider all these malignancies in detail, but it will provide the pathobiological background or a brief description of the most common and interesting of cases.

In the first instance we will consider the historical classification of lymphoid malignancies in greater detail.

Learning outcomes

After studying this chapter you should confidently be able to:

- Compare and contrast the historical attempts to classify lymphoid malignancies.
- Demonstrate a critical appreciation of the importance of the revised European and American classification of lymphoid neoplasms (REAL)/World Health Organization (WHO) classification systems for lymphoid malignancies.
- Distinguish between the French American British (FAB) and WHO classification systems for acute leukaemias.

■ Outline the main differences between precursor neoplasms and mature cell neoplasms.

■ Describe the key recurrent cytogenetic abnormalities associated with precursor lymphoid neoplasms.

■ Critically discuss some of the common mature B-cell neoplasms and outline the key cytogenetic findings of each.

■ Critically discuss the role of immunoglobulin variable heavy-chain gene (*IGVH*) somatic hypermutation in the pathogenesis of CLL/SLL.

■ Differentiate between the main plasma cell neoplasms and explain the key clinical and laboratory findings in each.

■ Discuss the pathogenesis of plasma cell myeloma-related bone disease.

■ Describe the common T-lineage malignancies and provide an outline of the role of ALK dysregulation.

■ Outline the laboratory findings associated with T-prolymphocytic leukaemia.

12.1 The history of lymphoid classification

Since the 1950s a number of systems have been in use for the classification of lymphoid malignancies in an attempt to standardize the way in which they were diagnosed and reported. At the time, there was very little understanding about the immune system, and in particular the differences between innate and adaptive immunity were still to be recognized. An interesting quote attributable to Yoffey, dating back to 1956, demonstrates the lack of understanding at the time when he describes the lymphocyte as '*a somewhat inconspicuous cell with no particular striking functional or morphological characteristics*'. It is certainly understandable with views such as these why it was so problematic in devising an appropriate classification system for lymphoid malignancies.

Let us now look at some of the important classification systems in more detail.

The Rappaport system

The first truly successful classification system of lymphoid tumours was developed by Rappaport in 1956 and updated in 1966. It focused firstly on the architectural pattern of the cells within their originating tissue, i.e. whether cellular distribution was nodular or diffuse, and secondly on cytology—according to cell type. Small cells were called lymphocytic, whilst larger cells were called **histiocytic**. Table 12.1 shows an outline of the Rappaport classification system. The Rappaport system was easy to use and generally provided reproducible results which were shown to provide prognostically important information.

histiocyte
A type of macrophage found within connective tissue.

Cross reference
Cellular distribution and infiltration were considered in greater detail in Chapter 10.

TABLE 12.1   **Rappaport classification of non-Hodgkin lymphoma.**

Diffuse
Well differentiated lymphocytic
Nodular or diffuse
Poorly differentiated lymphocytic
Mixed (lymphocytic–histiocytic)
Undifferentiated

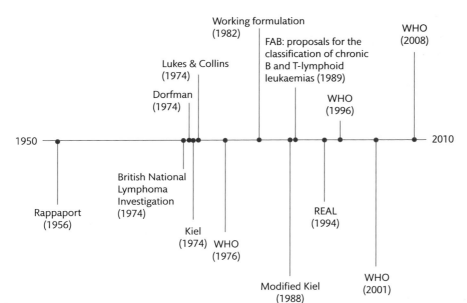

FIGURE 12.1
A timeline showing the major lymphoid classification systems introduced since 1950.

In 1974, following major advances in the understanding of lymphoid malignancies with the development and increasing availability of immunological and molecular techniques, a number of classification systems were developed by various groups to try to introduce an up-to-date, relevant system for classifying lymphoid malignancies. These classification systems included Lukes and Collins, Dorfman, the British National Lymphoma Investigation (BNLI), and Kiel. Having so many classification systems released in the same year resulted in chaos, with clinicians largely unsure of which system to use and the relative merits of each. The main systems will be considered in more detail below. Figure 12.1 provides a timeline summary showing the publication dates for the key classification systems for lymphoid malignancies of the last 60 years.

Lukes and Collins

Lukes and Collins based their classification on immunological indicators, allowing differentiation between B and T cells to be determined morphologically. For any cases failing to fit into B- and T-cell categories according to immunological markers, an *undefined* category was recommended. Lukes and Collins suggested the undefined category would be an appropriate place to include lymphoblastic disorders or those of stem cells, rather than placing this aggressive group of 'blastic' diseases on their own. An unclassifiable section was provided to enable the classification of lymphoid malignancies which could not be assigned an appropriate lineage due to technical limitations. However, it was questionable whether this system was clinically relevant in determining the behaviour of the malignancy thereby allowing accurate prognostication. Table 12.2 provides an outline of the Lukes and Collins classification system.

Kiel

The Kiel classification, which was largely subscribed to by the European medical community was also published in 1974, and used morphological, cytochemical, and immunological methods for identifying and classifying lymphoid malignancies.

The Kiel classification recognizes low- and high-grade diseases based on cellular morphology and attempts to associate malignant cells with their 'normal' cell counterpart. Until the

TABLE 12.2 Lukes–Collins classification of non-Hodgkin lymphoma.

U (undefined)-cell
T-cell
Small lymphocyte
Convoluted lymphocyte
Sézary cell–mycosis fungoides
Immunoblastic sarcoma
Lennert's lymphoma
B-cell
Small lymphocyte
Plasmacytoid lymphocyte
Follicular centre cell
Small cleaved
Large cleaved
Small non-cleaved
Large non-cleaved
Immunoblastic
Histiocytic
Unclassifiable

introduction of the revised version, released in 1988, the Kiel classification did not stratify the malignancies into T-cell or B-cell as the authors believed too little was known about T-cell malignancies at that time.

Cells with a typical blast appearance, determined through the evaluation of cell and nuclear size, density of chromatin, and the number of proliferating cells (proliferation fraction) formed the main cellular component of *high-grade* disease, whereas more mature, smaller cells were considered *low-grade* disease.

The updated classification in 1988 followed technical advancements, making the identification and classification of a range of additional lymphoid malignancies possible. Table 12.3 shows a comparison between the 1974 and 1988 versions of the Kiel system. However, the Kiel classification failed to include all but one of the primary extranodal lymphomas, mycosis fungoides. It also failed to represent the heterogeneity of follicular lymphoma.

Cross reference

Mycosis fungoides and follicular lymphoma are discussed later in this chapter.

The Working Formulation

The publication of the Working Formulation in 1982 was the product of a major effort by the National Cancer Institute to try to reconcile the differences in diagnosis, classification, and treatment caused by the wide array of classification systems in place at that time. The analysis of survival data from the examination of six different classifications—including: BNLI, Rappaport, Lukes and Collins, Kiel, Dorfman, and the WHO of 1976—demonstrated that each was equally as good as the other in predicting survival, i.e. the classification systems were all clinically valid. The Working Formulation, which was largely subscribed to by the Americans, integrated the components of the six different classifications to provide an easy to use, clinically viable method of classifying lymphoid neoplasms by taking into account tumour aggressiveness and morphological appearance.

TABLE 12.3 Kiel classification. The original version is shown in the left hand column, with the revised version shown to its right. Note that the updated version is subdivided into B-cell and T-cell diseases.

1974 Kiel classification	1988 Updated Kiel classification	
	B-cell	**T-cell**
Low grade malignancy	**Low-grade malignant lymphoma**	**Low-grade malignant lymphoma**
Lymphocytic, chronic lymphocytic leukaemia	Lymphocytic	Lymphocytic
Lymphocytic, other	Chronic lymphocytic leukaemia	Chronic lymphocytic leukaemia
Lymphoplasmacytoid	Prolymphocytic leukaemia	Prolymphocytic leukaemia
Centrocytic	Hairy cell leukaemia	
Centroblastic–centrocytic, follicular without sclerosis		Small cell, cerebriform
Centroblastic–centrocytic, follicular and diffuse, without sclerosis		Mycosis fungoides, Sézary syndrome
Centroblastic–centrocytic, follicular and diffuse with sclerosis	Lymphoplasmacytic/ – cytoid (immunocytoma)	Lymphoepithelioid (Lennert's lymphoma)
Centroblastic–centrocytic, diffuse	Plasmacytic	Angioimmunoblastic (ALD, LgX)
Low-grade malignant lymphoma, unclassified	Centroblastic–centrocytic	
	Follicular +/– diffuse	
	Diffuse	
	Centrocytic (mantle cell)	Pleomorphic, small cell (HTLV-1 +/–)
	Monocytoid, including marginal zone	
High-grade malignancy	**High-grade malignant lymphoma**	**High-grade malignant lymphoma**
Centroblastic	Centroblastic	Pleomorphic, medium sized and large cell (HTLV-1 +/–)
Lymphoblastic, Burkitt type		
Lymphoblastic, convoluted cell type	Immunoblastic	Immunoblastic (HTLV-1 +)
Lymphoblastic, other (classified)	Burkitt lymphoma	
Immunoblastic		
High-grade malignant lymphoma, unclassified	Large cell anaplastic (ki-1+)	Large cell anaplastic (Ki-1 +)
Malignant lymphoma, unclassified (unable to specify 'high grade' or 'low grade').	Lymphoblastic	Lymphoblastic
Composite lymphoma	Rare types	

TABLE 12.4 Working Formulation of lymphoma.

Low grade
    A. Small lymphocytic
    B. Follicular, predominantly small cleaved cell
    C. Follicular, mixed, small cleaved and large cell

Intermediate grade
    D. Follicular, predominantly large cell
    E. Diffuse, small cleaved cell
    F. Diffuse, mixed small and large cell
    G. Diffuse, large cell

High grade
    H. Diffuse, large cell immunoblastic
    I. Lymphoblastic
    J. Small, non-cleaved cell

The Working Formulation was not a classification system in its own right, although it enabled clinicians using one of the composite classification systems to be able to translate their findings to other classification systems, allowing for agreement between clinicians and pathologists. Each of the categories provided in the working formulation relate to descriptions of cells, rather than particular disease entities. The working formulation was based on the assessment of 1175 cases of lymphoid neoplasms, resulting in a classification comprising three main grades—low, intermediate, and high—and ten disease entities, labelled A-J. Table 12.4 outlines the Working Formulation.

The Working Formulation lost favour as the component classifications were gradually replaced; the notion of a system that integrates a range of classification systems, where the systems it describes are considered no longer valid, becomes unviable. Additionally, the evaluation of patient material to formulate a diagnosis was based on H&E- stained slides. Advances in lymphoma research at the time of the development of the REAL system enabled this system to be based around immunological data as well as that provided by special cytochemical stains. A new classification system needed to be devised to replace the Working Formulation that would incorporate this 'new knowledge' and be firmly grounded in technical advancement.

SELF-CHECK 12.1

Provide a brief overview of the role of the Working Formulation in the classification of lymphoid neoplasms.

Proposals for the classification of chronic (mature) B- and T-lymphoid leukaemias

The French–American–British (FAB) group were instrumental in providing classification systems for acute leukaemias (both myeloid and lymphoid) and myelodysplastic syndrome, and in 1989 they published proposals to develop the classification of mature lymphoid leukaemias. This classification was based on cytology and the cell membrane immunophenotype of mature lymphoid malignancies within the bone marrow and peripheral blood. This system recognized several well-defined, leukaemic-phase disease entities, but did not incorporate solid lymphoid tumours.

The revised European and American classification of lymphoid neoplasms (REAL)

The development of the revised European and American classification of lymphoid neoplasms (REAL), published in 1994 as an expansion of the Kiel classification, included further clinical and biological criteria following research based on the updated Kiel system of 1988.

A group of 19 international haematologists, each a recognized expert in the area of lymphoma diagnosis, convened in order to establish a new classification system that would be clinically relevant to all haematologists. The group recognized some functional overlap between the main classifications; the Kiel, the Lukes–Collins, and the Working Formulation, although different names and diagnostic requirements were utilized by each. The main intention of the REAL classification was to standardize classification for lymphoid malignancies, whilst making the outcome of the classification process clinically relevant.

The REAL classification was based on morphology, but also included immunophenotypic, cytogenetic, clinical features, and normal cell counterpart—if known. For the first time, a unified classification system was presented that included both Hodgkin and non-Hodgkin lymphoma, demonstrating a degree of commonality between the two conditions—they are both lymphoid malignancies. Table 12.5 shows the lymphoid diseases recognized as discrete disease entities by REAL.

REAL was subscribed to by the Europeans and the Americans, ensuring a unified approach in the diagnosis of lymphoid neoplasms across the Atlantic.

The World Health Organization (WHO) classification of tumours of haematopoietic and lymphoid tissues

The World Health Organization (WHO) classification enhanced the already popular REAL classification. Now in its fourth edition, this system is considered to be the most comprehensive and clinically representative classification to date. The WHO classification utilizes the following data in order to enable the appropriate classification of malignancies, although it recognizes that, in most cases, using a combination of morphology and immunophenotype should be sufficient to provide an accurate diagnosis:

- *Morphology*—is still the cornerstone of lymphoma diagnosis, although it is important to recognize that lymphomas of different origin may share morphological features, whilst demonstrating different clinical behaviour.

- *Immunophenotype*—is an important adjunct to morphology and provides quantitative information useful in determining B-, T-, or NK-cell lineage. Immunophenotype also helps identify the maturational stage of the lymphoma cells; for example pre-germinal centre, germinal centre, or post-germinal centre. As we have previously established, immunophenotype can also identify surrogate markers (e.g. Zap-70 in B-CLL) which help us predict disease outcome.

- *Genotype*—a large number of non-random translocations are identifiable in lymphoma, some of which are diagnostic for particular subtypes; for example, follicular lymphoma

TABLE 12.5 Revised European–American classification of lymphoid neoplasms (REAL) 1994.

B-cell neoplasm

  I. Precursor B-lymphoblastic leukaemia/lymphoma

 II. Peripheral B-cell neoplasms

    1. B-cell chronic lymphocytic leukaemia/prolymphocytic leukaemia/small lymphocytic leukaemia/lymphoma

    2. Lymphoplasmacytoid lymphoma/immunocytoma

    3. Mantle cell lymphoma

    4. Follicular centre lymphoma, grades I, II, III

        Provisional subtype: diffuse, predominantly small-cell type

    5. Marginal zone B-cell lymphoma

        Extranodal (MALT-type +/– monocytoid B cells)

        Provisional subtype: nodal (+/– monocytoid B cells)

    6. Provisional entity: splenic marginal zone lymphoma (+/– villous lymphocytes)

    7. Hairy cell leukaemia

    8. Plasmacytoma/plasma cell myeloma

    9. Diffuse large B-cell lymphoma

        Subtype: primary mediastinal (thymic) B-cell lymphoma

   10. Burkitt lymphoma

   11. Provisional entity: high-grade B-cell lymphoma, Burkitt-like

T-cell and putative NK-cell neoplasms

  I. Precursor T-cell neoplasm: precursor T-lymphoblastic lymphoma/leukaemia

 II. Peripheral T-cell and NK-cell neoplasms

    1. T-cell chronic lymphocytic leukaemia/prolymphocytic leukaemia

    2. Large granular lymphocyte leukaemia:

        T-cell

        NK-cell type

    3. Mycosis fungoides/Sézary syndrome

    4. Peripheral T-cell lymphomas, unspecified

        Provisional cytologic categories: medium sized cell, mixed medium and large cell, large cell, lymphoepithelioid cell

        Provisional subtype: hepatosplenic γδ T-cell lymphoma

        Provisional subtype: subcutaneous panniculitic T-cell lymphoma

    5. Angioimmunoblastic T-cell lymphoma

    6. Angiocentric lymphoma

    7. Intestinal T-cell lymphoma (+/– enteropathy associated)

    8. Adult T-lymphoma/leukaemia (ATL/L)

    9. Anaplastic large cell lymphoma (ALCL), CD30[+], T- and null-cell types

   10. Provisional entity: anaplastic large-cell lymphoma, Hodgkin-like

Hodgkin disease

  I Lymphocyte predominance

 II Nodular sclerosis

 III Mixed cellularity

 IV Lymphocyte depletion

 V Provisional entity: lymphocyte rich classical-HD

is associated with t(14;18). A section entitled *B-lymphoblastic leukaemia/lymphoma with recurrent genetic abnormalities* describes aggressive conditions with typical cytogenetic characteristics that define particular disease entities.

- *Normal cell counterpart*—is important to recognize because we can predict the behaviour of the disease, to a certain extent, by knowing the properties of the normal counterpart.

- *Site of origin*—should be considered when reporting the lymphoma findings. Is the lymphoma of nodal or extranodal origin (gastrointestinal tract, central nervous system, skin, etc.)? This information can help predict clinical outcome through disease behaviour.

- *Clinical aggressiveness and prognosis*—are also considered and play an important role in choosing the appropriate therapy and keeping the patient informed of their condition.

The WHO classification of lymphoid neoplasms is outlined in Table 12.6.

TABLE 12.6 The WHO system, 4th edition, for malignant lymphoproliferative diseases. Acute lymphoblastic lymphomas and leukaemias are incorporated into precursor lymphoid neoplasms. Malignancies associated with mature cell morphology and phenotype are classified as mature B- or T-cell and NK-cell neoplasms. Hodgkin disease is also included. All provisional entities have been removed for clarity.

Precursor lymphoid neoplasms
B lymphoblastic leukaemia/lymphoma
B lymphoblastic leukaemia/lymphoma, not otherwise specified
B lymphoblastic leukaemia/lymphoma with recurrent genetic abnormalities
  B lymphoblastic leukaemia/lymphoma with t(9;22)(q34;q11.2); *BCR-ABL1*
  B lymphoblastic leukaemia/lymphoma with t(v;11q23); *MLL* rearranged
  B lymphoblastic leukaemia/lymphoma with t(12;21)(p13;q22); *TEL-AML1* (*ETV6-RUNX1*)
  B lymphoblastic leukaemia/lymphoma with hyperdiploidy
  B lymphoblastic leukaemia/lymphoma with hypodiploidy (hypodiploid ALL)
  B lymphoblastic leukaemia/lymphoma with t(5;14)(q31;q32); *IL3-IGH*
  B lymphoblastic leukaemia/lymphoma with t(1;19)(q23;p13.3); *E2A-PBX1* (*TCF3-PBX1*)

T lymphoblastic leukaemia/lymphoma
Mature B-cell neoplasms
Chronic lymphocytic leukaemia/small lymphocytic lymphoma
B-cell prolymphocytic leukaemia
Splenic marginal zone lymphoma
Hairy cell leukaemia
Lymphoplasmacytic lymphoma
Waldenström macroglobulinaemia
Heavy chain diseases
  Alpha heavy chain disease
  Gamma heavy chain disease
  Mu heavy chain disease
Plasma cell myeloma
Solitary plasmacytoma of the bone
Extraosseous plasmacytoma of the bone
Extranodal marginal zone lymphoma of mucosa associated lymphoid tissue (MALT lymphoma)
Nodal marginal zone lymphoma

(Continued)

TABLE 12.6 (Continued)

Follicular lymphoma

Primary cutaneous follicle centre lymphoma

Mantle cell lymphoma

Diffuse large B-cell lymphoma (DLBCL), not otherwise specified

    T-cell histiocyte rich large B-cell lymphoma

    Primary DLBCL of the central nervous system

    Primary cutaneous DLBCL, leg type

DLBCL associated with chronic inflammation

Lymphomatoid granulomatosis

Primary mediastinal (thymic) large B-cell lymphoma

Intravascular large B-cell lymphoma

ALK+ large B-cell lymphoma

Plasmablastic lymphoma

Large B-cell lymphoma arising in HHV8-associated multicentric Castleman disease

Primary effusion lymphoma

Burkitt lymphoma

B-cell lymphoma, unclassifiable, with features intermediate between diffuse large B-cell lymphoma and Burkitt lymphoma

B-cell lymphoma, unclassifiable, with features intermediate between diffuse large B-cell lymphoma and classical Hodgkin lymphoma

Hodgkin lymphoma

Nodular lymphocyte predominant Hodgkin lymphoma

Classical Hodgkin lymphoma

    Nodular sclerosis classical Hodgkin lymphoma

    Lymphocyte-rich classical Hodgkin lymphoma

    Mixed cellularity classical Hodgkin lymphoma

    Lymphocyte-depleted classical Hodgkin lymphoma

Mature T-cell and NK-cell neoplasms

T-cell prolymphocytic leukaemia

T-cell large granular lymphocytic leukaemia

Aggressive NK-cell leukaemia

Systemic EBV+ T-cell lymphoproliferative disease of childhood

Hydroa vacciniforme-like lymphoma

Adult T-cell leukaemia/lymphoma

Extranodal NK/T-cell lymphoma, nasal type

Enteropathy-associated T-cell lymphoma

Hepatosplenic T-cell lymphoma

Subcutaneous panniculitis-like T-cell lymphoma

Mycosis fungoides

Sézary syndrome

Primary cutaneous CD30+ lymphoproliferative disorders

    Lymphomatoid papulosis

    Primary cutaneous anaplastic large cell lymphoma

Primary cutaneous gamma-delta T-cell lymphoma

Peripheral T-cell lymphoma, not otherwise specified

Angioimmunoblastic T-cell lymphoma

Anaplastic large cell lymphoma, ALK+

TABLE 12.6 (Continued)

Post transplantation lymphoproliferative disorders (PTLD)
Early lesions
    Plasmacytic hyperplasia
    Infectious mononucleosis-like PTLD
Polymorphic PTLD
Monomorphic PTLD (B- and T/NK-cell types)
Classical Hodgkin lymphoma type PTLD

This chapter aims to outline some of the most commonly encountered or interesting lymphoid disease entities, but does not attempt to provide a comprehensive review of all the conditions outlined in the WHO classification.

The WHO has also included a number of 'provisional disease entities' within the lymphoid group, although these are not considered in this book. These diseases have been allocated the 'provisional status' due to a lack of scientific and clinical literature that can provide an appropriate evidence-base for their distinctive classification. Further research should address this deficiency of data, and attempt to provide much needed clarity in these areas.

It is important to recognize that, since 1976, the FAB group classified acute lymphoblastic leukaemias separately, combining them in a classification of acute leukaemias. The replacement of the FAB classification by that of the World Health Organization ensures that *all* lymphoid malignancies are classified in the same manner.

First we will consider acute lymphoblastic leukaemias and lymphoblastic lymphomas before moving on to the specific criteria used by FAB and the WHO for the classification of this diverse range of diseases.

SELF-CHECK 12.2

Outline the features considered important by the WHO for the classification of lymphoproliferative diseases.

12.2 **Acute lymphoblastic leukaemias (ALL)**

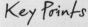

Key Points

In American texts, acute lymphoblastic leukaemia is referred to as acute lympho*cytic* leukaemia. This terminology is largely considered inaccurate in the United Kingdom and should be avoided. ALL is associated with an accumulation of lymphoblasts rather than mature lymphocytes, and its name should reflect this.

Lymphoblastic malignancies are thought to be derived from haemopoietic stem cells which harbour mutations ultimately leading to maturation arrest, self-renewal, and failure of

Cross references

Cancer stem cells were outlined in Chapter 9.

CD34 was outlined in Chapter 9.

Cytogenetic techniques and immunophenotyping were both outlined in Chapter 10.

Common features of patient presentation were outlined in Chapter 10.

apoptosis. In the context of ALL the concept of the cancer stem cell seems to be controversial, with recent studies suggesting that some lymphoblastic cells possess stem cell characteristics, although fail to express the stem cell marker CD34.

Using molecular techniques we can identify clonal rearrangements in immunoglobulin or T-cell receptor genes demonstrating differentiation into a particular lymphoid lineage. Additional identification of cellular subtype or normal cell counterpart is of limited value in the selection of therapies, and so immunophenotypic analysis should often focus on identifying the following key features:

- T-cell phenotype
- Mature B-cell phenotype
- B-cell precursor phenotype

Approximately 88% of lymphoblastic malignancies are of B-cell lineage, with the remainder being of T-cell lineage.

It is important to identify the aberrant expression of myeloid antigens on malignant lymphoid cells as these can be useful in differentiating this clone from the normal lymphoid population following treatment, thus enabling the appropriate assessment of minimal residual disease.

The accumulation of lymphoblasts showing minimal differentiation in the bone marrow and peripheral blood is the key finding to the diagnosis of ALL. In the majority of patients, in excess of 20% lymphoblasts will be found in the peripheral blood. Immunophenotyping and cytogenetic analysis are crucial in providing an accurate diagnosis, especially in the light of the WHO classification, and are important in the process of prognostication.

ALL is much more common in children than in adults, and age is an important factor in prognostication. Less than 5% of children have a heritable predisposition to lymphoblastic malignancies, with the remainder demonstrating a range of acquired genetic abnormalities implicated in the pathogenesis and progression of ALL and lymphoblastic lymphoma (LBL).

The highest incidence of ALL occurs in children between 2 and 5 years of age. There is a subsequent gradual decline followed by an increasing incidence after the age of 40 years and another peak between 80 and 84 years. Children between the ages of 1 and 9 years have the best prognosis, with approximately 80% of patients within this age group being cured.

Overall, leukaemia-free survival in adults is approximately 34%, although this can be further stratified according to particular age brackets, and, as we shall see later on in the chapter, by cytogenetic composition. Between 35 and 40% of patients aged 20–50 years can expect a leukaemia-free survival, but this drops significantly to 10–20% in patients aged over 60 years. Complete remission rates are as high as 95% in children and 40–60% in adults over 50 years of age.

Clinical findings are diverse, with the majority associated with bone marrow failure. There is a risk of testicular involvement in males and the development of central nervous system (CNS) disease in both sexes. A lumbar puncture followed by cytological investigation of cerebrospinal fluid for the presence of lymphoblasts is an important additional investigation to identify CNS involvement.

The WBC is variable in childhood cases. Approximately 45% of patients have a white cell count less than 10×10^9/L and 50% of cases have a WBC in excess of 50×10^9/L. Thrombocytopenia is present in approximately 70% of patients, and this can be associated with bleeding complications. Anaemia is atypical at presentation in younger patients. In adults, the WBC is raised in over 60% of cases and approximately 80% of patients are anaemic.

We will now look at the FAB classification for ALL before considering the WHO system in depth.

FAB: acute lymphoblastic leukaemia

According to the FAB classification system, ALL can be divided into three groups (L1, L2, and L3) based on cellular morphology. Apart from their importance in differentiating between myeloid and lymphoblastic leukaemias, cytochemical stains are of little value in distinguishing between the three classes of ALL. By differentiating these three groups of acute leukaemia according to blast size, nucleocytoplasmic ratio and cytoplasmic coloration using Romanowsky stain, we do not really gain an understanding of the disease process.

L1 and L2 can be either B- or T-lineage, whereas L3 is only B-lineage. From a clinical perspective, there is no difference between L1 and L2, but it was always essential to be able to separate L3, now considered the leukaemic phase of Burkitt lymphoma, from the others, since Burkitt lymphoma has a worse prognosis than L1 or L2 and requires a different therapeutic regimen.

The main types of ALL recognized by FAB are:

ALL–L1

L1 is associated with small homogeneous lymphoblasts. Although the nucleocytoplasmic ratio is high, the scanty cytoplasm demonstrates variable basophilia. Approximately 80% of ALL cases are classified as L1.

ALL–L2

L2 is associated with much larger, heterogeneous lymphoblasts. Although variable in size, the cytoplasm tends to be more abundant, therefore the nucleocytoplasmic ratio is lower. Approximately 18% of cases of ALL are classified as L2.

Clinically, there is very little difference between the L1 and L2 categories.

ALL–L3

L3 constitutes approximately 2% of all cases of ALL. It is essential that all cases of L3 are correctly classified as this particular subtype is associated with specific therapeutic treatment. The cells are large, but homogeneous, and have abundant, highly basophilic cytoplasm. L3 morphology is commonly associated with cytoplasmic vacuolation, which, although sometimes present in L1 and L2, is prominent in L3. The immunophenotype of L3 lymphoblasts correlates with that of a mature B cell.

Let's now have a look at the updated classification of ALL by examining the way in which the WHO have differentiated between the subgroups.

SELF-CHECK 12.3

Describe the different morphological features associated with acute lymphoblastic leukaemia in the FAB classification.

WHO classification of precursor lymphoid neoplasms

The classification of ALLs, and their division into appropriate subgroups, has become possible through the use of immunophenotyping and molecular biological techniques. The specificity and reproducibility of immunophenotyping to distinguish between myeloid and lymphoid lineages, and the ability to further differentiate lymphoid lineages into B and T lineages, relies upon the identification of particular **lineage-restricted** CD markers.

The WHO classification system includes a 'recurrent genetic abnormalities' section, mirroring that included for the myeloid malignancies. This section recognizes non-random, reproducible cytogenetic translocations which can be used to predict disease behaviour. Not all recognized translocations are included in this section, as the vast majority are not associated with disease behaviour, morphology, or prognosis.

Based on a cell's immunophenotype, the WHO separates lymphoblastic leukaemias according to B-cell, T-cell and NK-cell neoplasms. ALL previously classified as L1 or L2 would now be classified as precursor B-cell or precursor T-cell lymphoblastic leukaemia/lymphoma, whilst L3 correlates with the mature B-cell neoplasm, Burkitt lymphoma. If you look at Table 12.7 you will see the way in which immunophenotyping can help differentiate between these conditions.

lineage-restricted

Refers to CD markers expressed by only one cell lineage. Lineage restriction allows us to confidently identify malignant cells. An example is CD20, a B-lineage restricted marker.

TABLE 12.7 The key immunophenotypic features used to distinguish between the acute lymphoblastic leukaemias as recognized by the WHO and cross referenced to the morphological features recognised by FAB.

WHO classification	FAB classification	Immunophenotype
B-lymphoblastic leukaemia/lymphoma	L1 / L2	TdT+ HLA-DR+ CD79a+/− CD10+
T-lymphoblastic leukaemia/lymphoma	L1 / L2	TdT+ cytoplasmic CD3+ CD2+/− CD4+/− CD5+/− CD7+/− CD8+/− CD10+/−
Mature B-cell (Burkitt lymphoma/ leukaemia)	L3	CD19+ CD20+ CD 22+ CD10+ CD5− CD23− TdT− BCL6+ BCL2−

Key: TdT = Terminal deoxynucleotidyl transferase.

The WHO system does not attempt to stratify these conditions any further than these broad groups since further subclassification has no therapeutic value. If you look at Table 12.6, you will see that acute lymphoblastic leukaemias are now considered as lympho-blastic leukaemias/lymphomas and not distinct entities—as previously devised by the FAB group.

12.3 Precursor lymphoid neoplasms

The WHO has divided precursor lymphoid neoplasms into two broad groups based on whether the cells are characterized as B-lineage or T-lineage. Included within this section are lymphoblastic leukaemias and lymphoblastic lymphomas. These two entities have been combined because these diseases are clinically very similar. Lymphoblastic leukaemias are associated with an accumulation of lymphoblasts within the bone marrow and peripheral blood whereas lymphoblastic lymphomas tend to be site-restricted as a lymphomatous lesion.

In Chapter 11, we examined the classification of myeloid malignancies and established the role of classification, where possible, according to the presence of defined recurrent genetic abnormalities. The WHO has adopted this system for lymphoblastic leukaemias/lymphomas of B-cell lineage where these genetic abnormalities can predict clinical outcome. Named cyto-genetic aberrations are considered under the overarching section *B-lymphoblastic leukaemia/ lymphoma with recurrent genetic abnormalities*.

Cross reference
AML with recurrent genetic abnormalities was discussed in detail in Chapter 11.

B-lymphoblastic leukaemias or lymphomas failing to demonstrate any of the named recurrent genetic abnormalities are combined within another group—*B lymphoblastic leukaemia/lymphoma not otherwise specified*. Whilst this group should not be used to classify inadequately investigated patients, it is likely that the composition of cases within this group will change in subsequent editions of the WHO classification as more is discovered about this particular group of lymphoid malignancies.

At the time of writing, T-lymphoblastic leukaemias and lymphomas have no defining cytogenetic abnormalities that can be used for classification purposes, and therefore these T-lineage lympho-blastic conditions are combined under the heading of *T lymphoblastic leukaemia/lymphoma*.

We will now consider the WHO classification of the range of lymphoblastic leukaemia/ lymphoma entities in some detail.

B-lymphoblastic leukaemia/lymphoma with recurrent genetic abnormalities

In this section, seven cytogenetic abnormalities are recognized as recurrent, disease-defining entities. Where appropriate, the molecular basis of these translocations in leukaemogenesis is discussed.

B-lymphoblastic leukaemia/lymphoma with t(9;22)(q34;q11.2); BCR–ABL1

The fusion protein BCR–ABL1 is associated with 30% of cases of adult ALL and 3% of childhood cases. This translocation is uniformly associated with a poor prognosis in cases of ALL, even though in CML t(9;22) is associated with a good prognosis. The size of the BCR–ABL1 peptide

breakpoint cluster region
An area of a gene where chromosomal breakages are particularly common and well defined.

Cross reference
The translocation t(9;22) was discussed in greater detail in Chapter 11.

is 190 kDa in childhood ALL due to breakpoints occurring in the minor **breakpoint cluster region (BCR)**, with a larger product of 210 kDa associated with adult ALL and CML. Abnormal signalling initiated by the mutated ABL tyrosine kinase is responsible for dysregulated cell growth, differentiation, and failure of apoptosis.

The cell surface expression of CD25 has been linked with cases of ALL harbouring t(9;22), although the presence of CD25 should not be used as a surrogate marker for this transloca-tion. The frequent aberrant expression of the myeloid antigens CD13 or CD33 has also been reported in cases harbouring t(9;22)(q34;q11.2).

As in CML, the use of imatinib mesylate has shown some success in targeting the tyrosine kinase activity of the BCR-ABL1 peptide.

B-lymphoblastic leukaemia/lymphoma with t(v;11q23); MLL rearranged

This group only contains 11q23 rearrangements. Cases involving MLL (mixed lineage leukaemia) deletion are not included in this category as they have not consistently been associated with predictable disease behaviour.

MLL rearrangements are associated with a poor prognosis, with age also seeming to be an important factor. In paediatric cases of ALL, patients under the age of one year harbouring MLL rearrangements have a worse prognosis than patients over the age of one year.

Interestingly, in the research arena, cases of ALL harbouring MLL abnormalities have a distinc-tive gene expression profile that seems to enable these MLL-related diseases to be identified without the need for cytogenetic analysis. Whilst this finding has only been reported in a handful of cases, replacing cytogenetic analysis *should not* be considered appropriate in the classification of cases suspected of harbouring MLL rearrangement at present. However, in the future, classification according to gene expression profile may well be important in identify-ing and reporting these conditions. The most common of the 11q23 rearrangements, t(4;11) (q21;q23), results in the fusion of MLL to AF4. Cases harbouring 11q23 abnormalities tend to be associated with a higher white cell count and CNS involvement.

B-lymphoblastic leukaemia/lymphoma with t(12;21)(p13;q22); TEL–AML1 (ETV6–RUNX1)

Cross reference
AML with recurrent genetic abnormalities was discussed in Chapter 11.

This is the most common cytogenetic abnormality associated with ALL, occurring in up to 25% of childhood cases. As a consequence of t(12;21)(p13;q22) TEL (translocation ETS leukaemia; now ETV6), a member of the ETS family of transcription factors, is fused to AML1 (now called RUNX1)—a component of the core binding factor complex. This translocation has similar molecular consequences to t(8;21)(q22;q22), one of the recognized translocations associated with AML outlined in *AML with recurrent genetic abnormalities*.

ETV6 contains a **helix–loop–helix domain**, essential for homodimerizing with other ETV6 proteins and heterodimerizing with other members of the ETS family. An ETS domain enables ETV6 to bind to DNA.

ETV6 can bind to a number of transcriptional repressors including histone deacetylase (HDAC), thereby suppressing target gene transcription and translation and functioning as a likely tumour suppressor. The fusion of ETV6 with RUNX1, results in the production of a fusion protein containing the ETV6-derived helix–loop–helix domain and repressor binding regions combined with the entire RUNX1 structure. The net result of this translocation is the inappro-priate localization of transcriptional repressors and co-repressors to RUNX1-inducible genes.

This in itself is insufficient to be oncogenic, but additional genetic lesions could lead to a malignant phenotype.

Additional evidence suggests that the helix–loop–helix region can bind the wild-type ETV6 inhibiting ETV6's tumour suppressor function. In the vast majority of cases, however, the wild-type ETV6 located on the other chromosome 12 is deleted.

Generally t(12;21)(p13;q22) is associated with a good prognosis, with over 90% of children cured.

B-lymphoblastic leukaemia/lymphoma with hyperdiploidy

These cases possess in excess of 50 chromosomes per cell and are associated with a good prognosis. Commonly within the 1–10 age range, the white cell count is low and the cells are predisposed to undergo spontaneous apoptosis.

In excess of 90% of children with hyperdiploidy may be cured.

B-lymphoblastic leukaemia/lymphoma with hypodiploidy (hypodiploid ALL)

In cases of hypodiploid ALL, chromosome number is less than 45 per cell and is associated with a poor prognosis. As the chromosome count approaches haploidy (23 chromosomes) the prognosis considerably worsens.

B-lymphoblastic leukaemia/lymphoma with t(5;14) (q31;q32) (IL3–IGH)

This is a particularly rare entity accounting for less than 1% of cases of ALL. The translocation t(5;14)(q31;q32) is considered a discrete entity as it is associated with an increased number of circulating eosinophils. These eosinophils are not part of the malignant clone, but rather the consequence of an induced inflammatory response secondary to the translocation. The *IL3* gene, localized on 5q31, is translocated to the IgH locus on 14q32, resulting in the upregulation of IL-3 expression as a consequence of the stronger IgH promoter. IL-3 then stimulates eosinophil differentiation from common myeloid precursors, resulting in a peripheral blood eosinophilia. At the time of writing, there is no conclusive survival data for this particular subtype.

B-lymphoblastic leukaemia/lymphoma with t(1;19)(q23;p13.3); E2A–PBX1 (TCF3–PBX1)

TCF3 encodes two transcription factors E12 and E47 which bind to the regulatory elements of a range of genes, including *IGK*—the gene encoding Igκ. E12 and E47 are essential for normal lymphopoiesis and control the rate of transcription of a number of important genes actively involved in the process of lymphocyte development. *PBX1* is a **homeobox** gene, encoding a transcription factor essential for lymphopoiesis from the haemopoietic stem cell stage to the pro-B cell stage of maturation.

The E12 and E47 transcriptional activation domains are kept intact in this fusion product, and are localized to the PBX1 DNA-binding domain. It is likely that the fusion of these proteins results in the expression of atypical proteins within cells harbouring this translocation, leading to maturational arrest and leukaemogenesis.

Generally, t(1;19)(q23;p13.3) is associated with a good prognosis.

homeobox

genes encode transcriptional regulators which are expressed at particular times and in particular places within an organism—for example during embryonic development, or in cell differentiation.

Outline the reasons why eosinophilia occurs in cases of leukaemia harbouring t(5;14)(q31;q32).

T-lymphoblastic leukaemia/lymphoma

T-ALL is an aggressive form of leukaemia, accounting for approximately 15% of childhood and 25% of adult ALLs. T-LBL accounts for 85–90% of lymphoblastic lymphomas.

There is often significant bone marrow and peripheral blood involvement, commonly accompanied by an apparent mass within the thoracic cavity (**mediastinum**), hepatosplenomegaly, and lymphadenopathy. In excess of 25% blasts are usually found within the bone marrow in T-ALL, although this is not the case in T-LBL where the blasts are usually confined to a bulk lesion outside of the bone marrow microenvironment.

Immunophenotyping can often be used to identify the normal cell counterpart based on the expression of different combinations of T-cell antigens on the cell surface.

A variety of genetic and chromosomal abnormalities are associated with T-lymphoblastic leukaemia/lymphomas although these are not related to particular disease subgroups at the time of writing.

Now that we have considered the precursor neoplasms, we should go on to look at the mature B-cell neoplasms.

mediastinum

This defines the area within the thorax between the lungs containing the heart, trachea, oesophagus, and thymus.

12.4 Mature B-cell neoplasms

Mature B-cell neoplasms demonstrate the expression of lineage-specific markers and follow a less aggressive course than the precursor lymphoid neoplasms. It is important to recognize that, in these cases, these diseases can still be aggressive and are associated with significant morbidity and mortality.

An understanding of the concept of the germinal centre is important in understanding the pathogenesis of these diseases. Recognizing the terms *centroblast*, *centrocyte*, *mantle zone*, *marginal zone*, *memory B cell*, and *plasma cell* is important in understanding the origin of the normal cell counterpart. In this section, the normal cell counterpart has not been explicitly outlined, as is the case in the WHO publication, although where critical in understanding the basic concepts of the disease, the normal cell counterpart has been included.

Cross reference

Germinal centres were outlined in Chapter 8.

The role of cytogenetic analysis is critical in understanding B-cell lymphoid neoplasms, the majority of which are associated with discrete non-random chromosomal translocations. The mechanisms in place for controlling somatic hypermutation and immunoglobulin class-switching often become dysregulated in B-cell neoplasms, and it is thought that dysregulation of this normal mutational machinery is responsible for the large numbers of cytogenetic abnormalities associated with lymphoid malignancies. Where appropriate, the genetic or cytogenetic basis of mature B-cell neoplasms will be discussed in relation to discrete disease entities.

This section outlines some of the most common and interesting cases of mature B-cell neoplasm, beginning with chronic lymphocytic leukaemia and its solid tumour counterpart, small lymphocytic lymphoma.

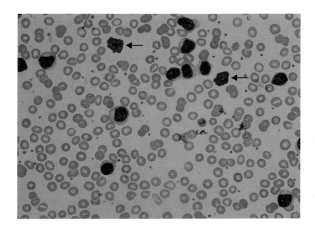

FIGURE 12.2
A case of chronic lymphocytic leukaemia. Note the increased number of mature lymphocytes. The cytoplasm is pale blue and the nucleus is composed of clumped chromatin. Two smear cells are apparent (see arrowheads). Image courtesy of Jackie Warne, Haematology department, Queen Alexandra Hospital, Portsmouth.

Chronic lymphocytic leukaemia/small lymphocytic lymphoma

Chronic lymphocytic leukaemia (CLL) and small lymphocytic lymphoma (SLL) are considered variations of the same disease. CLL, as its name suggests, is composed of malignant lymphocytes in leukaemic phase (i.e. within the peripheral blood), whereas SLL is composed of malignant lymphocytes in one or more bulk lesions. The morphology of the lymphocytes and their immunophenotype is identical in each case. CLL/SLL is a disease of the elderly, occurring predominantly in Westernized societies. In the UK, the incidence is approximately 3 per 100 000, occurring mainly in those over 50 years of age.

The diagnosis of CLL is largely dependent on a lymphocyte count in excess of 5×10^9/L for three months or more. Malignant lymphocytes appear homogeneous or monomorphic, with a thin rim of cytoplasm and a nucleus containing clumped chromatin. **Smear cells**, cells that have ruptured and smeared across the slide in response to mechanical damage from producing the blood film, are frequent features. Figure 12.2 is a photomicrograph of a typical case of B-CLL. In the vast majority of cases, with lymphocyte counts in excess of 30×10^9/L, immature lymphocytes called **prolymphocytes** will account for up to 5% of the white cells.

Key Points

A common complication of CLL is the production of autoantibodies directed against red cells. During the diagnostic process it is important that patients should have a direct antiglobulin test (DAT) performed to determine whether or not red cell autoantibodies are present. It is important that the DAT is monitored throughout the duration of the disease. Direct antiglobulin tests are performed within blood transfusion laboratories and use antihuman globulin (AHG) to cause agglutination of red cells sensitized with antibodies or complement components.

The presence of red cell agglutination following incubation of the patient's red cells with the patient's plasma in the presence of AHG suggests autoantibodies have been produced against the patient's red cells.

Autoantibodies directed against neutrophils and platelets can also occur in patients with CLL.

Cross reference
The direct antiglobulin test is illustrated and described in Chapter 6.

Approximately 50% of cases of CLL are diagnosed following a full blood count for an unrelated full blood count referral.

As CLL progresses, a normocytic normochromic anaemia may be found, but patients may also develop an autoimmune haemolytic anaemia following the production of autoantibodies directed against red cells or their precursors. Red cell aplasia can occur as a consequence of human parvo-virus infection, leading to a profound anaemia requiring blood transfusion support.

CLL/SLL is typified by the immunophenotype: CD5+, CD19+, CD20+, CD23+, CD22–. Surface membrane immunoglobulin (smIg), FMC7, and CD79b may or may not be expressed. Other causes of malignant lymphocytosis, including mantle-cell lymphoma and splenic marginal-zone lymphoma, may appear morphologically identical, but can be distinguished on the basis of their immunophenotype. A scoring system, using immunophenotyping outlined in Table 12.8, has been developed in order to help differentiate CLL from other lymphoproliferative disorders. CLL will achieve a score of three or above, whereas other lymphoproliferative diseases should score less than three.

Cross references

Characteristic immunophenotyping results for CLL can be found in the immunophenotyping section of Chapter 10.

Examination of a bone marrow trephine is an essential component of the diagnostic process and indicates the level of bone marrow infiltration by malignant lymphocytes. A diffuse pattern of infiltration is associated with a poor prognosis as it indicates advanced disease. The sheets of malignant lymphocytes occupying the bone marrow compromise haemopoiesis leading to anaemia, neutropenia, and thrombocytopenia.

Significant progress has been made in correlating disease behaviour and patient survival with the molecular and cytogenetic events occurring within CLL/SLL. The identification of two distinct CLL pathologies based around *IGVH* mutational status has aided our understanding of disease behaviour. One CLL subgroup shows evidence of *IGVH* somatic hypermutation, whilst the other possesses unmutated *IGVH*. *IGVH* hypermutated cases are associated with a better prognosis than those cases failing to demonstrate hypermutated *IGVH*.

Zeta associated protein 70 (ZAP-70) is a tyrosine kinase signalling molecule not usually found in normal circulating B lymphocytes. The association of ZAP-70 with unmutated *IGVH* has enabled routine laboratories to quantify ZAP-70 using immunophenotyping technologies to provide data in the absence of performing complex and expensive *IGVH* sequencing. However, this is still a relatively demanding technique to set up, and many laboratories have opted not to test ZAP-70 using their own equipment.

Cytogenetic studies have demonstrated that up to 80% of patients exhibit chromosomal abnormalities, the majority of which can be used for prognostication.

TABLE 12.8 **CLL immunophenotyping score.**

CD marker	Score	
	1	0
CD5	positive	negative
CD23	positive	negative
FMC7	negative	positive
SmIg	weak	moderate/strong
CD22/CD79b	weak/negative	moderate/strong

Key: score >3 = CLL; <3 = other B-cell malignancy.

BOX 12.1 *Guidelines*

The British Committee for Standards in Haematology (BCSH) has guidelines for the diagnosis and management of CLL published on its website http://www.bcshguidelines.com.

Del13q14.3, occurring in approximately 35% of cases, is associated with a good prognosis. Patients with this deletion, as an isolated genetic abnormality, have been shown to have a better prognosis than patients demonstrating a normal karyotype. Patients with del13q14.3 have a reported survival of 132 months compared with 120 months for patients with a normal karyotype.

Deletion of 17p13 and loss of p53 occurs in approximately 7% of cases and is universally associated with a poor prognosis, with survival as low as 36 months in these patients. In addition, the loss of 11q23, the locus for the tumour suppressor gene ataxia telangiectasia mutated (*ATM*), is also associated with a poor prognosis and is reported in approximately 20% of cases. Isolated 11q23 abnormalities are associated with a survival of approximately 84 months.

Other important prognostic markers that will be assessed in the routine diagnostic laboratory include CD38. CD38 expression is associated with a poor prognosis, but expression of CD38 is thought to vary over the course of the disease. Lymphocyte doubling time (LDT) is an important indicator of disease progression and prognosis. CLL/SLL lymphocytes have a low proliferative rate, with high lymphocyte numbers being a consequence of accumulation following the failure of apoptosis rather than rapid proliferation. However, patients with an LDT of less than 12 months have a worse prognosis than those with an LDT in excess of 12 months. Beta 2-microglobulin (β_2m) and lactate dehydrogenase (LDH) can easily be measured by the clinical biochemistry department, and patients showing a raised β_2m and LDH have a worse prognosis than those with a normal β_2m and LDH. β_2m forms part of the MHC class I structure expressed on B cells, whilst LDH is a useful marker of cell turnover and tumour size.

Recent evidence suggests that the measurement of serum-free light chains in CLL/SLL will also aid in prognostication. Recent research by Pratt *et al.* published in the *British Journal of Haematology* shows that abnormal serum-free light chain ratios ($\kappa : \lambda$) can be used as a prognostic indicator, especially when combined with *IGVH* mutational status. Although more research needs to be completed in this area, patients with unmutated *IGVH* and an *elevated* $\kappa : \lambda$ ratio had a worse prognosis than those with a normal ratio. Patients demonstrating mutated *IGVH* and a reduced $\kappa : \lambda$ ratio also had a worse prognosis than those with normal $\kappa : \lambda$ ratios.

SELF-CHECK 12.5

Describe how CLL has been subdivided into two different pathologies.

B-cell prolymphocytic leukaemia

B-cell prolymphocytic leukaemia (B-PLL) is a rare, aggressive, B-cell lymphoproliferative disorder compared with CLL/SLL and accounts for 1–2% of all chronic lymphoid leukaemias. Patients present at a mean age of 70 years, with splenomegaly, absence of lymphadenopathy, and a very high WBC count (>100 × 10^9/L). The threshold for the diagnosis of B-PLL is 55% prolymphocytes in the peripheral blood, although in most cases patients will have in excess of 90% prolymphocytes. Figure 12.3 shows typical prolymphocytes in a case of B-PLL.

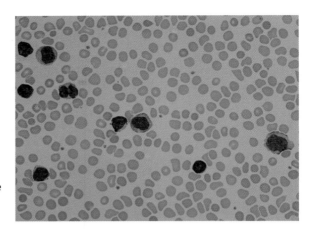

FIGURE 12.3

Prolymphocytic leukaemia. The lymphocytes here are pleomorphic, with typical prolymphocytes present. The chromatin is not as clumped in these cases as in CLL. Many of the cells contain prominent nucleoli. Image courtesy of Jackie Warne, Haematology department, Queen Alexandra Hospital, Portsmouth.

The bone marrow from many of these patients shows a marked infiltration by prolymphocytes with either an interstitial/diffuse or diffuse distribution pattern which disrupts normal haemopoiesis. This infiltrative pattern is present in excess of 50% of patients at the time of diagnosis and manifests itself clinically as anaemia and thrombocytopenia. Other patients may show a nodular distribution of prolymphocytes within the bone marrow, which does not disrupt normal haemopoiesis.

The B-PLL immunophenotype is strongly positive for: CD19, CD20 and CD22, smIg; and FMC7; and CD79b, CD5, and CD23 are variably expressed.

Cytogenetically, a number of abnormalities are associated with B-PLL. Mutations involving chromosome 14 occur in excess of 50% of cases, and t(11;14)(q13;q32) has been described. It is now believed that cases resembling B-PLL but harbouring t(11;14) are actually a variant of mantle cell lymphoma rather than B-PLL. Other mutations include the deletion of 17p13, 13q14.3, and 11q23 as noted in B-CLL/SLL.

There is no correlation between prognosis in B-PLL and the prognostic indicators in B-CLL/SLL. Examination of *IGVH*, CD38, ZAP-70 and del(17p) in cases of B-PLL are not associated with an adverse prognosis. Overall survival is in the range of 30–50 months from diagnosis.

Splenic marginal zone lymphoma

Splenic marginal zone lymphoma (SMZL) is invariably associated with splenomegaly in the absence of lymphadenopathy, and occurs in approximately 2% of patients diagnosed with a lymphoid malignancy. The median age of patients at presentation is 65 years. The bone marrow always shows signs of infiltration, with any of the patterns of infiltration occurring— nodular, interstitial, paratrabecular, or diffuse. Characteristically, an intrasinusiodal pattern of infiltration, that is, malignant cells within the verais sinuses, is noted, helping to differentiate SMZL from all other types of low-grade lymphoma. A bone marrow trephine is usually more useful for the diagnosis of SMZL than a bone marrow aspirate, and often, because the malignant B cells express CD20, anti-CD20 should be used to visualize the extent of bone marrow infiltration by SMZL cells.

Cross reference

Bone marrow assessment was discussed in Chapter 10.

The peripheral blood contains variable numbers of malignant lymphocytes with an increase in the absolute lymphocyte count occurring in approximately 75% of cases. Villous lymphocytes are apparent in 15% of cases and are demonstrated in Figure 12.4.

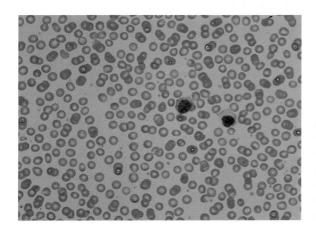

FIGURE 12.4

Splenic marginal zone lymphoma. Heterogeneous cells with villous protrusions of the cell membrane are typical features. The nucleus contains clumped chromatin and has a rounded appearance. Note the presence of rouleaux, suggesting an increased paraprotein concentration. Image courtesy of Jackie Warne, Haematology department, Queen Alexandra Hospital, Portsmouth.

Signs and symptoms of anaemia occur in approximately 64%, and severe thrombocytopenia features in 15% of patients. Neutropenia is also often apparent, leading to an increased risk of opportunistic infections. Reduction in the platelet, neutrophil, and red cell counts may be a consequence of splenic sequestration, bone marrow infiltration, or autoimmunity.

Approximately 50% of patients demonstrate a monoclonal band—usually IgM, IgG, or, very rarely, IgA—using serum electrophoresis, but with serum concentrations generally <20 g/L. Serum lactate dehydrogenase is usually within the reference range, whereas β_2m tends to be raised.

Immunophenotypically, CD19, CD20, CD22, CD79b, and FMC7 are all positive. There is always evidence of light-chain restriction, and variable expression of surface immunoglobulins. The majority of patients express both IgM and IgD with a minority expressing IgM but not IgD (IgM+IgD-). IgG surface expression is more frequent than IgA expression but not as common as IgM/IgD expression. CD5, CD10, and CD23 are not generally expressed on SMZL cells.

Cytogenetically, there are no characteristic chromosomal abnormalities diagnostic for SMZL, although the most common features involve the rearrangement or loss of chromosome 7 and trisomy 3. Mutations of *TP53* have been variably reported, but only occur in advanced disease.

Clinically, SMZL is a stable disease, with median survival between 8 and 13 years. Approximately 10% of patients transform to an aggressive lymphoma.

Follicular lymphoma

Follicular lymphomas comprise approximately 30% of all non-Hodgkin lymphomas and, as its name suggests, in the vast majority of cases cell growth follows a follicular pattern. In some cases a combination of follicular and diffuse cell growth is present. Within the diffuse regions of growth, sclerosis will often be present.

As with normal lymphoid follicles, in follicular lymphoma, a combination of large, non-cleaved highly proliferative centroblasts are present accompanied by smaller, cleaved, non-proliferative centrocytes.

Sometimes there will be evidence of follicular lymphoma cells within the peripheral blood. These cells are often small with pale cytoplasm, with a proportion of cells showing a nuclear cleft. Figure 12.5 shows an example of follicular lymphoma cells in the peripheral blood of a patient in leukaemic phase. Note the small cell size and the distinctive nuclear clefts.

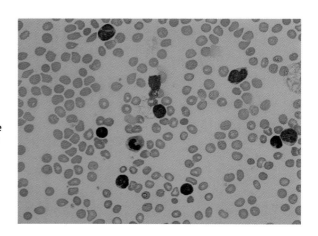

FIGURE 12.5

Follicular lymphoma. Predominantly composed of small lymphocytes; a thin rim of cytoplasm is a typical feature. Some nucleoli are apparent, see top left hand cell. Nuclear clefts are characteristic features of centrocytes, from which follicular lymphoma originates. Please also note variations in red cell shape and size called aniso-poikilocytosis. Image courtesy of Jackie Warne, Haematology department, Queen Alexandra Hospital, Portsmouth.

Follicular lymphoma is graded according to the number of centroblasts and centrocytes found in the biopsy, as measured when examining the tissue using high-power fields (hpf). Grading ranges from 1 to 3, based on the number of centroblasts preset per high power field. Grade 3 in further subdivided into 3A and 3B according to the presence or absence of centrocytes in the assessed follicles. The greater the number of centroblasts, the higher the assigned grade. Cases demonstrating largely diffuse growth accompanied by occasional follicles and large numbers of centroblasts should be considered *diffuse large B-cell lymphoma with follicular lymphoma*.

Cross reference

Diffuse large B-cell lymphoma is outlined later in this chapter.

The immunophenotype of follicular lymphoma cells is CD19+, CD5–, CD10+. If there is any doubt as to the diagnosis from morphology alone, CD10-positivity distinguishes follicular lymphoma from the other main types of B-cell lymphoma.

The translocation t(14;18)(q32;q21) is present in 70–95% of cases of follicular lymphoma. This translocation leads to the overexpression of the anti-apoptotic protein BCL2. Following translocation, *BCL2* is moved from its original locus 18q21 to the *IGH* locus at 14q32. BCL2 is now under the transcriptional control of the *IGH* promoter, leading to BCL2 upregulation resulting in continued cell survival.

In normal B cells, BCL2 is often over-expressed during Ig rearrangement, meaning that apoptosis is not initiated, ensuring the cells survive. Following Ig rearrangement, BCL2 should be repressed enabling apoptosis of poorly functional/non-functional B cells to occur.

Key Points

t(14;18)(q32;q21) has been identified in B cells of normal individuals, implying that this translocation alone is insufficient to cause lymphomagenesis, conforming to Knudson's hypothesis. The frequency of t(14;18) appears to increase with age, and higher levels of this translocation are seen in smokers compared to non-smokers.

Disease progression is common in follicular lymphoma and although delaying the beginning of treatment in some patients in favour of a watch-and-wait policy is common practice, at autopsy up to 70% of patients show evidence of high-grade transformation. These high-grade malignancies are very aggressive and often fail to respond to therapy. The majority of patients survive for less than 12 months following transformation.

SELF-CHECK 12.6

Outline the role of t(14;18)(q32;q21) in the pathogenesis of follicular lymphoma.

Hairy cell leukaemia

Hairy cell leukaemia (HCL) accounts for approximately 2% of all lymphoid leukaemias, with patients presenting at a median age of 50 years. HCL is associated with the accumulation of malignant lymphocytes with a mature B-cell phenotype.

Patients present invariably with splenomegaly and the FBC shows pancytopenia. Even though the patient is pancytopenic, an absolute monocytopenia is a typical finding in HCL. HCL is often a difficult disease to diagnose because low numbers of leukaemic cells are found in the peripheral blood. Morphologically, these B cells have an oval or indented nucleus and fine hair-like projections protruding from the cell surface—the defining morphological feature of the disease. Figure 12.6 shows a typical peripheral blood film from a patient diagnosed with HCL.

The spleen, liver and bone marrow become infiltrated by hairy cells, but the lymph nodes tend to be spared. Synthesis and secretion of basic fibroblast growth factor (bFGF) and tumour growth factor-β1 (TGFβ1) stimulate fibroblast proliferation within the bone marrow, resulting in marrow fibrosis. This bone marrow fibrosis can lead to the aspirate producing a dry tap, so a trephine biopsy is a useful diagnostic tool in cases of HCL. The combination of bone marrow infiltration and fibrosis is thought to be predominantly responsible for pancytopenia at presentation, although cell sequestration by the enlarged spleen accompanied by haemodilution is also likely to reduce peripheral blood counts, contributing to anaemia, bruising, and opportunistic infection.

In over 85% of cases, HCL cells show evidence of somatic hypermutation, indicating these cells have progressed through the germinal centre; and HCL cells express IgM, IgG, and IgA on the cell surface in 40% of patients. This unusual expression of surface immunoglobulin is found in no other lymphoproliferative disorder, and suggests HCL is derived from cells undergoing isotype-switching. Gene expression profiling suggests that HCL cells are actually derived from mutated memory B cells and as such have completed their transit through the germinal centre.

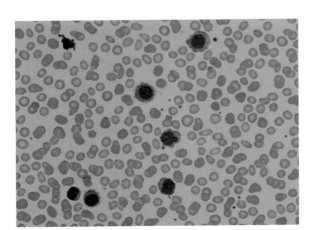

FIGURE 12.6

Hairy cell leukaemia. Numerous large lymphocytes, each with villous projections. The cytoplasm in this case is deeply basophilic. The nuclei in most cases are round or oval. One nucleus shows a small protrusion (centre), and another (bottom centre) appears folded. Image courtesy of Jackie Warne, Haematology department, Queen Alexandra Hospital, Portsmouth.

The 10-year survival of HCL patients is over 90% following successful therapy with interferon-α and the purine analogues cladribine or pentostatin. The anti-CD20 monoclonal antibody, rituximab, has proven beneficial in treating HCL when combined with one of the purine analogues.

SELF-CHECK 12.7

What is the normal HCL cell counterpart? Explain how you have made this determination.

Lymphoplasmacytic lymphoma

Lymphoplasmacytic lymphoma (LPL) is a heterogeneous lymphoid malignancy associated with the accumulation of small B lymphocytes, plasmacytoid cells, and plasma cells within the bone marrow, lymph nodes or spleen. It is derived from a mutated post-germinal centre B cell prior to differentiation into a plasma cell. Figure 12.7 shows a blood film containing a number of small lymphocytes in a case of LPL. A subtype of LPL called Waldenström **macroglobulinaemia** (WM) is diagnosed following cytological findings associated with LPL infiltration of the bone marrow, often accompanied by mast cell infiltration, and evidence of an IgM paraprotein.

> **macroglobulinaemia**
> Large amounts of big proteins circulating in the blood, for example, IgM antibodies.

Studies examining the *IGVH* genes associated with LPL/WM have shown that somatic hypermutation has occurred and therefore these cells have passed through the germinal centre. Furthermore, there is a lack of intraclonal *IGVH* sequence variation in individual tumours—suggesting the cells, rather than being of a late germinal centre origin, are of a post-germinal centre origin.

Complicating features occur in patients expressing high levels of IgM paraprotein, where this can result in an increased blood viscosity (called **hyperviscosity**), and associated with cardiovascular complications in some patients. Occasionally, the paraprotein precipitates and aggregates at low temperatures forming **cryoglobulins**. In some cases, the paraproteins have autoreactivity with host antigens leading to autoimmune complications.

Immunophenotypically, these cells express CD19, CD20, and surface immunoglobulin. In WM, this is restricted to IgM, although IgG or, rarely, IgA may be expressed in other LPL. CD138 expression represents plasmacytic differentiation and should be positive in a subset of cells in LPL/WM.

Cytogenetically, deletions of chromosome 6q21 are found in approximately 42% of patients, whilst trisomy 4 is found in approximately 20% of patients. On a number of occasions,

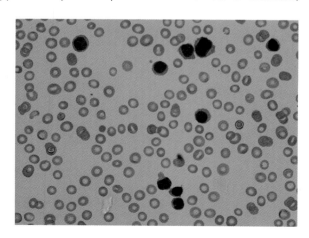

FIGURE 12.7
Lymphoplasmacytic lymphoma. Lymphocytes are numerous and demonstrate cytoplasmic basophilia. Image courtesy of Jackie Warne, Haematology department, Queen Alexandra Hospital, Portsmouth.

t(9;14)(p13;q32) has been reported to be associated with LPL/WM, but it now appears that t(9;14) (p13;q32) is associated with a range of lymphoid malignancies.

LPL/WM is associated with a median survival of approximately 60 months.

We should now consider a range of other post germinal centre malignancies, the plasma cell neoplasms.

Plasma cell neoplasms

Plasma cells are post-germinal centre antibody-secreting cells. A wide range of plasma cell neoplasms are recognized, and in this section we will look at some of the most common. Figure 12.8 provides a brief summary of the range of plasma cell neoplasms recognized by the WHO. Only plasma cell myeloma and related disorders, monoclonal gammopathy of undetermined significance, extraosseous plasmacytoma and solitary plasmacytoma of bone are discussed in this section.

Plasma cell myeloma

Plasma cell myeloma, also called multiple myeloma, is a malignancy of plasma cells with a median age at presentation of 70 years, and a survival between 3 and 5 years.

Patients usually present with bone pain or pathological fractures, and demonstrate signs and symptoms of anaemia, recurrent infections and renal failure. Serum electrophoresis demonstrates a monoclonal band, called an **M-protein** (monoclonal protein) or paraprotein, within the electrophoretogram. M-proteins are either whole immunoglobulins or just the free

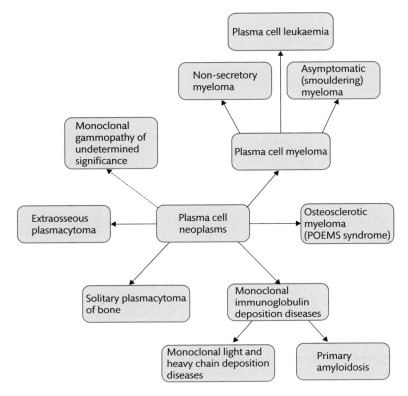

FIGURE 12.8

A chart to show the different types of plasma cell neoplasm and the way in which some of these conditions inter-relate. These conditions are all represented in the WHO classification system although are not all discussed in this text.

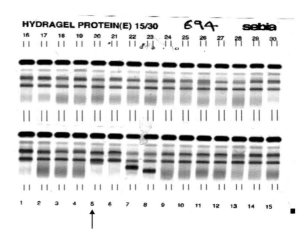

FIGURE 12.9

Serum electrophoresis. Of particular interest are patients 5, 7 and 8, all of whom show additional bands. Patient 5 shows a band within the β-region and patients 7 and 8 show distinctive bands within the γ region. Densitometry and immunofixation is performed to attempt to quantify and identify the species of abnormal proteins. Image courtesy of Rajee Goswami, Southampton General Hospital.

light-chain component. Urinary analysis shows paraproteins, called **Bence-Jones proteins**, in approximately 80% of cases.

Figure 12.9 shows an electrophoretogram for serum electrophoresis for a wide range of patients. If you look along the bottom row you will see patients 5, 7 and 8 all show distinct bands. Patient 5 has an additional band within the β-region, whilst patients 7 and 8 have dark bands within the γ-region. These bands are paraproteins. Figure 12.10 shows the densitometric analysis of the electrophoretogram for patient 5. Densitometry is used to quantify the size

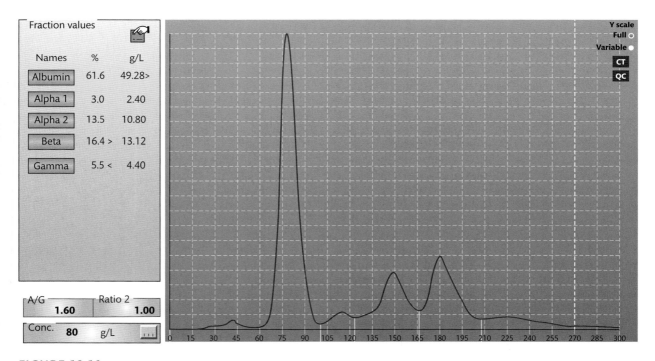

FIGURE 12.10

Results of densitometric analysis. Patient 5 showed a total protein concentration of 80g/L. The major species, albumin, gives a large peak at position 80. The beta region (position 150) is increased in size whereas the gamma region (position 180) is reduced, as indicated in the fraction values on the left. The increased protein band visualized on the electrophoretogram (Figure 12.9) is confirmed within the beta region using this technique. Higher levels of paraprotein are expected in myeloma, and it is likely this patient is receiving treatment. Image courtesy of Rajee Goswami, Southampton General Hospital.

BOX 12.2 Bence-Jones proteins

Although Bence-Jones proteins (BJP) in multiple myeloma were first described by Dr Henry Bence-Jones in 1847, the nature of BJP was first investigated and reported by Edelman and Gally in 1962. BJP were identified as the light-chain components of immunoglobulin, comprising the M-protein. Heavy chains are too large to pass through the glomerular filter.

Identification of BJP can be performed from urinary samples, and the monoclonal nature of these proteins can be established using immunofixation.

Paraproteins are excreted in the urine before accumulating in the plasma. Only when renal excretion is compromised do paraproteins accumulate in the plasma.

of the protein bands. As you can see, peak size matches the banding pattern. In this patient, the paraprotein is hidden within the β-region.

Figure 12.11 demonstrates the result of immunofixation for patient 5. The electrophoretic strip on the left demonstrates a match to the original in Figure 12.9. We can identify from this immunofixation that this patient has an IgA κ paraprotein.

Investigation of suspected plasma cell myeloma should include the following:

- Full blood count
- Urea and electrolytes (U&Es)
- Serum calcium
- Serum creatinine
- Serum electrophoresis
- Erythrocyte sedimentation rate (ESR)
- Blood film
- Bone marrow biopsy

In addition, radiographic investigations should be included, especially in regions of bone pain to identify the presence of **osteolytic lesions**.

The full blood count may show a low haemoglobin concentration and a normal mean cell volume, the typical findings of a normocytic normochromic anaemia. Neutropenia may also be present, which may explain the occurrence of recurrent infections in a proportion of these patients.

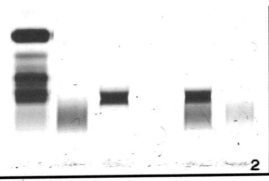

ELP G A M K L

FIGURE 12.11

Using immunofixation, a distinct monoclonal band is identified as IgA, also demonstrating κ light chain restriction. The electrophoretic strip (labelled ELP) on the left shows the distribution of proteins in the patient's plasma. Image courtesy of Rajee Goswami, Southampton General Hospital.

Prior to the microscopic examination of a blood film, the macroscopic examination of the blood film following Romanowsky-staining is usually the first indication of increased protein content in the plasma. The blood smear will have a deep-blue coloration—a consequence of the Romanowsky stain interacting with the fixed paraprotein on the blood film. Microscopically, paraprotein will be apparent as **background staining**. In cases with a paraprotein, rouleaux (red cells stacking upon one another) formation will be apparent on the blood film. Absence of these staining characteristics does not exclude a diagnosis of myeloma as these are all a consequence of raised serum paraprotein levels.

In patients with a raised plasma paraprotein concentration, the ESR will be raised.

Biochemical analysis will show a raised serum calcium concentration, called **hypercalcaemia**—caused by increased bone degradation in a number of these patients (discussed later in this section). Serum creatinine will be raised in patients with renal impairment, secondary to increased paraprotein concentrations and hypercalcaemia. In addition, serum electrophoresis demonstrates an M-protein which can be present within any region. The frequencies of the different M-proteins is outlined in Table 12.9. The use of immunofixation—a technique used to identify proteins within a sample using monoclonal antibodies—will enable the monoclonal or polyclonal nature of the proteins to be established. Total protein levels may be increased in patients with plasma cell myeloma. Conversely, there may also be a decrease in the other immunoglobulins—**immune paresis**. Immune paresis can be seen in up to 90% of patients with plasma cell myeloma.

background staining
The uptake of Romanowsky stain by plasma-derived paraprotein fixed on the microscope slide

immune paresis
This describes the reduction of all immunoglobulins in a patient's serum, except for the paraprotein.

SELF-CHECK 12.8

Outline the key laboratory findings associated with plasma cell myeloma.

Cytogenetic changes in plasma cell disorders

Cytogenetic abnormalities demonstrated by FISH are found in more than 90% of patients. Approximately 40–50% of cases possessing chromosomal translocations involve 14q32, combining the IgH locus with:

- 11q13—*CCND1*—cyclin D1
- 4p16.3—FGFR3/MMSET (fibroblast growth factor receptor 3/multiple myeloma SET domain)
- 16q23—*CMAF*—cellular **musculoaponeurotic fibrosarcoma** proto-oncogene
- 6p21—*CCND3*—cyclin D3
- 20q11—*MAFB*—c-MAF-related gene

musculoaponeurotic
Pertaining to a fibrous or membranous sheath that connects muscle to bones.

fibrosarcoma
Tumour developing in the fibrous connective tissue.

Monosomy 13 or del(13q14) occurs in approximately 15–40% of patients and trisomy 3, 5, 7, 9, 11, 15, 19, and 21 are also common features. Up to 10% of patients with an abnormal karyotype demonstrate gains of chromosome 1q. In approximately 30–40% of cases, patients demonstrate *RAS* mutations, p16 gene methylation in 20–30%, *MYC* rearrangements in 10–15%, and *TP53* mutations in 5–10%. These mutations either induce an increase in proliferative capacity within the malignant cells, or a dysregulated range of tumour suppressor proteins.

Myeloma-related bone disease

A frequent finding in patients with plasma cell myeloma and related diseases is bone disease, with areas containing osteolytic or 'punched-out lesions' apparent on X-ray analysis. This bone

TABLE 12.9 M-proteins identified in plasma cell myeloma.

M-protein	Frequency (%)
IgG	53
IgA	22
Light chain	20
Non secretory	3
IgD/IgE	1.5
IgM	0.5

disease is responsible for the bone pain often experienced by patients, and also accounts for the high frequency of pathological fractures associated with plasma cell neoplasms.

Malignant plasma cells are often associated with areas of active bone resorption. Bone remodelling is an essential process for maintaining bone architecture, involving both bone resorption and bone deposition through the balanced action of osteoclasts and osteoblasts, respectively. Increased activity of osteoclasts, and a relative reduction in osteoblast numbers and activity during the later stages of myeloma, leads to a loss of localized bone density and the accumulation of osteolytic lesions.

Secretion of osteoclast activating factors (OAFs) is essential in the development of myeloma-associated bone disease. Chemical signalling between plasma cells and normal osteoclasts results from localization of these plasma cells to areas in close proximity to osteoclasts. There are two important processes involved in myeloma-related bone disease, including the upregulation of macrophage inflammatory protein-1α (MIP-1α) and dysregulation of the *osteoprotegerin/Receptor activator of nuclear factor κB ligand/Receptor activator of nuclear factor κB* (OPG/RANKL/RANK) pathway. These processes are illustrated in Figure 12.12.

MIP-1α is a chemokine thought to be responsible for the proliferation of osteoclasts in regions occupied by malignant plasma cells. MIP-1α levels increase in two ways:

- MIP-1α is synthesized by malignant plasma cells.
- MIP-1α synthesis and secretion can be induced from osteoblast-like cells in response to interleukin 1 (IL-1) and tumour necrosis factor-α (TNFα)—both synthesized and secreted by malignant plasma cells.

MIP-1α binds to the chemokine receptors CCR1 and CCR5 on the surface of osteoclasts, and induces proliferation and activation of these cells and uncoupling of the bone remodelling balance.

RANK is a member of the TNF superfamily of receptors and is expressed on osteoclasts. The binding partner for RANK—RANKL (RANK ligand)—is expressed on the surface of osteoblasts, and interaction between RANKL and RANK results in:

- Increased osteoclast differentiation
- Increased osteoclast activity
- Inhibition of osteoclast apoptosis
- Increased bone resorption

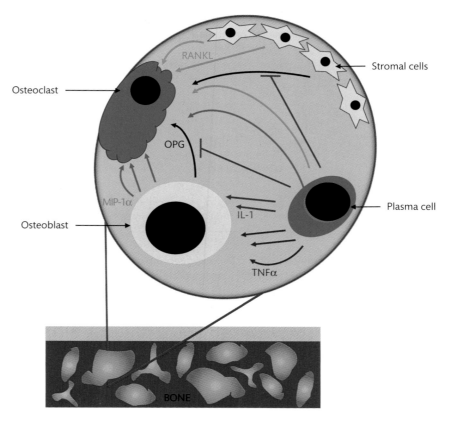

FIGURE 12.12

Pathogenesis of myeloma-related bone disease. Malignant plasma cells accumulate within the bone marrow and interact with a variety of cells. The secretion of IL-1 (brown arrows) and TNFα (purple arrows) stimulates osteoblasts to synthesize and secrete macrophage inflammatory protein -1α (MIP-1α) (blue arrows). MIP-1α is also synthesized by the plasma cells and increases osteoclast proliferation. Receptor activator of nuclear factor κB ligand (RANKL) (green arrows) is secreted by malignant plasma cells and bone marrow stromal cells resulting in an increase in the number of osteoclasts and their activity in the local area. Osteoprotegerin (OPG) (black arrows), a negative regulator of RANKL secreted by osteoblasts and bone marrow stromal cells, is inhibited in myeloma. The net result is an increase in irreversible bone resorption.

The expression of soluble OPG by bone marrow stromal cells and osteoblasts inhibits the interaction between RANK and RANKL, thereby limiting the differentiation and activation of osteoclasts. In plasma cell myeloma there is a decrease in the synthesis of OPG and, importantly, an increase in the expression of RANKL, not only by bone marrow stromal cells, but also by the malignant plasma cells. This upregulation of RANKL and downregulation of OPG favours the osteolytic activity of osteoclasts leading to a net loss of bone density in those areas.

The diagnosis of plasma cell myeloma must be considered in all patients demonstrating an M-protein. There are two distinct types of myeloma: symptomatic plasma cell myeloma and asymptomatic (or smouldering) plasma cell myeloma. The most important feature in discriminating between the two is the presence of organ or tissue damage, including hypercalcaemia, renal insufficiency, anaemia, and bone lesions—described by the acronym **CRAB**. It is important to recognize that these symptoms are not specific to plasma cell myeloma and patients must be fully investigated prior to a diagnosis and subsequent treatment.

SELF-CHECK 12.9

Describe the process through which myeloma-related bone disease develops.

Symptomatic plasma cell myeloma

Patients show evidence of CRAB and harbour a clonal population of plasma cells, either in the bone marrow or as a plasmacytoma. In most patients, at least 10% of the nucleated cells within the bone marrow are plasma cells, but this figure is not considered an important diagnostic threshold. Specific threshold concentrations of M-protein within the plasma or urine are not considered as part of the classification requirement because these are so variable between patients. Depending on the type of paraprotein produced by the plasma cells, many patients will have plasma IgG levels in excess of 30 g/L or an IgA concentration greater than 25 g/L. Some patients present with CRAB but do not fulfil these paraprotein criteria.

Asymptomatic (smouldering) myeloma

Approximately 8% of patients are diagnosed with asymptomatic plasma cell myeloma. The diagnostic requirements of asymptomatic myeloma are much more prescriptive than those required for symptomatic plasma cell myeloma, primarily because there are no overt signs of organ or tissue damage. In order for the diagnosis of asymptomatic myeloma to be made, a serum concentration of M-proteins in excess of 30 g/L should be present with or without the presence of a clonal population of plasma cells within the bone marrow.

Patients with asymptomatic plasma cell myeloma may progress to symptomatic plasma cell myeloma.

Non-secretory myeloma

This occurs in approximately 3% of cases of myeloma and is associated with a lack of M-protein secretion. Using immunohistochemical analysis, a distinction should be made between cases showing cytoplasmic M-protein and cases in which no M-protein is synthesized. The behaviour and treatment of these variants is identical. Careful consideration of a diagnosis of non-secretory myeloma should be given for patients demonstrating clinical signs of myeloma with absence of an M-protein. Bone marrow biopsy and histochemical investigations are indicated to ensure this diagnosis is not missed.

Plasma cell leukaemia

Plasma cell leukaemia (PCL) is defined by the presence of:

- 2×10^9/L plasma cells or more in the peripheral blood.
- Plasma cells comprising 20% of the total white blood cell count—which is particularly important to consider in patients with a low WBC count.

PCL can be either a primary or secondary disease. Primary PCL occurs in about 5% of patients from presentation with no previous medical history or evidence of plasma cell myeloma. Secondary PCL is the leukaemic phase of an established plasma cell myeloma. Primary PCL is considered to be a separate disease entity due to its different disease behaviour, cytogenetic, and immunophenotypic profile. PCL is associated with considerable extramedullary infiltration and aggressive behaviour.

The peripheral blood cell morphology for a patient with PCL can be seen in Figure 12.13.

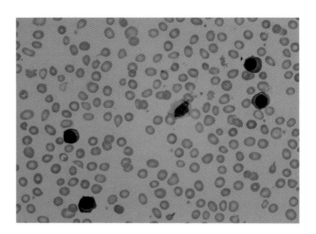

FIGURE 12.13

Plasma cell leukaemia. The presence of circulating plasma cells showing distinctive eccentric nuclei with a pale Golgi zone called the perinuclear halo. Cytoplasm is deeply basophilic. The blood film also shows an apparent thrombocytopenia and tear drop poikilocytes. Image courtesy of Jackie Warne, Haematology department, Queen Alexandra Hospital, Portsmouth.

Monoclonal gammopathy of undetermined significance (MGUS)

MGUS is a frequently encountered plasma cell disorder within haematology, and is not really considered to be a plasma cell neoplasm as it does not always progress to an overt malignancy. MGUS is found in approximately 3% of all individuals over the age of 50 years rising to 5% of individuals aged 70 years and over.

The vast majority of patients are diagnosed following investigation for a completely unrelated disorder; these patients have an M-protein of less than 30 g/L identified and no evidence of Bence-Jones proteinuria. There should be an absence of CRAB and full blood count indices should be normal.

Approximately 46% of patients demonstrate 14q32 translocations, the most common of which is t(11;14)(q13;q32)—which result in the overexpression of cyclin D1.

The risk of transformation to a malignant disease is approximately 1% per year for IgG MGUS, rising to approximately 1.5% a year for MGUS secreting IgA. Deranged serum free light-chain ratios (κ:λ) may help predict the risk of progression.

To date, two forms of MGUS have been identified based on the following paraproteins:

- IgM paraprotein
- IgG or IgA paraprotein

IgM-related MGUS is thought to be derived from a B-cell population failing to undergo Ig class-switching, although there is evidence of somatic hypermutation. Conversely, IgG- and IgA-related cases are derived from a post-germinal centre plasma cell.

IgG paraproteins are the most common, occurring in approximately 75% of cases, followed by IgM (15%) and IgA (10%). Should transformation occur, IgM-secreting cells are likely to transform to lymphoplasmacytic lymphoma or Waldenström macroglobulinaemia, whilst IgG or IgA MGUS may progress to plasma cell myeloma or amyloidosis.

In cases where MGUS is diagnosed, a watch-and-wait strategy is employed, ensuring patients are monitored every six months to determine whether the disease remains stable or the paraprotein concentration is increasing.

BOX 12.3 *UK Myeloma Forum guidelines*

The British Committee for Standards in Haematology have newly published guidelines (2009) entitled 'UK Myeloma Forum (UKMF) and Nordic Myeloma Study Group (NMSG): Guidelines for the investigation of newly detected M-proteins and the management of Monoclonal Gammopathy of Undetermined Significance (MGUS)'.http://www.bcshguidelines.com.

Solitary plasmacytoma of bone and extraosseous plasmacytoma

A plasmacytoma is an accumulation of malignant plasma cells within a particular tissue type. As their names suggest, the malignancy is restricted to skeletal areas in solitary plasmacytoma of the bone, but can be found at any site except the bone in extraosseous plasmacytoma. The prognosis for both sets of diseases is reasonable to good, with one-third of patients surviving beyond 10 years with bony disease and 70% surviving beyond 10 years in extraosseous cases. An M-protein is found in a variable number of cases. There is a risk of pathological fractures at the site of the plasmacytoma in bony disease, otherwise neither disease is associated with myeloma-related symptoms.

Now we have concluded our section on plasma cell neoplasms we should continue our discussion of mature B-cell malignancies. The next range of diseases we should consider are the marginal zone lymphomas.

Marginal zone lymphomas

Marginal zone lymphomas (MZL) are a diverse group of lymphoid malignancies, and according to the WHO, can be subdivided into:

- Extranodal marginal zone lymphoma of mucosa associated lymphoid tissue (MALT lymphoma)
- Nodal marginal zone lymphoma

Each of these conditions will be considered in turn.

Extranodal marginal zone lymphoma of mucosa associated lymphoid tissue (MALT lymphoma)

Extranodal MALT lymphomas account for 5–8% of non-Hodgkin lymphomas and develop as a consequence of:

- The transformation of pre-existing previously normal MALT tissue, for example in the **Peyer's patches** in the gut.
- The acquisition of MALT in unusual sites.

A significant number of cases are attributable to chronic antigenic stimulation, by infection or inflammation, leading to the hyperproliferation of B cells and lymphomagenesis. Infectious agents associated with the development of extranodal MALT lymphoma include:

Peyer's patches
A group of lymph nodes in the wall of the ileum.

cutaneous
Pertaining to the skin.

ocular adnexa
The accessory structures of the eye; they include the eyelids, lacrimal glands, orbit and paraorbital areas.

- *Helicobacter pylori*—gastric MALT lymphoma
- *Borrelia burgdorferi*—**cutaneous** MALT lymphoma
- *Chlamydia psittaci*—**ocular adnexal** MALT lymphomas
- *Camphylobacter jejuni*—immunoproliferative small intestine disease (IPSID)/α-chain disease

and may also occur in autoimmune conditions such as:

- Hashimoto's thyroiditis
- Sjögren's syndrome

Following the isolation of the causative pathogen, treating patients with specific antibiotics can, in a significant number of cases, induce regression of the MALT lymphoma and lead to cure.

Typically, marginal zone lymphoma cells are morphologically heterogeneous—representing a wide variety of marginal zone-derived B-lineage cells responding to antigen. Immunophenotypically, these cells express surface and cytoplasmic immunoglobulin. IgM is more frequently expressed than IgG. B-cell antigens CD19, CD20, CD22, CD79a, and CD79b are expressed, whilst CD3, CD5, CD10, CD11c, and CD23 are not expressed in these malignancies.

Approximately 60% of cases of extranodal MALT lymphoma demonstrate cytogenetic abnormalities. The most frequent translocation, occurring in approximately 30% of cases, is t(11;18)(q21;q21), although t(1;14)(p22;q32) and t(14;18)(q32;q21) are also found. We will now look at each of these translocations in turn.

t(11;18)(q21;q21)

This translocation fuses the *API2* (apoptosis inhibitor-2) gene, located at 11q21 with the *MALT* gene, locus 18q21—leading to the production of the fusion gene *API2–MALT1*. API2 is a member of the inhibitor of apoptosis (IAP) gene family, whilst MALT1 has been identified as a **paracaspase**, activated following the formation of a complex with BCL10. As a consequence of the activation of MALT1 via BCL10-binding, **ubiquitination** of the inhibitor of nuclear factor κB (IκB) occurs, leading to increased NFκB signalling. This in turn results in the overexpression of a number of NFκB regulated genes, many of which are involved in apoptotic inhibition. Interestingly, one of the downstream targets of NFκB is API2, the expression of which is increased following signalling via API2–MALT1. In addition, increased NFκB signalling via API2–MALT1 mimics B-cell receptor signalling, which usually follows an encounter with antigen. In this case increased NFκB signalling leads to an upregulated proliferative drive, clonal growth, and survival of B cells.

paracaspase
A caspase-related protein.

ubiquitination
Involves the addition of ubiquitin monomers to a peptide which allows for degradation of the peptide via the proteasome.

SELF-CHECK 12.10

Outline the relationship between NFκB and API2–MALT1.

t(1;14)(p22;q32)

The translocation t(1;14)(p22;q32) is encountered less frequently than t(11;18) but has a similar biological role in tumour progression. The gene encoding BCL10 is situated at locus 1p22 and, as explained above, is *normally* associated with the activation of NFκB following the formation of a BCL10–MALT1 complex. In t(1;14), *BCL10* fuses with the immunoglobulin heavy-chain gene (*IGH*)—*IGH-BCL10*, resulting in the upregulation of BCL10 through the control of the strong IGH promoter. BCL10 has an important role in promoting B-cell survival following signalling via the BCR.

t(14;18)(q32;q21)

Translocation t(14;18)(q32;q21) involves the fusion of *MALT1* with *IGH* leading to the overexpression of MALT1 and the localization of BCL10 within the perinuclear region of malignant B cells. Occurring in 15–20% of cases, the consequence of IGH–MALT1 is the constitutional activation of NFκB signalling as described for t(11;18).

Key Points

MALT lymphoma-related t(14;18)(q32;q21) should not be confused with the translocation involving the same chromosomal breakpoints in follicular lymphoma. In follicular lymphoma BCL2 is involved, whereas in MALT, MALT1 is rearranged. BCL2 is located approximately 5 Mb telomeric to MALT1, but is still considered the same region according to banding pattern.

Nodal marginal zone lymphoma

Nodal marginal zone lymphoma is a rare malignancy, accounting for less than 2% of all lymphoid malignancies, and is most frequently found in patients aged 50–62 years. Largely restricted to lymph nodes, nodal marginal zone lymphoma cells are rarely found in the bone marrow or peripheral blood. The majority of patients present with disseminated disease involving cervical and abdominal lymph nodes. The 5-year survival is between 50 and 70%.

Mantle cell lymphoma

Mantle cell lymphoma (MCL) was originally described in 1992, comprising approximately 5% of all non-Hodgkin lymphomas. MCL is associated with a poor prognosis, with a survival of 3–5 years. In patients with a largely leukaemic form of mantle cell lymphoma, with little evidence of bulky nodal disease, median survival is approximately 6 years.

Most patients present with bone marrow involvement, hepatosplenomegaly, and lymphadenopathy with evidence of malignant B cells within the peripheral blood. Figure 12.14 demonstrates the typical appearance of a mantle cell in the peripheral blood of a patient in leukaemic phase. Immunophenotypically, MCL cells express a phenotype very similar to the CLL phenotype: CD5+, CD19+, CD20+; but FMC7, CD10, CD20, CD23, and BCL6 are

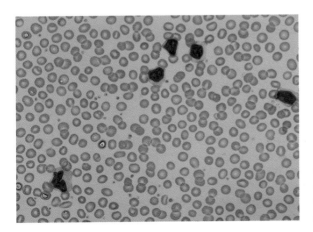

FIGURE 12.14

Mantle cell lymphoma. Large B cells within the peripheral blood during leukaemic phase. The mantle cells each have a large nucleus with a prominent nucleolus and pale cytoplasm. Image courtesy of Jackie Warne, Haematology department, Queen Alexandra Hospital, Portsmouth.

(a)

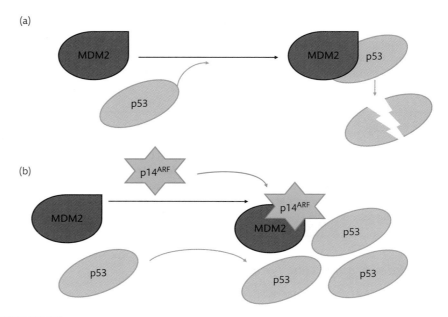

(b)

FIGURE 12.15

Regulation of p53 by MDM2 and p14ARF. (**a**) MDM2 is a negative regulator of p53.
Interaction between MDM2 and p53 leads to the inhibition and degradation of p53.
(**b**) p14ARF inhibits MDM2, allowing p53 to accumulate within the cell. Inhibition of p14ARF
by deletion or epigenetic silencing, allows MDM2 to accumulate—inhibiting
p53-dependent tumour suppressor functions.

typically not expressed. IgM and IgD are present on the MCL cell surface, helping to identify
the pre-germinal centre origin of these cells.

SELF-CHECK 12.11

Compare and contrast the immunophenotype of CLL and MCL.

Approximately 95% of cases harbour t(11;14)(q13;q32), fusing *CCND1*, encoding cyclin D1,
with the IgH gene. Cyclin D1 is important in controlling the G1 phase of the cell cycle. Patients
failing to express t(11;14) demonstrate translocations involving the other G1 cyclins, cyclin D2
or cyclin D3, leading to their overexpression. Overexpression of the D-type cyclins pushes these
malignant cells through G1 to S phase of the cell cycle, resulting in increased cell proliferation.

Additional genetic mutations involving the tumour suppressor ATM, occur in 40–75% of cases.
The ARF/MDM2/p53 and p16INK4A/CDK4 pathways have also been shown to be dysregulated
in MCL. Figure 12.15 outlines the interactions between p14ARF, p53, and MDM2.

In a normal situation, MDM2 is responsible for the sequestration and degradation of p53. p14ARF
is a negative regulator of MDM2, and the homozygous deletion of p14ARF removes the negative regulator of MDM2, increasing MDM2/p53 interactions. The net result of this interaction
between MDM2 and p53 is a loss of p53 activity within p14ARF mutated cells. In addition, the loss
of p16INK4A results in the uncontrolled interaction between cyclin D1 and its associated kinase
CDK4. The association of cyclin D with CDK4 leads to progression of the cell cycle through G1
into S phase. Mutations in these tumour suppressors are largely associated with an increased
proliferation rate, more aggressive disease, poor response to therapy, and reduced survival.

Diffuse large B-cell lymphoma

Diffuse large B-cell lymphoma (DLBCL) is a heterogeneous group of B-cell malignancies, accounting for up to 40% of all cases of NHL. This group of disorders is so broad, containing both common and rare DLBCL variants, that they cannot all be discussed in depth within this textbook. Included is a broad summary of each type, but you are encouraged to read around the subject using current literature reviews and research articles to further your knowledge.

These malignancies are designated as large B-cell lymphomas because they demonstrate large B-cell morphology. The B cells are approximately twice the size of normal B-lymphocytes and grow in a diffuse pattern when examined using histological techniques. Approximately 50% of cases are nodal with the remainder occurring extranodally.

DLBCL appears to be derived from antigen-experienced cells that have had some association with the germinal centre. The vast majority of cases show evidence of *IGVH* somatic hypermutation, and some cases (especially the germinal centre type outlined below) show intraclonal variation of *IGVH*, suggesting ongoing somatic hypermutation. Intraclonal variation of *IGVH* sequences is consistent with the intra germinal centre phenotype. Molecular profiling of DLBCL lymphocytes has allowed scientists and clinicians to allocate malignant cells to one of three DLBCL groups:

- Germinal-centre like (GCB)
- Activated B-like (ABC)
- Primary mediastinal DLBCL

Particular chromosomal and molecular abnormalities, survival profiles, and cells of origin have been established for each of these conditions, and these are summarized in Table 12.10.

The WHO classification has successfully stratified DLBCL into a number of well-recognized variants and subgroups to help the clinician with diagnosis, treatment, and prognostication, and it also recognizes the molecular variants highlighted above. Unfortunately, the vast majority of cases, although subdivided to an extent, are still classified as *DLBCL not otherwise specified*.

Other DLBCL disease entities include:

T-cell/histiocyte-rich large B-cell lymphoma—accounting for approximately 10% of all DLBCL, it is associated with a poor prognosis;

TABLE 12.10 Chromosomal translocations and five year survival figures associated with the three molecular subtypes of DLBCL.

Molecular subtype of DLBCL	Origin	Typical chromosomal abnormalities	5-year survival
Germinal centre B-cell	GC	t(14;18)(q32;q21) Genomic gains of 2p and 2q 6q21–22 abnormalities	59%
Activated B-cell	Post GC	Gains of 3q and 18q21–22 Loss of 6q21–q22 Constitutive activation of NFκB	30%
Primary mediastinal	Thymic B cell	Gains of 18q21–22 and 9q21 Constitutive activation of NFκB	64%

Primary diffuse large B-cell lymphoma of the CNS (CNS DLBCL)—This is a particularly interesting subtype as it occurs within the brain, spinal cord, or eye, but systemic disease is not evident. As lymphoid tissue is absent in the brain, and the malignant lymphocytes show evidence of *IGVH* somatic hypermutation, it remains unknown how these tumours develop and from where the malignant cells originate. Associated with a poor prognosis, CNS DLBCL can be stratified according to the immune status of the patient. Immunocompromised patients—most commonly those with HIV—have an Epstein–Barr virus (EBV) -positive tumour. In contrast, immunocompetent patients possess tumours driven by a different, currently unknown mechanism.

Primary cutaneous DLBCL, leg-type—A rare disease occurring predominantly in the elderly, this is a typically aggressive disease with only 50% of patients surviving beyond 5 years.

EBV-positive diffuse large B-cell lymphoma of the elderly—Always EBV-driven, it occurs in patients over the age of 50 years. This malignancy is uncommon in the West with survival of up to 2 years.

DLBCL associated with chronic inflammation—This form of DLBCL only seems to occur following a period of 10–20 years' chronic inflammation. The proliferation of transformed B cells seems to be driven by EBV-infected cells in these cases. This is an aggressive lymphoma with mortality approaching 50% at 5 years.

Lymphomatoid granulomatosis—Is an EBV-driven B-cell malignancy primarily affecting the lung, although other sites may also be involved. The median survival is approximately 2 years.

Primary mediastinal (thymic) large B-cell lymphoma (PMBL)—This is considered a disease in its own right, although it is still consistent with the DLBCL classification. PMBL *has* been outlined as a distinctive molecular entity along with GC- and ABC-type DLBCL as listed above.

Intravascular large B-cell lymphoma—An aggressive disease associated with a poor prognosis. Malignant B cells accumulate within the lumen of blood vessels in a variety of organs, although infrequently malignant cells may be identified in an FBC and peripheral blood film.

Cross reference

ALK is discussed in greater detail in relation to anaplastic large cell lymphoma, ALK-positive in the mature T-cell and NK-cell neoplasms section of this chapter.

ALK-positive large B-cell lymphoma—The presence of anaplastic lymphoma kinase (ALK) protein defines this rare DLBCL subtype first described in 1997 by Delso *et al.* in the journal *Blood*. This disease is associated with mutations of 2p23—the ALK locus commonly expressed as t(2;17)(p23;q23). Although typically aggressive, variable survival patterns have been reported—especially when paediatric cases are considered, as these appear to have a more favourable prognosis than adult cases.

Plasmablastic lymphoma—A very rare and aggressive form of DLBCL occurring predominantly in immunocompromised patients, especially those harbouring HIV. EBV tends to be co-expressed with HIV in most cases, and survival is reported to be less than 12 months from presentation.

Large B-cell lymphoma arising in HHV8-associated multicentric Castleman disease (HHV8 MCD)—An aggressive DLBCL, which, as its name suggests, is associated with human herpesvirus-8 (HHV8) and frequently demonstrates EBV co-infection. Rarely seen in the full blood count and peripheral blood film, this condition is typically found in patients with HIV, or elderly immunocompetent patients with HHV8. Multicentric Castleman disease is a lymphoproliferative disorder thought to occur following an aggressive immune response to HHV8 and is associated with anaemia, fever, and lymphadenopathy. Survival is considered to be less than 6 months following the development of HHV8 MCD.

Primary effusion lymphoma—A rare malignancy commonly arising in body cavities such as the pleural, peritoneal, and pericardial spaces, it is predominantly associated with HIV-positive individuals, the immunocompromised, and the elderly. All cases are associated with human herpesvirus-8 (HHV8), although in immunocompromised patients EBV may also be co-expressed. Symptoms are dependent upon the site of the lymphoma. Patients with peritoneal localization present with abdominal distension, whilst those with pericardial or pleural disease exhibit dyspnoea. Typically, there is no evidence of lymphadenopathy. Prognosis is poor, and the majority of patients die within 6 months from initial presentation.

SELF-CHECK 12.12

List the subtypes of DLBCL associated with viral infection.

Burkitt lymphoma

Burkitt lymphoma (BL) was first identified by Denis Burkitt, working in Uganda. He noted the presence of a significant deformity in the jaws and abdomen of a number of children. Following contact with Anthony Epstein in 1961, the herpesvirus, later named the Epstein–Barr virus (EBV), was identified within the tumour cells. BL became the first human malignancy to be associated with an oncogenic virus.

The BL identified in these cases was certainly endemic BL, although we can now recognize three subtypes as outlined below:

Endemic BL—Occurs mainly in children aged between 4 and 7 years in equatorial Africa and Papua New Guinea, and presents as large tumours of the jaw or abdomen which are invariably EBV-positive. Endemic BL accounts for up to 75% of all malignancies in children in Equatorial Africa or 40% of all childhood cases of non-Hodgkin lymphoma worldwide.

Sporadic BL—Again, this occurs mainly in children but has a weaker association with EBV, with up to 20% of cases in the West demonstrating evidence of EBV within tumour cells. Geographically, poorer, tropical countries have a higher association with EBV in sporadic BL and

BOX 12.4 *Burkitt lymphoma*

In 1972 Denis Burkitt published the paper describing his findings of an unusual sarcoma in 38 children during 7 years based at Mulago hospital, Kampala, Uganda. Although Christiansen published a paper describing a patient with similar clinical features in 1938, Burkitt and colleagues did an exceptionally thorough investigation of these children, leading to the recognition of a discrete disease entity which later bore his name. (See Burkitt (1958) in the Reference list at the end of this book.)

it should, therefore, be considered a heterogeneous disease. The incidence of sporadic BL is approximately two per million.

Immunodeficiency BL— This, the most common BL, occurs most in approximately 30–40% of cases of non-Hodgkin lymphoma in patients infected by HIV. In approximately 30% of cases, EBV will be identified in tumours. Development of immunodeficiency BL is indicative of progression to AIDS.

BL tumour cells typically have a very rapid proliferation rate, with the tumour cells often having a doubling time of 24–48 hours. Immunostaining using the proliferation marker Ki-67 provides a Ki-67 index of 95% (see Ki-67 box below for an explanation), demonstrating that the majority of cells are actively proliferating. Accompanying this high proliferative behaviour is an increased rate of cell death, leading to an increase in the number of macrophages within the tumour. These macrophages scavenge the cellular debris produced by the high rate of cell death. Histological investigation of the tumour reveals large numbers of macrophages interspersed with tumour cells—demonstrating what has often been described as a 'starry sky appearance'.

Key Points Ki-67

Ki-67 is a protein marker used for determining the number of cells within a tissue progressing through the cell cycle. Visualization of Ki-67 can be accomplished by immunostaining utilizing monoclonal antibodies. The most commonly used monoclonal antibody for the purposes of Ki-67 identification is called MIB-1 (Molecular Immunology Borstel-1). G1, S, G2, and M phases all express Ki-67, and only quiescent cells (those in G_0) fail to express the Ki-67 antigen. The percentage of cells within a tissue expressing Ki-67 provides the 'Ki-67 index' or the proliferation fraction. Ki-67 is useful to measure because it tells us how quickly cells divide and enables us to predict tumour growth. The Ki-67 index can also be used as a prognostic marker.

Occasionally BL presents as an acute lymphoblastic leukaemia, previously classified as L3 by the FAB group. Figure 12.16 shows an example of typical Burkitt lymphoma cells within the peripheral blood. Note the presence of cytoplasmic vacuoles and deeply basophilic cytoplasm.

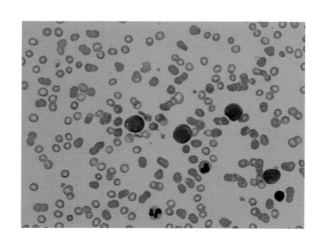

FIGURE 12.16
Burkitt lymphoma. Also called L3 by the FAB group, the lymphoblasts have a high nucleocytoplasmic ratio with deep cytoplasmic basophilia and vacuolation. The nucleus contains fine open chromatin, with numerous nucleoli. The lymphoblasts are much larger than the two neutrophils on this slide. The patient appears thrombocytopenic. Please note macrocytic hypochromic red cells and rouleaux apparent in this slide. Image courtesy of Jackie Warne, Haematology department, Queen Alexandra Hospital, Portsmouth.

The tumour cell immunophenotype includes surface expression of IgM and is accompanied by the B-cell markers CD19, CD20, CD22, and CD79a. In addition, the germinal centre markers BCL6, CD10, and CD38 are expressed and are accompanied by molecular evidence of somatic hypermutation. The immunophenotypic data coupled with evidence of somatic hypermutation indicate that BL is caused by mutated GC-derived B cells.

Typical cytogenetic findings in Burkitt lymphoma

Cytogenetically, three translocations are associated with BL, all involving the upregulation of the proto-oncogene *MYC*. These translocations are t(8;14)(q24;q32), t(8;22)(q24;q11), and t(2;8)(p12;q24). Accounting for up to 80% of cases of BL, t(8;14) utilizes the *IGH* promoter whereas the kappa and lambda genes are located on chromosomes 22 (5%) and 8 (15%), respectively. Variable breakpoints occur within these translocations, although the end result—the upregulation of c-Myc—is a constant finding.

Although the vast majority of cases of BL harbour translocations involving *MYC*, these translocations are not exclusively found in BL, and are therefore *not* diagnostic for BL.

The role and dysregulation of c-MYC

The role of c-Myc in cellular control is both complex and diverse. c-Myc has been implicated in the control of cell growth, proliferation, induction of apoptosis, and metabolism. Dysregulation of c-Myc following mutation or translocation can lead to modification of all of these functional properties.

Research has shown that in non-malignant cells, the tumour suppressors p14^{ARF} and p53 are up-regulated following the overexpression of c-Myc. Up-regulation of these tumour suppressors leads to cell cycle arrest and the induction of apoptosis in cells where c-Myc is dysregulated. Overexpression of c-Myc and inactivating mutations of p53 are common findings in patients with BL, facilitating oncogenesis by removing this important negative feedback mechanism.

Interestingly, the overexpression of c-Myc downregulates the activity of the CDK inhibitor p27. Cyclin E-CDK2 activity is controlled by p27, resulting in the progression of the cell cycle through G1 into S-phase. c-Myc also activates CDK4. When accompanied by cyclin D, cyclin D-CDK4 phosphorylates pRb, releasing the transcription factor E2F-1 leading to the increased synthesis of cyclin E.

The overexpression of c-Myc is thought to be a prerequisite for BL lymphomagenesis, although the mutation of *MYC* alone is not thought to be sufficient to induce malignant transformation. *TP53* mutations are also common in BL as is the epigenetic silencing of a range of other tumour suppressor genes. Therefore, a number of events, including *MYC* dysregulation, seem important.

Cross reference
The cell cycle and its regulation are outlined in Chapter 9.

Burkitt lymphoma prognosis

The prognosis for patients with BL is very good. Largely, endemic BL is considered to have the highest mortality, but this is due to endemic BL occurring in Africa and equatorial regions where a poor standard of healthcare is expected. The use of high-dose combination chemotherapeutic agents leads to rapid cell lysis, and the risk of **tumour lysis syndrome**. Up to 90% of individuals with BL can be cured using appropriate combination chemotherapy.

Key Points

Tumour lysis syndrome is considered to be a medical emergency and is a consequence of the release of a number of intracellular components following the lysis of tumour cells. Patients will have raised plasma potassium (hyperkalaemia), phosphate (hyper-phosphataemia), and uric acid (hyperuricaemia) concentrations accompanied by reduced calcium (hypocalcaemia) levels and often acute renal failure.

An overlap condition sharing both morphological and cytogenetic characteristics of Burkitt lymphoma and diffuse large B-cell lymphoma is called *B-cell lymphoma, unclassifiable, with features of diffuse large B-cell lymphoma and Burkitt lymphoma*. Although recognized by the WHO classification, this will not be considered any further here.

T-cell malignancies are far less frequently encountered than B-cell malignancies and do not have the same cytogenetic or molecular predictability as associated with the development of malignant B cells. However, on occasion, working in a haematology laboratory you will encounter T-cell malignancies and you should be aware of some of the important features of the most frequently occurring.

The WHO subdivides the T-cell malignancies into *precursor lymphoid neoplasms* and *mature T-cell and NK-cell neoplasms*. So far we have considered the important precursor neoplasms and the mature B-cell neoplasms, and now we should move on to look at the most common of the mature T-cell and NK-cell neoplasms.

SELF-CHECK 12.13

Describe the role of Ki-67 in evaluating BL cell behaviour. Describe the molecular mechanisms that might be responsible for the typical Ki-67 index.

12.5 Mature T-cell and NK-cell neoplasms

The diseases considered below are of a mature T-cell origin and are clearly defined using the WHO guidelines. Only the most frequently encountered T-cell neoplasms are outlined here.

T-cell prolymphocytic leukaemia (T-PLL)

This is an aggressive T-cell malignancy which used to be considered the T-cell counterpart to B-CLL, although this is no longer the case. Approximately 75% of patients present with splenomegaly, and 50% of cases will show signs of hepatomegaly or lymphadenopathy. Importantly for laboratory haematologists, these cells will be found in the full blood count and on the peripheral blood film, as seen in Figure 12.17. The white cell count is usually greater than 100×10^9/L, with the full blood count demonstrating a normocytic normochromic anaemia and thrombocytopenia, both caused by a diffuse bone marrow infiltration of malignant T cells.

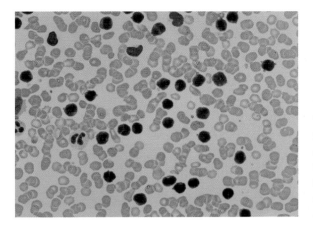

FIGURE 12.17
T-cell prolymphocytic leukaemia. A high WBC count showing small-sized prolymphocytes. The cells have scant basophilic cytoplasm, with many unusually shaped nuclei. This image was taken from a relatively thick region of the blood film, resulting in the considerable red cell stacking apparent in this image. Image courtesy of Jackie Warne, Haematology department, Queen Alexandra Hospital, Portsmouth.

The most frequently encountered cytogenetic feature is an inversion or translocation of chromosome 14. Immunophenotypically, T-PLL demonstrates surface expression of CD2, CD3, and CD7, but CD1a and TdT are not expressed.

Response to chemotherapy is generally poor and median survival is less than 12 months.

T-cell large granular lymphocytic leukaemia (T-LGL)

T-LGL is associated with an increased number of circulating large granular lymphocytes co-expressing CD3 and CD8. Although a number of patients will be diagnosed following a full blood count for an unrelated medical complaint, approximately 50% of patients present with splenomegaly, and hepatomegaly occurs in 20%. A common feature is an isolated neutropenia which increases the risk of opportunistic infections for patients with this malignancy. Occasionally anaemia and thrombocytopenia may be found, but these are rare complications. The blood film frequently shows large granular lymphocytes, as shown in Figure 12.18. Autoimmunity is a common complication, with rheumatoid arthritis frequently reported.

Median survival has been reported to be 13 years following diagnosis.

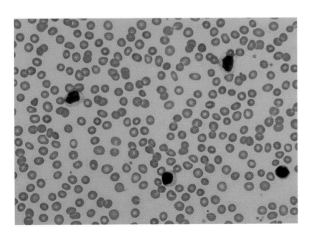

FIGURE 12.18
T-cell large granular lymphocytic leukaemia. Circulating large granular lymphocytes (NK cells) can be seen dominating this blood film. The cytoplasm is light blue, almost clear in places except for some large granules scattered throughout the cytoplasm. Image courtesy of Jackie Warne, Haematology department, Queen Alexandra Hospital, Portsmouth.

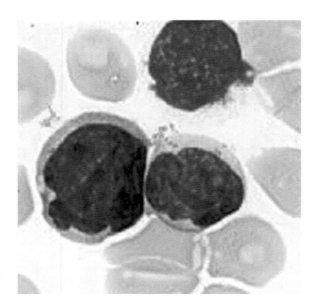

FIGURE 12.19

Sézary syndrome. The large lymphocyte on the left contains a cerebriform nucleus with condensed chromatin. The cytoplasm is moderately basophilic and vacuoles can be seen in the lymphocyte in the top right of the image. Reproduced from Provan *et al. Oxford Handbook of Clinical Haematology*, 2nd edn 2004. By permission of Oxford University Press.

Mycosis fungoides and Sézary syndrome

Although these diseases are considered as *separate entities* by the WHO, they are related and will be considered as variations of a single pathology in this text. Mycosis fungoides (MF) is the most frequently occurring cutaneous T-cell lymphoma, accounting for over 50% of all lymphomas of the skin, where it usually remains restricted. In contrast, Sézary syndrome accounts for only 5% of cutaneous T-cell lymphomas, does have a leukaemic phase, and, as a consequence, can become easily disseminated. Morphologically Sézary syndrome is readily identified within the peripheral blood film. Typically the cells for both conditions are cerebriform—meaning the nucleus of the cell looks 'brain-like', as demonstrated in Figure 12.19. Sézary syndrome is also associated with **erythroderma** and lymphadenopathy, demonstrating the broad effects this malignancy can have on a range of tissues.

erythroderma

Red and scaling skin caused by inflammation.

Immunophenotypically, both MF and Sézary cells express T-cell markers CD2, CD3, and CD5, but generally fail to express CD8. An increased population of CD4-positive, CD7-negative cells is characteristic of the Sézary phenotype with peripheral blood immunophenotyping.

Depending on the stage of the disease, patients with mycosis fungoides have been reported to survive for over 33 years following diagnosis, compared with a 5-year survival of 20% for patients diagnosed with Sézary syndrome.

Peripheral T-cell lymphoma, not otherwise specified

These diseases account for the majority of cases of T-cell lymphoma and are incorporated into the *not otherwise specified* category due to a lack of predictable features of morphology, immunophenotype and cytogenetics. The diseases included in this section are highly aggressive, with the majority of patients dying within 5 years following diagnosis. Previously, this group also included three rare cutaneous tumours, but now, following comprehensive research, the neoplasms listed below have been assigned discrete subtypes in their own right:

- Primary aggressive **epidermotropic** CD8+ cytotoxic T-cell lymphoma
- Cutaneous γ-δ T-cell lymphoma
- Primary cutaneous CD4+ small/medium-sized **pleomorphic** T-cell lymphoma

These variants will not be discussed further in this text.

epidermotropic
A preference to existing within the epidermis.

pleomorphic
Variations in the appearance of a particular type of cell.

Angioimmunoblastic T-cell lymphoma (AITL)

Originally considered to be a reactive process, AITL is the most common of the T-cell lymphomas, accounting for up to 70% of reported cases. Occurring most frequently in the elderly with a median age at diagnosis of 65 years, clinical indicators include hepatosplenomegaly, autoimmune haemolytic anaemia, skin rash, eosinophilia, and a polyclonal hypergammaglobulinaemia.

Lymph node examination reveals tumour cells on a background of neutrophils, eosinophils, plasma cells and epithelioid histiocytes, typically accompanied by **atrophied** lymphoid follicles. Proliferating high endothelial venules are also seen in lymph node biopsies.

atrophy
Wasting of a structure with subsequent change in function.

Coexisting EBV-infected B cells are apparent in the majority of cases. In addition, following the immunosuppression and dysregulation encountered in AITL, the unchecked re-emergence of EBV can occur, leading to an EBV-driven population of immortalized B cells.

Overall 5-year survival is approximately 30%, with a median survival reported in most publications of approximately 3 years.

Anaplastic large cell lymphoma, ALK-positive (ALCL, ALK+)

Accounting for 10–20% of childhood lymphomas and 12% of mature T/NK-cell malignancies, this is a relatively uncommon T-cell malignancy associated with heterogeneous morphology. The defining features of ALCL, ALK+ include the presence of horseshoe-shaped cells (called hallmark cells) independent of the other morphological features, CD30+ immunophenotype, and cytoplasmic expression of anaplastic lymphoma kinase (ALK).

The most common cytogenetic feature, occurring in 40–60% of patients, is a translocation involving chromosomes 2 and 5– t(2;5)(p23;q35)–resulting in the fusion of the *ALK* and (*NPM*) nucleophosmin genes. Currently, nine *ALK* fusion partners have been described, with the second most common being tropomyosin 3 (*TPM3*) as a consequence of t(1;2)(q21;p23). The chimeric product of t(2;5)(p23;q35), NPM–ALK, has **constitutionally** active tyrosine kinase activity leading to enhanced signalling through the JAK3–STAT3 transduction pathway.

constitutionally
Pertaining to an entity's composition.

NPM is important for the shuttling of ribonucleoproteins from the cell nucleus to the cytoplasm, and is found in both the nucleus and the cytoplasm in cases harbouring t(2;5)(p23;q35). NPM contains an oligodimerization domain which is conserved in the NPM–ALK fusion protein enabling NPM–ALK dimers to form and constitutional activation of ALK.

Overall 5-year survival rates in ALCL, ALK+ are reported to be around 80%.

Now that the most common of the non-Hodgkin lymphomas have been considered, we will go on to examine Hodgkin lymphomas.

SELF-CHECK 12.14

Describe the role of ALK in lymphomagenesis.

12.6 **Hodgkin lymphoma**

Hodgkin's disease, later renamed Hodgkin lymphoma (HL), was first identified as a specific disease entity in 1832 by Thomas Hodgkin. In 1898 and 1902, respectively, Reed and Sternberg independently described the mononucleated 'Hodgkin cell' and the multinucleated cells characteristic of HL; these were later described as 'Reed–Sternberg cells' (HRS cells). Hodgkin lymphoma is a lymphoid malignancy commonly associated with young adults.

The incidence of Hodgkin lymphoma has remained steady in comparison with other types of lymphoma, and is considered to be relatively treatable. Up to 70% of patients diagnosed with HL can be considered cured following intensive chemotherapy and radiotherapy.

Hodgkin lymphoma is not considered a single disease entity, but rather a composite of two disorders—classical HL and nodular lymphocyte predominant HL—subdivided according to the morphology and immunophenotype of the malignant cells and the nature of the cellular infiltrate around the malignant cells within lymphoid tissue. Figure 12.20 demonstrates how Hodgkin lymphoma can be subdivided.

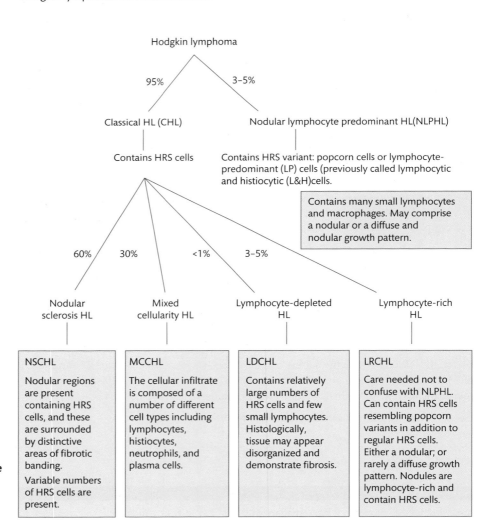

FIGURE 12.20

Hodgkin lymphoma and the subdivision into classical and nodular lymphocyte-predominant diseases.

Classical HL is further subdivided into four distinct entities; importantly, all classic HLs can be treated in the same way. In contrast, nodular lymphocyte-predominant type requires correct identification, as its higher rate of relapse is an indication for specific therapy.

Compared with other haematological malignancies, the cancer cells in HL only comprise between 0.1% and 1% of the total number of nucleated cells in the affected tissue. The majority of cells within the tumour mass are inflammatory cells as described in mixed cellularity HL.

HL is associated with dissemination to nearby (contiguous) lymph nodes. Adjacent lymph node regions are rarely uninvolved as the lymphoma spreads throughout the lymphatic vessels.

What are HRS cells?

HRS cells are derived, in about 98% of cases, from germinal-centre B cells that have undergone somatic hypermutation of *IgV* genes. In approximately 2% of cases, HRS cells are of T-cell origin. Somatic hypermutation is dysregulated in HRS cells, leading to the incorporation of nonsense mutations in immunoglobulin genes in about 25% of cases. As a consequence of these nonsense mutations, B-cell receptors are not expressed on the cell surface. Failure of B-cell receptor expression should induce apoptosis, but in these cells the apoptotic mechanism fails, leading to the survival of dysregulated B cells.

The expression of most B-cell immunophenotypic markers is lost in HRS cells, making their origins difficult to establish in initial scientific investigations. Expression of CD45, CD19, CD20, and CD22 is completely absent from the majority of HRS cells. Furthermore, analysis using DNA microarrays has shown that gene expression is decreased in HRS cells, resulting in difficulty in assigning a normal cell counterpart to HRS cells. In the vast majority of cases, HRS cells continue to express MHC class II, CD40, and other molecules, which facilitate interaction with T_H cells—the most numerous of the infiltrative cells. The expression of CD30 is important in facilitating the interaction between eosinophils and mast cells commonly seen in the HL infiltrate.

A number of cytogenetic and molecular events have been reported in HRS cells, leading to an overexpression of transcription factors and overactivity of signalling pathways. Probably the most important event is increased NFκB signalling, leading to apoptotic failure. In addition, increased signalling through the JAK–STAT pathway increases the number of transcription factors within the nucleus of these cells. Translocations involving the germinal centre regulator BCL-6 are often found in B-cell lymphomas, but are not associated with HRS cells. Studies have identified BCL-6 translocations in some cases of HL expressing LP cells. LP cells and their association with Hodgkin lymphoma are outlined in Figure 12.20. Overexpression of MDM2, the negative regulator of the tumour suppressor protein p53, is found in approximately 60% of cases of HL. Inhibiting p53 through altered MDM2 expression has the potential to increase the number of additional mutations occurring within HRS cells, leading to increased genomic instability within these cells and diverse progression.

In the Western world, EBV can be identified in approximately 40% of classic HL cases, of which the mixed cellularity type has the greatest association. NLPHL is very rarely associated with EBV. The following important EBV-derived proteins are expressed in classic cases: latent membrane protein (LMP)1, LMP2A, Epstein–Barr (virus) nuclear antigen-1 (EBNA-1), and Epstein–Barr (virus) encoded RNAs (EBERs)-1 and -2.

LMP1 suppresses apoptosis by increasing NFκB signalling through the direct activation of the NFκB pathway, and the inhibition of the NFκB inhibitor IκB via phosphorylation events. LMP2A acts as a surrogate B-cell receptor, ensuring that B cells can survive in the absence of a functional BCR. EBNA-1 is a maintenance protein allowing the replication of viral DNA, whilst EBERs are non-essential proteins which induce the synthesis of IL-10, thought to inhibit cytotoxic T cells.

An overlap syndrome called *B-cell lymphoma, unclassifiable, with features intermediate between diffuse large B-cell lymphoma and classical Hodgkin lymphoma* is recognized by the WHO classification, but will not be considered further in this text.

SELF-CHECK 12.15

Describe the cell of origin for HRS.

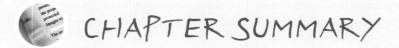

CHAPTER SUMMARY

- A diverse range of classification systems have historically been implemented to try to aid understanding of the complexity associated with lymphoid neoplasms.

- The REAL classification, the first internationally recognized system for classifying lymphoid malignancies, was used as a foundation for the WHO classification.

- The WHO classification takes into account a wide range of investigative techniques in order to classify distinct clinicopathological entities.

- Clear cytogenetic abnormalities have been identified and used, where appropriate, to outline distinctive pathologies.

- As scientists and clinicians, we have a vast knowledge of the molecular basis of a number of these diseases which allows us to predict disease behaviour.

- Viruses—including HIV, EBV, and HHV8—are important in the pathogenesis of a number of lymphoid malignancies.

- Hodgkin lymphoma is still considered a discrete disease entity, but has been incorporated into the lymphoid classification following recognition of the cellular basis of Hodgkin/Reed–Sternberg cells.

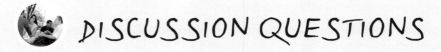

DISCUSSION QUESTIONS

12.1 How can knowledge of the germinal centre improve our understanding of malignant B-cell behaviour?

12.2 Why is the classification of lymphoid malignancies such a medical minefield?

12.3 Critically discuss the role of IgH translocations in lymphoid malignancies.

FURTHER READING

● Degos L, Linch DC, Löwenberg B. (ed.). *Textbook of Malignant Haematology*, 2nd edn. Taylor & Francis, Oxon, 2005.

● Hoffbrand AV, Catovsky D, Tuddenham EGD (ed.). *Postgraduate Haematology*, 5th edn. Blackwell Publishing Ltd, Massachusetts–Oxford–Carlton, 2005.

● Jaffe ES, Harris NC, Stein H, Isaacson PG. Classification of lymphoid neoplasms: the microscope as a tool for disease discovery. *Blood* 2008:**112**;4384–99.

● Norton J. Classification of non-Hodgkin's lymphomas. *Baillière's Clinical Haematology* 1996:**9**(4);641-652.

● Rezk SA, Weiss LM. Epstein–Barr virus-associated lymphoproliferative disorders. *Human Pathology* 2007:**38**;1293–1304.

● Swerdlow SH, Campo E, Harris NL, Jaffe ES, Pileri SA, Stein H Thiele J, Vardiman JW (ed.). WHO Classification of Tumours of Haematopoietic and Lymphoid Tissues. IARC, Lyon, 2008.

Answers to self-check questions, case study questions, and discussion questions are provided in the book's Online Resource Centre, visit www.oxfordtextbooks.co.uk/orc/moore

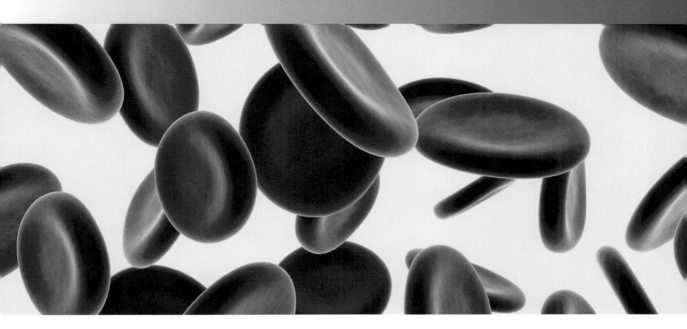

PART 4

Haemostasis in Health and Disease

13

Normal haemostasis

Gary W. Moore

In this chapter we will outline the processes that cause blood to clot in a controlled manner and present an overview of the interplay between the various components.

Learning objectives

After studying this chapter you should confidently be able to:

- Explain the importance of effective haemostasis.
- List the major components of haemostatic mechanisms.
- Describe the mechanisms of primary haemostasis.
- Describe the mechanisms of secondary haemostasis.
- Describe the mechanisms of fibrinolysis.
- Outline the interplay between the elements of haemostasis.

13.1 Introduction to haemostasis

The mechanisms of haemostasis have a number of crucial functions:

1. Under normal physiological conditions, to maintain blood contained within the vasculature in a fluid state.
2. Upon vessel trauma/injury, to limit and arrest bleeding by the formation of a blood clot, whilst at the same time maintaining blood flow through the damaged vessel.
3. Removal of the blood clot upon completion of wound healing.

Mechanisms of haemostasis

In health, the haemostatic mechanisms maintain the fluidity of circulating blood and are essentially anticoagulant in nature—that is, they retard or prevent clotting. Upon damage to blood vessels, a variety of **procoagulant** mechanisms are initiated which involve a complex interplay between vessel endothelium, circulating platelets and coagulation factors. A fine balance exists between maintaining blood fluidity and preventing excessive activation of procoagulant pathways that may lead to thrombosis and vascular occlusion. This balance is controlled by

procoagulant
Physiological or pharmacological mechanism that promotes clotting processes.

positive and negative feedback pathways, localization mechanisms, and inhibitory pathways. In this chapter we will describe the haemostatic mechanisms as three distinct phases:

- **Primary haemostasis**, which involves interactions between blood vessels, platelets, and von Willebrand factor (VWF, leading to formation of the initial barrier to blood loss, the primary haemostatic plug.
- **Secondary haemostasis**, whereby the pathways of coagulation biochemistry act in concert to generate fibrin strands which strengthen the clot.
- **Fibrinolysis** is a separate biochemical system that degrades the fibrin clot to prevent vascular occlusion and ultimately remove the clot once the wound has healed.

Although we will describe haemostasis under these discrete headings, it is important to recognize that the different phases are in fact integrated, many of the processes occurring simultaneously.

Cross reference

Primary haemostasis, secondary haemostasis and fibrinolysis are all covered in more detail in dedicated sections of this chapter.

SELF-CHECK 13.1

What are the main roles of haemostasis and what are the mechanisms involved?

13.2 **Primary haemostasis**

The initial responses after vessel injury are mediated by interactions between the vessel wall and circulating platelets to begin the formation of a clot. In order to understand the events of primary haemostasis we will first consider some relevant details of the main players: blood vessels, VWF, and platelets.

General blood vessel structure

The walls of the larger blood vessels (i.e. arteries and veins) consist of three layers: the intima, media, and adventitia. The intima is the inner layer which is lined by a single continuous layer of endothelial cells that rests on a basement membrane of subendothelial microfibrils. These microfibrils predominantly consist of different types of **collagen** and also some elastin. The middle layer, or media, contains mainly circularly arranged smooth muscle cells which allow contraction and relaxation of the vessel. The media is separated from the outer layer, the adventitia, by the external elastic lamina which allows the vessel to stretch and recoil. The adventitia comprises collagen fibres and fibroblasts that protect the vessel and anchor it to its surroundings. It also contains smaller blood vessels and nerves. The structure of large blood vessels is shown in Figure 13.1.

collagen

A long protein fibre that connects and strengthens numerous tissues.

Small blood vessels (i.e. capillaries, post-capillary venules, and arterioles) are also lined by a single layer of endothelial cells surrounded by a continuous basement membrane. Pericytes (or Rouget cells) provide support and stability by surrounding the endothelial layer, which is encircled by the adventitia.

Haemostatic roles of blood vessels

The vessel wall has many important haemostatic functions. Blood flow contributes to effective haemostasis, the flow conditions in a given vessel being a direct function of its diameter. Higher flow rates are encountered in the centre of the vessel lumen and can be significantly lower at the endothelium surface. As a result, the relatively larger erythrocytes are more concentrated in the centre of a vessel and the smaller platelets circulate in areas of lower flow

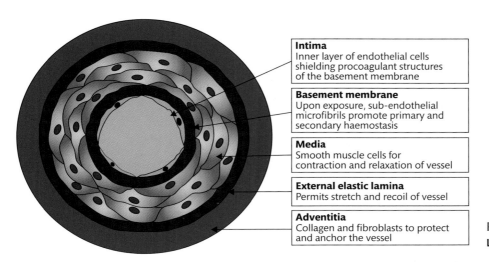

| Intima |
| Inner layer of endothelial cells shielding procoagulant structures of the basement membrane |

| Basement membrane |
| Upon exposure, sub-endothelial microfibrils promote primary and secondary haemostasis |

| Media |
| Smooth muscle cells for contraction and relaxation of vessel |

| External elastic lamina |
| Permits stretch and recoil of vessel |

| Adventitia |
| Collagen and fibroblasts to protect and anchor the vessel |

FIGURE 13.1
Large blood vessel structure.

near to the vessel wall. **Shear forces** induced by blood flow affect the reactivity of cells and the crucial haemostatic protein VWF.

Under normal physiological conditions, where there is no vessel trauma or disease, the endothelial layer of the intima is **antithrombotic**. This layer enlists a variety of mechanisms that actively maintain blood fluidity by the synthesis and secretion of agents that inhibit clotting processes. Upon vessel injury, or as a result of certain disease states, endothelial cells switch to functions that actively promote blood clotting: they become **prothrombotic**. The main haemostatic contributions of endothelial cells and the basement membrane are summarized in Table 13.1.

Once exposed to circulating blood, the subendothelium of the intima is strongly **thrombogenic** as it contains structures that promote both primary and secondary haemostasis. Vascular injury causes endothelin-1, which acts as a potent vasoconstrictor, to be released from endothelial cells. **Vasoconstriction** is brought about by the smooth muscle cells of the media and is an important mechanism for reducing or preventing blood loss, especially in the microvasculature. Cells of the adventitia express tissue factor, which is crucial to the initial reactions of the coagulation biochemistry of secondary haemostasis.

SELF-CHECK 13.2

How do blood vessels contribute to haemostasis?

von Willebrand factor (VWF)

VWF is a large adhesive glycoprotein produced constitutively in endothelial cells and megakaryocytes. Unlike many of the activated coagulation factors we will encounter in the section on secondary haemostasis, it is not an enzyme. The primary functions of VWF involve binding to cells and molecules and are outlined below:

- Binding to subendothelial collagen exposed due to vessel injury.
- Binding to a **receptor** on the surface of non-activated platelets, the glycoprotein Ib (GPIb) complex.
- Binding to a receptor on the surface of activated platelets, the GPIIbIIIa complex.
- Binding to factor VIII (FVIII) to protect it from proteolytic degradation in the plasma.

shear forces

Forces produced when surfaces are pressed together or move over each other.

thrombogenic

Causing blood to clot; causing thrombosis.

vasoconstriction

Narrowing of the diameter of a blood vessel.

receptor

A molecule on the surface of (or in) a cell that acts as a recognition site for other molecules that bind in order to promote specific functions.

Cross references

The significance of these functions will be discussed later in this chapter in the section covering the events of primary haemostasis, and also in Chapter 14 when we consider disorders of primary haemostasis.

TABLE 13.1 Haemostatic functions of the vessel intima.

Function	Properties	
	Anticoagulant	**Procoagulant**
Synthesis/secretion	Prostacyclin and nitric oxide inhibit platelet function and act as vasodilators	von Willebrand factor is integral to platelet function
	Tissue plasminogen activator promotes clot lysis	Tissue factor initiates coagulation reactions
	Thrombomodulin, endothelial protein C receptor, and heparan sulphate contribute to the inhibition of coagulation	Factor V and factor VIII are essential cofactors in coagulation biochemistry
		Plasminogen activator inhibitor-1 inhibits clot lysis
		Thrombospondin and endothelin-1 promote platelet aggregation
Protein & cell binding	Binding of coagulation inhibitors (see below)	Adhesion molecules for neutrophils
		Exposure of sub-endothelial microfibrils to promote platelet binding via VWF
		Binding of some coagulation factors (see below)
Coagulation biochemistry	Endothelial protein C receptor binds protein C to allow its activation by the thrombin–thrombomodulin complex, leading to inactivation of activated factors V and VIII	Thrombin–thrombomodulin complex activates a fibrinolysis inhibitor
	Heparan sulphate enhances the inhibition of activated clotting factors by antithrombin	Tissue factor binds factor VII to begin coagulation

monomer
A molecule that can combine with others to form a polymer; the smallest repeating unit of a polymer.

domain
A discrete section that is part of the structure of a protein.

dimer
A molecule composed of two linked subunits.

Structure and assembly of VWF

The basic VWF **monomer** consists of 2050 amino acids containing distinct **domains** that have specific functions. The A1 domain binds GPIb and heparin and the A3 domain specifically binds collagen. Binding to GPIIbIIIa is via the C1 domain and the domain for FVIII binding is D'/D3, which can also bind with heparin. This pre-pro-VWF molecule is formed in the endoplasmic reticulum where the monomers are then linked via C-terminal disulphide bonds to form **dimers**, which are termed the pro-VWF molecules.

Post-translational glycosylation then occurs in the Golgi, and it is interesting to note that this results in VWF being one of few proteins that carry ABO antigens. This has clinical relevance as populations with blood group O have lower mean levels of VWF than those with blood groups A, B, and AB, which is a result of altered VWF survival *in vivo*.

Processing of the dimers continues in the Golgi where the formation of N-terminal disulphide bonds facilitates **multimerization** of the dimers—that is, formation of an aggregate of multiple molecules joined by non-covalent bonds. **Multimers** vary in size and the larger forms are functionally more effective. Processing of the pro-VWF into mature VWF is carried out by the enzyme furin, which also cleaves the propolypeptide known as von Willebrand antigen II (VW AgII) from the pro-VWF dimers. VW AgII is required for multimer formation and also chaperones VWF into storage granules, which in endothelial cells are the **Weibel–Palade bodies**, and in platelets are the α-granules.

VWF is constitutively released into the plasma from endothelial cells and can also be released from the Weibel–Palade bodies in response to stimuli such as exercise, adrenergic stimulation, and certain drugs such as **desmopressin**. Constitutive secretion only occurs from endothelial cells as platelets do not release α-granule contents until activated.

Vascular endothelial cells and platelets contain ultra-large VWF multimers that are highly adhesive. However, they are only transiently detectable in plasma as they are cleaved by a circulating protease called **ADAMTS-13**, the acronym for **A** zinc- and calcium-dependent **D**isintegrin and **M**etalloprotease with **T**hrombo**S**pondin type 1 motifs, member 13 (also known as VWF-cleaving protease). ADAMTS-13 degrades the ultra-large multimers into smaller forms ranging in size from 500 kDa to ~20 000 kDa.

SELF-CHECK 13.3

How does von Willebrand factor contribute to primary haemostasis?

Platelets

As you saw in Chapter 3 on haemopoeisis, platelets are anucleate fragments of megakaryocyte cytoplasm, each megakaryocyte producing between 2000 and 3000 platelets. Platelets circulate in a dormant state, and, as we will see, are capable of a rapid and dramatic response to vessel injury. This is crucial to effective haemostasis as they form the platform for a number of essential haemostatic mechanisms.

The main functions of platelets are to:

- Interact with VWF to form the initial barrier to blood loss.
- Allow platelet–platelet interactions to propagate the thrombus.
- Provide a negatively charged lipid surface to support key reactions of coagulation biochemistry.
- Deliver a variety of haemostatically active molecules to increase their local concentration.
- Localize thrombus formation.
- Promote vasoconstriction.
- Promote vessel repair.
- Maintain the molecular integrity of endothelial cell junctions.

Relative to leucocytes and erythrocytes, platelets are small and discoid in shape, are approximately 3.0 μm by 0.5 μm, and have a volume of 7.5–11.5 fL. The shape and small size of

Cross references

Details of blood groups and their antigens are covered in the *Transfusion and Transplantation Science* volume in this series.

You will meet α-granules later in this chapter when we look at platelet structure and function.

multimer
A protein composed of more than one peptide chain.

desmopressin
Synthetic antidiuretic drug that stimulates the release of FVIII and VWF.

platelets, together with conditions of blood flow, result in them circulating towards the edges of blood vessels where they are ideally placed to rapidly respond to vessel damage. To achieve the functions listed above, platelets have a highly specialized structure which we will now consider in more detail. Figure 13.2 shows you the general structure of a platelet and organization of the features covered in the following sections.

Key Points

Localization mechanisms are important to ensure that a clot forms only where it is needed. We will see the pathological consequences of breakdown of localization processes in Chapter 14.

Platelet membrane

glycoproteins

Proteins with carbohydrate chains.

The platelet membrane is a complex structure containing a variety of components crucial to effective haemostasis. The external coat of the membrane, or glycocalyx, is rich in anchored **glycoproteins**. Some of these glycoproteins act as receptors for molecular stimuli which trigger

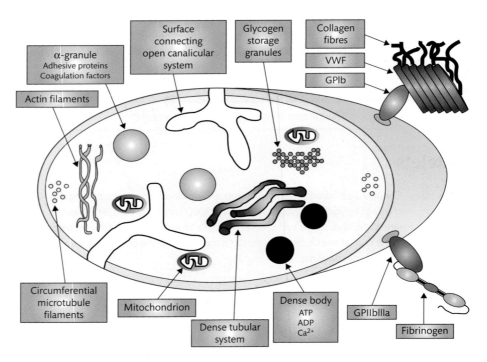

FIGURE 13.2

Platelet ultrastructure. The two main glycoprotein (GP) receptors are shown binding to their main ligands, GPIb binding to VWF and GPIIbIIIa binding to fibrinogen. Dense bodies containing adenine nucleotides and calcium, and α-granules containing adhesive proteins and coagulation factors are present in the cytoplasm. The surface-connected open canalicular system forms channels to allow molecules in and out of the platelet, and the dense tubular system regulates platelet activation. Actin filaments and the microtubules maintain platelet shape, and change shape upon activation. Mitochondria and glycogen-storage granules provide energy.

platelet activation, whilst others facilitate platelet adhesion to subendothelium via VWF or platelet aggregation. The middle layer is rich in asymmetrically distributed phospholipids that act as a surface for the interaction with specific components of coagulation biochemistry, such as factor II and factor X. The inner layer takes part in translating signals received on the outer coat into chemical messages and physical alterations in platelet structure that accompany activation. Figure 13.3 depicts a schematic of the platelet membrane showing the main receptors you are about to meet in the following sections. Note that some are directly connected to components of the cytoplasm (see Figure 13.2).

The **surface-connected open canalicular system** (SCOCS) is a network of channels throughout the interior of the platelet formed from invaginations of the membrane. These channels, or canaliculi, are continuous with the external membrane and significantly increase the surface area of platelet exposed to plasma. This provides a route for molecules to reach deep within the platelet. The canaliculi also serve as conduits for the extrusion of substances from within platelets once activated.

A separate internal membrane system is the **dense tubular system** (DTS), which is derived from the endoplasmic reticulum of the parent megakaryocyte. The channels of this system also pervade the cytoplasm. The DTS regulates platelet activation by sequestering or releasing calcium, and is also the site of prostaglandin synthesis.

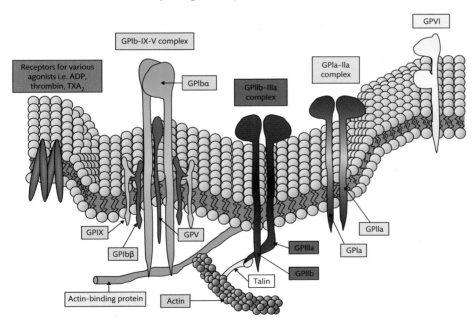

FIGURE 13.3

Platelet membrane receptors. Platelets have receptors for each of the agonists capable of activating resting platelets, such as ADP, thrombin, and thromboxane A$_2$ (TXA$_2$). The GPIb-IX-V complex that is responsible for binding platelets to VWF consists of two molecules each of GPIbα, GPIbβ and GPIX flanking a single molecule of GPV. The GPIIbIIIa complex, responsible for binding to fibrinogen to facilitate platelet to platelet aggregation, consists of one molecule of each GP with GPIIIa anchored to actin via talin. The GPIaIIa complex and GPVI are involved in binding platelets to collagen. Note that some are directly connected to components of the cytoplasm, such as GPIbα molecules anchored to an actin-binding protein and GPIIIa anchored to actin via talin. GP, glycoprotein.

actin-binding protein
Proteins that bind actin

talin
Ubiquitous cytoskeletal protein linking integrins to the actin cytoskeleton

Cytoskeleton

Three cytoskeletal systems maintain the discoid shape of resting platelets as they encounter the shear forces generated in flowing blood:

1. The membrane skeleton
2. The cytoplasmic actin network
3. The microtubule coil

The membrane skeleton is composed of elongated spectrin strands that are connected to the membrane. Actin is the most abundant platelet protein, forming 2000–5000 linear actin polymers that exist as a network of filaments filling the cytoplasm of a resting platelet. Rigidity of the actin network is enhanced by interconnections formed of filamin and α-actin. The spectrin strands are interconnected through binding to the ends of actin filaments originating from the cytoplasm, so the spectrin lattice and actin network essentially form a single continuous ultrastructure. Each platelet contains a single microtubule that exists as a coil just below the plasma membrane at its widest circumference. This circumferential microtubule coil, a hollow polymer consisting of 12–15 subfilaments of αβ-tubulin dimers, is the major support for maintaining the discoid shape. The arrangement of the subfilaments is shown in Figure 13.4.

Cytoplasm contents

Platelet cytoplasm contains mitochondria and glycogen stores for energy. Important to the haemostatic functions of platelets are three main types of storage granules which rapidly release their contents upon activation.

1. Alpha-granules
2. Dense bodies
3. Lysosomes

The α-granules are the most numerous platelet organelle, about 80 per platelet, and the main secretory granule, containing a vast array of predominantly large molecules necessary for haemostasis and wound healing. Upon platelet activation the molecules are carried to the cell surface for release, some of which adhere to the platelet surface whilst others are incorporated in the platelet membrane or diffuse into the extracellular fluid.

The **dense bodies**, also termed dense granules or δ-granules, are the smallest platelet granule with a frequency of 5–7 per platelet. They are so-called because when viewed with an electron microscope they are electron-dense, which means that they are impermeable to the electron beam in the microscope. They are the storage and secretory organelles for small non-protein molecules necessary for effective haemostasis. The main contents of these organelles, and their functions, are detailed in Table 13.2. Note that some constituents have multiple functions.

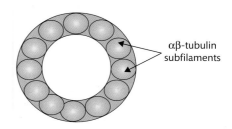

FIGURE 13.4

Substructure of platelet microtubule. The coil consists of 12–15 subfilaments of αβ-tubulin dimers circularly arranged to form a hollow tube.

αβ-tubulin
subfilaments

TABLE 13.2 Platelet α-granule and dense body–constituents and their functions.

Function	Constituents
α-Granules	
Adhesive proteins	VWF (platelet adhesion)
	Fibrinogen (platelet aggregation)
	Fibronectin, vitronectin, fibrinogen (wound healing)
Membrane proteins	GPIIbIIIa, GPIb, P-selectin
Coagulation biochemistry	FV, FVIII, fibrinogen
Fibrinolysis	Plasminogen
Inhibition	TFPI, protein S, α_2-macroglobulin, α_1-antitrypsin, protease nexin II (inhibit coagulation)
	α_2-antiplasmin, PAI-1 (inhibit fibrinolysis)
	Thrombospondin-1 (inhibits angiogenesis)
Chemokines for leucocyte attraction	Platelet factor 4, β-thromboglobulin
Cellular mitogens	PDGF (smooth muscle proliferation)
	VEGF-A, VEGF-C (angiogenesis)
Dense bodies	
Vasoconstriction	Serotonin
Platelet activation	ADP, serotonin (weak activator)
Coagulation biochemistry	Calcium ions
Energy for platelet biochemistry	ATP
Membrane proteins	GPIIbIIIa, GPIb, P-selectin
Integrin regulation	Calcium ions, magnesium ions

This table outlines the main constituents of α-granules and dense bodies but is not exhaustive.
Abbreviations: VWF, von Willebrand factor; GP, glycoprotein; TFPI, tissue factor pathway inhibitor; PAI-1, plasminogen activator inhibitor-1; PDGF, platelet-derived growth factor; VEGF, vascular endothelial growth factor; ADP, adenosine diphosphate; ATP, adenosine triphosphate.

Lysosomes are organelles that contain digestive enzymes and are found in most cells. In platelets they are also termed λ-granules and are few in number. They contain acid hydrolase enzymes which are assumed to facilitate the digestion of blood clots when they are no longer needed.

The events of primary haemostasis

Primary haemostasis comprises a series of events involving the activation of platelets and their interplay with VWF and subendothelium. These events lead to the formation of a plug of platelets and set the stage for secondary haemostasis.

Adhesion

The primary haemostatic response begins with vessel injury, which results in disruption of the vessel wall and the consequent exposure of procoagulant stimuli. The initial event following vessel damage is that of **platelet adhesion** to the collagen components of the subendothelium. Platelet adhesive events are mediated by two groups of glycoprotein (GP) surface membrane receptors, the integrin family and the leucine-rich motif (LRM) family. The integrin family consists of GPs comprising non-covalently associated αβ-heterodimers that mediate attachment to the subendothelium and/or platelet-to-platelet cohesion. LRM proteins are defined by the presence of a 24-residue structural motif. Four members of this family—GPIbα, GPIbβ, GPIX, and GPV—form the GPIb–IX–V complex which serves as the main VWF receptor. This complex is depicted in Figure 13.3.

At the low-shear stress conditions encountered in the venous circulation, platelets adhere to collagen directly via interactions with specific receptors, predominantly GPIaIIa (integrin $\alpha_2\beta_1$) and GPVI.

Under the intermediate- to high-shear conditions that exist in arteries, arterioles, capillaries, and stenosed (narrowed) vessels, platelet adhesion to collagen is indirect and dependent on the interaction between VWF and the GPIb–IX–V complex, the VWF providing a molecular bridge between the platelet surface and exposed collagen. This interaction can support adhesion in the venous circulation.

Circulating VWF is immobilized via the collagen within the exposed subendothelium and promotes *tethering* of platelets, which you can see in Figure 13.5. Resting platelets (i.e. non-activated) express GPIb–IX–V on their surface, but binding to VWF either does not occur or occurs with low affinity in the normal circulation. This is because the GPIb–IX–V binding section of circulating VWF is masked. Immobilization of VWF on the collagen surface allows the shear forces of flowing blood to unravel VWF and expose the binding section thus facilitating binding to GPIb–IX–V and consequent capture of platelets circulating at the edges of the vessel.

Look at Figure 13.6 and you will see that once tethered, platelets *roll* over immobilized VWF in the direction of blood flow as a result of the progressive formation of new VWF–GPIb–IX–V interactions as subsequent sections of the platelet membrane come into contact with the VWF, beginning at the site of tethering.

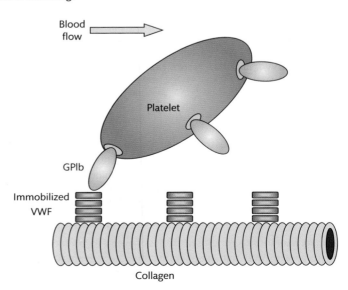

FIGURE 13.5

Platelet tethering via collagen, VWF and GPIb. VWF anchors to exposed collagen and blood flow facilitates unravelling of VWF to expose the GPIb-binding site. Platelets circulating at the edge of the vessel are then captured and tethered by VWF via binding to the constitutively expressed GPIb.

Blood flow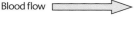

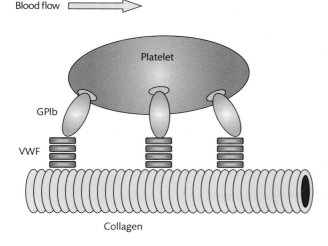

FIGURE 13.6
Platelet rolling. Once tethered via initial VWF–GPIb interactions, blood flow forces the platelet to roll over from the tethering point and promote further VWF–GPIb interactions.

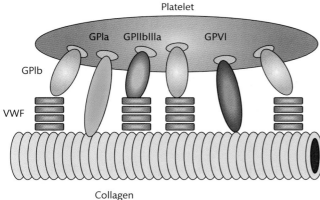

FIGURE 13.7
Stable adhesion of platelets. Stabilization of platelet adhesion to exposed sub-endothelium occurs via binding to glycoproteins additional to GPIb. GPIa and GPVI bind directly to collagen and GPIIbIIIa binds via VWF.

Interaction with VWF is not stable due to a fast dissociation rate so *stable adhesion* of platelets to the subendothelium also involves the collagen receptors GPIaIIa and GPVI, the **fibronectin** receptor GPIc′-IIa (integrin $\alpha_5\beta_1$), and the fibrinogen receptor GPIIbIIIa (integrin $\alpha_{IIb}\beta_3$), the latter being able to bind VWF at high-shear rates, and also fibronectin and **vitronectin**. The main interactions are shown in Figure 13.7.

Interaction of GPVI with collagen triggers signalling responses that lead to platelet activation, including elevation of cytosolic calcium ions, cytoskeletal actin-filament rearrangements, activation of enzymes (i.e. tyrosine kinases) and activation of GPIIbIIIa. Circulating platelets express GPIIbIIIa on the surface but there is no binding to plasma fibrinogen or VWF as the integrin maintains very low affinity for these **ligands** in resting platelets. Signalling responses resulting from collagen adhesion that activate GPIIbIIIa via tyrosine kinases are termed *inside-out signalling*. They modulate the adhesive activity of GPIIbIIIa by two distinct processes:

1. Activation of GPIIbIIIa via its cytoplasmic tails causes a conformational change in the extracellular domain that increases its affinity for ligands.

2. Clustering of GPIIbIIIa receptors to increase their local concentration, thereby promoting binding to multivalent ligands such as fibrinogen.

fibronectin
A multifunctional glycoprotein involved in cell adhesion, differentiation, growth, and wound healing.

vitronectin
A multifunctional protein that stabilizes plasminogen activator inhibitor 1, contributes to binding of platelets to vascular cell walls and promotes adherence, migration, proliferation, and differentiation of many different cell types.

ligands
Binding molecules.

Binding of fibrinogen and VWF to the extracellular domain of GPIIbIIIa causes further clustering and also conformational changes in the cytoplasmic domains that promote *outside-in signalling*. Signalling cascades are triggered in the cytoplasm that influence cytoskeletal re-organization, full platelet aggregation, granule secretion, and availability of procoagulant phospholipid activity. We will meet other GPIIbIIIa activators shortly when we explore platelet aggregation.

SELF-CHECK 13.4

What are the main events of platelet adhesion?

Shape change and platelet spreading

Once activated, platelets undergo a change in shape, transforming from discoid to a spherical centre with cytoplasmic extensions that enable closer physical interactions with each other and allow attachment to the vessel wall.

Transition from disc to sphere is mediated by the contraction of platelet myosin. Upon activation, the microtubule depolymerizes and the actin filaments of the cytoskeleton undergo a rapid disassembly and reorganization into new structures. This is under the control of a number of actin regulatory proteins, primarily gelsolin, which is activated by the significant increase in intracellular calcium ions mediated by phospholipase C. The re-assembly of actin filaments forms two types of cytoplasmic extensions. The first to appear are the needle-shaped *filopodia* which grow from the periphery of the platelet, and the larger and flatter *lamellipodia* which fill in the area between the filopodia. Extending these protuberances has the effect of flattening and spreading the platelet which squeezes granules and organelles into the centre of the platelet, giving the characteristic 'fried egg' appearance when viewed microscopically. The stages of transformation from disc to 'fried egg' are shown diagrammatically in Figure 13.8.

The process of adhesion generates a platelet monolayer that is sufficient to initiate platelet plug formation, but the single layer of cells itself is insufficient to prevent bleeding. We will now turn our attention to events that work towards extension of the forming thrombus.

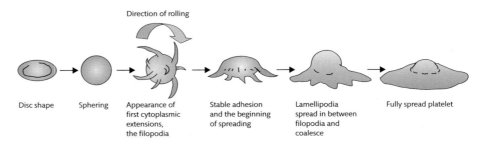

Direction of rolling

| Disc shape | Sphering | Appearance of first cytoplasmic extensions, the filopodia | Stable adhesion and the beginning of spreading | Lamellipodia spread in between filopodia and coalesce | Fully spread platelet |

FIGURE 13.8

Platelet shape change and spreading. Once platelets are activated, myosin contraction converts their shape from discoid to spherical. Disassembly and reorganization of actin filaments first results in the formation of thin, needle shaped filopodia while the platelet is rolling. At the stage of stable adhesion the platelet can begin spreading by forming lamellipodia which flatten and spread the platelet. Spreading squeezes cytoplasmic granules into the centre of the platelet.

Release reaction

Centralization of the α-granules and dense bodies, in the presence of elevated levels of calcium ions, leads to fusion of the granules with the membranes that line the SCOCS. The SCOCS acts as a conduit system of internal membrane leading to external secretion of the granule contents into the surrounding medium or onto the surface of platelets. Several of the haemostatic proteins within α-granules are present in relatively higher concentrations in platelets than in plasma. VWF and fibrinogen are 3–4 times more concentrated, and factor V is nearly 30 times more concentrated. The release of granule contents serves to increase their concentration in the area of the forming thrombus, one of the important localization mechanisms of the haemostatic response.

In addition to secretion, fusion of α-granules to the SCOCS and platelet membrane provides a number of crucial surface receptors, in particular, GPIIbIIIa and P-selectin. Although activated platelets already express functional GPIIbIIIa, this fusion provides a significant increase in GPIIbIIIa that magnifies its functions in relation to platelet spreading and aggregation. P-selectin binds to a receptor on leucocytes that initiates the leucocyte adhesion cascade, an essential step in inflammation.

Key Points

Inflammation (the process by which white blood cells and an array of biochemicals protect from infection and foreign substances) and tissue repair are directly linked to haemostasis. Activated platelets release inflammatory mediators such as histamine to increase capillary permeability. Substances such as platelet factor 4 and adenine nucleotides modulate white cell function, whilst others (such as platelet-derived growth factor) contribute to repair mechanisms. You will meet other instances of cross-over with inflammation and repair later in this chapter.

The **serotonin** released from dense bodies functions mainly as a vasoconstrictor, but it is also a weak platelet activator. The prime function of ATP is for energy, although it also has a role in platelet activation by triggering calcium influx. You will see in the next section that ADP plays a major role in platelet activation.

serotonin
Also known as 5-hydroxytryptamine (5-HT), a hormone that acts as a neurotransmitter in the brain and contributes to haemostasis by initiating vasoconstriction.

Platelet agonists and aggregation

Platelets express surface receptors for a number of ligands that will activate them as they arrive at the scene of vessel damage. This allows activated platelets to be recruited to accumulate on the platelet monolayer. These ligands, often referred to as **agonists** in this context, become available as part of the haemostatic response and contribute to one or more of three main platelet signalling processes:

agonists
Molecules that activate platelet functions via surface receptors.

1. Increase in cytoplasmic calcium ions
2. Reorganization of the actin cytoskeleton
3. Suppression of cyclic adenosine monophosphate synthesis

We have already covered the roles of the first two responses when we considered activation via GPVI, and these ligands provide alternative routes to platelet activation. Cyclic adenosine monophosphate (cAMP) is formed in platelets from ATP and inhibits platelet signalling, and so needs to be suppressed for platelets to become activated.

The main agonists are ADP, thrombin, and **thromboxane A₂** (TXA$_2$). Thrombin plays a pivotal role in haemostasis and we will meet it in more detail in the section on coagulation biochemistry. TXA$_2$ is produced from membrane arachidonic acid as part of the cyclooxygenase pathway, which is initiated upon platelet activation.

Cross reference

The cyclooxygenase pathway is shown in Figure 16.12 of Chapter 16.

Platelet aggregation is the formation of platelet-to-platelet linkages through the binding of mainly fibrinogen to activated GPIIbIIIa on adjacent cells, allowing the thrombus to grow beyond the initial platelet monolayer.

You can see in Figure 13.9 that the VWF- and collagen-mediated events of platelet adhesion generate the platform for the recruitment of resting platelets, which once activated, provide the platform for secondary haemostasis.

SELF-CHECK 13.5

What are the main platelet events following adhesion?

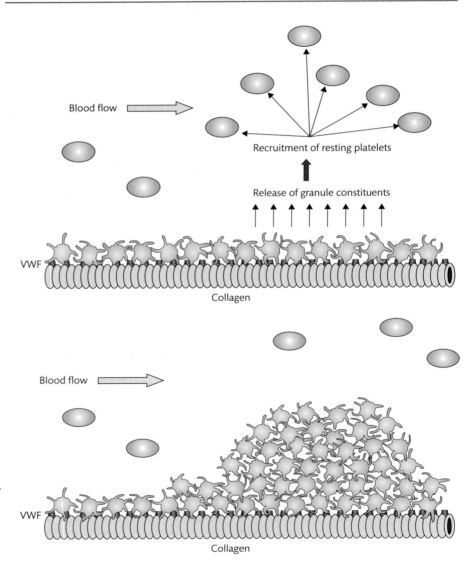

FIGURE 13.9

Activation and recruitment of platelets. Platelets forming a monolayer on the surface of exposed collagen are activated and release agonists into the local circulation to activate platelets arriving at the scene. Once activated, these platelets change shape to promote greater physical interactions and express surface GPIIbIIIa to facilitate aggregation via the formation of fibrinogen bridges.

Procoagulant activity

Critical to an effective haemostatic response is the presentation of negatively charged phospholipids on the surface of activated platelets which act as a platform for the assembly of two multiprotein complexes that are vital to coagulation biochemistry. Strong platelet activation or potent shear stress can induce the release of fragments of platelet membrane called *platelet microparticles*. These fragments express GPIb, GPIIbIIIa, and also phosphatidyl serine, which may play a role in supporting coagulation by providing an additional surface for the formation of the multiprotein complexes.

Additionally, exposed vessel adventitia cells and epithelial cells of surrounding tissues constitutively express **tissue factor** (TF) on their surfaces, which can also be expressed on platelet microparticles. TF is crucial to the activation of coagulation biochemistry and we will now turn our attention to that compartment of haemostasis.

13.3 **Secondary haemostasis**

In the microcirculation, a platelet plug alone is normally sufficient to stem blood loss, but it needs to be reinforced when forming in larger vessels if it is to be haemostatically effective. This is where the biochemical reactions of coagulation come into play. They converge on soluble fibrinogen to convert it into a meshwork of insoluble fibrin that intertwines with the cellular components of the forming thrombus to form a supporting scaffold.

The terms 'haemostasis' and 'coagulation' are often used interchangeably, yet the latter is but a part of the former. The processes of coagulation comprise a tightly regulated orchestration of coagulation factors, cofactors, and inhibitors that result in the controlled formation of the pivotal enzyme thrombin, which, in addition to activation and regulatory functions, initiates fibrin formation. The main players and their principal roles are outlined in Table 13.3.

Coagulation factors

The coagulation factors are a group of **zymogens** which cooperate in an integrated system of enzyme activation (and inactivation) steps. The substrate(s) of a given activated coagulation factor will be the zymogen of a different coagulation factor which becomes activated after part of the molecule, the activation peptide, has been cleaved to expose the active site.

zymogen
Inactive precursor of an enzyme, also called a proenzyme.

Coagulation factors are numbered using roman numerals in the order they were discovered and not in the order they were first thought to work. As indicated in Table 13.3, convention has it that zymogens are abbreviated to the letter F plus the roman numeral, and the activated forms are then subscripted with lower case a, e.g. FX and FXa. The majority of the activation reactions are confined to membrane surfaces because the coagulation factors or their precursors have specific binding sites for phospholipids, calcium ions, or specific receptors or cofactors expressed on cell surfaces, which contribute to the concentration and localization of the haemostatic response.

All the coagulation factors that function as activation enzymes belong to a class of **peptidases** called serine proteases, which are characterized by the presence of a serine residue in the active site of the enzyme.

peptidases
Enzymes that cleave **peptide** bonds in proteins.

Many of these enzymes require the presence of cofactors to maximize their rate of substrate activation. Examples of cofactors are tissue factor and the activated forms of the coagulation factors V and VIII. Strictly speaking they are coenzymes as they are organic (cofactors are inorganic), but it is common for them to be referred to as cofactors and we adopt that convention in these chapters.

TABLE 13.3 Key proteins of coagulation biochemistry.

Common name	Abbreviation	Vitamin K-dependence	Mean plasma level (µg/mL)	Half-life (h) in plasma	Main roles of active form
Factor II	FII	Yes	90	60–70	Converts fibrinogen to fibrin, activate PC and FXI
Factor V	FV	No	10	12–15	Cofactor for FXa
Factor VII	FVII	Yes	0.5	3–6	Activates FIX & FX (& FVII)
Factor VIII	FVIII	No	0.1	8–12	Cofactor for FIXa
Factor IX	FIX	Yes	5	18–24	Activates FX
Factor X	FX	Yes	8	30–40	Activates FII
Factor XI	FXI	No	5	45–52	Activates FIX
Fibrinogen	Fib/FGN	No	3000	72–120	Converts to insoluble fibrin clot
Factor XIII	FXIII	No	10	200	Stabilizes fibrin clot
Tissue factor	TF	No	NA	Cellular	Cofactor for FVII/FVIIa
Tissue factor pathway inhibitor	TFPI	No	NA	Cellular	Inhibits FVIIa activation of FX
Antithrombin	AT	No	140	72	Inhibits FIIa, FIXa, FXa & FXIa
Protein C	PC	Yes	4	6	Inactivates FVa & FVIIIa
Protein S	PS	Yes	10	42	Cofactor for activated PC
Protein Z	PZ	Yes	2.2	60	Cofactor for ZPI
Protein Z-dependent protease inhibitor	ZPI	No	Unknown	60	Inhibits FXa & FXIa
Heparin co-factor II	HCII	No	90	60	Secondary FIIa inhibitor
Alpha-1-antitrypsin	α1AT	No	250	120	Inhibits FXIa
α_2-macroglobulin	α_2M	No	2000	36	Backup to AT in certain conditions
Thrombomodulin	TM	No	NA	Cellular	Activation of PC
Endothelial protein C receptor	EPCR	No	NA	Cellular	Activation of PC

TF, TFPI, TM, and EPCR are membrane bound and do not have plasma levels or half-lives. Subscript a to a clotting factor denotes an active form.

Vitamin K-dependence

A group of the coagulation factors, FII, FVII, FIX, and FX, are termed vitamin K-dependent. During their biosynthesis in the liver, a series of post-translational enzymatic reactions include a step that requires vitamin K to function as a cofactor to a carboxylase enzyme. The enzyme+cofactor add carboxyl groups to the γ-carbon of a number of specific glutamic acid (Glu) side chains

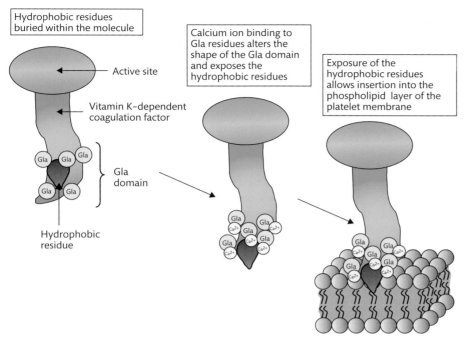

Hydrophobic residues buried within the molecule

Active site

Vitamin K–dependent coagulation factor

Gla domain

Hydrophobic residue

Calcium ion binding to Gla residues alters the shape of the Gla domain and exposes the hydrophobic residues

Exposure of the hydrophobic residues allows insertion into the phospholipid layer of the platelet membrane

FIGURE 13.10

Gla-domain function in vitamin K-dependent coagulation factors. Gla domains mask hydrophobic residues that are exposed upon binding of calcium ions to the Gla domains. The hydrophobic residue facilitates insertion of the coagulation factor into the phospholipid of the platelet membrane, which ensures localization of the coagulation reactions. Gla = γ-carboxyglutamic acid.

converting them to γ-carboxyglutamic acid (Gla). The section of the molecule containing them is termed the **Gla domain**.

The Gla residues bind calcium ions and are necessary for the activity of these coagulation factors. Figure 13.10 shows that binding of calcium alters the conformation of the Gla domain, which exposes hydrophobic phospholipid binding sites, thus enabling them to interact with membrane surfaces by direct binding to phospholipids.

Key Points

Naming the vitamin K-dependent factors is a common examination question so worth committing to memory. Note in Table 13.3 that protein C, protein S and protein Z are also vitamin K dependent. You will meet them in more detail when we look at coagulation inhibitors.

The events of coagulation

The generation of fibrin is essential to stabilize clots in larger vessels. Coagulation begins with an initiation phase, which is then amplified to set the stage for a burst of thrombin generation during a propagation phase.

Initiation

The events that start coagulation biochemistry via tissue factor and activated factor VII are referred to as the **initiation** phase. The sole initiator of coagulation is the membrane-bound protein tissue factor (TF). It is constitutively expressed at biological boundaries such as skin and organ surfaces, where it forms a protective envelope immediately available to initiate blood coagulation in the event of injury or blood loss. It is found in almost all tissues, although, interestingly, not in joints, where severe haemophiliacs have their worst bleeding episodes. TF is not expressed on vascular endothelial surfaces but is abundant in the vascular adventitia.

Initiation of coagulation begins with exposure of subendothelium after vessel damage which brings circulating blood into contact with the TF of the adventitia and surrounding tissues. TF binds FVII and functions as a cofactor in the activation of FVII, the formation of the TF–FVII complex also serving as a localization mechanism.

Unique amongst the serine proteases of coagulation, not all of FVII circulates as a zymogen: approximately 1% circulates in the active state (FVIIa). Plasma FVIIa has an inefficient active site and thus little **proteolytic** activity unless bound to TF, so at normal blood levels has no significant activity towards its substrates and is unreactive with circulating inhibitors. Both FVII and FVIIa bind to TF, the FVII remaining enzymatically inactive until autoactivated by TF–FVIIa, which induces a conformational change resulting in activation to the functional serine protease. The stages of FVII activation are shown in Figure 13.11. This TF–FVIIa complex is anchored on the cell surface in close proximity to negatively charged phospholipids, facilitating optimal positioning for its substrates. Tissue factor expressed on the surface of macrophages, monocytes, fibroblasts and platelet microparticles can also bind FVII/FVIIa.

Figure 13.12 shows that the TF–FVIIa complex then binds FX forming the so-called **extrinsic tenase complex** which activates the FX to FXa on the subendothelial surface. It also converts some factor IX to factor IXa. The complex is more efficient at catalysing the conversion of FX so FXa is the initial product.

At this stage the cofactor for FXa is unavailable so its reaction rate is relatively slow. Nonetheless, the FXa is able to cleave its main substrate, FII (prothrombin), to generate trace amounts of FIIa, otherwise known as thrombin, which is shown in Figure 13.13. Whilst insufficient to initiate significant fibrin formation, this thrombin generation is pivotal to amplification of the coagulation response.

Only small amounts of FXa are formed as its generation by this mechanism is rapidly downregulated by **tissue factor pathway inhibitor** (TFPI), which first binds to the active site of FXa and inhibits it. The TFPI–FXa complex then binds with high affinity to the FVIIa within the TF–FVIIa complex. This results in a fully inhibited quaternary complex of TF–FVIIa–TFPI–FXa preventing further activation of factor X via TF–FVIIa, as depicted in Figure 13.14.

proteolytic
Enzymes that digest or lyse proteins into smaller sections or amino acids.

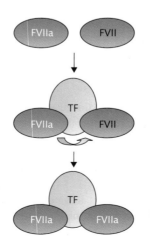

FIGURE 13.11
Stages of FVII activation. Activated and non-activated FVII bind to tissue factor (TF) that is exposed upon vessel damage. Binding of FVIIa to TF, its cofactor, bestows full enzymatic activity whereby it can activate zymogen FVII to FVIIa.

Approximately 1% of FVII circulates in the active state but it has little enzymatic activity unless bound to tissue factor

• Vessel damage leads to exposure of tissue factor
• FVII and FVIIa bind to the tissue factor
• FVII remains inactive until activated by the FVIIa which is now fully functional as it is bound to tissue factor

All the bound FVII becomes fully activated and available to activate FIX and FX

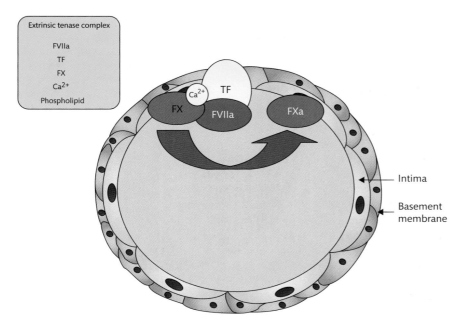

Extrinsic tenase complex

FVIIa
TF
FX
Ca²⁺
Phospholipid

Intima

Basement
membrane

FIGURE 13.12
Formation of the extrinsic tenase complex. The tissue factor–FVIIa complex is bound to the exposed vessel subendothelium and combines with FX to form the extrinsic tenase complex. The product of this reaction is FXa.

TFPI is predominantly produced in the endothelium and there are three pools:

- Approximately 90% is bound to the endothelium
- Between 5 and 10% resides in platelet α-granules
- A small amount circulates in plasma associated with lipoproteins.

Despite rapid inhibition of the initiation phase via TFPI, sufficient FXa is generated to further the coagulation response before it is shut down.

SELF-CHECK 13.6

How is secondary haemostasis initiated?

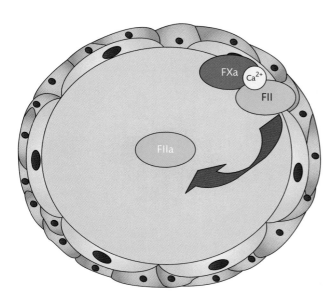

FIGURE 13.13
Generation of trace thrombin. FXa bound to phospholipid via calcium-ion interactions combines with FII (prothrombin) and converts it to FIIa (thrombin). At this stage, the cofactor for FXa (FVa) is unavailable so the reaction rate is slow and only trace amounts of thrombin are formed.

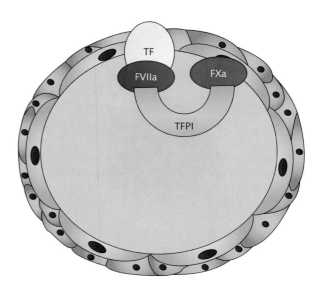

FIGURE 13.14

Down regulation of initiation by tissue factor pathway inhibitor (TFPI). Only small amounts of FXa are formed at the initiation stage because the tissue factor pathway is downregulated by the inhibitor TFPI, which first binds FXa and then the TF–FVIIa complex.

Amplification

The small amount of thrombin (FIIa) generated during initiation then enters an **amplification** phase to facilitate the availability of important cofactors. The trace amount of thrombin is able to activate the protein cofactors FV and FVIII and also platelets. FVa is the cofactor for FXa (the cofactor that was unavailable during the initiation phase), and FVIIIa is the cofactor to FIXa. Activation of more platelets results in exposure of the procoagulant phospholipid surface on a large scale. The availability of FVa and FVIIIa to significantly accelerate the reaction rates of their partner enzymes, together with the abundant platelet phospholipid, set the stage for large-scale thrombin generation sufficient to form fibrin clots and initiate important feedback mechanisms. The FIXa generated during initiation diffuses onto the platelet surface to facilitate the final phase of coagulation, that of propagation. The key elements of the amplification phase are depicted in Figure 13.15. Note that coagulation is transferred from one cell surface, the exposed subendothelium, to another, the membrane of activated platelets.

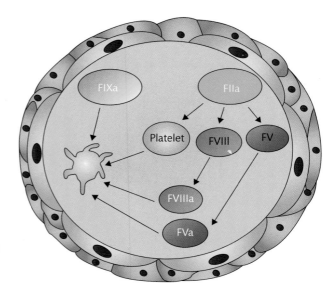

FIGURE 13.15

Amplification phase of secondary haemostasis. The small amount of thrombin generated at initiation is sufficient to activate circulating FV and FVIII and some platelets. The FIXa generated at initiation migrates to the surface of activated platelets to begin the propagation phase of coagulation.

What are the three haemostatic components that are activated by thrombin during amplification? Why is only a trace amount of thrombin generated at this stage?

Propagation

The shut-down of FX activation via TF–FVIIa means that an alternative route is required if thrombin generation is to continue. This comes predominantly in the form of the **intrinsic tenase complex** which comprises FIXa as the enzyme, FVIIIa as the cofactor, and FX as the substrate. FIX and FX are vitamin K-dependent proteins and so anchor the complex to the platelet phospholipid surface as a result of their interaction with calcium ions via their Gla domains. Activated platelets undergo a membrane re-orientation which affects the distribution of phospholipids, the activation process leading to a greater availability of phosphatidyl serine to promote the binding of activated coagulation factors. Assembly of the intrinsic tenase complex is shown in Figure 13.16.

The initial source of FIXa comes from the activation of FIX by TF–FVIIa during the initiation phase. Additionally, some of the membrane-bound FXa formed via this route will have activated FIX. Once FVIIIa is formed during the amplification phase, the intrinsic tenase complex becomes the major activator of FX. Binding of FIXa to FVIIIa induces a 10^6-fold increase in its ability to activate FX, the complex being 50 times more efficient than TF–FVIIa in FXa generation. Consequently, more than 90% of FXa is ultimately produced by the intrinsic tenase complex.

FXa combines with its cofactor and substrate, FVa and FII respectively, anchored to the platelet surface via calcium ions and phospholipid, to form the **prothrombinase complex**, which is shown in Figure 13.17. Along with the FVa generated in plasma, activated platelets provide another source of FV which is secreted from α-granules and is partially activated, becoming fully activated once in contact with thrombin.

Cross reference
You met the role of Gla domains in Figure 13.10.

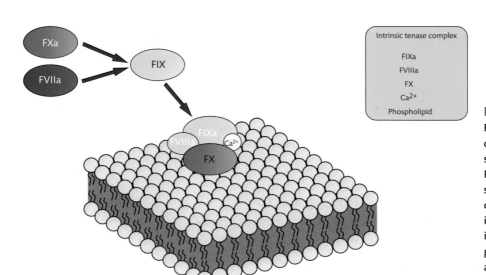

Intrinsic tenase complex

FIXa
FVIIIa
FX
Ca^{2+}
Phospholipid

FIGURE 13.16
Formation of the intrinsic tenase complex on the phospholipid surface of an activated platelet. FIXa binds to the phospholipid surface of the platelet via Gla domain–calcium ion interactions, and associates with its cofactor, FVIIIa, which was generated during amplification, and its substrate, FX. The product of the reaction is FXa.

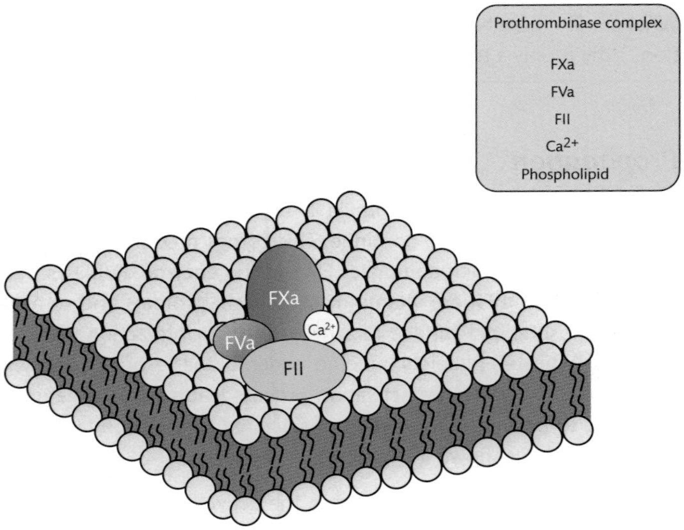

Prothrombinase complex

FXa
FVa
FII
Ca^{2+}
Phospholipid

FIGURE 13.17

Formation of the prothrombinase complex on the phospholipid surface of an activated platelet. FXa binds to the phospholipid surface of the platelet via Gla domain–calcium ion interactions, and associates with its co-factor, FVa, which was generated during amplification and released from platelet α-granules, and its substrate, FII. The product of the reaction is FIIa (thrombin).

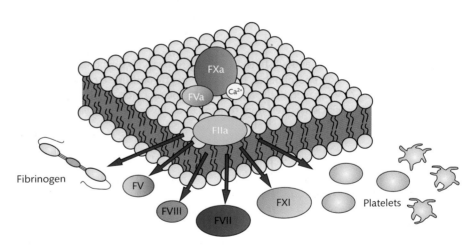

FIGURE 13.18

Burst of thrombin generation. The thrombin generated via the prothrombinase complex activates further components of haemostasis, allowing a positive feedback loop that leads to further thrombin generation. More platelets are activated by thrombin, and fibrinogen can now be converted to fibrin to stabilize the forming clot.

You can see in Figure 13.18 that the product of the prothrombinase complex is thrombin. This enzyme has multiple functions, mainly integral to haemostasis. Its main roles are listed below:

1. Proteolysis of fibrinogen
2. Activation of FV, FVII, FVIII, FXI, and FXIII
3. Activation of platelets via protease-activated receptor-1 (PAR-1)
4. Activation of protein C
5. Activation of thrombin-activatable fibrinolysis inhibitor (TAFI)
6. Tissue repair and development

Key Points

Key to the processes detailed above is that each step involves the assembly of multiprotein complexes onto cell surfaces, primarily the phospholipid-rich surface of activated platelets. Each complex comprises an enzyme, a cofactor, and a substrate:

- For extrinsic tenase, they are FVIIa, TF, and FX, respectively
- For intrinsic tenase they are FIXa, FVIIIa, and FX, respectively
- For prothrombinase, they are FXa, FVa, and FII, respectively

The substrates are serine protease zymogens, the product of one reaction becoming the enzyme of another. FIX is an alternative substrate for FVIIa + TF.

Note that the enzyme in each complex is a vitamin K-dependent factor and thus capable of binding to phospholipid surfaces via calcium ions to localize coagulation at the site of injury where appropriate surfaces are exposed.

With thrombin now being produced via the intrinsic tenase and prothrombinase complexes, it is available to enter into positive feedback loops to propagate coagulation. More FV and FVIII will be activated, and this is where FXI enters the process as another activator of FIX. FXI circulates in complex with high-molecular-weight kininogen (HMWK) which is required for binding FXI to phospholipid surfaces. In the presence of calcium ions and HMWK, FXIa activates FIX and can also autoactivate FXI to form more FXIa to propagate this route of FIX activation.

Despite the shutting down of FVII activation by TFPI during the initiation phase, FIXa, FXa, and thrombin are all capable of activating FVII and provide a route for introducing FVIIa into the propagation phase to generate more FIXa, FXa, and of course, FVIIa. Ultimately though, TF availability is reduced as the initial vessel breach is obscured by the forming clot, and thrombin generation continues without TF–FVIIa.

Key Points

You saw in Figure 13.16 how assembly of the intrinsic tenase complex on the surface of an activated platelet localizes the formation of its product, FXa, which then participates in assembly of the prothrombinase complex on the same surface to generate the pivotal enzyme thrombin.

Formation of thrombin via the intrinsic tenase complex and subsequent positive feedback mechanisms produce a burst of thrombin generation sufficient to cleave fibrinogen to form fibrin, and also to continue the feedback processes.

Key Points

Thrombin triggers inflammatory responses such as the production of chemokines to attract white cells to the site of injury.

SELF-CHECK 13.8

Name the three multiprotein complexes of coagulation biochemistry and their component enzymes, substrates, and cofactors.

Fibrinogen

hepatocytes
Liver cells involved in protein synthesis and storage.

Fibrinogen is a glycoprotein synthesized in **hepatocytes** and is present in a high concentration in plasma, (approximately 3.0 g/L), in marked excess to the minimal requirements necessary for normal haemostasis. It is also found in platelet α-granules where it is not synthesized but taken up from plasma by receptor-mediated endocytosis. Fibrinogen is a symmetrical dimer composed of two identical subunits, each of which consists of three non-identical polypeptide chains that are intricately folded together, these being:

- Aα chains
- Bβ chains
- γ chains

Fibrinogen was the first biological macromolecule to be visualized by electron microscopy. The molecular architecture was revealed to be trinodular, comprising two roughly spherical modules termed the D-domains, connected to a central E-domain. The E-domain contains the N-termini of all six chains tethered to each other via disulphide bonds. Two thin coiled coil regions stretch out on either side of the E-domain, each consisting of one Aα, one Bβ, and one γ polypeptide. Each coil ends in a globular D-domain which contains the C-termini of the Bβ and γ chains and part of the Aα chain. The remainder of the Aα chain protrudes from the D-domain as a long strand. Look at Figure 13.19 to see how the polypeptide chains are arranged and that they are linked at various positions by disulphide bonds. Figure 13.19 translates polypeptide arrangement into domainal structure for ease of interpreting the subsequent related diagrams.

In approximately 15% of circulating fibrinogen molecules one of the γ-chains is a minor variant termed γ′, and molecules where both are γ′-chains comprise about 1%. Molecules containing γ-chains are called fibrinogen 2.

Fibrinogen is a multi-functional molecule with roles in haemostasis, inflammation, and wound healing that are summarized in Table 13.4. We have covered its role in primary haemostasis and will now look at its function in secondary haemostasis.

Fibrin formation

Fibrin is formed from fibrinogen via the action of thrombin, which cleaves small peptide fragments from the N-terminal ends of the Aα and Bβ chains, which are termed **fibrinopeptide A** (FPA) and **fibrinopeptide B** (FPB), respectively. The fragments are small and constitute just 3% of the mass of fibrinogen. The fibrinopeptides shield polymerization sites on the parent molecule and prevent interaction with complementary structures in other fibrinogen molecules, sometimes referred to as 'knobs' and 'holes' respectively.

Figure 13.20 shows FPA release from a single fibrinogen subunit exposing the E_A polymerization site in the E-domain which joins non-covalently with the unshielded D_a binding site on the γ chain of the outer D-domain of another fibrin monomer/fibrinogen molecule. Note that

Fibrinogen polypeptide arrangement

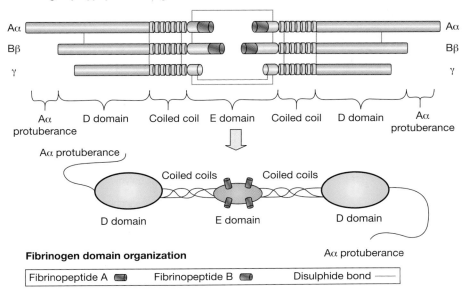

FIGURE 13.19

Fibrinogen structure. Symmetrical dimer structure composed of two identical sub units, each containing three non-identical polypeptide chains: the Aα, Bβ, and γ chains. The N-termini of all six chains are tethered together via disulphide bonds in the E domain. Two coiled coil regions stretch out on either side of the E domain, each consisting of one each of the Aα, Bβ, and γ chains. Each coil ends in a globular D-domain which contains the C-termini of the Bβ and γ chains and part of the Aα chain. The remainder of the Aα chain protrudes from the D domain as the Aα protuberance.

TABLE 13.4 Functions of fibrinogen.

Process	Functions
Haemostasis	Supports platelet aggregation
	Parent molecule for fibrin in the formation of an insoluble fibrin clot
	Clot dissolution
Inflammation	Bridging molecule in cell–cell interactions during inflammatory cell trafficking
Wound healing	Modulates cellular responses
	Structural support of adhesive cell–cell / cell–extracellular provisional matrix interactions
	Fibrinogen (and fibrin) found in tumour matrices to support angiogenesis
	Matrices provide structural scaffold to bind growth factors and support: cell adhesion, spreading, migration, and proliferation

one portion of the E_A site is at the N-terminus of the Aα chain and the other on the Bβ chain. FPB release, which is slower than FPA release, exposes the separate E_B polymerization site of the Bβ chain in the central E-domain which joins non-covalently with an inherently expressed

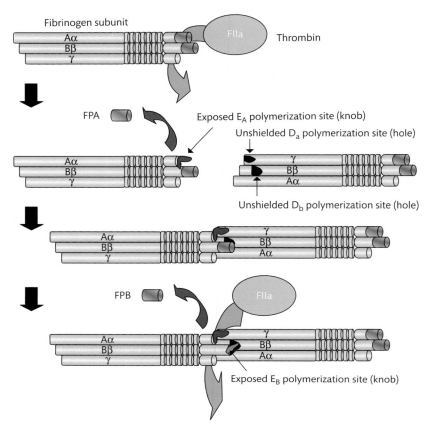

FIGURE 13.20

Fibrinopeptide release. Thrombin cleaves FPA from a fibrinogen sub-unit to expose the E_A polymerization site in the E domain, which joins with an unshielded D_a binding site on the γ chain of the outer D-domain of another molecule. Thrombin also cleaves FPB to expose a separate E_B polymerization site on the Bβ chain in the central E-domain, which joins with the unshielded D_b binding site of a Bβ chain in the D-domain of another molecule. The differing chain lengths and positions of the 'holes' result in the molecules overlapping to form the half-staggered overlap.

D_b-binding site of a Bβ chain in the D-domain of another molecule. Note that the differing chain lengths and positions of the 'holes' result in the molecules overlapping—the so-called half staggered overlap.

Fibrin molecules can link together through the interaction of the E-domain on one fibrin molecule to the D-domains on up to four other fibrin molecules. Fibrinopeptide release converts fibrinogen molecules to fibrin monomers and initially leads to the formation of fibrin dimers. The fibrin dimers are characterized by the overlap structure and are stabilized by the non-covalent interactions between the knobs and holes on the central and outer domains, which you can see represented in domain form in Figure 13.21. At this stage, the fibrin remains soluble. As the thrombin-catalysed fibrinopeptide cleavage continues, rapid polymerization ensues to generate two-stranded fibrin polymers called protofibrils. The fibrin molecules align in the staggered overlap end-to-middle domain arrangement which facilitates the formation of twisting fibrils. Multi-stranded fibrils are formed as a result of lateral association. Fibril

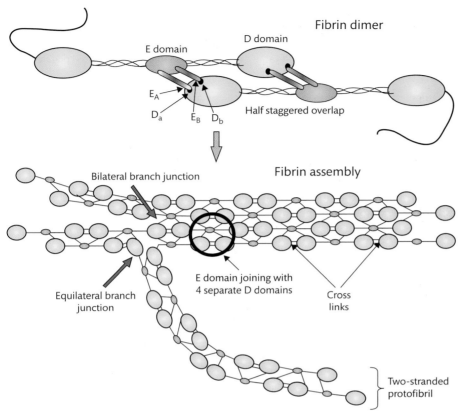

Fibrin dimer

E domain

D domain

E_A

D_a E_B D_b

Half staggered overlap

Fibrin assembly

Bilateral branch junction

Equilateral branch junction

E domain joining with 4 separate D domains

Cross links

Two-stranded protofibril

FIGURE 13.21

Domainal representation of fibrin formation. Fibrin dimer formation represents the start of fibrin polymerization; the diagram depicts the associations you met in Figure 13.20 in terms of E-domain and D-domain interactions. Formation of lateral fibrin polymers occurs when E-domains join with four separate D-domains, indicated by the thick circle. Branching occurs upon formation of bilateral or equilateral junctions.

branching to form a clot network is facilitated by formation of bilateral and equilateral branch junctions, which you can see in Figure 13.21.

The initial interactions forming the staggered overlaps are via E_A–D_a associations, release of FPB contributing to lateral associations. After a certain molecular size is reached, fibrin solubility is significantly reduced, leading to formation of an insoluble polymer.

SELF-CHECK 13.11

Outline the molecular events of fibrin formation.

Fibrin stabilization

Despite the intricacies of fibrin formation, the clot requires stabilization if it is to withstand higher blood pressure and shear forces and become fully haemostatically effective. The fibrin clot is stabilized and rendered mechanically stronger by the action of the activated form of FXIII.

Plasma FXIII circulates in the form of a tetramer composed of two A subunits, which are the catalytic component, bound to two stabilizing carrier B subunits. The plasma FXIII circulates bound by its B subunits to fibrinogen 2. FXIII also occurs intracellularly in platelets in the form of a homodimer of the two A subunits.

Activation of cellular or plasma FXIII is by calcium-dependent thrombin cleavage of the A chains. In the case of plasma FXIII, the A chains dissociate from the B chains, the active enzyme being a calcium-dependent transglutaminase that catalyses the formation of intermolecular covalent glutamine–lysine bonds between fibrin molecules (and between fibrin and other proteins). These links are commonly referred to as **cross links**. Intracellular FXIII can also be activated without cleavage by the elevated calcium levels in thrombin-activated platelets.

In the early stages of fibrin assembly, FXIIIa catalyses the formation of cross-links between the D-domains of the assembling fibrin molecules via γ chains. After the majority of γ chains have been paired, a slower process of cross link formation between α chains proceeds. Cross-linking can also occur between α chains and γ chains. The stabilized fibrin mesh strengthens the clot by binding platelets together and contributing to their attachment to the vessel wall, mediated by binding to platelet receptors and interactions with other adhesive proteins. FXIIIa cross-links fibrin γ chains to the platelet membrane.

FXIIIa also binds to α_2-**antiplasmin**, the main inhibitor of the enzyme plasmin which is responsible for dissolution of the clot.

The adhesive protein fibronectin comprises approximately 4% of the proteins in a fibrin clot and is subject to cross-linking by FXIIIa, connecting fibronectin molecules to each other or fibrin. Fibronectin contributes to increased fibre size, density, and strength. FXIII also plays an important role in wound healing, cell adhesion, and cell migration.

SELF-CHECK 13.12

What is the haemostatic role of FXIIIa?

SELF-CHECK 13.13

What are the main roles of fibrinogen in primary and secondary haemostasis?

Clot retraction

Over a time course of minutes to hours, blood clots draw in by a process termed clot retraction, which serves two crucial functions:

1. Helping platelet-rich thrombi withstand high shear forces.
2. Compacting the clot to facilitate continued blood flow whilst the wound repairs.

The process of clot retraction is driven by forces within platelets. GPIIbIIIa is integral to this function as it acts as a link between cytoplasmic actin filaments and surface-bound fibrin polymers. Additionally, GPIIbIIIa generates the intracellular signals that trigger retraction through activation of tyrosine kinases, which lead to the assembly of an intracellular complex of actin-binding proteins resulting in tethering of the actin to GPIIbIIIa. FXIIIa also cross-links actin to fibrin and to myosin. Once tethered, actin interacts with cytoplasmic myosin, which is the molecular motor that applies the contractile force on actin filaments.

Regulation of secondary haemostasis

Although localization mechanisms exist to restrict clot formation to the site of injury, the generation of potentially lethal enzymes such as thrombin in the circulation requires additional regulatory mechanisms. Left unchecked, the thrombin that could be generated from 20mL of blood could (theoretically) clot all circulating fibrinogen in less than a minute. This does not happen due to the existence of localization mechanisms and a group of physiological anticoagulant substances that co-operate to inhibit coagulation.

Once the coagulation reactions have been activated, a separate series of reactions occur that bring inhibitory mechanisms into play to limit and control the clotting processes. The **naturally occurring inhibitors** of coagulation fall into three main subtypes:

- Kunitz-type inhibitors
- Serine protease inhibitors (serpin)
- Components of the protein C system

We will now look at each of these inhibitors in turn.

Kunitz-type inhibitors

These inhibitors are so-termed because they contain biochemical modules called Kunitz domains. These domains are found throughout nature in many proteins that are usually inhibitors of specific serine proteases. The general mechanism of inhibition is the insertion of a looped structure from the inhibitor into the serine protease module of the enzyme where it occupies and disrupts the active site.

The two Kunitz-type inhibitors of importance to coagulation are TFPI, which we met earlier, and **protease nexin-2** (PN-2), which has inhibitory activity against FXIa and also FIXa and FXa in the prothrombinase complex. PN-2 circulates at low concentrations in plasma so has little inhibitory activity against any free FXIa, and the FIXa and FXa in the prothrombinase complex are membrane-bound anyway. However, PN-2 is present in platelet α granules and this is the likely route for its contribution to the inhibition of coagulation.

Serpins

As most TFPI is membrane-bound and therefore present in low concentrations in plasma, it can only delay the coagulation reactions, and so other inhibitors must come into play to regulate clot formation during subsequent stages. As well as FVIIa, the other main enzymes of coagulation are serine proteases, and human plasma contains a number of serpins that perform anticoagulant functions.

Serpins inhibit their target enzymes using a suicide substrate-inhibition mechanism. The reactive centre sequence of the serpin is recognized by the target enzyme as a substrate-like sequence and cleaves a peptide bond in the serpin. This leads to the formation of a covalent bond between the enzyme and the serpin and results in a massive conformational change in the serpin, and, to a lesser extent, of the enzyme too, which is consequently inactivated. The resultant enzyme–inhibitor complex is irreversible.

The plasma serpins vary in their specificity, some having almost incidental activity against activated coagulation factors with their main physiological roles being elsewhere in human biochemistry. The serpins that act predominantly as coagulation inhibitors are antithrombin (AT), heparin cofactor II (HC II), and protein Z-dependent protease inhibitor (ZPI).

Antithrombin

There were originally thought to be six antithrombins, but subsequent research has proven all but one to be other entities; thus, what has been termed antithrombin III in many publications is now referred to as just antithrombin.

AT is an important endogenous coagulation inhibitor, its name being something of a misnomer as it has inhibitory activity towards FIXa, FXa, and FXIa as well as thrombin. It also possesses activity against FVIIa in the FVIIa–TF complex, but not free FVIIa.

AT forms stable 1:1 complexes with its target enzymes; that is, one molecule of inhibitor binds to one molecule of target enzyme and neither takes any further part in haemostasis. It is an inefficient inhibitor in the absence of activating cofactors, and so complex formation without cofactors is progressive. Cofactor activity is provided *in vivo* by heparan sulphate, a glycosaminoglycan anchored to the vessel wall by a proteoglycan core and present on the surface of most eukaryotic cells and in the extracellular matrix. It serves to localize and concentrate activated AT on or in the vessel wall. Heparan sulphate binds AT via a unique pentasaccharide sequence, inducing a conformational change in the reactive centre of AT that potentiates its ability to bind and inhibit serine proteases. Once the inactive complexes are formed, heparan sulphate's affinity for AT decreases, allowing dissociation and subsequent rapid clearance of the complexes by the liver.

AT inhibits free FXa and thrombin more efficiently than FXa and thrombin which are bound to activation assemblies or clots as they are resistant to AT inactivation in those forms. In this case AT acts as a scavenger of FXa and thrombin molecules which diffuse away from complexes and clots, thus playing a crucial role in localizing and limiting coagulation and preventing unnecessary fibrin formation and deposition.

AT plays an important role in regulating the low-level activation of coagulation that occurs normally in the uncompromised circulation. In direct contrast to the protection afforded FXa when part of platelet surface complexes, FVIIa when in complex with TF on a cell surface is more susceptible to AT inactivation and provides a route for AT to regulate TF-induced coagulation.

AT circulates in two isoforms, α-AT and β-AT, the latter being less glycosylated. β-AT has enhanced affinity for heparan sulphate and is more effective than α-AT at inhibiting the thrombin appearing on the wall of injured vessels. The fact that 90% of circulating AT is the α-isoform is probably a reflection of the increased binding capacity and increased vessel wall consumption of β-AT.

AT also adopts non-anticoagulant functions. Its action on thrombin results in regulation of the enzyme's own non-coagulant functions, and thus has anti-proliferative and anti-inflammatory properties. Cleaved and latent forms of AT have potent anti-angiogenic properties.

SELF-CHECK 13.14

How are the anticoagulant roles of AT split between the two isoforms?

Heparin cofactor II

Heparin cofactor II (HC II) inhibits thrombin by forming 1:1 complexes, but it has no activity against other coagulation serine proteases. Binding to dermatan sulphate enhances the inhibitory action of HC II towards thrombin. AT is present in plasma in a two-fold molar excess over HC II, and it appears that the latter has different physiological roles related to thrombin inhibition in extravascular lesions and thrombin regulation during pregnancy.

Protein Z-dependent protease inhibitor

Protein Z-dependent protease inhibitor (ZPI) inhibits FXa via assembly of a calcium ion-dependent tertiary complex containing FXa, ZPI, and the vitamin K-dependent cofactor protein Z (PZ) at the phospholipid surface. PZ enhances the rate of FXa inhibition by ZPI more than 1000-fold. A portion of plasma ZPI circulates in complex with PZ. ZPI also inhibits FXIa, independently of calcium ions, phospholipids, and protein Z, by competing with other FXIa inhibitors and FIX for the active site of FXIa. The interaction between ZPI and FXIa generates cleaved, inactive ZPI, which reduces the amount of ZPI available for FXa inhibition.

ZPI can also inhibit FXa contained within the prothrombinase complex although its effect is negated at high prothrombin concentrations and so occurs either prior to FV activation or after local prothrombin consumption. Thus it seems that ZPI has a role in dampening coagulation by delaying initiation and reducing thrombin generation.

Alpha 2-macroglobulin

Alpha 2-macroglobulin (α_2M) is not strictly speaking a member of the serpin superfamily as its effects are not restricted to serine proteases, its binding to activated coagulation factors being away from the serine-active centre. In a normal adult it contributes to no more than 20% of the inhibition of thrombin and 10% of FXa inhibition. In coagulation, α_2M functions as a 'back-up' or 'fail-safe' serine protease inhibitor, particularly in times of pathological stress when some of the main inhibitors are overwhelmed. α_2M levels in children can be double those of adults, suggesting a compensatory role for the lower levels of AT in children. Other physiological roles for α_2M include the inhibition of non-coagulation proteinase enzymes and the regulation of growth factors and immune function.

Other serpins

α_1-antitrypsin is the main inhibitor of FXIa and also exhibits some activity against FXa, although it does not have a major impact in the regulation of thrombin generation. Its prime physiological role is the inhibition of neutrophil elastase. C1-esterase inhibitor plays a minor role in FXIa inhibition, its primary role being inhibition of the complement pathway. The final serpin of relevance to haemostasis is one of the main fibrinolysis inhibitors, α_2-antiplasmin (α_2AP), which we will meet in more detail later in this chapter.

The protein C anticoagulant system

We have seen that the generation of the cofactors FVa and FVIIIa during the amplification phase of coagulation is a pivotal point in clot formation as their presence facilitates assembly of the tenase and prothrombinase complexes on phospholipid surfaces. As AT has a limited inhibitory effect on FXa and thrombin bound to activation assemblies, the protein C pathway plays a crucial role in the regulation of coagulation on phospholipid surfaces by directly limiting the procoagulant activity of FVa and FVIIIa, and indirectly, thrombin. There are six key players in the pathway.

Protein C

Protein C (PC) is the circulating vitamin K-dependent zymogen of the serine protease **activated protein C** (APC), the enzyme responsible for inactivating FVa and FVIIIa.

SELF-CHECK 13.15

Which clotting factors are inhibited by activated protein C?

Thrombomodulin and thrombin

Thrombomodulin (TM) is a transmembrane receptor present on the endothelial cells of most arteries, veins, capillaries, and lymphatic vessels as well as most other tissues. The ratio between endothelial cell surface and blood volume is at its highest in the capillaries, so the TM concentration in the microcirculation is >1000-fold higher than in the major vessels. A fascinating paradox in haemostasis is that the pivotal procoagulant molecule, thrombin, when in complex with TM, loses its procoagulant activity and becomes anticoagulant in nature by activating protein C. Thrombin binds with high affinity for TM, which functions as a cofactor for thrombin, producing a >1000-fold increase in the rate of PC activation. Thrombin and TM bind in a 1:1 complex.

Endothelial protein C receptor

Endothelial protein C receptor (EPCR) is a transmembrane receptor on endothelial cells that is abundantly expressed in the larger arterial vessels and at lower levels in veins and capillaries. Although TM enhances activation of PC by thrombin, the conversion is a relatively low-affinity reaction. EPCR augments the activation of PC, providing a further 20-fold increase in the rate of PC activation by the thrombin–TM complex.

Protein S and factor V

APC requires the presence of two cofactors to exert its full anticoagulant effect: **protein S** (PS) and the intact form of FV.

PS is a vitamin K-dependent factor but is not a serine protease. Approximately 60% of circulating PS is associated in a 1:1 complex with C4b-binding protein (C4bBP) and is unavailable for APC cofactor functioning. The remaining 40% is termed free PS and it is this pool that is available to act as an APC cofactor. Free PS has little or no intrinsic inhibitory activity against FVa and FVIIIa; it acts by binding strongly (via the Gla domain) to negatively charged phospholipids on the surface of activated platelets, and then forming a calcium ion-dependent complex with APC. Whilst the presence of PS alone is sufficient for APC to inactivate FVa, regulation of FVIIIa within the tenase complex requires the synergistic APC cofactor activities of PS and FV.

PS does possess some intrinsic (APC-independent) inhibitory activity against FVa and FXa thereby affecting prothrombin activation, although the physiological significance is unclear. PS has a role in programmed cell death by binding to phospholipid exposed on apoptotic cells and stimulating phagocytosis.

Activation and function of protein C

The protein C pathway is brought into play as a direct consequence of the generation of thrombin. As the thrombin concentration rises its high affinity for TM results in much of it binding to TM, primarily on the endothelial surface. This binding promotes three important anticoagulant functions.

1. Occupation of a specific area of the thrombin molecule by TM prevents the binding of thrombin to its procoagulant substrates and activated platelets.

2. Binding to TM causes a conformational change in thrombin, altering its substrate specificity, and allowing it to activate PC.

3. When bound to TM, thrombin is more susceptible to inhibition by AT than free thrombin, so once thrombin generation ceases, the activation complex stops activating PC. A chondroitin sulphate side chain of TM stimulates this inhibition.

The Gla domains of PC/APC allow binding to negatively charged phospholipids; they are also the site of binding to EPCR. Figure 13.22 shows that PC is localized to the endothelial surface by EPCR which then moves laterally on the cell surface to locate a thrombin–TM complex. Here, PC is aligned by EPCR for optimal cleavage of an activation peptide thereby converting the serine protease domain to its active conformation. The platelet α-granule protein platelet factor 4 (PF4) that is released from activated platelets enhances PC activation by binding to the Gla domain and causing a **conformational change** that enhances PC affinity for the

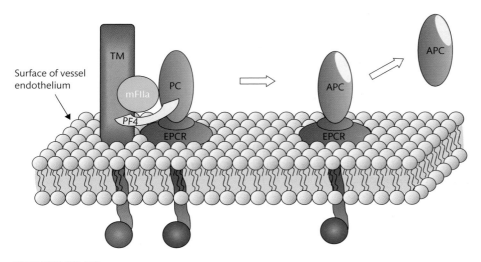

FIGURE 13.22

Activation of protein C on the surface of the vessel endothelium. Protein C (PC) is first localized on the endothelial surface by attachment to endothelial protein C receptor (EPCR) via Gla domains and then locates a thrombin–thrombomodulin complex. Binding of platelet factor 4 (PF4) enhances the affinity of PC for the thrombin–thrombomodulin complex, which activates PC to activated protein C (APC). The APC–EPCR complex then dissociates from the thrombin–thrombomodulin complex but APC does not exert any anticoagulant effect until it subsequently dissociates from EPCR. Note that thrombomodulin (TM) and EPCR are transmembrane proteins. mFIIa: thrombomodulin-modified thrombin.

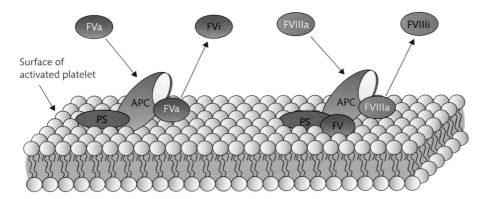

FIGURE 13.23

Inactivation of FVa and FVIIIa by activated protein C on the platelet membrane surface. Activated protein C (APC) released from the vessel surface forms a membrane-bound complex with protein S (PS), which orientates the active site of APC above the platelet surface to increase activity against FVa and FVIIIa. The APC–PS complex inactivates FVa and FVIIIa by cleaving a small number of peptide bonds, but it needs the zymogen FV and PS to work in synergy as cofactors for the cleavage of the bonds in FVIIIa.

thrombin–TM complex. APC is unreactive with its substrates whilst part of the activation complex, and so dissociates. You can see in Figure 13.22 that APC initially remains bound to EPCR, where it is able to contribute to cell signalling processes related to inflammation. APC must also dissociate from EPCR and onto the platelet surface in order to exert its anticoagulant effects.

PS binds with high affinity to negatively charged phospholipids and forms a membrane-bound complex with the APC on the surface of activated platelets. Notice in Figure 13.23 that assembly of this complex orients the active site of APC above the platelet surface, thereby enhancing its activity against FVa and FVIIIa within the forming clot. Without this mechanism, FVa and FVIIIa are protected from APC inactivation by FXa and FIXa, respectively. APC is a highly specialized enzyme that inactivates membrane-bound FVa and FVIIIa by cleaving just a small number of peptide bonds in these homologous molecules, so preventing further participation in effective thrombin generation.

The concentration of FV in plasma is about 100 times greater than that of FVIII, so APC is more likely to inactivate FVa than FVIIIa and mechanisms are required to ensure the inactivation of FVIIIa. The synergistic cofactor effect of FV and PS contributes to this, the effect also being required as the tenase complex is highly efficient and APC + PS alone is insufficient to regulate it. Also, FVIIIa is the preferred substrate for APC.

SELF-CHECK 13.16

Outline the interplay of the components of the protein C system.

Inhibition of the protein C pathway

APC is slowly and progressively inhibited by the protein C inhibitor (PCI; a serpin) through the formation of 1:1 complexes. Free thrombin can cleave free PS and abolish its ability to bind phospholipid and APC.

SELF-CHECK 13.17

Name the vitamin K-dependent factors in haemostasis.

13.4 **Fibrinolysis**

Fibrin clots cannot grow unchecked or remain in place indefinitely. They are degraded by enzymatic proteolysis through the multi-component mechanisms of fibrinolysis. Like coagulation, it includes zymogen precursors, activators, cofactors, and inhibitors and is a localized, surface-bound process. The main roles of fibrinolysis are:

- To act as the principal defence mechanism against vascular occlusion by preventing fibrin formation in excess of that required to prevent blood loss or rapidly removing excess fibrin.
- Removal of a fibrin clot as part of the process of tissue remodelling.

Fibrinolytic activity is always present in plasma, playing a role in the control of the normally occurring low-level activation of coagulation. Fibrin will only accumulate when its production exceeds its destruction.

Components of the fibrinolytic system

The pivotal enzyme that degrades fibrin (and fibrinogen) is **plasmin**, which is formed from its zymogen **plasminogen**. Several activators of plasminogen are known, and the system is regulated by inhibitors of plasmin and plasminogen activators.

The interplay between the main players of fibrinolysis is shown in Figure 13.24, which you can refer to as you meet each player in more detail in the following sections.

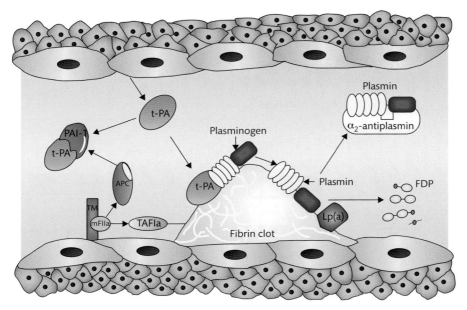

FIGURE 13.24

Interplay of components of fibrinolysis. t-PA released from vessel endothelium rapidly complexes with its inhibitor PAI-1. In the presence of a fibrin clot, t-PA and plasminogen assemble on the fibrin surface via attachment to lysine residues whereby t-PA undergoes a conformational change to facilitate the activation of plasminogen to plasmin, the enzyme that degrades fibrin to its breakdown products. Plasmin activity is regulated by its inhibitor α_2-antiplasmin. Lp(a) acts as a competitive inhibitor by competing for lysine-binding sites on the fibrin surface. The thrombin–thrombomodulin complex activates TAFI and protein C. TAFIa acts as an inhibitor by removing lysine binding sites but activated protein C impairs the inhibition of t-PA by PAI-1. t-PA, tissue plasminogen activator; PAI-1, plasminogen activator inhibitor type 1; TM, thrombomodulin; mFIIa, modified thrombin; APC, activated protein C; TAFIa, activated thrombin activatable fibrinolysis inhibitor; Lp(a), lipoprotein (a); FDP, fibrin degradation products.

Plasminogen and plasmin

Plasminogen is a single-chain glycoprotein. In its native form, plasminogen has a glutamic acid residue at the N-terminus and is referred to as Glu-plasminogen. Important to the localization of the fibrinolytic response are five looped structures, or kringles (named after a Scandinavian pastry that has a knotted appearance). The kringles contain lysine binding sites that promote binding to lysine residues on the surface of a fibrin clot.

Glu-plasminogen is activated mainly by **tissue plasminogen activator** (t-PA) to form two-chain Glu-plasmin, which you can see in Figure 13.25. However, Glu-plasmin is fibrinolytically ineffective as its lysine-binding sites are masked. Glu-plasmin converts Glu-plasminogen to single-chain Lys-plasminogen which has a higher affinity for fibrin. Lys-plasminogen is then converted by t-PA to two-chain Lys-plasmin, which is the active serine protease enzyme as it can bind to fibrin. Lys-plasmin can also convert Glu-plasminogen to Lys-plasminogen, and Glu-plasmin can also autocatalyse to Lys-plasmin.

Plasmin can hydrolyse a variety of substrates by cleaving lysine–arginine bonds. Its main substrates are fibrinogen and fibrin but it can also hydrolyse FV and FVIII. Plasmin also has a role in inflammation by activating the complement protein, C3.

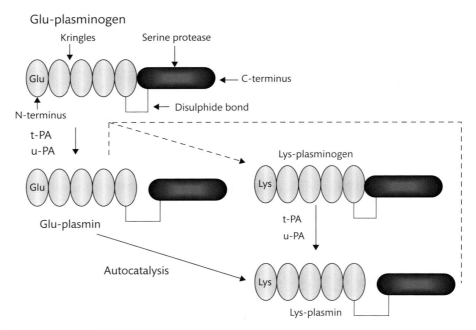

FIGURE 13.25

Plasminogen activation. Glu-plasminogen is activated by t-PA to the two chain Glu-plasmin, which has masked lysine-binding sites. Glu-plasmin converts Glu-plasminogen to single chain Lys-plasminogen which is then converted by t-PA to two-chain Lys-plasmin, the active form of the enzyme. Lys-plasmin converts Glu-plasminogen to Lys-plasminogen and Glu-plasmin autocatalyses to Lys-plasmin.

Tissue plasminogen activator

t-PA is a serine protease and its only known substrate is plasminogen. It is secreted into the circulation by endothelial cells as a single-chain form, and quickly cleared by the liver or inactivated by formation of a 1:1 complex with the fast acting inhibitor, **plasminogen activator inhibitor type 1** (PAI-1). Most circulating t-PA is bound to PAI-1.

The rate of t-PA release is markedly increased by a variety of physical and biochemical stimuli, including venous occlusion, strenuous exercise, diet, hypercoagulability, thrombin, vasopressin or its analogues, and some antidiabetic drugs. Free t-PA, however, is an inefficient activator of plasminogen in the absence of fibrin. Assembly of t-PA and plasminogen onto the fibrin surface to form a ternary complex is shown in Figure 13.24, which causes a conformational change in the t-PA, so facilitating plasminogen activation. The resultant plasmin not only digests the fibrin but cleaves t-PA into a two-chain form which enhances the formation of t-PA–plasminogen–fibrin complexes. Conversion of fibrinogen to fibrin exposes cryptic binding sites for t-PA–plasminogen, so free t-PA has minimal affinity for plasma fibrinogen. The requirement of fibrin as a cofactor for the t-PA–plasminogen complex is a localization mechanism, and demonstrates that fibrin colludes in its own destruction.

SELF-CHECK 13.18

How is the action of plasmin localized?

Urinary plasminogen activator

Sometimes called urokinase, the **urinary plasminogen activator** (u-PA) is synthesized predominantly in the kidneys and also by fibroblast-like cells in the gastrointestinal tract. It is secreted as a single-chain zymogen termed pro-urokinase and becomes a two-chain serine protease upon activation by kallikrein and plasmin. The one kringle module in u-PA has no fibrin affinity, and u-PA binds instead to its cell-associated receptor, u-PAR. Thus, its main functions are within tissues where it plays a role in the cellular events of differentiation, mitogenesis, wound healing and inflammation, and also has a minor role in clot lysis.

Other plasminogen activators

A number of exogenous activators of human plasminogen from animals and microorganisms have been described. Various strains of the bacterium *Streptococcus* produce an extracellular protein called **streptokinase** (SK), purified versions of which have been used to treat life-threatening thrombotic events such as myocardial infarction by activating plasminogen to destroy the clot. Staphylokinase (SAK) from the bacterium *Staphylococcus aureus* also has thrombolytic properties. SK and SAK form 1:1 complexes with plasminogen, but there is no activation in the absence of fibrin.

A number of snake venoms contain plasminogen activators to exacerbate bleeding in their prey by digesting clots. Examples include TSV-PA from the Chinese green tree viper (*Trimeresurus stejnegeri*), LV-PA from the Bushmaster pit viper (*Lachesis muta muta*), and Haly-PA from the Siberian pit viper (*Agkistrodon halys*).

The saliva of the vampire bat (*Desmodus rotundus*) has a highly potent plasminogen activator (DS-PA) to keep blood in a fluid state while it feeds. DS-PA has a higher affinity for fibrin than t-PA so there is virtually no plasminogen activation without it and it can be used therapeutically.

Inhibitors of plasmin

Similar to thrombin generation, the plasmin-generating potential of plasma is considerable and requires regulatory mechanisms to prevent build up of a potentially lethal enzyme. The inhibitors affect either plasmin itself or its activators.

α_2-antiplasmin and α_2-macroglobulin

The primary inhibitor of plasmin is the serpin α_2-antiplasmin which exerts its effect in two ways:

- Formation of a stable 1:1 complex with plasmin which completely inactivates the enzyme.
- Retardation of fibrinolysis by masking lysine-binding sites on Glu-plasminogen and thus interfering in the binding to fibrin. Lys-plasmin(ogen), however, has a higher affinity for the fibrin surface and is less susceptible to this effect of α_2-antiplasmin.

The cross-linking of α_2-antiplasmin to the fibrin clot by FXIIIa is a mechanism to resist premature clot destruction. In plasma, the concentration of plasminogen exceeds that of α_2-antiplasmin, which is not the case in a fibrin clot where the latter is concentrated as a result of the cross-linking. The small amount of plasmin generated during normal physiology is rapidly neutralized by α_2-antiplasmin, but under pathological conditions of extreme fibrinolytic activation (i.e. snake bite, streptokinase therapy) it can become swamped. This is where **α_2-macroglobulin** comes into play, acting as a scavenger inhibitor by forming 1:1 complexes with excess plasmin that retain weak enzymatic activity but are cleared rapidly by the liver.

Thrombin activatable fibrinolysis inhibitor

Also known as carboxypeptidase B, **thrombin activatable fibrinolysis inhibitor** (TAFI) reduces fibrin's ability to act as a cofactor by removing lysine binding sites for plasminogen and t-PA. Interestingly, TAFI is activated by thrombin only when the thrombin is in complex with thrombomodulin.

SELF-CHECK 13.19

What are the main mechanisms of plasmin inhibition?

Other plasmin inhibitors

Histidine-rich glycoprotein (HRG) regulates fibrinolysis due to its capacity to bind and block the high-affinity lysine binding sites of plasminogen. Approximately 50% of circulating plasminogen is reversibly bound to HRG.

Lipoprotein (a) has striking structural homology with plasminogen and acts as a competitive inhibitor for binding sites on fibrin, fibrinogen, and t-PA.

Thrombospondin is a platelet α-granule constituent that has activity against plasmin.

Inhibitors of plasminogen activators

Activators of plasminogen are regulated by their own set of inhibitors. Plasminogen activator inhibitor type 1 (PAI-1) is principally synthesized and secreted by endothelial cells and is present in platelet α-granules and adipocytes (fat cells). Platelets are the major pool of PAI-1. Endothelial synthesis is upregulated by many compounds, including thrombin, lipoproteins, insulin and pro-insulin. PAI-1 functions as a fast-acting inhibitor of t-PA, u-PA, and, to a lesser extent, plasmin, all of which cleave the same bond in PAI-1 and are subsequently inhibited by the formation of a 1:1 complex.

Approximately 80% of plasma PAI-1 is in complex with t-PA; the remaining free PAI-1 is functionally active and stabilized by association with vitronectin. Plasma PAI-1 levels exhibit diurnal fluctuations with an early morning peak that can halve by the afternoon.

Plasminogen activator inhibitor type 2 (PAI-2) exists in both an intracellular form and a secreted form that vary with respect to glycosylation. Very little PAI-2 is detectable in plasma, except during pregnancy where it is produced by the placenta. This is because villous cells are the main source of PAI-2 so the presence of a villous-rich organ like the placenta results in increased plasma levels. It is more effective against u-PA than t-PA but is less effective than PAI-1 against both activators. Its main roles are intracellular where it can alter gene expression and influence the rate of cell proliferation and differentiation.

APC forms a tight complex with PAI-1 whereby it can no longer inhibit t-PA. It also has an indirect inhibitory effect on TAFI as it downregulates thrombin generation which, in turn, leads to reduced TAFI activation. Interestingly, PCI, the APC inhibitor, is also referred to as **plasminogen activator inhibitor type 3** (PAI-3).

Fibrinogen and fibrin degradation by plasmin

Fibrinogen and fibrin are degraded in a sequential fashion by plasmin to soluble degradation products. Figure 13.26 shows that the first stage of fibrinogen proteolysis is the symmetrical

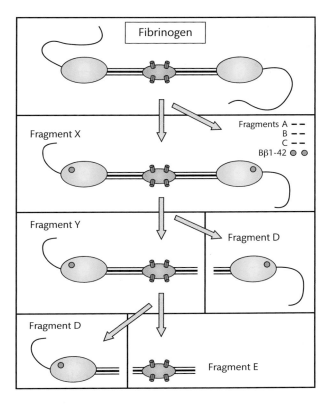

FIGURE 13.26

Fibrinogen degradation by plasmin. The first stage of the plasmin mediated proteolysis of fibrinogen is the cleavage of fragments A, B, and C from the C terminal of the Aα chains, followed by cleavage of the Bβ1–42 fragments from the Bβ chains. The remainder of the parent molecule is termed fragment X. The next plasmin attack point leads to the removal of one D fragment; the remainder of the parent molecule is referred to as fragment Y. Removal of the second D fragment from fragment Y leaves the tethered N-termini of all six chains, fragment E.

removal of three small peptides from the C-terminal of the Aα chains, termed fragments A, B and C. This is followed by cleavage of the first 42 amino acids of the Bβ chains generating the Bβ1–42 fragments, the remainder of the parent molecule being fragment X. You can see in Figure 13.26 that fragment X is little different to an intact fibrinogen molecule. Still looking at the figure, it shows that fragment X is then asymmetrically degraded by the removal of a section from its C–terminal end comprising parts of all three chains linked by disulphide bonds, which is termed fragment D. The remainder of the parent molecule is fragment Y, from which another fragment D is removed, leaving the N-terminal portion of all six, disulphide-linked chains, termed fragment E.

Plasmin degradation of cross-linked fibrin initially generates large aggregates of fragments termed X and Y **oligomers**. The progressive degradation of these large complexes to the terminal derivatives, DD–E, DD, and E, which occurs in solution after their release from the clot, is depicted in Figure 13.27. Of particular diagnostic interest are the **D-dimer** derivatives. Note that each D-fragment has a different parent molecule and they remain joined due to cross-linking, so the detection of D-dimers in plasma indicates the presence of an *in situ* clot, whereas detection of single D-fragments from fibrinogen lysis can result from other conditions.

Cross reference

You will meet the use of D-dimers in the diagnosis of thrombotic disease in Chapter 16.

SELF-CHECK 13.20

How do the D-fragments of fibrin degradation differ from the D-fragments of fibrinogen degradation?

Cross-linked fibrin strands

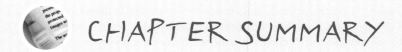

FIGURE 13.27

Fibrin degradation by plasmin. Plasmin degrades fibrin in a similar way to fibrinogen, although the presence of cross links results in differing products. Degradation of fibrin initially generates large aggregates of fragments termed X and Y oligomers, which are further digested by plasmin to the terminal derivatives DD–E, DD, and E.

Key Points

Inflammation promotes the production of increased levels of a group of proteins called acute-phase reactants, such as the complement proteins. Many of the haemostatic proteins you have met in this chapter are acute-phase reactants, such as FVIII, VWF, fibrinogen, PAI-1, t-PA, and plasminogen.

CHAPTER SUMMARY

Roles

- Haemostasis exists to maintain blood fluidity and to limit and arrest blood loss resulting from injury.

- Mechanisms exist to remove clots once they have served their purpose.

Components

- Vascular integrity
- Platelets
- Blood coagulation
- Fibrinolysis
- Inhibitory mechanisms

Primary haemostasis

- Damaged blood vessels expose structures that promote clotting mechanisms.
- VWF is immobilized on collagen fibres and facilitates the adhesion of platelets.
- Adhered platelets become activated and recruit more platelets via the release reactions and aggregation.

Secondary haemostasis

- Damaged blood vessels expose tissue factor, which initiates coagulation biochemistry via FVII/FVIIa to activate FIX and FX.
- Trace levels of thrombin are generated that activate FV, FVIII, and platelets before the pathway is shut down by TFPI.
- FVIIIa acts as cofactor to the FIXa, which moves to the phospholipid surface of activated platelets to activate more FX, which once activated and linked to cofactors, generates more thrombin.
- The thrombin back-activates the coagulation system and converts soluble fibrinogen to insoluble fibrin strands, which are stabilized by cross-linking and then intertwine between platelets to consolidate the clot.

Fibrinolysis

- t-PA activates plasminogen to plasmin once they have both bound to the fibrin surface.
- Plasmin degrades fibrin, generating soluble fragments.

Inhibitory mechanisms

- AT forms 1:1 complexes with thrombin and FXa.
- APC inhibits phospholipid-dependent reactions in the presence of PS and FV by cleaving FVa and FVIIIa.
- PAI-1 inhibits t-PA to regulate plasmin generation.
- α_2-antiplasmin inhibits plasmin.
- TAFI removes binding sites for plasmin on the fibrin surface.

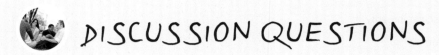

DISCUSSION QUESTIONS

13.1   How do localization mechanisms contribute to effective haemostasis?

13.2   What might be the physiological advantages of having multiple-component enzyme systems for coagulation and fibrinolysis in preference to the direct generation of fibrin and plasmin?

13.3   Which came first, the coagulation factor or the inhibitor?

13.4   Platelets are the platform for haemostasis; discuss.

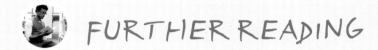

FURTHER READING

- **Colman RW, Hirsh J, Marder VJ, Clowes AW, George JN (ed.)** *Hemostasis and Thrombosis: Basic Principles & Clinical Practice*, 4th edn. Lippincott Williams & Wilkins, Philadelphia, 2001.

  Detailed chapters on different components of haemostasis.

- **Hoffbrand AV, Catovsky D, Tuddenham EGD (ed.)** *Postgraduate Haematology*, 5th edn. Blackwell Publishing Ltd, Massachusetts–Oxford–Carlton, 2005.

  Good overview of haemostasis and a separate chapter on platelet function.

- **Hoffman M, Monroe DM. A cell-based model of haemostasis.** *Thrombosis and Haemostasis* 2001:**85;**958–65.

  One of the first review articles covering the cell-based model of haemostasis.

- **Michelson AD (ed.)** *Platelets*. Elsevier Science, California–London, 2002.

  Extensive coverage of platelets in health and disease with coverage of laboratory techniques.

- **Mosesson MW. Fibrinogen and fibrin structure and functions.** *Journal of Thrombosis and Haemostasis* 2005:3;1894–904.

  Excellent detail of current knowledge of fibrinogen.

Answers to self-check questions, case study questions, and discussion questions are provided in the book's Online Resource Centre, visit www.oxfordtextbooks.co.uk/orc/moore

14

Bleeding disorders and their laboratory investigation

Gary W. Moore and David A. Gurney

In this chapter you will be introduced to bleeding disorders that arise from hereditary or acquired abnormalities of coagulation factors, von Willebrand factor (VWF), platelets, and blood vessels. We will then look at the main laboratory tests available to biomedical scientists to identify and characterize bleeding disorders.

Learning objectives

After studying this chapter you should confidently be able to:

- Name a number of bleeding disorders and describe their causes.
- Describe the principles and interpretation of coagulation screening tests.
- Describe the principles of factor assays and raw data assessment.
- Describe the principles of inhibitor screening and measurement.
- Describe the laboratory investigation for von Willebrand's disease and outline the subclassification.
- Describe screening tests for primary haemostatic disorders.
- Describe the principles and interpretation of platelet function analysis.

14.1 Bleeding disorders

Bleeding disorders occur when components of haemostasis are deficient to an extent that confers a tendency to bleed excessively. The phrase *deficiency* is used as an all-encompassing term relating to the biological activity of a given substance. Some patients make molecules with normal function, but the deficiency exists because the molecules are manufactured in lower amounts than normal. Other patients manufacture the molecules in normal amounts but with impaired function, so the biological activity is deficient even if the concentration of the molecule is not.

Patients with more severe disorders will experience bleeding episodes that begin in early childhood, often with no obvious precipitating event—these are called spontaneous bleeds. Those with mild disorders are more likely to exhibit excessive bleeding following trauma, surgery, or dental extraction. Common symptoms of bleeding disorders include the following:

- **Epistaxis (nosebleeds)**
- Gingival (gum) bleeds
- Bruising
- Purpura (skin haemorrhages appearing as purple spots or patches)
- Petechiae (small skin haemorrhages appearing as minute red or purple spots)
- Menorrhagia (heavy menstrual bleeding)
- Joint bleeds leading to arthritic complications
- Muscle bleeds
- Chronic anaemia

The type, site, and severity of haemorrhage can give important clues to whether a haemostatic disorder is present, and if so, the areas of haemostasis that are affected. Easy bruising, epistaxis and menorrhagia are common, but unless persistent and severe, do not necessarily indicate a haemostatic abnormality. Broadly speaking, there are differences between the clinical manifestations of defects in primary and secondary haemostasis. In the former, bruises are small, epistaxis is common and often severe, bleeding from cuts and abrasions can be prolonged and profuse, and bleeding after dental extraction or surgery is immediate. Conversely, patients with factor deficiencies can present with large bruises at unusual sites, epistaxis is uncommon, bleeding from cuts and abrasions is not severe, and bleeding after dental extraction or surgery tends to be delayed. **Haematuria** is common in factor deficiencies as is **haemarthrosis** in severe haemophilia, but they are rare in primary haemostatic disorders. Haemostatic abnormalities leading to bleeding disorders can involve any area of haemostatic function and can be hereditary or acquired.

haematuria
Presence of blood in urine.

haemarthrosis
Bleeding into joint spaces that can lead to joint damage and disability.

Hereditary bleeding disorders

Probably the most well known are the haemophilias, yet the most common hereditary bleeding disorder is **von Willebrand's disease** (VWD), which you will meet later in this chapter.

Haemophilia

Deficiency of FVIII is referred to as **haemophilia A** and deficiency of FIX is **haemophilia B**, the latter sometimes referred to as Christmas disease as it is named after the first boy described with it, Stephen Christmas. Both are X-linked disorders and so occur almost exclusively in males. You will remember from Chapter 13 that the function of FVIII and FIX are directly linked, FVIIIa being a cofactor for FIXa, so deficiencies of one or the other have virtually identical clinical signs and symptoms. Many different genetic mutations have been described that give rise to deficiencies of varying clinical severity and bleeding frequency, which are inversely correlated with the FVIII or FIX level of activity. Haemophilia A is subclassified according to FVIII activity, as shown in Table 14.1, which can also be applied to FIX levels in haemophilia B.

Haemophilia A occurs at a frequency of approximately 1 : 10 000 males, of which about 30% are spontaneous mutations where no family history of a bleeding disorder will be apparent. Haemophilia B has an approximate frequency of 1 : 50 000 males.

TABLE 14.1 Sub-classification of haemophilia A.

Classified as	Severe	Moderate	Mild
FVIII level (IU/dL)	<1.0	1.0 – 5.0	>5.0
Age at presentation	Infancy	<2 years	>2 years
Bleeding symptoms & frequency	Frequent spontaneous bleeds into joints, muscles and internal organs. Severe bleeding after trauma.	Much fewer spontaneous bleeds than patients with severe disease. Minor trauma can precipitate a bleed.	No spontaneous bleeds. Bleeding after significant trauma/ surgery
Approximate percentage of cases	50	30	20

Reference range for FVIII: 50–150 IU/dL.

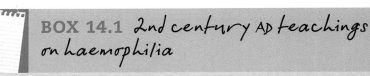

BOX 14.1 *2nd century AD teachings on haemophilia*

The earliest known description of haemophilia and the recognition that it affects males can be found in the Babylonian *Talmud*, a book of Jewish laws, ethics customs and history. The *tana'im*, who were Rabbinic sages, taught that 'If she circumcised her first son and he died, and a second son and he died, she must not circumcise a third one.'

A third haemophilia exists, **haemophilia C** (or Rosenthal's disease), which is due to a deficiency of FXI. It is an autosomal disorder of variable clinical severity where the bleeding manifestations do not correlate with FXI levels. It is predominantly, but not exclusively, found in patients of Ashkenazi Jewish heritage. About 8% of Ashkenazi Jews have FIX deficiency.

Haemophilia in females

Some carrier females have a sufficient reduction in FVIII/FIX to require treatment prior to invasive procedures or after major trauma. The main causes of markedly reduced FVIII/IX levels in females are listed below:

- Extreme **lyonization** of the FVIII or FIX gene in a carrier
- Hemizygosity (unpaired genes) of X chromosome with mutant FVIII/FIX gene (i.e. XO in Turner syndrome)
- Female with Normandy variant VWD (see below)
- True haemophiliac female (parents are a male haemophiliac and a female carrier who are often cousins)
- Female with acquired haemophilia (see below)

lyonization
The process by which one copy of the X chromosomes in a female is inactivated.

> **BOX 14.2 Lyonization**
>
> Only one X chromosome is necessary to generate sufficient levels of the gene products. Lyonization occurs to prevent females having twice the levels of males, who only possess one copy of the X chromosome. The inactivation is random in all mammals except marsupials where it occurs only in the X chromosome derived from the male parent. A clear manifestation of lyonization is seen in tortoiseshell cats, which have black and orange alleles for fur colour on their X chromosomes. Every patch of orange fur occurs because the X chromosomes in those areas that carry the black allele have been inactivated, and vice versa. If a woman haemophilia carrier undergoes extreme lyonization of her X chromosomes carrying normal genes for FVIII/FIX, she can have sufficiently low levels to present with a symptomatic bleeding disorder.

SELF-CHECK 14.1

What are the main differences between haemophilias A, B, and C?

14.2 von Willebrand's disease

This disease was first described in 1926 by Dr Eric Adolf von Willebrand in a population on the Åland Islands and termed 'pseudo-haemophilia', VWD is now known to be an autosomal bleeding disorder of variable clinical severity resulting from a variety of subtypes of VWF deficiency. It is present in about 1% of the population and classically presents as a mild to moderate bleeding disorder with symptoms such as epistaxes, bruising, excessive minor wound bleeding, heavy menstruation, and excessive, yet rarely life-threatening bleeding after trauma/surgery. Prolonged bleeding after a first dental extraction is often the first manifestation. Because primary haemostasis (i.e. VWF, platelet and vessel interactions) predominates in small vessels, patients with all but the most severe VWD do not suffer the crippling and painful joint and muscle bleeds seen in people with haemophilias A or B who are more dependent on effective secondary haemostasis.

In addition to the effects of VWD on primary haemostasis, the reduction in VWF leads to a concomitant reduction in FVIII levels because there is less VWF to protect FVIII from proteolytic degradation in the plasma. In the most severe form of VWD, where VWF is absent, this leads to FVIII levels similar to those of moderate or severe haemophiliacs and exacerbates the clinical condition. However, the FVIII level does not fall to zero as the patients have functional FVIII genes and continually produce enough FVIII to maintain a baseline of about 1.0–2.0 IU/dL. The full subclassification of VWD is detailed later in this chapter when we consider its laboratory investigation.

SELF-CHECK 14.2

What are the two mechanisms by which a deficiency of VWF can contribute to bleeding symptoms?

Other clotting factor deficiencies

Deficiencies of other clotting factors are much rarer than VWD or haemophilias A and B. Deficiency of FVII has an estimated prevalence of 1 : 500 000, whilst deficiencies of fibrinogen, FV, FX, and FXI are each about 1:1 000 000. Prothrombin and FXIII deficiencies are rarer still, each occurring with a frequency of about 1 : 2 000 000. They all demonstrate an autosomal-recessive pattern of inheritance, with the exception of dysfunctional fibrinogens, which tend to be autosomal-dominant. Population frequencies show geographical differences, the recessive disorders being more common in countries where consanguineous marriages are frequent.

An interesting autosomal-recessive disorder presenting as a combined deficiency of FV and FVIII is known, with a prevalence of about 1:1 million. It is not, as one might expect, the result of dual inheritance of FV and FVIII mutations, but the deficiency of a chaperone protein for these factors that is involved in their intracellular transport known as **lectin mannose binding protein 1** (LMAN1). The disorder can also be caused by deficiency of the cofactor molecule for LMAN1, **multiple coagulation factor deficiency 2** (MCFD2).

The clinical severity of these rarer disorders is variable. Most **dysfibrinogenaemias** (60%) are asymptomatic, whilst about 20% will have bleeding symptoms and 20% thrombotic episodes. **Hypofibrinogenaemia** is usually mild and often not detected until surgery or trauma. **Afibrinogenaemia** gives rise to a severe bleeding disorder. Prothrombin deficiency can be severe when levels are low and undetectable prothrombin levels are probably incompatible with life. Combined FV and FVIII deficiency is usually clinically mild (the levels are not as low as seen in haemophilia itself), as is isolated FV deficiency. The clinical severity of FVII deficiency is variable and does not correlate well with plasma levels, probably because only a small amount of FVIIa is necessary to trigger coagulation. Deficiencies of FX and FXIII tend to be more severe, with patients often suffering the bleeding into joints and muscles seen in haemophilias A and B.

dysfibrinogenaemia
Functional deficiency of fibrinogen.

hypofibrinogenaemia
Low concentration of functionally normal fibrinogen.

afibrinogenaemia
Absence of plasma fibrinogen.

Treatment

The main treatment is replacement therapy with concentrates of the deficient factor. Concentrates can be derived from multiple donations of human plasma, or manufactured utilizing recombinant technology. Some patients are treated prophylactically, whilst others are treated when a bleed is recognized or suspected.

Treatment of VWD can involve concentrates, but some subtypes respond to a drug called **desmopressin**, which increases the release of VWF from endothelial cells.

Other primary haemostatic disorders

Other than VWD, primary haemostatic disorders occur as a result of a reduction in the numbers or function of platelets, which are covered later in this chapter, or the haemorrhagic vascular disorders.

Hereditary haemorrhagic telangiectasia (HHT) is an autosomal-dominant disorder characterized by fragile blood vessels which are prone to bleeding as they cannot support the mechanisms of primary haemostasis. Type 1 HHT is caused by a mutation in **endoglin**, which is involved in cytoskeletal organization, and Type 2 HHT by a mutation in **activin receptor-like kinase 1** (ALK-1), which controls the maturation phase of **angiogenesis**.

angiogenesis
Blood vessel formation.

Connective tissue disorders can result in fragile blood vessels, such as the collagen abnormalities seen in Ehlers–Danlos syndrome and osteogenesis imperfecta, or the elastic-fibre abnormality of Marfan syndrome.

Acquired disorders of haemostasis

A number of clinical situations exist where bleeding symptoms occur that are not due to hereditary haemostatic abnormalities but are secondary to other disorders, and are thus referred to as acquired bleeding disorders.

One potentially life-threatening condition is **disseminated intravascular coagulation** (DIC), which results from the excessive activation of coagulation plus loss of the control and localization mechanisms. The key triggering event is an increase in tissue factor (TF) expression, which occurs on monocytes and endothelial cells in response to cytokines, endotoxins, interleukin 1 (IL-1), or tumour necrosis factor in conditions such as sepsis and malignancy. DIC is often a presenting feature of acute promyelocytic leukaemia as the immature cells express TF. The tissue damage from trauma or surgery can induce the release of TF into the circulation. Some snake venoms induce DIC by directly activating specific coagulation factors, and, as we will see later in this book, they can be used as laboratory tools for diagnostic purposes. These triggers without localization cause inappropriate systemic activation of coagulation and platelets. This can lead to clots that cut off circulation to the extremities such that they may require amputation, and even to major organs, which can subsequently fail.

Eventually, clotting factors are consumed faster than they can be replaced and bleeding symptoms result. Bleeding is exacerbated by the consumption of inhibitors and platelets, and also the generation of excessive fibrin degradation products, which themselves are anticoagulant in nature as they impair fibrin formation and bind to platelet membranes. The severe nature of DIC has led some to refer to the acronym as 'death is coming'.

Look at Table 14.2 for a summary of the main causes of acquired bleeding disorders. Acquired thrombocytopenias are covered in Table 14.7.

SELF-CHECK 14.3

Describe the causes of acquired bleeding disorders.

14.3 Laboratory investigation of a suspected bleeding disorder

Diagnosis of a bleeding disorder is dependent on the presence of bleeding symptoms in the patient, yet compiling the bleeding history is subjective. Questionnaires are available where the examining clinician gives scores depending on the presence and severity of particular symptoms, the so-called bleeding score, which can aid diagnosis and choice of laboratory investigations. When there is clinical suspicion of a bleeding disorder, characterization of the presence and nature of any defect(s) begins with the performance by biomedical scientists of screening tests that will indicate the area(s) of haemostasis affected. Table 14.3 lists the commonly used tests.

TABLE 14.2 Acquired bleeding disorders.

Primary disorder	Acquired cause of bleeding
Sepsis, shock, obstetric calamities, trauma, surgery, some malignancies, transplant rejection, recreational drugs, snake bite	Acute DIC
Some malignancies, chronic infections, chronic kidney disease, Kasabach-Merritt syndrome	Chronic DIC (less severe than acute DIC)
Liver disease	Reduced synthesis of coagulation factors and thrombocytopenia
Renal disease	Uraemia and increased prostacyclin release impair platelet function
Vitamin K deficiency	Dietary deficiency or malabsorption reduces synthesis of vitamin K dependent factors. Newborns are vitamin K deficient and can present with haemorrhagic disease of the newborn.
Autoantibodies to coagulation factors or platelets	Reduction in affected coagulation factor or platelet numbers
Old age, prolonged steroid use, vitamin C deficiency	Compromised blood vessel integrity
Amyloidosis (extracellular protein deposition)	Impaired platelet function; amyloid binds FX causing plasma FX deficiency and can interfere with fibrin polymerization
Dilutional coagulopathy	Massive transfusion of stored blood products &/or volume replacement with blood substitutes (i.e. they do not contain coagulation factors and live platelets) can reduce platelet numbers and concentrations of circulating coagulation factors
Drug therapy	Anticoagulant therapy (see Chapter 16); various drugs impair platelet function (see later in this chapter)

TABLE 14.3 Screening tests for defects of haemostasis associated with bleeding.

Area of haemostasis	Tests	Result determinants
Platelets/vessels	Platelet count	Platelet numbers
	Blood film examination	Platelet morphology
	Platelet function screen	Platelet function; VWF
	Bleeding time	Platelet function; VWF; vessel abnormalities
Coagulation	Prothrombin time	Levels of factors II, V, VII, X & fibrinogen; inhibitors
	Activated partial thromboplastin time	Levels of factors II, V, VIII, IX, X, XI, XII, PK, HMWK & fibrinogen: inhibitors
	Mixing tests	Distinguish between factor deficiencies and inhibitors
	Thrombin time	Level of fibrinogen
	Reptilase time	Level of fibrinogen
	Fibrinogen activity	Direct measurement of fibrinogen
Fibrinolysis	D-dimers	Direct measurement of FDPs
	Dilute clot lysis time, euglobulin clot lysis time, fibrin plate	Mainly t-PA, PAI-1, plasminogen and α_2 antiplasmin

Coagulation screening

The investigation of platelets and fibrinolysis is discussed elsewhere, so we will now concentrate on **coagulation screening.** Before we consider the hows and whys of each test, we need to introduce the concept of the **cascade theory of coagulation**. This theory preceded the cell-based model that you saw in Chapter 13, and forms the basis of some screening test design. Briefly, two separate enzyme pathways were considered to each generate FXa which then began a third pathway culminating in fibrin generation. The coagulation factors in each pathway were considered to follow strict sequential order, one enzyme activating many more molecules of the next in sequence before being inactivated. The cascade theory is presented in Figure 14.1 where you will notice some factors that were not part of the coagulation model you met in Chapter 13—FXII, prekallikrein (PK), and high molecular weight kininogen (HMWK). These are involved in the contact activation of the **intrinsic pathway** where exposure to the collagen surface partially activates FXII, which becomes

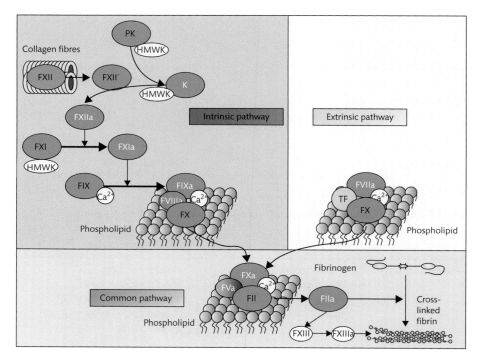

FIGURE 14.1

Coagulation cascade. The intrinsic pathway is activated by the contact of FXII with the negatively charged surface of collagen. This partially activates FXII to FXII′, which becomes fully activated by kallikrein, which is generated via its precursor prekallikrein in the presence of high molecular weight kininogen. FXIIa activates FXI in the presence of high molecular weight kininogen. FXIa activates FIX, which combines with FVIIIa, calcium, phospholipids, and FX to form the intrinsic tenase complex, whose product is FXa. The extrinsic pathway involves FVIIa, tissue factor, calcium, phospholipids, and FX, which form the extrinsic tenase complex, which also generates FXa. The FXa from these pathways begins the common pathway by forming the prothrombinase complex in tandem with FVa, calcium, phospholipids, and FII. The product is FIIa (thrombin), which converts fibrinogen to fibrin, which is stabilized by thrombin-activated FXIII.

fully activated via PK and HMWK before it activates FXI. Deficiencies of the three 'contact factors' do not cause bleeding disorders. As you saw in Chapter 13, they play little part in coagulation *in vivo* and in fact have other roles related to fibrinolysis and inflammation.

SELF-CHECK 14.4

Name and outline the 3 discrete pathways of the cascade theory of coagulation.

In contrast to the cell-based model, the cascade theory does not explain why subjects with contact factor deficiencies are free of bleeding problems, or why the haemophilias are so severe when there is apparently another pathway that can generate FXa. It does not account for why FXI deficiency is less severe than deficiencies of FVIII and FIX when FIX apparently relies on FXIa for its activation. Similarly, the cofactors FV and FVIII are activated by thrombin, yet generation of the latter occurs after FV and FVIII activation in the cascade model.

Screening tests

Coagulation screening tests are designed to isolate specific compartments of the cascade theory to give clues to where an abnormality exists. An hereditary or acquired abnormality of coagulation is termed a **coagulopathy**. You saw in Table 14.3 the coagulation factors that affect each test and we will now look at the design and use of each test.

Prothrombin time

The reagents detailed in Box 14.3 allow the patient's plasma to form a fibrin clot via the **extrinsic pathway** and **common pathway** and the time taken to clot is recorded as the **prothrombin time** (PT).

The patient's PT, measured in seconds, is compared to a reference range which will vary depending on the analytical technique and type of thromboplastin used. (There are more details on thromboplastin types in Chapter 16.) If the clotting time is elevated above the reference range, it may indicate one or more of the following:

- Deficiencies of factors II, V, VII, X or fibrinogen
- Autoantibodies against the above clotting factors

BOX 14.3 *Prothrombin time design*

- **Thromboplastin** contains tissue factor to 'activate' FVII, and also phospholipid for reactions involving vitamin K-dependent factors (which ones will operate here?).
- Manual methods add calcium ions subsequently, whereas automated methods use thromboplastins containing calcium.
- The intrinsic pathway is not activated as there is no contact factor activator. Although FVIIa can activate FIX, thromboplastin reagents provide such a powerful stimulus that the FXa generated will form a clot via the common pathway before FIX can exert any appreciable effect.

- Anticoagulant drugs affecting the production of vitamin K-dependent factors (i.e. warfarin)
- Anticoagulant drugs directly affecting thrombin (i.e. hirudin)
- Vitamin K deficiency
- Liver disease
- DIC
- Lupus anticoagulants, albeit rarely (see Chapter 15)

SELF-CHECK 14.5

Describe the principle of the PT, and the causes of elevated clotting times with this test.

Activated partial thromboplastin time

The reagents detailed in Box 14.4 allow a patient's plasma to form a fibrin clot via the intrinsic and common pathways—the time taken to clot, measured in seconds, is recorded as the **activated partial thromboplastin time** (APTT).

The patient's APTT is compared to a reference range, and if the clotting time is elevated above the reference range, it may indicate one or more of the following:

- Deficiencies of factors II, V, VIII, IX, X, XI, XII, PK, HMWK or fibrinogen
- Some subtypes of VWD (due to associated FVIII deficiency)
- Autoantibodies against the above clotting factors
- Anticoagulant drugs affecting the production of vitamin K-dependent factors, although the APTT is less affected than the PT because there are more non-vitamin K-dependent factors contributing to the clotting time
- Anticoagulant therapy with heparin
- Anticoagulant drugs directly affecting thrombin (i.e. hirudin)

BOX 14.4 *APTT design*

■ Patient plasma is incubated for a set time period, typically 2–5 minutes, with a contact activator to activate FXII and begin the intrinsic pathway. Commonly used contact activators are kaolin, silica, and ellagic acid.

■ Although not a significant reaction *in vivo*, FXII is used in this way to activate FXI independently of thrombin generated via the extrinsic pathway. Similarly, the activation of FIX and FX is independent of FVII.

■ The reagent also contains a 'partial' thromboplastin comprising phospholipids for reactions involving vitamin K-dependent factors (which ones will operate here?) but no tissue factor, thereby preventing activation of the extrinsic pathway.

■ Incubation with activator only allows the intrinsic pathway to proceed as far as FXIa generation. After the incubation period, calcium ions are added to allow coagulation to proceed to completion.

- Vitamin K deficiency
- Liver disease
- DIC
- Lupus anticoagulants

Describe the principle of the APTT and causes of elevated clotting times with this test.

Result interpretation—We can narrow down the *in-vitro* compartment of coagulation from where a deficiency involving a single factor exists based on whether one or both of the PT and APTT results are abnormal:

PT and APTT elevated: deficiency exists in the common pathway
PT only elevated: FVII deficiency
APTT only elevated: deficiency exists in the intrinsic pathway

Mixing tests

Factor deficiency can result from a reduced production/increased clearance of the factor, or the presence of antibodies that interfere with function (i.e. inhibitors). If you mix an equal volume of normal plasma with plasma from a patient who has a factor deficiency and repeat the screening test that was initially abnormal, the missing factor will be replaced by that present in the normal plasma and the result will correct into the reference range. However, if the patient has an **inhibitor**,

CASE STUDY 14.1 *Screening tests in a patient with a factor deficiency*

A 5-year-old boy presented with an intramuscular haematoma with no history of bleeding from minor cuts and abrasions.

The results of tests showed (RR, reference range):

PT (s)	11.9	(RR: 10.0–14.0)
APTT (s)	102.3	(RR: 32.0–42.0)
APTT 1:1 **mixing test(s)**	38.0	
TT (s) (see below)	9.3	(RR: 9.0–11.0)
Fibrinogen (g/L)	3.8	(RR: 1.5–4.0)
Platelet count ($\times 10^9$/L)	250	(RR: 150–400)

What is the probable diagnosis, and what further investigations would you perform to confirm the diagnosis?

it will interfere with the function of the normal plasma as well as the patient's plasma and the result will not correct. These simple follow-up tests assist biomedical scientists and medical staff in deciding on the next stages of the diagnostic process. We will meet assays for specific factors and inhibitors later in this chapter, and the *in vitro* inhibitors known as lupus anticoagulants are covered in Chapter 15. A word of caution: some inhibitors are time-dependent and may not manifest without prolonged incubation at 37 °C. There are more details about them later in this chapter.

Key Points

The diagnostic process involves marrying clinical and laboratory data.

Thrombin time and reptilase time

The **thrombin time** (TT) is a simple test, whereby thrombin is added to patient plasma to directly convert fibrinogen to fibrin and the time to clot measured in seconds. The patient's TT is compared to a reference range, and if the clotting time is elevated above the reference range, it may indicate one or more of the following:

- Hypofibrinogenaemia—acquired causes such as DIC are more commonly encountered than hereditary forms.
- Dysfibrinogenaemia—can be hereditary or acquired (i.e. liver disease)
- Afibrinogenaemia.
- Anticoagulant therapy with heparin.
- Anticoagulant drugs directly affecting thrombin (e.g. hirudin).
- Hypoalbuminaemia, amyloidosis, paraproteins, and elevated levels of fibrin/fibrinogen degradation products (FDP) can interfere with fibrin polymerization.

In clinical practice, there are occasions when the laboratory is inadvertently not informed that a patient is receiving therapeutic heparin and the biomedical scientist is presented with an unexpected elevated TT accompanied by an elevated APTT but normal PT. One way to confirm that the results are due to heparin therapy is to perform a **reptilase time** (RT). The RT is similar to TT except that the reagent is not thrombin but a thrombin-like enzyme purified from the venom of the Common Lancehead pit viper snake (*Bothrops atrox*). Heparin

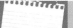

BOX 14.5 *Haemophilia B variants*

Haemophilia B Leyden is an interesting variant characterized by severe FIX deficiency at birth that is gradually ameliorated from the onset of puberty—probably by the action of testosterone on an androgen-responsive element in the FIX promoter.

The results above in Case Study 14.1 are typical for a patient with haemophilia. Mutations causing haemophilia Bm result in a FIX molecule with an inhibitory effect on the activation of FX by FVIIa–tissue factor—which is detectable *in vitro* when bovine thromboplastin is used for PT analysis, leading to an elevated PT as well as APTT. The 'm' stands for Martin, the surname of the family in which the variant was first described.

anticoagulates by markedly potentiating antithrombin, but because reptilase is a reptile enzyme it is unaffected by human antithrombin so the RT will be normal. RT can be elevated for the reasons stated above for TT, except for anticoagulant drugs directly affecting thrombin, and of course, heparins.

Since heparin is administered by continuous intravenous infusion, blood samples are often taken from the line in the vein so that the patient does not have to receive a separate venepuncture. Unless the line is properly flushed to remove heparin, blood samples can be contaminated such that the APTT, TT, and even PT (which is rarely affected by therapeutic levels of heparin), are incoagulable. A normal RT in this circumstance would indicate heparin contamination and a repeat sample should be requested.

Interestingly, the snake venom enzyme only removes fibrinopeptide A from fibrinogen, in contrast to thrombin that additionally removes fibrinopeptide B. Discrepancies between TT and RT can sometimes indicate a dysfibrinogenaemia if the mutation is in the Bβ chain as the TT will be abnormal but the RT normal.

SELF-CHECK 14.7

What are thrombin time and reptilase time used for in clinical laboratories?

Direct assays of fibrinogen

In the **Clauss fibrinogen assay**, plasma is diluted (usually one part plasma to nine parts buffer) to dilute out interfering substances like heparin and fibrin(ogen) degradation products (FDP). The diluted plasma is clotted with a strong concentration of thrombin so that the clotting times are independent of thrombin concentration over a wide range of clotting times. In view of the thrombin concentration, the dilution of the plasma also prevents clotting times being too short. The clotting time is read off a standard curve and converted to fibrinogen concentration. If the fibrinogen concentration is sufficiently high or low that the clotting time is beyond the linearity limits of the standard curve, the plasma is re-diluted to bring the clotting time into the measurable limits and the dilution taken into account in the calculation of the final result. This means that a plasma with a low fibrinogen level may need a 1:5 or 1:2 dilution, resulting in less dilution of interfering factors which can then generate an erroneous result that underestimates the fibrinogen level.

Automated analysers using photo-optical clot detection can derive a fibrinogen level from the patient's PT data. The optical density-changes for a range of dilutions of a plasma with a known fibrinogen level are used to generate a standard curve. The optical density-change from the patient's PT curve is read off the standard curve to produce the fibrinogen value. This derived fibrinogen assay is simple and ostensibly free because the result is derived from the raw data of another test. However, there is wide variation in results depending on the thromboplastin and analyser pairing used. The optical clarity and fibrinogen level of the standard can affect accuracy, many methods generating higher results than Clauss assays.

Immunological methods such as ELISA can be used to measure the total amount of fibrinogen antigen present irrespective of function. Dysfibrinogenaemias will have lower functional results than antigenic results whereas they will be concordant in patients with hypofibrinogenaemia.

SELF-CHECK 14.8

What tests can be used to assess fibrinogen levels?

BOX 14.6 *A false sense of security?*

It is important to remember that a coagulation screen (+ platelet count) will not identify all haemostatic abnormalities. A patient's positive clinical history of bleeding but normal coagulation screen and platelet count may be due to the following:

■ Bleeding not due to a haemostatic disorder (e.g. mechanical).

■ Disorders of platelet function.

■ Vascular disorders.

■ FXIII deficiency—stabilization by cross-linking is not necessary for clots to form and persist *in vitro*.

■ Mild factor deficiencies may not manifest because reagents tend to be sensitive to deficiencies in the region of 30–40% of normal and below, although this varies from one reagent to another. In some instances of FII, FV, and FX deficiencies this can result in *either* PT *or* APTT being elevated, which is not the expected laboratory presentation of a common pathway deficiency. For most patients, mild factor deficiencies are of little clinical significance.

■ Milder forms of VWD may not reduce FVIII levels sufficient to prolong an APTT.

■ Fibrinolytic disorders.

Key Points

All coagulation screening tests are performed at 37 °C

Pre-analytical variables

Unless care is taken to ensure that samples received in the laboratory are of suitable quality for analysis, performing the tests can generate results that are useless or even dangerous to the patient. A vital role of the biomedical scientist is ensuring that samples are fit for purpose, and Table 14.4 details the main areas that impact on sample quality.

Isolating a factor deficiency

If coagulation screening suggests a **factor deficiency**, assays can be performed to determine the plasma concentration of individual factors. The choice of factors to assay will be informed by the patient's clinical history and which of the screening tests was abnormal.

SELF-CHECK 14.9

If a young male patient presented with an intramuscular bleed and the only abnormal screening test was his APTT, which two clotting factors would you assay first and why?

TABLE 14.4 Pre-analytical variables in haemostasis analysis.

Variable	Effect on results
Phlebotomy	Venous samples should be used whenever possible. Capillary samples can be contaminated/diluted with tissue fluids and may require modified analytical techniques.
	Stress and exercise prior to venepuncture can increase FVIII, VWF, PAI-1 and t-PA.
	Venous occlusion with a tourniquet can activate platelets, some clotting factors and fibrinolysis.
	Difficult/traumatic venepuncture can activate some clotting factors and lead to shortened PT and/or APTT results that may mask an abnormality. Platelets may also be activated. Some samples may also contain small clots, or be completely clotted, and are unsuitable for analysis.
	Not checking patient identity can mean taking a good-quality sample but from the wrong patient.
Sample collection tube with correct anticoagulant	Tri-sodium citrate (usually 105 mmol/L) is the anticoagulant of choice because its removal of calcium is reversible.
	Heparin and EDTA directly inhibit coagulation and are unsuitable for coagulation testing.
Sample volume	Tri-sodium citrate is a liquid anticoagulant so there is a dilution factor. Nine parts blood is taken into one part citrate.
	If too much blood is put in the tube it will be under-anticoagulated and clot quicker when tested.
	If the sample is underfilled it will be over-anticoagulated which may generate erroneously elevated clotting times and falsely suggest an abnormality.
Sample age	Components of haemostasis deteriorate quite rapidly and coagulation screens should be performed within 4 hours of collection. FV and FVIII are particularly labile. Plasma for most other tests can be stored frozen until analysis. Platelet function analysis can only be undertaken on fresh blood.
Centrifugation	Insufficient centrifugation can result in platelets remaining in the plasma and compromise standardization of phospholipid composition in PT and APTT. Lupus anticoagulant testing is particularly reliant on platelet removal.
Properties of plasma	Haemolysed samples can activate coagulation factors and the colour can interfere with photo-optical clot detection. Similarly for the strong colour of icteric samples.
	Lipaemic samples can interfere with turbidity recognition in photo-optical clot detection. It can also increase viscosity and interfere with mechanical clot detection.
Interfering substances/ contamination	PT and APTT are used to monitor therapeutic anticoagulation but can interfere with other tests that attempt to isolate specific components based on the assumption that the patient's coagulation is otherwise normal, e.g. lupus anticoagulant testing, activated protein C resistance screening.
	Other drugs can interfere with specific tests; e.g. aspirin affects platelet function.
Storage	Frozen plasma can be stored between −40°C and −70°C for some weeks without significant loss of activities.
	Samples cannot be repeatedly frozen and thawed as this leads to progressive loss of activities.

CASE STUDY 14.2 *Grossly abnormal screening tests*

The following results were obtained on a sample of acceptable quality for analysis. No clinical details were available.

PT (s)	> 120	(RR: 10.0–14.0)
APTT (s)	> 120	(RR: 32.0–42.0)
TT (s)	> 120	(RR: 9.0–11.0)

Further investigations to explain the deranged results showed the following:

Fibrinogen (g/L)	5.9	(RR: 1.5–4.0)
RT (s)	13.3	(RR: 12.0–15.0)
Platelet count ($\times 10^9$/L)	321	(RR: 150–400)

What do the above follow-up results suggest? If, however, the follow-up tests had given the following results what would they indicate?

Fibrinogen (g/L)	0.2	(RR: 1.5–4.0)
RT (s)	> 120	(RR: 12.0–15.0)
Platelet count ($\times 10^9$/L)	25	(RR: 150–400)

Irrespective of whether a deficiency is due to a dysfunctional molecule or reduced synthesis/increased clearance of a normally functioning molecule, assays assessing biological function in coagulation-based systems will indicate a deficiency. Immunological methods do not detect dysfunction.

As well as investigating patients with a bleeding history, coagulation screens are commonly performed prior to surgery to check that coagulation status is sufficient to cope with the trauma of surgery. The unexpected and incidental preoperative finding of abnormal results may result in cancellation of the surgery until the cause is isolated.

One-stage coagulation factor assays

Bioassays for coagulation factors are usually performed with **one-stage coagulation assays**, so called because the fibrin clot endpoint is generated directly with one set of reagents. The assays use PT or APTT reagents to facilitate *in-vitro* coagulation of manipulated patient plasma as detailed in the Method box below and in Figure 14.2.

Assays for factors II, V, VII and X are usually performed using PT reagents to facilitate the coagulation reactions. Factors VIII, IX, XI, XII, PK and HMWK are assayed with APTT reagents.

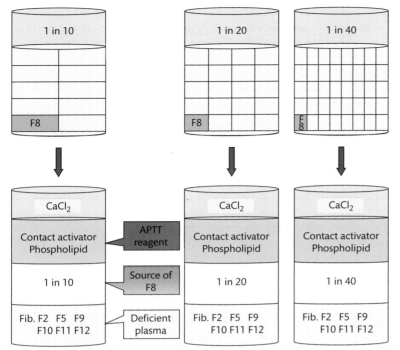

FIGURE 14.2

Principle of a one-stage FVIII assay. Test plasma is doubly diluted to gradually reduce the amount of FVIII present. One volume of each dilution is separately added to an equal volume of FVIII-deficient plasma and an APTT performed on each mixture. Full details are given in the Method Box below.

METHOD *One-stage factor assays*

- At least three doubling dilutions are made of patient plasma in buffer, typically 1:10, 1:20, and 1:40.

- In separate tubes, one volume of each dilution is added to an equal volume of a plasma that is totally deficient in the factor being tested but otherwise normal.

Manipulating the patient plasma like this means that the only source of the factor being assayed is the patient's plasma, so it becomes rate-limiting.

The levels of all the other coagulation factors will be constant in each tube so the clotting time of the 1:40 will be longer than the 1:20, which in turn will be longer than the 1:10 as a direct result of diluting the patient's plasma. Although all other coagulation factors will be present in the patient plasma, the dilution renders their contribution to coagulation capacity negligible in relation to that supplied by the deficient plasma.

- Clotting times are plotted against dilution factor on double-log graph paper and compared to those of a standard plasma, as shown in Figure 14.3.

Assessment of raw data

The plots for the patient and standard, and any controls, should form parallel straight lines. A patient's line that is to the right of that of the standard (i.e. the clotting times are longer at each dilution) indicates that the level of factor being measured is lower than the standard value, and if to the left, it is higher.

To calculate the actual result, the 1:10 dilution of the standard plasma is assigned a potency of 100%. Thus, the 1:20 and 1:40 become 50% and 25%, respectively, and so on if further dilutions are used. This means that if a 1:5 dilution is added, it adopts a value of 200%. Similar to the Clauss fibrinogen assay you met earlier, the standard curves are only linear within a certain range of clotting times and can vary from one batch of deficient plasma to another. Therefore, if the clotting times from a patient's dilutions are beyond those of the standard curve, the patient must be re-assayed using dilutions that generate clotting times within that range.

You can see in Figure 14.3 that the 1:10 dilution of the patient's plasma is read directly from the curve, the 1:20 is multiplied by 2 as it is the 50% dilution, and the 1:40 multiplied by 4 as it is the 25% dilution. Providing that the results for each of the patient's dilutions are within 10% of each other, the mean is calculated to generate the potency of the patient's factor.

Although we arbitrarily assign a value of 100% to the standard when plotting the data, its actual value may be more or less than that, which means that all we have done so far is assess the potency of the patient's factor as a percentage of the standard. If the actual value of the standard is indeed 100%, no further calculations are necessary. If the actual value is different, a further calculation is necessary as shown in the Method box below.

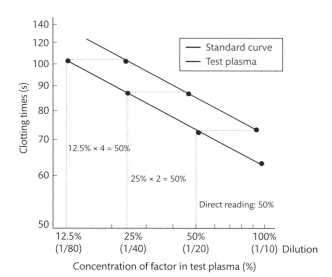

FIGURE 14.3
Graphical plot of standard and test plasma for a one-stage factor assay, a so-called 'parallel-line bioassay plot'.

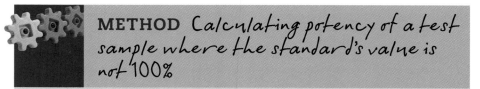

METHOD *Calculating potency of a test sample where the standard's value is not 100%*

If the standard had a true factor content of 92%, the final result for a patient whose potency from the standard curve was 50% would be calculated thus:

$$50 \times 92/100 = 46\%$$

If the standard had a true potency of 105%:

$$50 \times 105/100 = 52.5\%$$

Units

Plasma concentration of coagulation factors varies widely, so rather than measure factor levels in concentration units such as g/L, we report them in units that indicate enzyme potency relative to normality.

So, what exactly do we mean when we report a factor assay result as a percentage, that is to say, a percentage of what? Before the availability of standards with potency assigned as enzyme units, factor levels were reported merely as a percentage of the potency of a pooled normal plasma. Because the pools are prepared from a large number of healthy donors who would have a range of potencies of the factor being measured, the pools were assumed to have a potency of 100%, i.e. the theoretical mean.

Standards are now available with potency assigned as (enzyme) u/mL or u/dL, which have a theoretical equivalence to percentage values, thus: 100% of a given factor is considered equivalent to 1.00 u/mL or 100.0 u/dL.

International standards, or secondary standards calibrated against them, are available for most factors, the units designated as IU/mL or IU/dL.

Assay validity

The reason we assay the patient's plasma at more than one dilution is because there are situations where the line is not parallel to the standard. The main reasons why this occurs are:

- Presence of inhibitors
- Low but detectable levels
- Total absence of the factor being measured

Look at Figure 14.4 which illustrates typical results in the presence of an inhibitor. At the lowest dilution of 1:10, the inhibitor interferes with coagulation and significantly prolongs the clotting time. The inhibition remains in the 1:20 dilution, although you can see that the effect is less marked because the point on the graph is much closer to the standard line, and the point for the 1:40 is below the standard. The higher the dilution, the greater the loss of inhibitory effect, so the calculated factor potency gets higher with each dilution. Notice that this assay included a 1:80 dilution, which when married with the 1:40 dilution, generated a linear line parallel

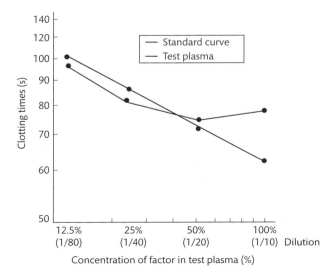

FIGURE 14.4

Graphical plot of standard and test plasma for a one-stage factor assay where the patient has an inhibitor that interferes with linearity and parallelism at low dilutions.

to the standard. This indicates that the inhibitor had been diluted to such a degree that it no longer interfered and the values from those dilutions can be used to report an accurate result.

The graph in Figure 14.5 has achieved linearity and parallelism at lower dilutions but not in the higher dilution. This is because the factor being measured is present but at a low concentration, so by the time it is diluted 1:40 it is virtually undetectable and linearity is lost. Performing the assay again using lower dilutions (e.g. 1:5) should provide a linear and parallel assay to allow calculation of the coagulation factor level.

The plot in Figure 14.6 is interesting because it is linear but not parallel. This is because the factor being measured is absent, so whatever dilution is used the clotting time is the same because each one is ostensibly a blank. This could also be due to an extremely potent inhibitor.

Factor assays can be performed manually or on automated analysers. Some of the latter perform all the dilutions and calculations for you and display the parallel line graph, allowing the operator to assess validity. Others will only assay a single dilution of patient plasma and/or not display the graph. You can see from Figures 14.4 and 14.5 that if the mean result

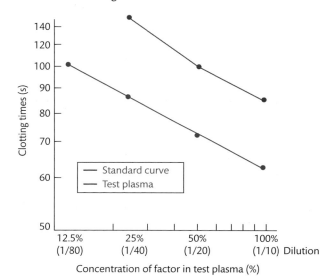

FIGURE 14.5

Graphical plot of standard and test plasma for a one-stage factor assay where a patient has a low level of the clotting factor, such that parallelism and linearity are lost at the higher dilution because the factor has been diluted to an undetectable level.

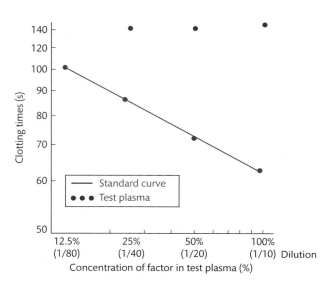

FIGURE 14.6

Graphical plot of standard and test plasma for a one-stage factor assay where a patient has undetectable levels of the factor being assayed.

from each dilution was calculated without reference to the graphical display for assay validity, erroneous results would be reported with the potential for inaccurate diagnosis and inappropriate treatment. *Scrutiny of factor assay graphs is a crucial part of the analytical process.*

Outline the principle of a one-stage clotting assay to measure FIX.

Two-stage coagulation factor assays

Also available for the measurement of FVIII are **two-stage factor assays**. The first stage involves the generation of FXa in a FVIII-dependent manner. In the second stage the FXa is either added to normal plasma, phospholipids, and calcium ions to form a clot, or allowed to react with a chromogenic substrate. Clotting-based two-stage assays are rarely used as they are technically demanding. The design for the chromogenic assay is shown in Figure 14.7.

An occasional problem with one-stage assays is that they are sensitive to sample pre-activation that can result from a difficult venepuncture. This is circumvented in two-stage assays as all the patient's FVIII is pre-activated in order to generate the FXa, which is then assayed separately.

Discrepancies between one-stage and two-stage FVIII assays

In the absence of interfering factors, most patients will generate equivalent results in both assay types. However, some mutations causing mild haemophilia A give rise to clinically significant discrepancies between the assay types. Mutations altering the stability of the activated molecule give rise to twofold, or higher, results from one-stage compared with two-stage assays, some even giving FVIII activity results within the one-stage assay reference range. The bleeding phenotype correlates with the two-stage result. Less common is the reverse discrepancy where two-stage results can be double the one-stage.

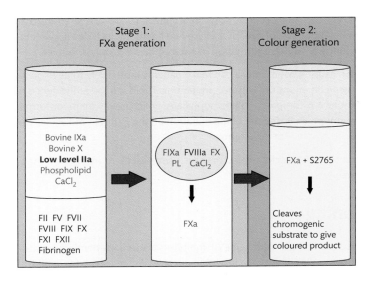

FIGURE 14.7

Principle of the chromogenic two-stage FVIII assay. FXa is generated in a FVIII-dependent manner in the first stage by activating the patient's FVIII and then reacting it with exogenous FIXa, FX, phospholipids, and calcium ions. The amount of FXa generated is directly proportional to the amount of FVIII in the patient's plasma. The FXa is reacted with a chromogenic substrate, the resultant colour intensity being directly proportional to the amount of FXa generated and thus the FVIII level.

Stage 1:
FXa generation

Stage 2:
Colour generation

Bovine IXa
Bovine X
Low level IIa
Phospholipid
$CaCl_2$

FII FV FVII
FVIII FIX FX
FXI FXII
Fibrinogen

FIXa FVIIIa FX
PL $CaCl_2$

FXa

FXa + S2765

Cleaves chromogenic substrate to give coloured product

Alternative factor assays

Alternatives to standard one-stage and two-stage techniques exist when exogenous enzymes are available that directly activate specific factors. We have met one of these already in the form of the reptilase enzyme that directly converts fibrinogen into fibrin. Venom from the Russell's Viper (*Daboia russelli*) contains a fraction that directly activates FX, and venom from the world's most dangerous land snake, the Coastal Taipan (*Oxyuranus scutellatus*), contains an FII activator. Directly activating a factor at different plasma dilutions in the presence of appropriate cofactors generates clotting times that can be plotted as parallel-line bioassays. A variation of the Russell's Viper venom FX assay allows the generated FXa to cleave a chromogenic substrate instead of generating a fibrin-clot endpoint.

Detection and characterization of inhibitors

Whilst most deficiencies of coagulation factors will be due to hereditary mutations or acquired causes of reduced production/increased consumption, some patients generate antibodies (inhibitors) that can interfere with coagulation function or facilitate immune-mediated clearance from the circulation of a specific factor.

The most commonly encountered inhibitors in clinical practice are lupus anticoagulants, which can be found incidentally during pre-operative screening in asymptomatic patients. These antibodies interfere with the phospholipid-dependent stages of some coagulation tests, but do not inhibit specific coagulation factors. In symptomatic patients they are clinically associated with thrombosis and are considered in depth in Chapter 15.

The most common antibodies to specific factors associated with bleeding are those directed against FVIII. Approximately 30% of patients with severe haemophilia A develop **alloantibodies**, which result from treatment with FVIII replacement products because their immune system considers FVIII to be a 'foreign' protein. One molecule of inhibitor combines with one FVIII molecule, the resulting complex having no FVIII activity. Such inhibitors are considered to possess simple kinetics. Approximately 8% of patients with mild or moderate haemophilia A develop inhibitors that are **autoantibodies** with complex kinetics. These inhibitors rapidly inactivate FVIII but the complex then dissociates leaving some FVIII activity, and adding further FVIII results in the same residual activity. These are considered complex kinetics and such antibodies can also occur in non-haemophiliacs, who are referred to as having 'acquired' inhibitors. About 12% of patients with severe haemophilia B develop inhibitors, but the overall incidence of inhibitor formation in haemophilia B is only about 3%.

The type of gene mutation causing haemophilia can make patients more likely to develop an inhibitor, such as major gene deletions or nonsense mutations. There is a lower incidence of such mutations in haemophilia B compared to haemophilia A, which is why inhibitor formation is less common in haemophilia B. The site of the mutation on the FVIII/FIX molecules can also influence the likelihood of inhibitor development.

Inhibitors directed against all the other clotting factors have been described, including fibrinogen and FXIII, but they are very rare.

Inhibitor screening

Most inhibitors are immediate acting *in vitro*, but FVIII inhibitors are time-dependent because the FVIII has to dissociate from VWF before the inhibitor can act. We can screen for inhibitors

---

alloantibodies

Antibodies directed against substances that are recognized as foreign to self.

autoantibodies

Antibodies directed against an organism's own tissues or native proteins.

BOX 14.7 *Acquired haemophilia due to autoantibodies*

Acquired haemophilia due to anti-FVIII antibodies is largely a disease of the elderly, but with a smaller peak associated with pregnancy or post-partum. It is a rare condition with an incidence of 2:1 million annually. There is a greater likelihood of developing acquired haemophilia in the presence of malignancy or an autoimmune disorder.

Patients present with prominent subcutaneous haematomas (and bleeding elsewhere). The bleeding is often more severe than suggested by the inhibitor titre, although haemarthroses are rare. Acute bleeds are treated with prothrombin concentrate or recombinant FVIIa, and the inhibitors are eliminated with steroids and intravenous immunoglobulin plus low-dose cytotoxic therapy.

Most elderly patients die within 2 years of diagnosis from comorbid conditions rather than from bleeding.

by mixing equal volumes of patient and normal plasma and testing immediately and then serially after incubation at 37 °C over two hours. Although this is normally done using APTT because most clotting factors contribute to the clotting time, it can also be done using PT and even Clauss fibrinogen.

The results shown in Table 14.5 are typical of a time-dependent inhibitor. At time 0, APTTs are performed on patient and normal plasma separately and on the mixture. Aliquots of each are incubated and tested again at 30-minute intervals, as well as a fresh mixture prepared from the separately incubated patient and normal aliquots. Results are interpreted as follows:

Tube 1—The normal plasma clotting times are equivalent throughout, indicating no appreciable deterioration over the test period for this plasma.

Tube 2—The patient at time 0 has an elevated clotting time because the inhibitor has already acted on the FVIII *in vivo* and remains elevated throughout.

Tube 3—The clotting time of the incubated mixture increases over time revealing the progressive nature of the inhibitor, which had no effect on the FVIII in the normal plasma at time 0 but a marked effect by completion of incubation.

TABLE 14.5 Inhibitor screening results for a progressive inhibitor in APTT.

Time point (min)	TUBE 1 Normal plasma clotting time (s)	TUBE 2 Patient plasma clotting time (s)	TUBE 3 Incubated 50:50 mixture clotting time (s)	TUBE 4 Fresh 50:50 mixture clotting time (s)
0	30	75	31	—
30	30	76	37	32
60	31	77	45	33
90	32	79	54	34
120	32	80	78	34

Tube 4—Performing APTTs on the fresh mixture proves that the abnormality is only expressed when patient plasma is incubated with normal plasma over time.

Key Points

Non-FVIII inhibitors would be demonstrated at time 0 in the mixture and no further incubation would be necessary.

Quantifying an inhibitor

If an inhibitor is suspected, factor assays will reveal which clotting factor is affected, where-upon biomedical scientists can perform a **Bethesda assay** that will measure inhibition of that factor. In haemophiliacs it will be obvious which factor is affected and it is important to moni-tor the inhibitor levels as they have a marked effect on treatment. The assay is detailed in the following Method box and in Figure 14.8.

In practice, you are rarely fortunate enough to get a result of exactly 50% FVIII. Therefore, the results for the dilutions whose results are closest to 50% are plotted, as shown in Figure 14.9, to estimate the dilution that would have given exactly 50% residual FVIII and hence the inhibitor level itself. The assay design assumes there is no FVIII in the patient plasma, which is not neces-sarily the case for inhibitors with complex kinetics. The Bethesda assay is also used to quantify FIX inhibitors where extended incubation is unnecessary.

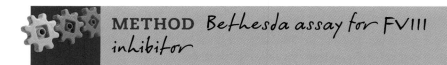

METHOD Bethesda assay for FVIII inhibitor

- Doubling dilutions are made of patient plasma in buffer to increasingly dilute out the inhibitor.

- One volume of each dilution is incubated with an equal volume of a normal plasma known to contain 100% FVIII (1.0 IU/mL), for 2 hours at 37 °C.

- The tubes are then put on ice to prevent any further antibody–antigen reactions, and each one assayed for FVIII.

If there is an inhibitor present, more residual FVIII will be present as the dilution factor increases

- One Bethesda Unit (BU) is the amount of inhibitor that will neutralize 50% of a normal plasma containing 100% FVIII after a 2-hour incubation at 37 °C. Thus, the dilution factor of the patient plasma dilution that has a residual FVIII of 50% can be used to calculate the inhibitor level in BU/mL; i.e. if the neat plasma had 50% residual FVIII, by definition it would contain 1.0 BU/mL. If however the inhibitor is more potent than that and the plasma needed diluting, say 1:10 to obtain 50% residual FVIII, the inhibitor level is 10×1.0 BU/mL.

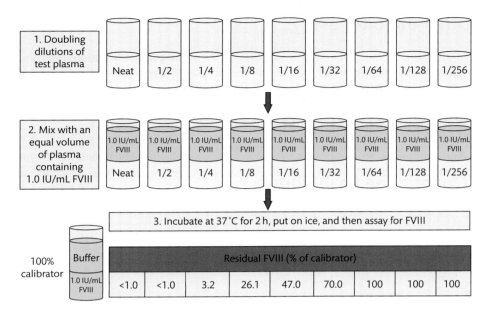

FIGURE 14.8

Principle of the Bethesda assay for FVIII inhibitor quantification. The inhibitor (if present) is increasingly diluted before each dilution is then reacted with an identical amount of FVIII during a 2-hour incubation at 37 °C. Antibody–antigen reactions are stopped by putting the tubes containing each dilution on ice. Each dilution is then assayed for residual FVIII.

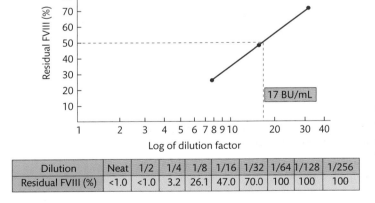

Dilution	Neat	1/2	1/4	1/8	1/16	1/32	1/64	1/128	1/256
Residual FVIII (%)	<1.0	<1.0	3.2	26.1	47.0	70.0	100	100	100

FIGURE 14.9

Graphical plot for Bethesda assay. The log of the three dilutions with residual FVIII closest to 50% are plotted against residual FVIII. The dilution that would have given exactly 50% residual FVIII is read off the curve and is reported as the Bethesda value.

You can see in Figures 14.8 and 14.9 that there was no residual FVIII in the neat plasma and the 1:2 dilution because the inhibitor was sufficiently potent to neutralize all the FVIII in the time frame. Between the 1:4 and 1:32 dilutions there is an increasing amount of FVIII as the effect of the inhibitor diminishes with increasing dilution. From the 1:64 dilution and above, the dilution of the inhibitor was sufficient to prevent it from acting within the time frame.

SELF-CHECK 14.11

Outline the methods used to detect clotting factor inhibitors.

Other inhibitor assays

A slightly altered version of the Bethesda assay is the **Nijmegen modification**. Here, the patient plasma is diluted in FVIII-deficient plasma instead of buffer, and the normal plasma is buffered directly. These modifications reduce pH drift which can otherwise cause a degree of FVIII inactivation and generate false-positive results when no inhibitor is present. The Nijmegen modification is now the recommended method for FVIII inhibitor testing by the International Society of Thrombosis and Haemostasis.

Some FVIII inhibitors are non-neutralizing and cause immune-mediated removal of FVIII from the circulation but will not inhibit FVIII activity in an inhibitor assay. These inhibitors are detected using ELISA-based assays.

Detection and classification of von Willebrand's disease

Approximately 70% of patients with VWD have a quantitative deficiency of normally functioning VWF (Type 1) and approximately 25% have a structural/functional defect (Type 2). The remainder have severe VWD where VWF is absent (Type 3).

The variable clinical and phenotypic expression of VWD means that standard screening tests generate limited information for the detection of VWF deficiencies:

- PT, TT, and fibrinogen are unaffected.
- APTT will be elevated only if the FVIII is sufficiently reduced.
- Platelet count is normal in most subtypes; platelet morphology may be useful when distinguishing from other primary haemostatic disorders

Other screening tests, the bleeding time, and analysers assessing high shear-dependent platelet function, are often abnormal in VWD but do not distinguish between subtypes. These are also abnormal in platelet disorders and can be normal in mild VWD. They are covered in more detail later in this chapter.

If VWD is suspected from the clinical history (with or without screening tests), biomedical scientists will then perform assays that assess VWF concentration, function, and structure:

- Patients with Type 1 VWD will have concordant functional and concentration assays because they produce low amounts of normally functioning VWF. Patients with Type 3 VWD will have concordant results insomuch as the VWF will be absent irrespective of how it is measured.
- Most patients with Type 2 VWD will have functional results <70% of the concentration result.

Measurement of FVIII activity is also included as it aids diagnosis and can have implications for treatment. The lower the FVIII, the more severe the VWD and the risk of bleeding. A normal FVIII level does not exclude VWD, whilst a reduced FVIII is not indicative in itself of VWD.

Assessing VWF concentration

Immunological assays that measure the total amount of VWF protein present irrespective of function are used to assess the overall VWF concentration as VWF antigen (VWF:Ag). The most commonly used methods are ELISA or LIA, the principles of which you met in Chapter 2.

Assessing VWF function

Three assays are used to assess different aspects of VWF function based on binding to platelets, collagen, or FVIII.

Platelet binding

Binding of VWF to the GPIb platelet receptor is measured in the **ristocetin cofactor assay** (VWF:RCo). Ristocetin A is an antibiotic isolated from the soil bacterium *Nocardia lurida* that promotes VWF–GPIb binding, as shown and described in Figure 14.10.

Dilutions of patient plasma are incubated at 37 °C in an aggregometer together with ristocetin and a suspension of platelets that have been washed to remove plasma and then fixed in formalin. The VWF in the patient plasma promotes platelet agglutination, and generates graphical traces with slope values that are directly proportional to the amount of VWF present in relation to its GpIb binding capacity.

Cross reference

You can find further detail about aggregometers later in this chapter in Section 14.4 on the investigation of platelet disorders.

Key Points

Binding of ristocetin on the platelet surface reduces the platelet's negative charge, and similarly on VWF. This reduces electrostatic repulsion between platelets and/or between platelets and VWF, thus allowing VWF to cause agglutination by bridging between platelets. This is in contrast to the platelet agonists you will meet in the following section that activate platelets to induce the aggregation processes you met in Chapter 13.

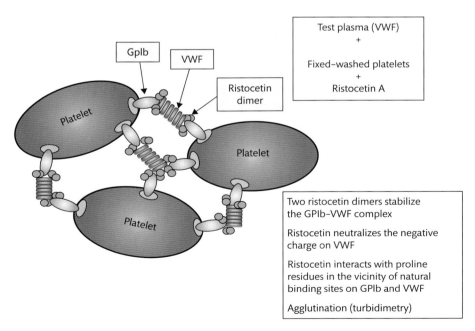

FIGURE 14.10

Principle of ristocetin cofactor assay. Patient plasma is mixed with fixed–washed platelets and ristocetin. Ristocetin dimers stabilize the GpIb-VWF complex by neutralizing the negative charge on VWF molecules and interacting with proline residues in the vicinity of natural binding sites, leading to agglutination of platelets. The amount of agglutination and slope of the resultant graph are proportional to the amount of VWF in the patient plasma.

Collagen binding

Integral to effective primary haemostasis is the ability of VWF to bind to subendothelial collagen that is exposed upon vessel trauma. This property is assayed in an indirect ELISA, where the patient VWF is captured on an ELISA plate using collagen itself to generate a **collagen-binding activity result** (VWF:CB).

FVIII binding

One subtype of VWD, Type 2N, has a normal VWF concentration and function with respect to both collagen and platelet binding. However, the VWF binds poorly to FVIII and results in circulating FVIII levels of around 15–30% in heterozygotes, thus mimicking mild haemophilia A.

A family history revealing affected females may be the only clue that it is not true haemophilia, prompting measurement of the **FVIII binding capacity** (VWF:FVIIIB). The principle of this ELISA-based assay is illustrated in Figure 14.11.

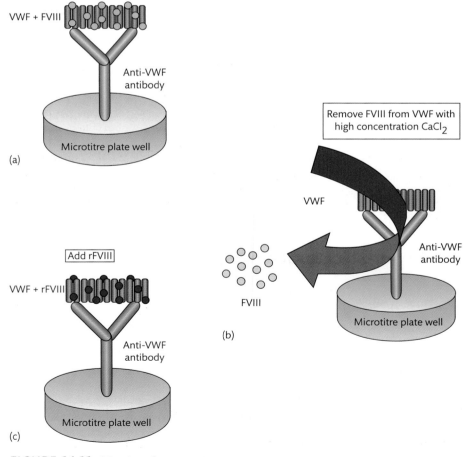

FIGURE 14.11 (*Continued*)

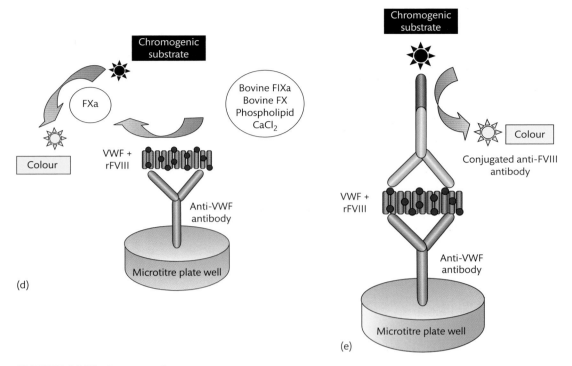

FIGURE 14.11 (Continued)
FVIII-binding assay (a) The patient's VWF is captured by an anti-VWF antibody. (b) Depending on whether the patient's VWF can bind FVIII, there may be some FVIII bound; however, this will vary between patients so it is removed with a high concentration calcium chloride solution. (c) Exogenous recombinant FVIII (rFVIII) is then added to standardize the amount of FVIII that is added to each patient's VWF. There are two methods available for determining the amount of FVIII that has bound to the patient's VWF. Figure 14.11 (d) shows the captured FVIII being reacted with FIXa, FX, phospholipids, and calcium ions to generate FXa, which is subsequently reacted with a chromogenic substrate. The intensity of the coloured product is proportional to the amount of FVIII that bound to the VWF. (e) Alternatively, an enzyme-linked antibody to FVIII (not VWF) is added and reacted with a substrate that produces a coloured product.

Identifying structural defects

You were introduced to the multimeric structure of VWF in Chapter 13. For diagnostic purposes, VWF can be split into its component multimers by heating the patient plasma to 56°C and then subjecting it to sodium dodecyl sulphate-polyacrylamide gel electrophoresis (SDS-PAGE), which separates the multimers according to size. The presence or absence of some or all multimers aids diagnosis and classification when assessing results in conjunction with those from the other assays. You can see in how VWD is classified in Table 14.6.

Distinguishing between Type 2B and pseudo-VWD

High molecular weight (HMW) multimers of VWF have the greatest effect on collagen and platelet binding, so VWF:RCo and VWF:CB assays are sensitive to their absence.

TABLE 14.6 Classification of VWD with typical laboratory findings.

Sub-type	PFA-100	FVIII	RIPA	VWF:RCo	VWF:CB	VWF:Ag	FVIII binding	VWF:RCo:VWF:Ag ratio	VWF:CB:VWF:Ag ratio	Multimer distribution	Further details
Type 1	N/↑	N/↓	N/↓	↓	↓	↓	N	>0.7	>0.7	All multimers present	Concordant activity and antigen. Partial quantitative deficiency of normally functioning VWF due to reduced production, defective release or increased clearance
Type 2A	↑	N/↓	↓	↓	↓	↓/N	N	<0.7	<0.7	HMW & intermediate forms absent	Discordant activity and antigen. Reduced platelet dependent function due to absence of HMW multimers
Type 2B	↑	N/↓	↑	↓	↓	↓/N	N	<0.7	<0.7	HMW forms absent	Discordant activity and antigen. Distinguish between pseudo VWD with RIPA studies. Variable thrombocytopenia
Type 2M	↑	N/↓	↓	↓	↓/N	↓/N	N	<0.7	>0.7	All multimers present	Discordant VWF:RCo activity and antigen. Decreased VWF-dependent platelet adhesion despite presence of HMW multimers i.e. dysfunctional HMW multimers
Type 2N	N	↓	N	N/↓	N/↓	N/↓	↓	>0.7	>0.7	All multimers present	Concordant activity and antigen. VWF-dependent platelet function is normal. VWF has reduced affinity for FVIII
Type 3	↓↓	↓↓	↓	↓↓	↓↓	↓↓	N/A	N/A	N/A	Multimers absent	(Concordant activity and antigen). Severe bleeding disorder due to markedly reduced or absent VWF. Markedly reduced FVIII (~2%)

N, normal; HMW, high molecular weight.

In Type 2B VWD, the HMW multimers are hyperresponsive and attach themselves to platelets *in vivo* causing the formation of microaggregates and moderate thrombocytopenia. In pseudo-VWD, sometimes called platelet-type VWD, the GPIb is hyperresponsive and removes HMW multimers from the circulation. It is important to distinguish between these subtypes because desmopressin treatment for Type 2B is contraindicated as it releases more hyperresponsive HMW multimers into the circulation and can lead to severe thrombocytopenia. This is done using the **ristocetin-induced platelet aggregation (RIPA) test**.

Subjecting a preparation of patient platelets, suspended in their own plasma, to a fixed concentration of ristocetin (1.2 mg/mL) will generate reduced agglutination compared to normal in most VWD subtypes. Both Type 2B and pseudo-VWD are over-responsive and cause agglutination at lower concentrations where even normal VWF levels are unreactive. To distinguish between Type 2B and pseudo-VWD, patient platelets are washed to remove plasma constituents, resuspended in a normal plasma, and then subjected to RIPA:

- If the RIPA remains over-responsive then the defect must lie in the patient's platelets, as their VWF has been removed and replaced with normal VWF.
- If the RIPA normalizes, the defect was in the patient's plasma. This can be double-checked by washing normal platelets, suspending them in patient plasma, and performing RIPA, which will be over-responsive.

SELF-CHECK 14.12

Outline the principles of assays used to detect and characterize VWD.

Reference ranges

You saw in Chapter 13 that VWF carries ABO blood group antigens which affect *in-vivo* survival. The effect is sufficiently significant that we cannot apply a single reference range to the entire population. Individuals with blood group O and no VWF mutation can have VWF:Ag levels as low as 35 iu/dL. For blood groups A and B, the lower thresholds are in the regions of 50 iu/dL and 55 iu/dL, respectively, and for individuals who are AB it is about 65 iu/dL.

Further notes on Type 1 VWD

Type 1 VWD classically presents in the laboratory with reduced but concordant activity and antigen results and normal multimer distribution, the VWF:Ag levels being in the region of 20–50%. Interestingly, only about 50% of these patients have a VWF mutation, the others having reduced levels for other reasons, such as blood group O. The advent of more sensitive multimer analysis techniques has revealed that many patients considered to have more severe Type 1 VWD (VWF:Ag <20%) have a slight decrease in HMW multimers or altered subunit structure and discordant activity and antigen results. The majority of these patients do have a VWF mutation and may be better classified as Type 2M.

An interesting variant of Type 1 VWD is the Vicenza subtype. The VWF has reduced survival in plasma, so the VWF:Ag and VWF:RCo levels are very low (<15 iu/dL) and concordant. However, the bleeding symptoms are milder than would be expected from these levels because the VWF in platelets is unaffected. The small amount of VWF that is detected in plasma contains ultra-high molecular weight multimers—because it has only just been released from endothelial cells and has yet to be subjected to cleavage by ADAMTS-13.

Acquired VWD

Acquired von Willebrand's disease (AVWD) is a rare bleeding disorder with similar clinical and laboratory findings to the inherited disorder. It can be caused by specific or non-specific antibodies, adsorption of VWF onto malignant cell clones, hypothyroidism, or loss of high molecular weight multimers under conditions of high shear stress such as in **aortic stenosis**. AVWD is usually diagnosed using standard laboratory tests for inherited VWD in the absence of a family history of bleeding. Inhibitors can be demonstrated in a modification of the VWF : RCo assay, in which the patient's plasma is mixed with normal plasma to facilitate inhibition of the VWF in the normal plasma by the antibody present in the patient's plasma.

aortic stenosis

Narrowing of the heart valve between the left ventricle and the aorta.

14.4 Diagnosis of platelet disorders

As you saw in Chapter 13, platelets are pivotal to an effective haemostatic response to injury, and comprise the platform for many crucial mechanisms. Thus, defects in both numbers and function, which can be hereditary or acquired, must be detected in the clinical laboratory. Inherited platelet disorders are rare, acquired abnormalities being more commonly encountered in clinical practice.

Thrombocytopenia

Even if platelet function is normal, reduced platelet numbers (thrombocytopenia) compromises both platelet plug formation and the availability of a phospholipid surface for coagulation biochemistry. Additionally, circulating platelets secrete **platelet-activating factor** (PAF) which contributes to the maintenance of endothelial cell junctions, so reduced PAF secretion in severe thrombocytopenia leads to 'unzipping' of endothelial junctions and bleeding due to compromised vascular integrity.

Thrombocytopenia is defined as subnormal numbers of circulating platelets, the reference range being $150-400 \times 10^9$/L of blood. In practice, platelet counts $>100 \times 10^9$/L rarely cause bleeding problems, whilst the risk of haemorrhage increases as the platelet count falls. Spontaneous bleeding commonly occurs when the platelet count falls below 20×10^9/L. The main causes of thrombocytopenia are outlined in Table 14.7 and are the result of one of three fundamental mechanisms:

- Impaired platelet production
- Increased platelet destruction/consumption
- Increased pooling of platelets in the spleen

Note in Table 14.7 that some disorders have reduced numbers and function and we will now look at disorders of platelet function in more detail.

Hereditary platelet function disorders

Disorders of platelet function are characterized by the area of function affected:

- Surface receptors
- Cytoplasmic granules
- Platelet biochemistry
- Phospholipid exposure

Key Points

Biomedical scientists need to be aware of the phenomenon of pseudothrombocyto-penia. The EDTA used to anticoagulate FBC samples can cause platelets to clump *in vitro* due to the presence of calcium-dependent antibodies that are present in approximately 0.1% of the population. The automated platelet count is low and platelet clumps can be seen on a stained blood film. The antibodies are not clinically significant and an accurate platelet count can be obtained by taking a new sample into a different anticoagulant such as tri-sodium citrate. This phenomenon can also be seen when patients receive therapeutic antibody preparations such as abciximab. Other antibodies can cause plate-lets to attach to white cells, typically neutrophils, and is termed platelet satellitism as they are seen to form rosettes around the periphery of the white cell.

Surface receptor disorders

The two most common receptor disorders are **Glanzmann's thrombasthenia** and **Bernard–Soulier syndrome**, which are amongst the most clinically severe of hereditary platelet function defects.

Glanzmann's thrombasthenia is characterized by a deficiency or functional defect of the GPIIbIIIa complex. It is classified into three subtypes:

- Type I has 0–5% of normal levels of GPIIbIIIa.
- Type II has 6–20% GPIIbIIIa.
- 'Variant' has 50–100% GPIIbIIIa but with reduced fibrinogen binding.

The most common clinical features are typical of a primary haemostatic disorder, such as epistaxis, purpura, petechiae, excessive bruising, gum bleeding, and menorrhagia. Platelet counts are normal. Bleeding after trauma/surgery can be severe and pregnancy/delivery mark-edly increase the risk of bleeding.

Bernard–Soulier syndrome results from the absence or decreased expression of the GPIb–V–IX complex on the platelet surface. Patients present with mild to moderate thrombocytopenia and enlarged or giant platelets. Bleeding symptoms are also typical of a primary haemostatic disorder, and are more severe than expected for the degree of thrombocytopenia alone because there is a concomitant functional defect.

Defects in the coupled ADP receptors $P2Y_1$ and $P2Y_{12}$, the collagen receptors GPVI and GPIaIIa, the thromboxane A_2 receptor, and the epinephrine receptor have been described in rare cases.

Key Points

Glanzmann's thrombasthenia and the Bernard–Soulier syndrome are both inherited as autosomal-recessive conditions. They have a higher incidence in populations where consanguineous partnerships are common. Heterozygotes tend to be asymptomatic.

SELF-CHECK 14.13

What are the two most common platelet receptor disorders and which receptors are affected in each?

TABLE 14.7 Thrombocytopenias.

Disorder	Features	Mechanism of thrombocytopenia	Associated with platelet function defect?
Inherited			
Fanconi's anaemia	Progressive bone marrow failure + other congenital anomalies	Impaired production	No
Thrombocytopenia with absent radius (TAR)	Skeletal anomalies + reduced or absent megakaryocytes	Impaired production	No
Bernard-Soulier syndrome	Abnormal GPIb + giant platelets	Impaired production	Yes
MYH9 disorders: May-Hegglin anomaly Sebastian syndrome Fechtner syndrome Epstein syndrome	MYH9 is the gene encoding for the heavy chain of non-muscle myosin White cell inclusions (Döhle-like bodies) + moderate thrombocytopenia and giant platelets	Impaired production	Yes
Grey platelet syndrome	Absent α-granules with mild to moderate thrombocytopenia and large platelets	Impaired production	Yes
Congenital amegakaryocytic thrombocytopenia	Almost complete absence of megakaryocytes leading to severe thrombocytopenia	Impaired production	No
Wiskott-Aldrich syndrome	X-linked immune deficiency + eczema + thrombocytopenia with small platelets	Impaired production	Yes
X-linked thrombocytopenia with dyserythropoiesis	Red cell abnormalities + marked thrombocytopenia with giant platelets	Impaired production	No
Montreal platelet syndrome*	Severe thrombocytopenia with giant platelets and spontaneous *in vitro* aggregation	Impaired production	Yes
Type 2B VWD	Abnormal VWF function causes platelet microaggregates leading to moderate thrombocytopenia**	Increased consumption	No
Platelet-type VWD	Abnormal GPIb function causes platelet microaggregates leading to moderate thrombocytopenia		Yes
Acquired			
Disseminated intravascular coagulation	Progressive activation and consumption of haemostatic components	Increased consumption	No

	Description	Mechanism	
Immune thrombocytopenic purpura (ITP)	Accelerated platelet destruction due to autoantibodies to platelets. Acute onset in children with spontaneous recovery. Insidious onset in adults where spontaneous recovery is rare.	Increased destruction	No
Neonatal alloimmune thrombocytopenia (NAIT)	Transplacental passage of maternal antibodies to platelet antigens not shared with the fetus	Increased destruction	No
Pregnancy-associated thrombocytopenia	Incidental; secondary to hypertension or fatty liver, ITP, HELLP syndrome (**h**aemolysis, **el**evated **l**iver enzymes and **l**ow **p**latelets)	Impaired production or increased destruction/consumption	No
Megakaryocytic aplasia	Autoimmune suppression of megakaryocyte development	Impaired production	No
Heparin-induced thrombocytopenia	Antibodies to the heparin–platelet factor 4 complex	Increased destruction	No
(Non-heparin) drug induced thrombocytopenia	Chemotherapy; many other drugs have been described to cause thrombocytopenia but not in every patient	Impaired production or increased destruction	No
Viral infections	Usually mild thrombocytopenia; can be seen in HIV, rubella, cytomegalovirus infections	Impaired production	No
Nutritional disorders	Deficiencies of vitamin B12 and folic acid; alcoholism	Impaired production	No
Thrombotic thrombocytopenic purpura	Autoantibodies to ADAMTS-13 lead to increased VWF function and formation of platelet aggregates. Rare hereditary form of TTP known as Upshaw–Schulman syndrome (ADAMTS-13 deficiency).	Increased consumption	No
Haemolytic uraemic syndrome	Childhood disorder with haemolytic anaemia, thrombocytopenia and acute renal failure		No
Bone marrow infiltration	Thrombocytopenia secondary to haemato-oncological disorders	Impaired production	No
Splenomegaly	Pooling of up to 90% of total body platelets in the spleen	Splenic pooling	No

* Recent reports suggest that Montreal platelet syndrome may be a manifestation of Type 2B VWD.

** Note that the thrombocytopenia itself is acquired as a result of the inherited Type 2B VWD.

Platelet granule disorders

Platelet function can be defective if granule numbers are reduced, granule contents are deficient, or if release mechanisms fail. Most of these disorders affect dense bodies or α-granules, but rarely affect both. Since the dense bodies and α-granules are storage sites, their defects are also referred to as storage pool disease.

Dense body disorders

Disorders of dense bodies are often part of a more complex congenital disorder, although isolated dense body defects are known. The bleeding phenotype associated with dense body disorders is usually of mild–moderate severity with significant bleeding associated with trauma/ surgery. Platelet counts and size are normal. There are three main disorders:

melanosome
Pigment-containing organelle.

Hermansky–Pudlak syndrome is a diverse autosomal-recessive disorder affecting a number of organelles, in particular, **melanosomes** and platelet dense bodies. Consequently, albinism and dense body deficiency are characteristic.

Chediak–Higashi syndrome is an autosomal-recessive disorder also associated with albinism and dense body deficiency. Additionally, the immune system is affected and large inclusion bodies are seen in white cell precursors in the bone marrow.

Primary dense body deficiency is a clinically heterogeneous disorder with an uncertain genetic basis that is not associated with other abnormalities.

Alpha-granule disorders

Defects of α-granules are extremely rare and so it is difficult to generalize about clinical features. There are three main disorders:

Grey platelet syndrome is the only disorder associated with a complete absence of α-granules, and thus the levels of their contents are reduced or absent. This results in the characteristic appearance of platelets on Romanowksy-stained blood films as agranular, misshapen grey blobs. The platelet count is often reduced and platelets can be slightly larger than normal.

Paris-Trousseau syndrome is characterized by thrombocytopenia together with other congenital abnormalities. There are giant α-granules in a percentage of the circulating platelet population that cannot release their contents, and a subpopulation of abnormally matured micromegakaryocytes that lyse upon maturation.

Quebec disorder is characterized by increased levels of platelet urinary plasminogen activator (u-PA), which activates platelet plasminogen that subsequently degrades α-granule contents.

SELF-CHECK 14.14

Outline the main platelet granule disorders.

Disorders of platelet biochemistry

Abnormalities in platelet biochemistry inevitably impair platelet function. Wiskott–Aldrich syndrome (WAS) is a rare X-linked disorder resulting from defects in the *WAS* gene that encodes for the WAS protein (WASp). WASp takes part in biochemical signalling and cytoskeleton maintenance. Children born with WAS present with bruising, small platelets, and purpura resulting from thrombocytopenia and abnormal platelet function. WAS is a complex disorder with eczema and immune deficiencies that can be severe.

Deficiencies of platelet enzymes such as cyclooxygenase have also been described.

Disorders of phospholipid exposure

Scott syndrome is an extremely rare bleeding disorder characterized by the reduced exposure of negatively charged phospholipids to facilitate tenase and prothrombinase formation. *Stormorken syndrome* is also rare and is almost the reverse of Scott syndrome. Non-activated platelets express full procoagulant activity but a reduced response to collagen.

Acquired platelet function disorders

Some systemic disorders affect platelet function, such as renal failure (due to the retention of platelet inhibitory substances), liver disease, and disseminated intravascular coagulation (DIC). Abnormal platelet function, as well as thrombocytopenia, is sometimes seen associated with the chronic myeloproliferative disorders, acute myeloid leukaemia and myelodysplastic syndromes you met in Chapter 11. Significant numbers of patients with myeloma and Waldenström macroglobulinaemia have impaired platelet function due to the interference of function by paraproteins.

Drugs are the most common cause of platelet dysfunction. The humble aspirin many of us use to alleviate headaches irreversibly inactivates the platelet cyclooxygenase pathway, thereby blocking aggregation. Aspirin can therefore be used as an effective anticoagulant drug. Many other drugs are known to affect platelet function to varying degrees, such as:

- Non-steroidal anti-inflammatory drugs (NSAIDs)—aspirin is also an NSAID
- Antibiotics
- Cardiovascular drugs
- Psychotropic drugs such as antidepressants
- Anaesthetics
- Chemotherapeutic drugs
- Anticoagulants

Not every drug within each category will affect platelet function and their effects tend to be concentration-dependent.

Some foods and food additives can also affect platelet function if ingested in sufficient amounts. Examples include fish oils, green tea, garlic, cumin, turmeric, chocolate, excessive use of vitamin supplements, and the black tree fungus used in Chinese takeaways. In sufficient amounts, these foodstuffs can generate abnormal results in platelet function testing that can complicate diagnostic interpretation. However, abnormal results due to foodstuffs alone are unlikely to translate into a genuine acquired bleeding disorder.

Name the main causes of acquired platelet dysfunction.

Laboratory investigation for platelet defects

Assessing a patient for a platelet function defect begins with taking a detailed history from the patient and should include the following:

- Personal and family history of bleeding episodes
- Severity, frequency, and type of bleeding episodes
- Drugs the patient is taking, detailing both prescribed and over-the-counter drugs
- Dietary intake
- Lifestyle choices such as smoking and exercise can affect platelet function.

Pre-analytical questionnaires are used to rationalize this process and assist the clinician. If they reveal that the patient's diet, lifestyle, or medication could significantly interfere with platelet function, laboratory testing may need to be postponed to allow for a period of abstinence prior to analysis. For an example of a pre-analytical questionnaire see Figure 14.13 which is used in the authors' laboratories.

Laboratory analysis

The first assays a biomedical scientist will undertake will be to check the size and number of the platelets. This is easily done on the current automated analysers that you met in Chapter 2, although their limitations must be recognized. Analysers that distinguish between cellular components based on size may erroneously place large platelets in the same sector as red cells, whilst small red cells would be placed in the platelet segment. This will lead to falsely reduced or elevated platelet counts.

Compare the platelet count histograms in Figure 14.12. In the normal histogram, you can see there is no cross-over between the population of particles counted as platelets and the threshold for inclusion in the erythrocyte count. The abnormal histogram is from a patient with

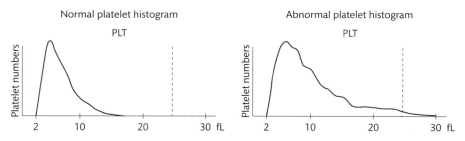

FIGURE 14.12
Platelet count histograms. The vertical dashed line indicates the cell-volume threshold for differentiating between platelets and red blood cells. Any cell above 25fL is counted as a red blood cell and below 25fL as a platelet.

Questionnaire for all platelet aggregation patients & controls

Question	Response
Are you taking?	
• Aspirin (within the last 14 days MINIMUM)	
• Over-the-counter cold relief medication e.g. Lemsip	
• Ibuprofen	
On any of the prescription medications below? COX1 inhibitors (indomethacin, sulfinpyrazone, naproxen), ADP receptor agonists (ticlopidine, clopidogrel), GPIIb/IIIa agonists (Reopro, tirofiban, eptifibatide, integrilin), prostaglandins (cliostazol), tri-cyclic antidepressants (imipramine, amitripyline)	
If the PATIENT has answered YES to the above please reschedule. If the CONTROL has answered YES please find another volunteer.	
On any other current prescription medication? Please circle relevant drugs. Penicillin, ampicillin, propranolol, atenolol, captopril, perindopril, anaesthesia	
Are you currently taking vitamin supplements? **If yes tick or circle if listed below** Vitamins B6, C, E all affect platelets	
Are you taking dietary supplements or herbal remedies? **If yes please tick or circle if listed below:** Starflower oil, fish oil, Ginko biloba and green tea all have platelet antagonistic ingredients	
Have you had a take-away within the last 48 hours? Elements in turmeric, cumin, onion, garlic, ginger, clove, black tree fungus & monosodium glutamate all affect platelets.	
Do you drink or smoke? Alcohol, caffeine & smoking have been known to affect platelets	
Was this a clean draw?	

FIGURE 14.13
Pre-analytical questionnaire for completion prior to platelet function analysis.

giant platelets, some of which are so large that they cross the threshold. When the histograms produced by the analyser indicate this is the case, an alternative method is required to obtain an accurate count. Flow cytometric counts can be performed and you will meet them later in this chapter. As you will see later in this section, platelet morphology on Romanowsky-stained peripheral blood films can aid diagnosis.

Assessment of platelet function—screening tests

Platelet function can be empirically assessed with a mildly invasive technique known as the *bleeding time*. A small uniform incision 1 mm deep is made in the skin of the underside of the forearm. Blood emerging from the wound is carefully removed with blotting paper at

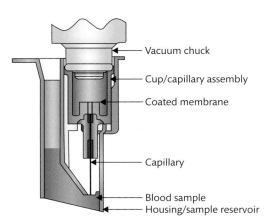

Vacuum chuck

Cup/capillary assembly

Coated membrane

Capillary

Blood sample
Housing/sample reservoir

FIGURE 14.14

PFA-100® cartridge. Anticoagulated whole blood is added to the reservoir in the cartridge. Pressure equivalent to that in the arteries passes the blood into a thin-bore capillary towards the agonist-impregnated collagen membrane. Blood passes through the pore in the membrane and the collagen–VWF–platelet interactions of primary haemostasis are initiated. The time taken for the clot to occlude the aperture is reported as the closure time.

30-second intervals and the time is noted when the bleeding stops. The procedure is partly standardized by using blades of a standard width and depth and using a sphygmomanometer to maintain a blood pressure of 40 mmHg in the arm being tested. However, the test is prone to operator variability and relies on the patient keeping still throughout. The small incision only induces trauma in the microcirculation and thus relies almost entirely on fully functioning primary haemostasis. Therefore, blood vessel disorders, platelet number, function abnormalities and some types of VWD will prolong the bleeding time—but haemophilia will not.

In response to the poor reproducibility of the bleeding time test, a number of instrument manufacturers have produced analysers that screen for abnormalities of primary haemostasis. The most widely used in the UK is the Platelet Function Analyser (PFA-100®) from Siemens Healthcare Diagnostics. The PFA-100 cartridge, shown in Figure 14.14, functions by using an equivalent pressure to that in the arteries to pass whole blood from a reservoir through a capillary. At the end of the capillary is a collagen membrane coated with either ADP or epinephrine (adrenaline) that contains a pore with a diameter of 150μm. The collagen reproduces the exposure of platelets to the subendothelial matrix and the agonists mimic localized activation. The analyser measures the time taken for enough platelets to adhere and aggregate that they occlude the pore in the membrane; the result is reported as closure time and is measured in seconds. Insufficient platelet numbers, reduced platelet function, and some forms of VWD will give elevated closure times, but, clearly, vessel abnormalities cannot be detected.

Other manufacturers have produced instruments employing differing technologies. The Impact-R™ analyser from DiaMed uses *cone and plate(let)* technology. Whole blood is applied to a polystyrene well under arterial flow conditions, whereupon fibrinogen and VWF adhere to the well surface. The flow conditions allow VWF to unravel, and platelets then adhere and

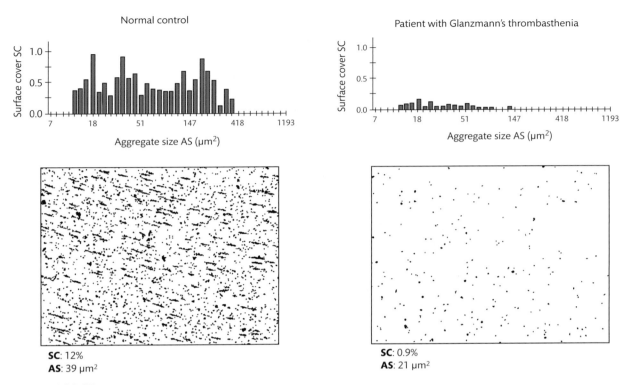

FIGURE 14.15

Result output from a DiaMed Impact-R analyser showing the surface coverage vs. aggregate size histograms and the images produced by the test well. In the example on the right the patient's platelets have largely failed to adhere to the test surface or to aggregate with each other. This gives poor surface coverage and very small aggregates indicative of a platelet function disorder: in this case, Glanzmann's thrombasthenia.

aggregate. Excess blood is washed off, and the adhered and aggregated platelets are stained. An image analyser quantifies the percentage of the well covered by the aggregates, which represents adhesion, and the average size of the aggregates themselves, representing aggregation. You can see platelet aggregates in a well in Figure 14.15.

Thromboelastography (TEG) is a measure of clot elasticity that assesses the whole dynamic process of haemostasis rather than isolating specific areas, and as such measures the strength of platelet interactions. Whole blood is activated via the contact pathway using Celite or kaolin and placed into a pre-warmed cuvette. A suspended rotating torsion wire is lowered into the cuvette and the blood is allowed to clot under a low-shear environment resembling sluggish venous blood flow. Fibrin strands interact with activated platelets and attach to the surface of the cuvette and torsion wire, resulting in the clot transmitting its movement to the wire. Changes in resistance are plotted and analysed on computer software to give distinctive 'fingerprints' for different disease states. A modification of this method exists where it is the cuvette and not the torsion wire that rotates. A graphical plot from a TEG analysis is shown in Figure 14.16.

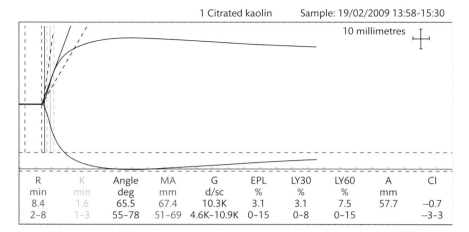

R	K	Angle	MA	G	EPL	LY30	LY60	A	CI
min	min	deg	mm	d/sc	%	%	%	mm	
8.4	1.6	65.5	67.4	10.3K	3.1	3.1	7.5	57.7	−0.7
2–8	1–3	55–78	51–69	4.6K–10.9K	0–15	0–8	0–15		−3–3

FIGURE 14.16

Output from a kaolin-activated normal whole blood sample processed on a Haemoscope TEG® analyser, showing: R, the value from addition of blood sample to clot formation; K, time taken to reach a given clot strength; G, measure of clot strength; Angle, a measure of the speed/strength of clot formation; MA, the maximum amplitude, which is when the clot formed is at its strongest. LY30 and LY60 measure clot lysis after 30 and 60 minutes respectively. EPL is the estimated clot lysis measured at a specific time point, and is equivalent to LY30 at 30 minutes and LY60 at 60 minutes. A is the amplitude of the tracing at the latest time point. CI (coagulation index) is a manufacturer's composite value taking into account R, K, MA, and Angle.

SELF-CHECK 14.16

What first-line screening tests are available when assessing platelet abnormalities?

Assessment of platelet function—diagnostic tests

Because the screening tests cannot distinguish between VWD and platelet function disorders, more specific analyses are required to isolate causes of platelet dysfunction.

Platelet function analysis

Platelet aggregation was devised by Gustav Börn and John O'Brien in the early 1960s. There are two main techniques:

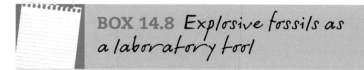

BOX 14.8 *Explosive fossils as a laboratory tool*

Celite is a brand name for a preparation of diatomaceous earth, which is composed of the fossilized remains of the hard-shelled algae called diatoms. It has various uses other than activating coagulation *in vitro*, such as a filtration aid, liquid absorbent, a component of cat-litter, and a component of dynamite.

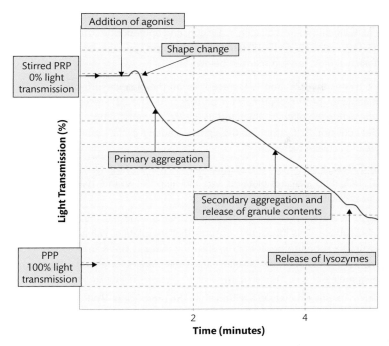

FIGURE 14.17

Platelet aggregation trace showing a normal response to the agonist ADP at a concentration of 2μmol/L. Assay performed on a BioData PAP-8E aggregometer. The analyser is set to recognize platelet-rich plasma (PRP) as zero light transmission. The patient's platelet-poor plasma (PPP) is used to set the analyser to recognize 100% light transmission. Addition of the agonist causes the platelets to initially change shape from a disc to a spiny sphere. They then enter a phase of primary aggregation where their altered shape promotes interaction by overlapping. This phase can reverse if the stimulus is not strong enough or the platelets are dysfunctional and cannot enter the secondary phase. The release reaction occurs in the secondary phase causing irreversible aggregation.

- The first involves producing *platelet-rich plasma* (PRP) by centrifuging the sample at a low speed for an extended time. The supernatant then contains plasma and platelets, the leucocytes and erythrocytes being spun down. PRP is placed in a cuvette in front of a light source. The PRP is constantly stirred to keep the platelets uniformly suspended. Addition of an agonist to the cuvette causes the platelets to aggregate, thus allowing more light to pass through the sample. A light detector situated on the other side of the cuvette transmits absorbance changes to a chart recorder. The amount and rate of fall of absorbance (i.e. increase in light transmission) are a function of agonist concentration and innate platelet function. You can see in Figure 14.17 that a normal aggregation response has different stages.

- The second involves placing a probe with two fine wires in the sample. A current is passed through the wires and as the platelets adhere to the wires in response to agonists the resistance changes. In accordance with Ohm's Law, the current changes and this change in electrical signal is converted to an aggregation value. As this method doesn't rely on light passage, whole blood can be analysed for aggregation.

A number of agonists are available that cause platelet activation, aggregation or agglutination via different mechanisms. Different platelet function abnormalities can be identified depending on the pattern of responses to the panel of agonists. The most common agonists used are ADP, arachidonate, collagen, ristocetin, and epinephrine. Thrombin-receptor agonist peptide (TRAP), U44619, and A23187 are used in more specialist laboratories. The modes of action of each agonist are summarized below:

- ADP activates the $P2Y_1$ and $P2Y_{12}$ receptors on the platelet surface. For ADP to function as an activator both receptors must be triggered. The $P2Y_1$ receptor triggers an enzyme cascade within the platelet which results in calcium mobilization. Calcium is a potent local platelet activator. $P2Y_{12}$ amplifies the signal via adenyl cyclase inhibition to increase aggregation and activate secretion.

- Arachidonate is converted into thromboxane A_2 (TXA_2) by intra-platelet cyclooxygenase (COX). TXA_2 then activates platelets and also activates an internal enzyme cascade which mobilizes calcium.

- Collagen activates GPIa and GPVI. When GPIa is activated the platelet adheres to the exposed surface. This interaction ensures that the platelet will adhere to exposed collagen from the subendothelial matrix, ensuring that any break in the vasculature is rapidly sealed. GPVI stimulation by collagen causes the platelet to release other activators stored in the granules.

- Ristocetin causes platelets to agglutinate in the presence of VWF. The VWF receptor complex GPIb–V–IX on the platelet needs divalent cations to bind VWF. When ristocetin is present there is a structural change in the VWF which causes it to bind to the receptor without the need for these cations. However this binding is temporary and only produces agglutination of platelets via VWF as opposed to true platelet aggregation.

- Epinephrine interacts with α–adrenergic receptors on the platelet surface, enhancing the effect of other agonists. Interestingly, epinephrine only aggregates platelets *in vitro* if the sample is anticoagulated with sodium citrate.

- TRAP activates protease-activated receptor (PAR) 1, the primary thrombin receptor on platelets. TRAP activates PAR1 without initiating fibrin formation, which would interfere with the assay.

- U46619 (9,11-dideoxy-9α,11α-methanoepoxy $PGF_{2\alpha}$) is a stable thromboxane **mimetic** and is useful for distinguishing between drug-induced defects of thromboxane generation and disturbances in arachidonate metabolism.

- A23187 is a calcium ionophore, enabling the study of calcium flux across platelet membranes.

These agonists activate enzyme cascades within the platelet that mobilize the surface receptor GPIIbIIIa (inside-out signalling), which, in turn, binds fibrinogen in a calcium-dependent fashion. Other agonists, such as those derived from snake venoms, are available but have limited use outside the research arena.

Mimetic
A compound that mimics properties of another.

SELF-CHECK 14.17

Outline the principles of platelet function analysis.

Identifying platelet disorders

Platelet aggregation studies are most commonly performed using the light-transmittance method with PRP. Table 14.8 details expected aggregation patterns encountered in the platelet function disorders.

TABLE 14.8 Typcial platelet aggregation response patterns in platelet disorders.

Condition	Platelets		Aggregation responses								Comment/further testing
	Count	Size	ADP	Coll	Ri	AA	Epi	TRAP	U46619	A23187	
Glanzmann's thrombasthenia	N	N	0	0	1	0	0	N	N	0	Flow cytometric analysis for glycoproteins IIbIIIa
Bernard-Soulier syndrome	Low	Large	N	N	0	N	N	R	N	N	Flow cytometric analysis for glycoprotein Ib
COX deficiency	N	N	1/N	R	N	R	N	N	N	R	COX analysis
Drug induced platelet defects; results shown are for aspirin	N	N	1	R	N	R/0	N	N	N	N/R	Stop aspirin (use of questionnaire reduces this)
Thromboxane deficiencies	N	N	1/N	R	N	R/0	N	N	N	N	Platelet nucleotides, receptor analysis, platelet biochemistry analysis
Thromboxane receptor deficiencies	N	N	1/N	N	N	R/0	N	N	R/1	N	Receptor analysis, platelet biochemistry analysis
P2Y$_{12}$ defects	N	N	R/0	N	N	N	N	N	N	N	Receptor analysis, platelet biochemistry analysis
MYH9 Disorders											
May Hegglin anomaly	Low	Large +++	N	N	N	N	N	N	N	N	Genetic analysis, film for neutrophil (Döhle) inclusions. Other associated clinical manifestations e.g. albinism, hearing loss, nephritis
Alport syndrome	Low	Large	R	R	N	N	N	N	N	N	Genetic analysis. Other associated clinical manifestations e.g. albinism, hearing loss, nephritis
Sebastian syndrome	Low	Large	N	N	N	N	N	N	N	N	Genetic analysis, film for leucocyte inclusions. Other associated clinical manifestations e.g. albinism, hearing loss, nephritis
Epstein syndrome	Low	Large	N/R	N/R	N	N	N	N	N	N	Genetic analysis
Eckstein syndrome	Low	Large	N	N	N	N	N	N	N	N	Genetic analysis
Misc. macrothrombocytopenias											
Montréal platelet syndrome	Low	Large	R	R	R	N	N	N/R	N	N	Spontaneous aggregation, autosomal dominant inheritance, prolonged bleeding time

(Continued)

TABLE 14.8 (Continued)

Condition	Platelets		Aggregation responses								Comment/further testing
	Count	Size	ADP	Coll	Ri	AA	Epi	TRAP	U46619	A23187	
Paris–Trousseau syndrome	Low	Large	N/R	N	N	N	N	R/1	N	N	Electron microscopy for giant alpha granules. Check for other physical/clinical features
Stormorken syndrome	Low	Large	N	R	N	N	N	N	N	N	Reduction in ATP secretion, spontaneous aggregation in whole blood. Flow cytometry annexin V analysis
Storage pool defects											
Grey platelet syndrome	Low	N	R/1	N/R	N	N	N	R	N	N	Electron microscopy, alpha granule content analysis such as beta-thromboglobulin and platelet factor 4 assays
Quebec platelet syndrome	N	N	N	N	N	N	0	N	N	N	Multimerin analysis, alpha granule content analysis such as beta-thromboglobulin and platelet factor 4 assays
Chediak–Higashi syndrome	N	N	R/1	R	N	N	R	N	N	N	Dense granule analysis, platelet nucleotide analysis. Other associated clinical manifestations e.g. albinism
Hermansky–Pudlak syndrome	N	N	R/1	R	N	N	R	N	N	N	Dense granule analysis, platelet nucleotide analysis. Other associated clinical manifestations e.g. albinism, prone to infections
Wiskott–Aldrich	Low	Small	R/1	R	N	N	R	N	N	N	Genetic analysis, WASp analysis
Scott's syndrome	N	N	N	N	N	N	N	N	N	N	Flow cytometry annexin V analysis
Montreal platelet syndrome	Low	Large	R	R	R	N	N	N/R	N	N	Spontaneous aggregation, autosomal dominant inheritance, prolonged bleeding time
Ehlers–Danlos syndrome	N	N	N	N	N	N	N	N	N	N	Genetic testing, other associated clinical manifestations eg albinism, hearing loss, nephritis
VWD	N	N	N	N	0/R/N	N	N	N	N	N	VWF: antigen, VWF: RCo activity, VWF: CBA, VWF RIPA, VWF multimer analysis

Key: N = normal, 0 = absent, 1 = primary wave only, R = reduced, Coll = collagen, Ri = ristocetin, AA = arachidonate, Epi = epinephrine, COX = cyclo-oxygenase. TRAP = Thrombin Receptor Agonist Peptide.

Further analyses can be performed to confirm and characterize diagnoses of glycoprotein defects and storage pool disorders.

Glycoprotein defects

Platelet glycoprotein receptors can be identified, or demonstrated to be reduced/absent, using the immunophenotyping method on a flow cytometer you met in Chapter 10 for identifying the cell types in haematological malignancies. The antibodies used are raised against the different platelet surface glycoproteins themselves.

Antibodies raised to the specific platelet receptors GPIb and GPIIbIIIa can be used to place a fluorescent 'tag' on normal platelets, and the number of 'tags' counted using a flow cytometer. This will then give an indication of the number of platelets within the sample that is more accurate than full blood count analysers which utilize the size gating system to count cells. Size gating suffers if the cells you are attempting to count are outside the set gates, such as small red cells or large platelets. Tagging platelets for flow cytometric counting means they are not dependent on size and a more accurate count is produced.

Storage granule defects

If defects in the dense bodies are suspected (δ-storage pool disorders) a luminosity technique can ascertain the quantity of the nucleotides ATP and ADP in the dense bodies. The nucleotides must be extracted from platelets by preparing PRP and then adding the following:

- EDTA to prevent any Ca^{2+}-dependent reactions
- The detergent Triton-X to disrupt platelet membranes and release the cytosol
- Ethanol to precipitate out membrane proteins and stabilize nucleotide concentrations

This is then centrifuged and the supernatant analysed. The supernatant is incubated with the enzyme *luciferase*, which is extracted from fireflies (*Photinus pyralis*), and its substrate *luciferin*. The following reaction occurs:

$$ATP + Luciferin \xrightarrow{\text{Luciferase} + Mg^{++}} Adenyl\ Luciferin + Light$$

The amount of light produced is measured and is directly proportional to the amount of ATP in the supernatant. This reaction only measures ATP. The nature of ADP is such that it is unstable and cannot be measured directly. In order to measure the ADP, it is converted to ATP in a separate aliquot of supernatant in the reaction below and the ATP is quantified again using the reaction above.

$$Phosphoenolpyruvate \xrightarrow[\substack{ADP \qquad ATP}]{\text{Pyruvate kinase}} Pyruvate$$

The ATP will be higher in the second result because the reaction tube will contain the ATP already present from the cytoplasm and dense bodies plus the converted ADP. The concentration of ADP is calculated by subtracting the result of the first reaction from that of the second.

About 30% of platelet ATP and most of the ADP are in the dense bodies, the ratio of total ATP:ADP in normal platelets being <2.5. The storage nucleotides are reduced in dense body defects, resulting in an increase in the ATP:ADP ratio. Up to 25% of patients with storage pool disorders may not manifest in standard platelet aggregation testing, so nucleotide quantification is an important part of the diagnostic armoury.

When a defect in α-granules is suspected (α-storage pool disorders), ELISA techniques are available to measure α-granule contents such as VWF, fibrinogen, beta-thromboglobulin, platelet factor 4, and P-selectin.

Lumi-aggregometry

Simultaneous analysis of both aggregation and the release of storage pool contents can be undertaken to detect enzyme defects. The analyser used is termed a lumi-aggregometer and contains two channels. One channel is for standard light impedance-based aggregometry and the other is for a luminometer that measures ATP release over time via the luciferase reaction. The analysis can be performed on whole blood or PRP. An enzyme defect that does not initiate dense body release will demonstrate normal measured levels of nucleotides and a normal ATP : ADP ratio but reduced release patterns by lumiaggregometry. Dense body defects will be abnormal in both analyses. Additionally, release defects will give a reduced response to arachidonate in aggregometry, whilst storage pool defects will be normal. Typical lumiaggregometer tracings are shown in Figure 14.18.

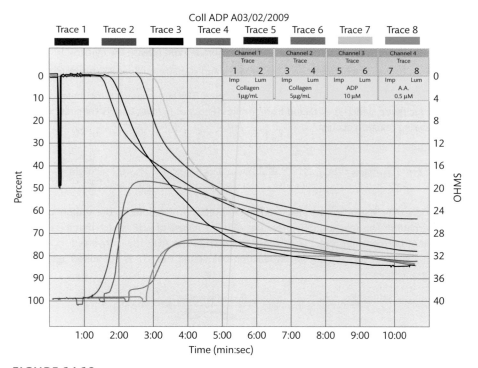

FIGURE 14.18

Normal traces from a Chronolog 700V whole-blood aggregation analyser showing both the whole-blood impedance aggregation trace (Imp) and the release of ADP detected by chemiluminescence (Lum). These traces show that the patient's platelets respond to the addition of varying agonists both by aggregation (top set of curves) and simultaneously releasing nucleotides (bottom set of curves), to initiate the second phase of aggregation.

Pitfalls of platelet function testing

As you saw earlier (and see Figure 14.13), many external factors interfere with platelet function. The patient should be made aware and requested to minimize their exposure to these elements before analysis takes place.

Most platelet function testing has to be done on fresh blood samples because platelets lose activity over time and cannot be stored. This means the patient must attend the clinic and the analysis be performed within three hours of venepuncture. Similar to coagulation screening, the quality of phlebotomy is important for the generation of clinically useful results. The needle must be of sufficiently wide bore so that it does not activate the platelets in the process of venepuncture. The venepuncture itself should not be traumatic for the patient, otherwise the platelets can become activated and mask a functional defect.

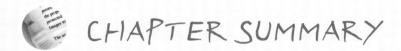

CHAPTER SUMMARY

Clinical considerations

- The nature and sites of bleeding symptoms give important clues to the type of bleeding disorder that may be present.

- Bleeding disorders can involve any area of haemostatic function and be hereditary or acquired.

Hereditary coagulation disorders

- Haemophilia A and B are rare X-linked deficiencies of FVIII and FIX, respectively, and can be life-threatening. Haemophilia C, deficiency of FXI, is a less severe disorder.

- VWD is a heterogeneous disorder of primary haemostasis resulting from VWF deficiency. In the more severe forms, the reduction in FVIII exacerbates the bleeding symptoms.

- Deficiencies of the other coagulation factors are much less common and vary in their clinical severity.

Acquired coagulation disorders

- A variety of primary disorders can cause secondary disturbances in haemostasis that lead to bleeding symptoms.

- Acquired coagulation disorders can result from an increased consumption or destruction of coagulation factors, decreased or impaired production, or via inhibitory mechanisms.

Laboratory investigation

- Investigation for a bleeding disorder begins with a coagulation screen and platelet assessment.

- Coagulation screening comprises PT and APTT and assessment of fibrinogen activity via TT and/or direct quantification.

- Interpretation of PT and APTT is based on the coagulation cascade theory. Although outmoded in terms of *in vivo* haemostasis, the cascade is used in the diagnostic setting in view of the test principles. PT assesses extrinsic and common pathway function, whilst APTT assesses intrinsic and common pathway function.

- Mixing studies can help direct diagnostic pathways by indicating the possible presence of either factor deficiencies or inhibitors.

- Coagulation screening does not detect all haemostatic abnormalities.

- Good-quality results can only be generated from good quality blood samples.

- Individual clotting factors are quantified by rendering the patient's clotting factor under investigation the rate-limiting factor in specialist assays based on PT or APTT. Scrutiny of the raw data is essential to ensure analytical validity and exclude interfering factors.

- Inhibitors of specific clotting factors are quantified by mixing a range of dilutions of the patient's plasma with a plasma of known factor content and incubating at 37°C for an appropriate length of time. The inhibitor will neutralize the factor to varying degrees because of the increasing dilutions and the value derived from this data.

- Most inhibitors act immediately, but FVIII inhibitors act progressively because the FVIII has to dissociate from VWF before the inhibitor can exert its effect.

- VWF is assayed using a variety of techniques in order to identify the subtypes. Activity is measured by platelet-binding and collagen-binding techniques and total VWF protein by immunological techniques. Some patients require ristocetin dose–response studies. VWF substructure is demonstrated by electrophoresis.

- Thrombocytopenia alone can cause bleeding symptoms, so the platelet count is crucial as an initial investigation.

- Disorders of platelet function can be detected in purpose-designed analysers that screen for abnormalities of primary haemostasis, which includes VWD but not vessel disorders.

- The mainstay for assessing hereditary platelet function disorders is aggregometry on platelet-rich plasma (PRP). Agonists that initiate platelet aggregation via different physiological mechanisms are added to separate PRP aliquots and the responses plotted graphically. The response patterns indicate the nature of any functional abnormalities.

- Follow-up investigations for platelet diagnostics include flow cytometry to indicate the presence/absence of surface glycoproteins, nucleotide quantification, and the release and measurement of α-granule contents.

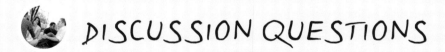 # DISCUSSION QUESTIONS

14.1 Why are the clinical symptoms of haemophilia A different to those of VWD, taking into account that the latter can be accompanied by reduced FVIII levels?

14.2 What do we gain by using coagulation screening tests that are based on an outmoded theory that does not fully mirror *in vivo* events?

14.3 What are the possible causes of finding an elevated PT and APTT in the presence of a normal TT and fibrinogen level? Justify your answer.

14.4   Assays to quantify FX tend to be based on PT analysis. Why might this be the case when an APTT-based assay would also work?

14.5   Surely a VWF:RCo assay tells us all we need to know about the clinical severity of any VWD subtype, so why bother with all the other tests?

14.6   If platelet function *in vivo* is inextricably linked to interactions with vessel endothelium, do the existing methods for assessing platelet function give clinically relevant information?

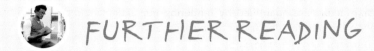

FURTHER READING

- Bolton-Maggs P, Chalmers EA, Collins PW, Harrison P, Kitchen S, Liesner RJ, Minford A, Mumford AD, Parapia LA, Perry DJ, Watson SP, Wilde JT, Williams MD. A review of inherited platelet disorders with guidelines for their management on behalf of the UKHCDO. *British Journal of Haematology* 2006:**135**;603–33.

- Chee YL, Crawford JC, Watson HG, Greaves M. Guidelines on the assessment of bleeding risk prior to surgery or invasive procedures. *British Journal of Haematology* 2008:**140**;496–504.

- Colman RW, Hirsh J, Marder VJ, Clowes AW, George JN (ed.). *Hemostasis and Thrombosis: Basic Principles & Clinical Practice*, 4th edn. Lippincott Williams & Wilkins, Philadelphia, 2001. Detailed chapters on different components of haemostasis.

- Harrison P. Assessment of platelet function in the laboratory. *Hämostaseologie* 2009:**29**;25–31.

- Lewis SM, Bain BJ, Bates I. (ed.). *Dacie and Lewis Practical Haematology*, 10th edn. Churchill Livingstone, Elsevier, 2006. Includes sections on coagulation screening, factor and inhibitor assays, and platelet function analysis.

- Peyvandi F, Cattaneo M, Inbal A, De Moerloose P, Spreafico M. Rare bleeding disorders. *Haemophilia* 2008:**14**(Suppl. 3);202–10.

Answers to self-check questions, case study questions, and discussion questions are provided in the book's Online Resource Centre, visit www.oxfordtextbooks.co.uk/orc/moore

15

Thrombophilia

Gary W. Moore and Ian Jennings

In this chapter we will define thrombophilia, look at the causes of thrombophilia and discuss the methods used to identify the defects which may be involved.

Learning objectives

After studying this chapter you should confidently be able to:

- Understand what is meant by the term 'thrombophilia'.
- Know the main causes of thrombophilia.
- Distinguish between hereditary and acquired causes of thrombophilia.
- Outline the tests used to investigate thrombophilia.
- Understand how the presence of one thrombophilia can interfere with the testing for some others.
- Understand the importance of accurate result interpretation in thrombophilia diagnosis.

15.1 Introduction

In Chapter 13 you met the normal function of the haemostatic processes which make up the balanced system between pro- and anticoagulant mechanisms to keep the blood flowing through intact vessels, cause a clot to form at the site of vessel damage to prevent blood loss, and to prevent extension of the clot beyond the region of damage. You learnt in Chapter 14 that a reduction in the quantity or quality of the procoagulant clotting factors could lead to a tendency to bleed, such as the haemophilias. In a similar way, defects or deficiencies of the anticoagulant system can lead to a predisposition to thrombosis, which is termed **thrombophilia**, which translates literally to 'clot-loving'. The consequence of thrombophilia for the individual is an *increased risk* of venous thrombosis. This is in contrast to the more severe bleeding disorders where bleeding symptoms are inevitable.

Thrombophilia may be either hereditary or acquired. Some defects which are thought to cause thrombophilia are of uncertain **aetiology**; that is, we do not know whether or not they are caused by some genetic changes, or acquired, or possibly both. These hereditary, acquired and uncertain causes of thrombophilia are listed in Table 15.1, and will be discussed in detail later.

TABLE 15.1   Causes of thrombophilia.

	Loss of function	Gain of function
Congenital/inherited causes	Protein S deficiency Antithrombin deficiency Protein C deficiency	FV Leiden Dysfibrinogenaemia Prothrombin G20210A
Mixed/uncertain	Elevated levels of FIX, XI, TAFI Hyperhomocysteinaemia Elevated levels of FVIII APC resistance in the absence of FVL	
Acquired	*Persistent*: antiphospholipid syndrome, age, malignancy, history of venous thromboembolism *Transient*: surgery, immobilization, pregnancy, hormone therapy/oral contraceptive use	

The mechanisms involved in keeping blood in an anticoagulated (fluid) state were introduced in Chapter 13. Figure 15.1 is a reminder of some of the key proteins involved in this process. Central to both procoagulant and anticoagulant mechanisms is the key enzyme thrombin.

15.2 **Natural anticoagulants**

When produced in large amounts from the cleavage of prothrombin, thrombin will in turn cleave fibrinogen to form fibrin, will activate FXIII to stabilize the fibrin clot, and will feed back into the coagulation mechanism to produce further amounts of thrombin. However, when produced in smaller quantities, two mechanisms act to have a negative feedback on the procoagulant system.

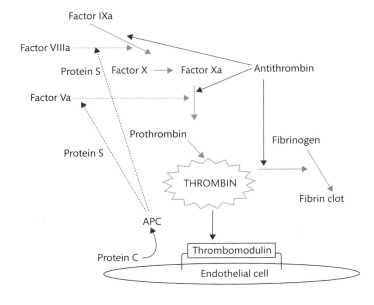

FIGURE 15.1

The central role of thrombin in procoagulant and anticoagulant mechanisms.

Key - ⟶ **Procoagulant activity**
       ⋯⋯⋯▶ **Anticoagulant/inhibitory activity**

Firstly, thrombin will bind to the endothelial membrane-bound protein thrombomodulin to activate protein C. Activated protein C then proteolytically cleaves active factor V and factor VIII, converting these two procoagulant proteins into inactive forms. In addition, antithrombin binds in a 1:1 **stoichiometric** complex with thrombin, rendering it inactive.

Key Points

Thrombophilia is generally taken to relate to venous thrombosis—thrombi forming in the venous system—which can cause **deep vein thrombosis** (DVT) and **pulmonary embolism** (PE). Thrombosis may also occur in the arterial system, where a thrombus may cause a myocardial infarction (MI) or stroke. The mechanisms and causes are different in the two systems. Arterial thrombosis will be discussed later.

Deficiency of the natural anticoagulants

Deficiency of the natural anticoagulants antithrombin, protein C, and protein S may be as a result of a mutation causing a reduced concentration of the normally functioning protein in the circulation (**type I defect**), or a mutation affecting the function of the protein (**type II defect**). Deficiencies of these anticoagulants are sometimes termed *loss-of-function* defects.

Antithrombin deficiency

Antithrombin is a naturally occurring inhibitor of several components of the procoagulant system, including thrombin, FIXa, FXa, FXIa and FVIIa–tissue factor (TF) complex.

In *type I antithrombin deficiency*, the concentration of antithrombin in the circulation is reduced. Antithrombin deficiency is an autosomal-dominant disorder, with levels in heterozygous individuals typically being about 50% of normal. Homozygous type I antithrombin deficiency is not encountered, and is thought to be incompatible with life. Heterozygous deficiency is associated with an up to 10-fold increased risk of **venous thromboembolism** (VTE) compared to normal. Mutations may cause a reduction in the amount of antithrombin produced, or increased destruction; point mutations, frameshift deletions or insertions, and major gene deletions have all been described.

Type II antithrombin deficiency occurs when a mutation in the antithrombin gene affects the function of the molecule. Here, assays which measure the activity of antithrombin in plasma will be affected, but normal concentrations of protein may be measured by immunological assays. Type II defects are further subdivided depending on the site of the mutation and the effect on function.

To understand the different subgroups of type II defects, it is necessary to review the function of antithrombin. In Chapter 13 you were introduced to antithrombin as an inefficient inhibitor of target enzymes in the absence of cofactors. The antithrombin molecule contains a heparin-binding region (D-helix) and a reactive site loop; this loop contains a **scissile** P1–P1′ (Arg393–Ser394) reactive site which binds to thrombin and other serine proteases. When heparin (added *in vitro* or administered as an anticoagulant) binds to the antithrombin molecule, the reactive site loop undergoes conformational change and exposes the P1–P1′ reactive centre, which then inhibits its target proteases approximately 1000 times more efficiently than in the absence of heparin. *In vivo*, the heparin is provided by heparan sulphate on the surface of endothelial cells which line the blood vessel.

Mutations causing type II antithrombin defects may affect the heparin-binding site (**type II HBS defects**), or the reactive site (**type IIRS**), or different mutations in other regions of the antithrombin gene may be having varied effects on antithrombin function (**type II pleiotropic defects**).

Laboratory assays for antithrombin

In order to distinguish between defects of concentration and function, two types of assays are required: immunological and functional.

Immunological assays for antithrombin

Since type II defects will not be detected with assays measuring the amount of protein present in plasma (immunological assays), these assays are generally only useful to distinguish type I and type II antithrombin deficiency.

Radial immunodiffusion assays, Laurell Rocket Electrophoresis, enzyme-linked immunosorbent assays (ELISA), and latex bead-based immunoassays can all be used to measure antithrombin antigen. Figure 15.2 shows the principle of the Laurell Rocket Electrophoresis method. Examples of latex-based and ELISA methods are shown later in this chapter (Figures 15.5 and 15.6, respectively).

Antithrombin circulates at a concentration of approximately 125 mg/L (2.3 µmol/L) in normal plasma, although measurement is more frequently determined as a percentage of antithrombin compared to normal.

1. A gel plate is prepared containing antibodies against the target antigen
2. Plasma is added to wells prepared in the gel and a current is applied to the plate.

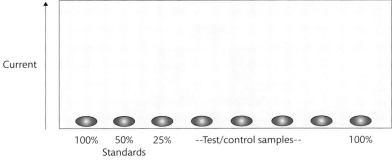

3. Proteins move across the plate and the antigen is captured and precipitated by the antibody. The distance travelled by the antigen is proportional to the quantity of antigen present in the plasma.
4. This can be visualized by staining the plate after drying, and the peak height can be plotted against the percentage of protein present.

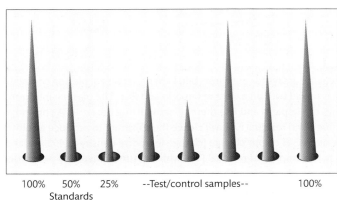

FIGURE 15.2
Principle of immunoelectrophoresis (Laurell Rocket Electrophoresis).

chromogenic substrate

A substrate that mimics the natural substrate of an enzyme, to which a dye, paranitroaniline (pna) is added. The enzyme will cleave the substrate to release the dye, causing a measurable colour change.

Antithrombin Cambridge II

An antithrombin variant arising from an alanine 384–serine (A384S) substitution, with a prevalence of up to 1.14 per 1000 individuals, and associated with a mild increase in thrombotic risk. The mutation modifies rather than abolishes serine protease inhibitory activity, and inhibits FXa more efficiently than thrombin.

Functional assays for antithrombin

The principle of antithrombin assays is based on the inhibition of thrombin or factor Xa; you can see how the assays work in Fig 15.3. When an excess of thrombin or factor Xa is added to plasma in the presence of heparin, antithrombin in the plasma will bind to heparin and inactivate some of the thrombin or factor Xa. The thrombin or factor Xa remaining free in the test system can be measured using a **chromogenic substrate**.

The amount of colour change that results from cleavage of the substrate is inversely proportional to the amount of antithrombin in the plasma sample.

Functional antihrombin assays can be performed using human thrombin, bovine thrombin, or factor Xa. The choice of assay is important. Human thrombin also reacts with heparin cofactor II (see Chapter 13); as this can interfere with the measurement of antithrombin, assays employing human thrombin are not usually used. Overincubation with heparin can mask some type II HBS defects. A relatively frequent, but clinically mild, antithrombin defect, **Antithrombin Cambridge II**, may not be detected with anti-Xa-based assays.

SELF-CHECK 15.1

What is the difference between type I and type II antithrombin deficiency?

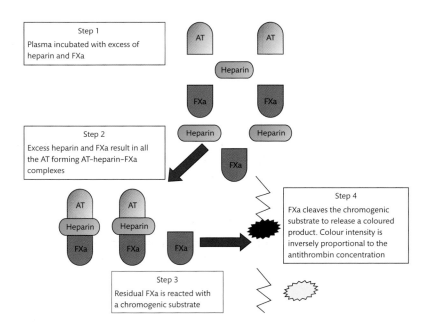

FIGURE 15.3

Functional (activity) assays for antithrombin. Patient or control plasma containing antithrombin is mixed with an excess of heparin and FXa. The plasma antithrombin complexes with the heparin and FXa thereby neutralizing the latter. A chromogenic substrate is added and residual FXa will cleave the substrate to produce a colour-change reaction. The degree of colour change (change in optical density at 405 nm) is directly proportional to the amount of residual FXa, which in turn is inversely proportional to the concentration of antithrombin in the plasma. Some assays use thrombin in place of the FXa.

AT, antithrombin; FXa, activated factor X.

What are the three subtypes of type II antithrombin deficiency?

Protein C deficiency

In Chapter 13 you were introduced to the function of protein C, which is activated by thrombin and then cleaves activated factors V and VIII to prevent these two factors acting to promote clotting. Deficiency of protein C means some of the negative feedback mechanisms in haemostasis are disrupted, and therefore deficiency is associated with an increased risk of thrombosis.

Mutations in the protein C gene can result in type I or type II defects. There is some debate about whether or not protein C deficiency is an autosomal-dominant or autosomal-recessive disorder. Some subjects with genetically confirmed protein C deficiency have protein C levels that fall within the reference range, which can complicate the diagnosis of this defect. Furthermore, age, sex and plasma lipids can affect plasma protein C levels. Homozygous deficiency of protein C is associated with massive thromboembolic complications shortly after birth, and characteristic symptoms such as **purpura fulminans**. Heterozygosity for protein C deficiency is associated with an up to 10-fold increase in the risk of VTE. In type I protein C deficiency, a concordant reduction in immunological and functional levels of protein C is seen, usually to about 50% of normal. The majority of protein C defects are type I defects, and approximately 60% are caused by missense mutations.

purpura fulminans

A life-threatening disorder characterized by cutaneous haemorrhage and necrosis (tissue death), and disseminated intravascular coagulation (DIC).

Laboratory assays for protein C

Similarly to identifying and subtyping AT deficiencies, assays measuring concentration and function are also required for protein C deficiency.

Immunological assays

Laurell Rocket Electrophoresis, ELISA, and radioimmunoassays have all been developed for measuring protein C, although for health and safety reasons, radioimmunoassays are less commonly employed. Concentrations of protein C in plasma are low, approximately 3–5 µg/mL, which makes some assays such as Laurell Rocket Electrophoresis quite difficult to interpret. For protein C deficiency, there seems to be little difference clinically between type I and II deficiency, so most laboratories only use a functional assay to diagnose a deficiency.

Functional assays: chromogenic and clotting

As we discovered in Chapter 13, protein C is activated by thrombin, and this process is accelerated when thrombin is complexed with membrane-bound thrombomodulin. Assays which measure the function of protein C also require protein C activation, but *in vitro* this is achieved by using a snake venom from the Southern Copperhead (*Agkistrodon contortrix contortrix*) which directly activates protein C in a similar way to thrombin. The function of activated protein C can then be measured using a chromogenic assay or an assay based on the clotting of plasma. You can see in Figure 15.4 how these two assays differ.

A small proportion (<5%) of type II defects will only be detected using a clot-based assay, such as mutations affecting the binding of protein C to calcium or protein S; however, the clot-based assay is also affected by a number of other factors, such as the presence of lupus anticoagulants or Factor V Leiden in plasma, or an increased concentration of Factor VIII.

What activates protein C *in vivo* and *in vitro*?

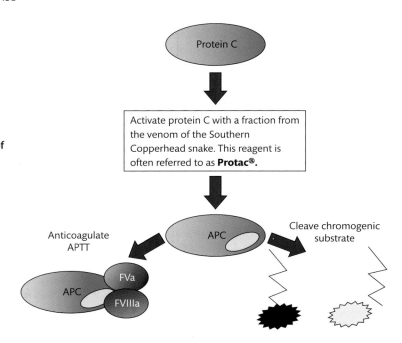

FIGURE 15.4

Functional (activity) assays for protein C. Addition of Protac to plasma causes activation of protein C; addition of a chromogenic substrate specific for protein C will result in cleavage of the substrate and a colour change which is directly proportional to the concentration of protein C in the plasma sample. Alternatively, the addition of APTT reagents will result in prolongation of the clotting time, also directly proportional to the concentration of protein C in the plasma sample.

APC, activated protein C; APTT, activated partial thromboplastin time; FVa, activated factor V; FVIIIa, activated factor VIII.

Within the figure: Protein C; Activate protein C with a fraction from the venom of the Southern Copperhead snake. This reagent is often referred to as **Protac®**. Anticoagulate APTT; APC; FVa; FVIIIa; APC; Cleave chromogenic substrate

Protein S deficiency

Protein S acts as a cofactor for protein C by helping to localize activated protein C on cell surfaces so that factors Va and VIIIa are more effectively inactivated, which you saw in Figure 13.23 in Chapter 13. However, protein S is a complex protein, in that approximately 60% of protein S in plasma is bound to **C4b-binding protein**, a component of the **complement system**, and this bound protein S has no significant anticoagulant role. Therefore, measurement of protein S in plasma must take into account the amount of total PS (both free and bound) and free PS.

Deficiency of protein S is caused by mutations in the gene for protein S, and can be subclassified on the basis of the plasma levels of total and free PS antigen and of PS function (also termed activity). This is slightly more complex than the type I and II deficiencies seen for PC and antithrombin deficiency. Table 15.2 shows you the levels of the different PS measurements for each subgroup. Heterozygosity for protein S deficiency is associated with an up to 10-fold increase in the risk of VTE, and homozygosity presents similarly to homozygous protein C deficiency.

> **complement system**
> An enzyme cascade triggered by antigen–antibody complex formation and resulting in the activation of a series of defence mechanisms, including inflammation and cell lysis.

Laboratory assays for protein S

Protein S can be also measured by Laurell Rocket Electrophoresis, ELISA, and radioimmunoassays. Latex-based assays have also been developed and are widely used to measure protein S in plasma. Total PS can be measured with no special treatment of the plasma. However, some assays used to measure free PS require bound protein S to be removed first. To do this, polyethylene

TABLE 15.2 Protein S levels in type I, II, and III deficiency.

	Total PS	Free PS	PS activity
Type I	Reduced	Reduced	Reduced
Type II	Normal	Normal	Reduced
Type III	Normal	Reduced	Reduced

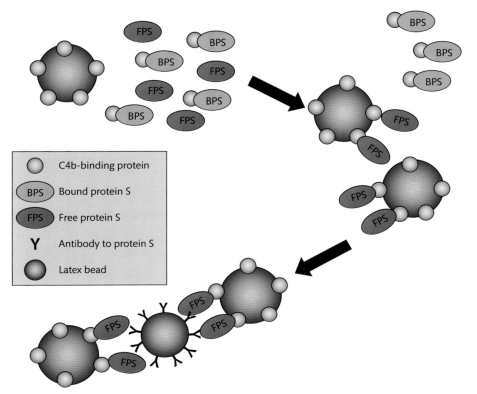

FIGURE 15.5

Free protein S latex immunoassay. Latex beads coated with C4b-binding protein (BP) are added to plasma. Only free protein S in the plasma which is not already bound to C4b-BP binds to the beads. Addition of a second set of beads coated with a monoclonal antibody to protein S results in further binding and agglutination of the beads, which can be measured optically. The turbidimetric changes are directly proportional to the amount of free PS in plasma.

glycol (PEG) is added to plasma, which precipitates the bound PS; after centrifugation, the supernatant will contain just free PS. Other immunological methods for PS utilize specific antibodies that allow direct measurement of the free PS without removing bound PS from the plasma. These assays may give greater precision as a layer of complexity has been removed from the assay. In Figures 15.5 and 15.6 you can see two approaches to the measurement of free PS in plasma.

Functional PS, or PS activity, cannot utilize a chromogenic assay method since protein S does not cleave a target substrate. Methods are therefore based on the ability of protein S to prolong the clotting time of plasma to which activated protein C has been added. Figure 15.7 shows you that this can be carried out using different activators of the clotting process. Functional protein S assays may be affected by activated protein C resistance, lupus anticoagulants, and increased levels of FVIII in the plasma.

SELF-CHECK 15.4

Why do we measure free protein S rather than total protein S?

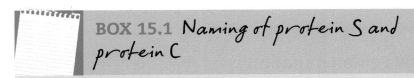

BOX 15.1 Naming of protein S and protein C

Protein S

Protein S is so-called because it was discovered in Seattle, USA. Protein C is so-called because it was the third vitamin K-dependent protein to elute from DEAE–Sepharose, a protein separation technique.

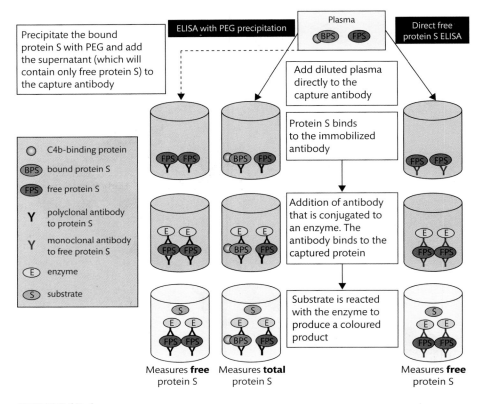

FIGURE 15.6

Protein S ELISA. A microtitre-well plate is coated with either a monoclonal antibody specific for free protein S, or a polyclonal antibody against protein S. Plasma is either added directly, or has bound protein S removed first by precipitation with polyethylene glycol (PEG). The amount of protein S bound to the antibodies in the wells of the plate is directly proportional to the concentration of protein S in the plasma. An enzyme-linked, anti-protein S antibody is then added, and binds to the protein S on the plate. A substrate is added and this is converted by the enzyme to a coloured product; the degree of colour change is directly proportional to the amount of enzyme-linked antibody bound to the protein S, and therefore to the concentration of protein S in the plasma.

Gain-of-function mutations

In contrast to deficiencies of the natural anticoagulants, some mutations in the genes coding for haemostatic proteins have been identified which either alter the interactions involving these proteins, or increase their concentration, causing an increased risk of thrombosis. These are sometimes termed **gain-of-function mutations**.

Factor V Leiden mutation

You saw in Chapter 13 that activated factor V (FVa) is a component of the procoagulant system, acting as a cofactor to FXa to enhance the activation of prothrombin. You also learnt that activated protein C (APC) is a naturally occurring anticoagulant which inactivates FVa. This inactivation occurs through cleavage of FVa at three specific sites on the heavy (aminoterminal) chain: Arg306, Arg506, and Arg679. Cleavage at Arg506 is required for efficient exposure of the other two cleavage sites.

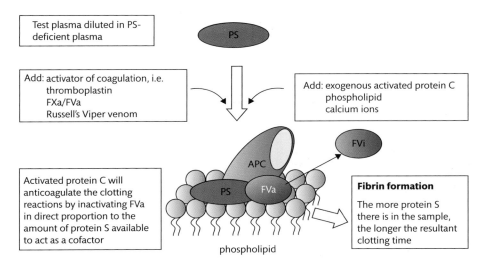

FIGURE 15.7

Functional protein S assays. Test or control plasma is mixed with protein S-deficient plasma (to ensure an excess of all other plasma proteins), and activated protein C is added. The plasma is then clotted by the addition of activators (thromboplastin, FXa, FVa, or Russell's Viper venom). The ability of the mixture to prolong the clotting time is directly proportional to the amount of protein S in the plasma sample.

PS, protein S; APC, activated protein C; FXa, activated factor X; FVa, activated factor V; FVi, inactivated FV.

A **point mutation** in the gene that codes for the intact factor V molecule, guanine to adenine at nucleotide position 1691, causes an amino acid change at position 506 from arginine to glutamine. You can see in Figure 15.8 that because this is the site that is recognized by activated protein C, the FV molecule formed when this mutation is present cannot be cleaved

point mutation

A type of mutation that causes a single base nucleotide in DNA to be replaced with another.

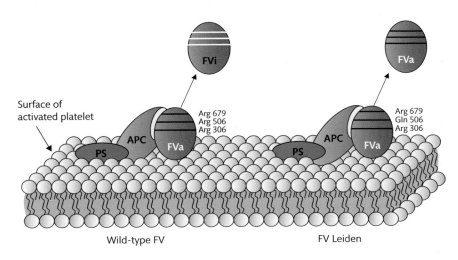

FIGURE 15.8

FV Leiden mutation. Wild-type (normal) factor Va is cleaved by activated protein C and cofactor protein S at positions Arg306, Arg506, and Arg679 to inactivate the active enzyme. Activated protein C is unable to cleave FV Leiden due to a substitution (Gln506) and cannot inactivate factor Va.

PS, protein S; APC, activated protein C; FVa, activated factor V; FVi, inactivated FV.

by APC. We term plasma that contains this mutant factor V 'APC resistant'. As this mutation was first identified in the town of Leiden in the Netherlands, the mutant factor V is called **factor V Leiden**. The mutation is very common, with about 3–5% of the Caucasian population heterozygous for FV Leiden, though it is virtually unknown in African and oriental populations. There is a 2.5-fold increased risk of thrombosis for carriers of the mutation; individuals who are homozygous for FV Leiden have an 80-fold increased risk of developing thrombosis.

Key Points

FV Leiden is the most common cause of unexplained DVT and PE in Caucasians.

Cross references

You will meet lupus anticoagulants later in this chapter.

Principles of PCR analysis are covered in Chapter 10.

Factor V Cambridge

Arg306Thr mutation in the factor V gene, rendering the FV molecule resistant to inactivation by activated protein C.

Factor V Hong Kong

Arg306Gly mutation in the factor V gene. It does not cause activated protein C resistance.

Factor V Liverpool

Ile359Thr mutation in the factor V gene, rendering the FV molecule resistant to inactivation by activated protein C.

In at least 90–95% of patients with APC resistance, FV Leiden is the cause. However, acquired APC resistance can occur in the absence of the FV Leiden mutation—found in individuals with increased levels of factor VIII and in pregnancy, with oral contraceptive use, and hormone-replacement therapy, as well as in subjects with lupus anticoagulants—and it is associated with increased risk of venous thrombosis.

Two rare mutations in the factor V gene, **FV Cambridge** and **FV Hong Kong**, have been described, which cause a change in the arginine at position 306. Both are associated with an increased thrombotic risk. Another rare mutation, **FV Liverpool**, causes a change in the isoleucine at position 359 and leads to mild APC resistance.

Testing for factor V mutations that confer APC resistance

A screening test for such FV mutations can be performed by measuring APC resistance in plasma. To do this, a clotting test, such as the APTT, can be performed in plasma with and without APC added. In normal individuals, activated protein C will cleave and inactivate FVa, and a prolonged clotting time will be obtained. In subjects with FV Leiden, activated protein C will be unable to cleave the FVa, and the clotting time with APC will not be as prolonged. Because a number of variables can affect this basic test, a modification using FV-deficient plasma can be used, to make the test almost 100% specific for FV mutations conferring APC resistance.

Screening the FV gene for the mutations should give a definitive result to show whether the patient is heterozygous or homozygous for a FV mutation, or does not have a mutation ('wild-type FV'). Polymerase chain reaction (PCR) and restriction enzyme (RE) digests have been used to detect the FV mutations, although many other techniques applicable to the detection of point mutations can also be used, such as melting curve analysis and fluorescence resonance energy transfer (FRET) techniques.

Prothrombin gene mutation

Soon after the discovery of FV Leiden, a mutation was described in the prothrombin gene that seemed to increase the risk of venous thrombosis. Here, the mutation is located not in the part of the gene that codes for the protein but in a non-translated part of the gene. The mutation, a guanine to adenine transition at position 20210 on the gene, causes increased levels of prothrombin in the circulation. As prothombin is the precursor of thrombin, it is probably not surprising that increases in the amount of prothrombin can cause a 2–3-fold increased risk of VTE in heterozygotes compared to normal. The increased risk for homozygous subjects is unknown as little data is available, although asymptomatic homozygotes have been described, indicating that this is a mild defect.

It is possible to measure the factor II (prothrombin) activity in patients with this mutation, but the increased level in affected individuals overlaps with the factor II level in normal subjects, so it can be difficult to diagnose on the basis of laboratory clotting methods. Instead, we can search for this mutation using the same genetic analysis methods as for FV Leiden; in some cases laboratories will use methods that can detect both mutations in the same system (multiplex methods).

Is APC resistance always caused by the factor V Leiden mutation?

Other thrombophilias

There are a number of other factors that have been implicated in thrombophilia; some are definitely heritable, others are definitely acquired, and for some it may be difficult to know whether genetics or environmental factors have caused the abnormality.

Fibrinogen—Mutations in the fibrinogen gene are rare, but some abnormalities cause dys-fibrinogenaemia with an associated increased risk of thrombosis, due to altered polymerization and/or resistance to plasmin digestion. In most cases, an abnormal thrombin time can suggest dysfibrinogenaemia, and an abnormal fibrinogen clotting activity : antigen ratio is confirmatory.

Homocysteine—Homocysteine is a non-protein sulphydryl amino acid derived from the metabolism of methionine. Homocysteine is subsequently remethylated to methionine, or undergoes trans-sulphuration to cysteine, depending upon methionine levels. Increased levels can occur in people with folate deficiency, and also in those with hereditary defects. The mechanism by which homocysteine increases thrombotic risk is not known, but it may relate to interference with endothelial cell function. A variety of laboratory methods are available to measure homocysteine, and it is important that plasma is removed from red cells within an hour of collection to avoid falsely raised plasma levels.

High levels of clotting factors—Some reports have shown that high levels of certain clotting factors, such as FVIII, FIX, and FXI, may increase the risk of thrombosis. In some cases, high levels of FVIII and thrombosis have been seen in the same family, suggesting there may be a genetic cause of the defect.

Antiphospholipid syndrome—This is an autoimmune disorder associated with both arterial and venous thrombosis, which is described in the next section of this chapter.

Fibrinolysis—In Chapter 13 you learnt about fibrinolysis, the mechanism by which a fibrin clot is broken down. In theory, failure of this system could lead to an extension of clots formed to repair small areas of vessel damage, and could lead to thrombosis. However, there are so many pre-analytical and analytical variables which affect tests for fibrinolysis, it has not been possible to demonstrate any definite association between a defect in the fibrinolytic system and thrombophilia, although there is evidence that a few PAI-1 polymorphisms, disturbances of t-PA release, and secondary disturbances (such as insulin resistance syndrome) may contribute to thrombophilia.

Pitfalls of thrombophilia testing

There are many considerations to be taken into account with thrombophilia screening. Sample collection and sample quality are important; as you will see later for lupus anticoagulant testing, some tests require plasma that is centrifuged twice to remove all residual platelets, some tests are very sensitive to the concentration of anticoagulant used, others require the separation of red cells from plasma within an hour of collection.

Interpretation of data is sometimes straightforward, as in the example in Case study 15.1. However, some defects will cause abnormal results in more than one test. For example, lupus anticoagulants and APC resistance can cause abnormal results in protein C and protein S clotting-based functional assays in individuals who actually have normal levels of protein C and protein S, which you can see in Case study 15.2. Testing patients soon after a venous

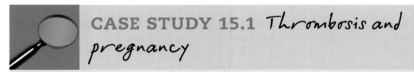

CASE STUDY 15.1 Thrombosis and pregnancy

A patient suffered a deep vein thrombosis during her first pregnancy, and reported a family history of thrombosis. Investigation for heritable thrombophilia gave the following results (RR = reference range):

PT (s)	11.1	(RR: 10.0–14.0)
APTT (s)	33.0	(RR: 32.0–42.0)
Fibrinogen (g/L)	3.7	(RR: 1.5–4.0)
Protein C antigen (u/dL)	82.0	(RR: 50–150)
Protein C activity (u/dL)	43.0	(RR: 50–150)
Total protein S antigen (u/dL)	98.0	(RR: 55–140)
Free protein S antigen (u/dL)	87.0	(RR: 53–135)
Antithrombin antigen (u/dL)	99.1	(RR: 75–125)
Antithrombin activity (u/dL)	88.5	(RR: 80–120)
APC resistance test (ratio)	2.25	(RR: >2.0)
Factor V Leiden mutation	Absent	
Prothrombin P20210A mutation	Absent	

What deficiency and subtype do these results indicate?

thrombosis, or whilst they are pregnant or receiving anticoagulant therapy, can complicate interpretation of the results. Therefore, knowledge of the problems and pitfalls of the tests used for thrombophilia screening is an important role of the biomedical scientist.

The mechanisms involved and the interpretation of results in antiphospholipid syndrome are particularly complex, and these are described in the following section.

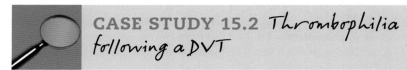

CASE STUDY 15.2 Thrombophilia following a DVT

A 49-year-old patient was investigated for thrombophilia following a first deep vein thrombosis. Laboratory investigation gave the following results (RR = reference range):

PT (s)	12.1	(RR: 10.0–14.0)
APTT (s)	37.0	(RR: 32.0–42.0)
Fibrinogen (g/L)	3.1	(RR: 1.5–4.0)
Protein C activity (u/dL) (clotting-based assay)	49.0	(RR: 50–150)
Protein S activity (u/dL)	51.0	(RR: 55–145)
Antithrombin activity(u/dL)	99.2	(RR: 80–120)
APC resistance test (ratio)	1.05	(RR: >2.0)

Comment: This laboratory only performed functional assays. These data suggest a combined protein C and protein S deficiency, together with an abnormal APC resistance which could be due to factor V Leiden. Combined deficiencies, though rare, markedly increase the risk of repeated thrombotic episodes.

However, APC resistance caused by factor V Leiden is known to interfere with clotting-based protein C and S assays. Further investigation at another site revealed the following results:

Protein C antigen (u/dL)	99.0	(RR: 50–150)
Protein C activity (u/dL) (chromogenic assay)	89.0	(RR: 50–150)
Total protein S antigen (u/dL)	128.0	(RR: 55-140)
Free protein S antigen (u/dL)	114.0	(RR: 53–135)
Antithrombin antigen (u/dL)	104.0	(RR: 75–125)
Factor V Leiden mutation	Homozygous	
Prothrombin P20210A mutation	Absent	

These data confirm that protein C levels by chromogenic assay and protein S antigen levels are normal, and the only likely abnormality is the homozygous FV Leiden mutation. It is possible that a type II protein S defect and/or a rare sub-type protein C defect are also present, but co-existence of all three defects is very unlikely.

15.3 Antiphospholipid antibodies

The **antiphospholipid syndrome** (APS) is an autoimmune disorder characterized by one or more episodes of arterial, venous or small vessel thrombosis, or pregnancy morbidity, accompanied by the persistent presence of one or more types of **antiphospholipid antibody** (APA). In the context of APS, pregnancy morbidity can take the form of unexplained intrauterine death, recurrent unexplained spontaneous abortions, or one or more premature births due to either **pre-eclampsia**, **eclampsia**, or **placental insufficiency**.

pre-eclampsia
Pregnancy-induced high blood pressure associated with protein in the urine. The only cure is delivery or abortion of the fetus.

eclampsia
One or more convulsions occurring during or immediately after pregnancy.

placental insufficiency
Placental failure to supply nutrients to the fetus and remove toxic waste.

Crucial to the diagnosis of APS is the laboratory detection of the different types of APA. The assays detect a heterogeneous group of antibodies that in fact target phospholipid-binding proteins such as **β₂-glycoprotein-I** (β_2GPI) and prothrombin, or protein–phospholipid complexes. Subclassification of APA is based on the assays that are used to detect them:

1. Antibodies detected in solid-phase assays, usually ELISAs, are **anticardiolipin antibodies** (ACA) and anti-β_2GPI antibodies (β_2GPI Ab).

2. Antibodies that interfere with phospholipid-dependent coagulation assays are termed **lupus anticoagulants** (LA).

Although APA have been shown to be significantly associated with thrombotic disease it remains unclear whether they are coincident, consequent, or causative. A variety of mechanisms have been proposed as potential causes of antibody-mediated thrombosis, which include the following:

*   Antibody-induced concentration of prothrombin on *in-vivo* phospholipid surfaces leading to enhanced thrombin generation
*   Interference with the (phospholipid-dependent) protein C pathway
*   Activation of specific clotting factors
*   Platelet activation
*   Endothelial cell activation

Similarly in pregnancy morbidity (although also unproven), APA-induced thrombosis in the placenta may be the cause of **infarction** resulting in placental insufficiency, yet this is not a ubiquitous feature. One hypothesis involves the development of antibodies to **annexin V**, a phospholipid-binding protein with potent anticoagulant activity necessary for the maintenance of placental integrity, leading to placental thrombosis. Early pregnancy loss may be related to the interference of **trophoblast** invasion/implantation by APA rather than a thrombotic mechanism.

Some patients, for whom the symptoms of APS and the presence of APA are the only manifestations of disease, are said to have primary APS, whereas for others, APS coexists alongside other conditions. Many of these are themselves autoimmune disorders, most patients with 'secondary' APS having a condition called **systemic lupus erythematosus** (SLE). It is possible the APS seen in SLE is not actually secondary but that both conditions represent different elements of the same process, or at least that SLE provides a pathophysiological setting for development of APS. Alternatively, APS and SLE may be two diseases coinciding in an individual patient.

An important criterion for the diagnosis of APS is the persistence of APA. This is because transient APA can be encountered as a consequence of other disease states and only persist for the duration of the primary disorder—these transient antibodies are very rarely associated with thrombosis. The only way to confirm that an antibody is persistent, and thus more likely to be involved in APS, is to repeat any positive test at least 12 weeks later. The transient antibodies can be associated with the following:

*   Viral infections, e.g. human immunodeficiency virus; hepatitis C
*   Bacterial infections, e.g. syphilis, leprosy
*   Parasitic infections, e.g. malaria
*   Lymphoproliferative disorders, e.g. lymphoma, chronic lymphocytic leukaemia
*   Drug exposure, e.g. some anticonvulsants and some antimalarials

A separate group of patients exists who do indeed possess persistent APA, yet they are clinically well and very few progress to the classic signs and symptoms of APS. In some cases, these patients may only be identified through abnormal coagulation screening tests performed for other reasons, such as preoperative screening.

Key Points

The vast majority of lupus anticoagulants detected in children are secondary to infections and are not associated with VTE.

The heterogeneous nature of APA and lack of standardization of the assays makes their detection an interesting diagnostic challenge. We will now turn our attention to the procedures available to the biomedical scientist in the identification of APA.

SELF-CHECK 15.6

What are the clinical criteria for a diagnosis of antiphospholipid syndrome?

Antibodies detected in solid-phase assays

ACA and β_2GPI Abs can be detected and quantified using **enzyme-linked immunosorbent assays (ELISA)**. The availability of international standards allows the calculation of ACA and β_2GPI Ab results to be reported in IgG or IgM (anti)phospholipid units—GPLU/mL and MPLU/mL, respectively—in relation to the concentration of the standards, which themselves are preparations of affinity-purified antibodies.

First isolated from heart tissue, **cardiolipin**, or biphosphatidyl glycerol, is a phospholipid that makes up about 20% of the inner mitochondrial membrane. It is found in high concentrations in metabolically active cells, such as heart and skeletal muscle, and has been found in some bacterial membranes. ACA produced as part of an autoimmune process, as in APS, are dependent on β_2GPI to bind to cardiolipin in the assay system. ACA are detected using an indirect ELISA using the design described in the Method box below.

METHOD Indirect ELISA for detecting anticardiolipin antibodies

Unlike a sandwich ELISA, where the antigen is captured by an antibody and then tagged with another, indirect ELISA captures the antigen with an immobilized substance that is known to bind with it.

- A 96-well microtitre is coated with purified cardiolipin and β_2GPI.

- Calibrators containing increasing amounts of purified standard are added to separate designated wells.

- Dilutions (in the region of 1 in 100) of the control and test samples are added to separate designated wells. The plate is left to incubate to allow binding of ACA, if present, to the immobilized cardiolipin/β_2GPI.

- The plate is washed three times with buffer to remove all unbound material and then coated with a solution of antibody to human immunoglobulins that is attached

to an enzyme (i.e. horseradish peroxidase), termed the conjugate. This is left to incubate to allow the conjugate to react with any antigen–antibody complexes that formed during the first stage.

- Unbound conjugate is then washed off.

- The enzyme is then provided with a substrate, the product of the reaction being coloured. The reaction is given time to generate sufficient colour that can be read spectrophotometrically and then stopped with dilute acid, causing a second colour change.

- The colour intensity (referred to as optical density) is in direct proportion to the amount of conjugate bound to the antigen–antibody complex, which itself is proportional to the initial concentration of the ACA in the control and test samples.

Despite the availability of purified standards, variations in reagent composition and details of methodology lead to only moderate inter-laboratory agreement. This is improved if results are stratified as weak, moderate, or strong positive in relation to the individual method and cut-off, rather than directly comparing quantitative results.

Non- β_2GPI-dependent ACA can be generated as part of the immune response to infection, such as seen in syphilis, but are still detected in standard ACA assays. To circumvent this potential for 'false-positive' ACA results, that is to say non-APS-related antibodies, assays using β_2GPI itself as the capture antigen have been developed and are widely available.

Consequently, assays for β_2GPI Ab show greater specificity than ACA for the diagnosis of APS. However, similar problems exist with both methodology and standardization, particularly in relation to the quality of β_2GPI used as the capture antigen.

The variation between assays means that some patients with β_2GPI-dependent antibodies may be detected in an ACA assay but not a β_2GPI Ab assay, and vice versa, so performing both types of assay increases the chances of detecting clinically significant antibodies. Persistent positivity in just one assay is sufficient to diagnose APS if accompanied by appropriate clinical signs and symptoms, although many patients will inevitably be positive in both.

Typically, the cut-off for normality is in the region of 10–15 G- or MPLU/mL, yet it is predominantly the medium to high titre antibodies that are associated with the clinical manifestations of APS. Assay variation makes it impossible to define a generic cut-off. Current expert opinion is that >40 G- or MPLU/mL should be used as a threshold for 'clinically significant' positivity or >99th percentile.

SELF-CHECK 15.7

How are ACA and β_2GPI Ab detected in the laboratory? What are the main problems with the assays?

Antibodies to prothrombin, or prothrombin in complex with phosphatidyl serine, are commonly present in patients with APS and can be detected by indirect ELISA. However, it is not yet clear whether the presence of these antibodies alone is sufficient for a diagnosis of APS and routine measurement is not recommended. Similarly, antibodies to specific phospholipids that are not complexed with protein have been demonstrated in the serum of APS patients, but their presence in isolation does not seem to be associated with thrombotic disease.

Lupus anticoagulants

A subgroup of APA, the lupus anticoagulants (LA), have the ability to interfere with phospholipid-dependent coagulation assays in an inhibitory manner. Their very name is a misnomer as they are present in patients other than those with SLE, the assays are not tests for the diagnosis of SLE, and their anticoagulant properties are purely an *in vitro* phenomenon.

Although ACA are five times more common than LA, it is the latter that have a greater association with thrombosis, pregnancy morbidity, and thrombosis in SLE. The LA can be dependent on β_2GPI or prothrombin for their *in-vitro* anticoagulant activity. Many patients have both types, although the β_2GPI-dependent antibodies have an even greater association with the above clinical manifestations.

BOX 15.2 *Discovery of lupus anticoagulants*

LA are so called because they were first described in 1952 in two patients with SLE who presented with bleeding and whose plasma exhibited *in-vitro* anticoagulant activity. It was suggested that the anticoagulant was associated with the bleeding, although it was in fact due to the thrombocytopenia frequently associated with SLE. A subsequent study in 1963 showed that the presence of this aspecific coagulation inhibitor was more frequently associated with thrombosis. The term lupus anticoagulant was proposed nine years later due to the frequency of the anticoagulants in patients with SLE, although we now recognize they are by no means confined to patients with SLE.

Patients with LA do occasionally present with bleeding symptoms, for the following reasons:

- Coexistence of antibodies to platelet glycoproteins, leading to thrombocytopenia.
- Coexistence of a separate prothrombin antibody that does not cause *in-vitro* inhibition but forms **immune complexes** with prothrombin resulting in its removal from the circulation, causing an acquired deficiency.
- Antibodies to other coagulation factors, such as FX, FVII, or FVIIa.

Immune complex
the combination of an antibody bound to its target antigen.

LA show significant heterogeneity and can even vary in their *in-vitro* behaviour over time in the same patient. Purified standards such as those used in solid-phase assays do not exist, so they are detected by inference due to their ability to inhibit phospholipid-dependent coagulation assays. Antibody heterogeneity and assay variability is considerable, and to such a degree that *no single test is capable of identifying all LA*.

Key Points

Some LA react better in certain types of clotting tests than others, or may be only detectable in one type of clotting test.

National (UK) and international expert guidelines suggest diagnostic strategies to maximize detection rates and include the recommendation to use at least two tests that are of different types. The four main criteria for the laboratory diagnosis of the presence of an LA are outlined in the Method Box below.

METHOD *Criteria for the laboratory detection of lupus anticoagulants*

- Prolongation of at least one phospholipid-dependent screening test.
- Evidence that the abnormality is phospholipid-dependent.
- Evidence that the abnormality is inhibitory in nature.
- Distinguish results from other coagulopathies that may mask, mimic, or co-exist with LA.

What are the usual presenting symptoms of patients with lupus anticoagulants and what other presentations are known?

LA screening tests

A variety of screening tests of different analytical designs are available for detecting LA (detailed in Table 15.3). Virtually all of them incorporate significantly diluted phospholipid to accentuate the inhibitory effect of the LA. They are all based on activating specific parts of the coagulation mechanisms and are thus susceptible to interference by other abnormalities that can lead to false-positive results, such as:

- Coagulation factor deficiencies
- Therapeutic anticoagulation
- Non-phospholipid-dependent inhibitors

Key Points

LA interfere with phospholipid-dependent coagulation tests because they act as competitive inhibitors by competing with coagulation factors for binding to phospholipid. Diluting phospholipid in the assay increases the competition as there are limited phospholipid molecules available, which therefore increases the likelihood of an LA prolonging the clotting time above the reference range.

Because we detect LA by inference, and because of potential interfering factors, the case studies in this section are provided to give an insight into the importance of the interpretive role of biomedical scientists in generating accurate and meaningful results and reports. You would not be expected to practise at this level until you reach more senior grades.

Which screening tests should you use?

You will see from Table 15.3 that the tests available to screen for LA fall into three categories, depending on whether the test design is based on directly activating the 'intrinsic', 'extrinsic' or the 'common' pathway. The recommendation to use at least two test types means that using, for instance, two different APTT reagents is insufficient as some LA are not reactive in assays of that design.

BOX 15.3 Snake venoms

You will see in Table 15.3 that a number of the assays use snake venoms to activate *in-vitro* coagulation at specific points in the pathways. Some of the snakes that provide the venom, which you can see in Figure 15.9, are amongst the most dangerous to man and possess some of the most potent venoms known.

TABLE 15.3 Screening tests for the detection of lupus anticoagulants (LA).

Screening test	Assay principle/design	Interfering factors	Further information
Activated partial thromboplastin time (**APTT**)	• 'Intrinsic pathway'-based assay • Coagulation activated by the action of a contact activator on FXII • Phospholipid is usually diluted but not the contact activator • Ca²⁺-dependent	False-positives can be due to: • Oral anticoagulant therapy • Unfractionated heparin therapy • Non-phospholipid dependent inhibitor • Deficiencies of FII, FV, FVIII, FIX, FX, FXI, PK, HMWK, FXII, or fibrinogen False-negatives can occur with weak LA in the presence of elevated FVIII	• Routine APTT reagents do not contain dilute phospholipid and can miss weak/moderate LA • Variation in phospholipid composition leads to inconsistent sensitivity between reagents • Normal result with a routine APTT reagent is insufficient to exclude the presence of an LA • Dilute APTT with LA-sensitive phospholipid composition should be used to screen for LA • Rarely affected by fractionated heparin
Kaolin or silica clotting time (**KCT/SCT**)	• 'Intrinsic pathway'-based assay • Coagulation activated by the action of a contact activator (kaolin or silica) on FXII • No phospholipid added at all • Ca²⁺-dependent	As for APTT	• Residual plasma lipid and platelets are the sources of phospholipid • Performed on neat plasma and a 1:4 mixture of test : normal plasma (which can dilute LA and lead to false-negative results) • Rarely performed with confirmatory test
Dilute prothrombin time (**DPT**)	• 'Extrinsic pathway'-based assay • Coagulation activated by the action of thromboplastin on FVII/FVIIa • Dilution of phospholipid achieved by diluting the entire thromboplastin reagent • Ca²⁺-dependent	False-positives can be due to: • Oral anticoagulant therapy • Unfractionated heparin therapy • Non-phospholipid dependent inhibitor • Deficiencies of FII, FV, FVII, FX, or fibrinogen	• Dilution of thromboplastin results in dilution of both activator and phospholipid • Considerable reagent variation • Recombinant thromboplastins tend to be more sensitive to LA than those from brain/placenta • Poor specificity relative to other assays

(Continued)

TABLE 15.3 (*Continued*)

Screening test	Assay principle/design	Interfering factors	Further information
Activated seven lupus anticoagulant (**ASLA**) assay	• 'Extrinsic pathway'-based assay • Coagulation activated by the action of recombinant human FVIIa on FX • Recombinant FVIIa used in supraphysiological concentration and works independently of thromboplastin (as it is already activated) • Phospholipid is diluted • Ca²⁺-dependent	False-positives can be due to: • Oral anticoagulant therapy • Unfractionated heparin therapy • Non-phospholipid dependent inhibitor • Deficiencies of FII, FV, FX, or fibrinogen	• Recombinant FVIIa is produced in baby hamster kidney cells and is structurally very similar to human FVIIa • More specific for LA than the other 'extrinsic pathway'-based assay, the DPT • Not widely used because the recombinant FVIIa is expensive
Dilute Russell's Viper venom time (**DRVVT**)	• 'Common pathway'-based assay • Coagulation activated by the action of a purified FX activator from the venom of Russell's Viper (*Daboia russelli* sp.) • Venom is diluted • Phospholipid is diluted • Ca²⁺ dependent	As for ASLA	• Most widely used assay for LA in the UK • Reagent variation does exist, although less marked than for APTT • Reagent variation due to phospholipid composition and venom heterogeneity (there are seven subspecies of Russell's Viper)
Taipan snake venom time (**TSVT**)	• 'Common pathway'-based assay • Coagulation activated by the action of a purified FII activator from the venom of the Coastal Taipan (*Oxyuranus scutellatus*) • Venom is diluted • Phospholipid is diluted • Ca²⁺ dependent	False-positives can be due to: • Unfractionated heparin therapy • Non-phospholipid dependent inhibitor • Deficiencies of FII or fibrinogen	• Taipan venom can activate the PIVKA form of FII and is thus insensitive to the effects of oral anticoagulation • Textarin venom from the Australian Eastern Brown Snake (*Pseudonaja textilis*) works similarly but is additionally FV-dependent. Can be used to screen for LA using the Textarin time

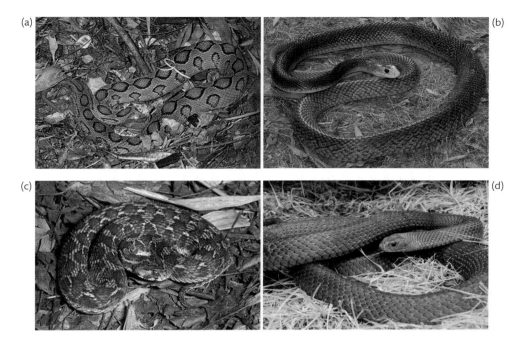

FIGURE 15.9

Snakes whose venom is used in lupus anticoagulant detection. (a) Russell's Viper (*Daboia russelli*), © Muhammad Sharif Khan. (b) Coastal Taipan (*Oxyuranus scutellatus*), © Stewart Macdonald/Ug Media. (c) Saw-scaled Viper (*Echis carinatus*), © Muhammad Sharif Khan. (d) Australian Eastern Brown Snake (*Pseudonaja textilis*) © Roger Michael Lowe. Russell's Viper is the second largest venomous snake in the world and responsible for thousands of human deaths every year across Southern Asia. The Coastal Taipan is an Australian snake related to cobras and considered the most dangerous of all land snakes to humans. The Saw-scaled viper is found in Africa and Asia and gets its name from the sawing sound it makes by rubbing scales from either side of its body together as a warning sign—it is highly dangerous to man. The Australian Eastern Brown Snake is also related to cobras and is one of the few snakes that both poisons and constricts its prey.

The most common pairing of tests in the UK is APTT and dilute Russell's Viper venom time (DRVVT). This combination has been shown to have high detection rates but will not detect all LA, the main reasons for which are listed below:

- Some laboratories use their routine APTT in the reagent pairing for LA detection. Many of these have poor sensitivity to LA compared to APTT reagents specifically formulated to detect LA.

- LA that are potentially detectable in a given assay type (i.e. DRVVT) may not be reactive to the reagents/methodology in local use for that type.

- Some LA are detectable only in extrinsic pathway-based assays.

In cases where the clinical suspicion of APS is high despite negative results, it is good practice to have alternative assays available. Where APTT and DRVVT are the first-line assays, appropriate second-line tests would be an 'extrinsic pathway'-based assay and using APTT/DRVVT reagents from different manufacturers to those used initially. There are resource implications for such a strategy so a common approach is to send samples to another laboratory which uses different tests/reagents. Some workers prefer APTT and dilute prothrombin time (DPT) as first-line assays. They both incorporate the 'common pathway' to form the fibrin clot endpoint, yet LA exist that will react in neither assay but are revealed in, for instance, DRVVT.

Results are often expressed as ratios that are derived from dividing the patient's clotting time by that of the normal control. This is preferable to using raw clotting times as it accounts for changes in reagent stability, variation in the clotting time of normal plasma and operator/analyser variability.

Confirmatory tests

As you saw in Table 15.3, a screening test may be prolonged for reasons other than the presence of an LA. Thus, we cannot stop the diagnostic process at the stage of an elevated screening test and must progress to other procedures to confirm the nature of the abnormality.

There are two aspects of LA *in-vitro* behaviour that we assess in order to confirm that an abnormal screening test is due to an LA, those of *inhibition* and *phospholipid dependence*.

Inhibition

Inhibition is demonstrated by mixing the patient's plasma with an equal volume of a normal plasma and then repeating the assay. If the patient's plasma contains an inhibitor it should continue to interfere with the phospholipid-dependent stages of *in-vitro* coagulation, whereas if the abnormality is due to a factor deficiency, the normal plasma will correct it and generate a normal result.

In practice, there is an unavoidable dilution of the LA antibodies in this process which leads to false negative mixing studies in a considerable number of cases. One response to this problem is to use a different ratio of test to normal plasma, such as four parts test to one part normal. This will still correct most factor deficiencies and reduce the possibility of diluting the LA to undetectable levels. However, the smaller amount of normal plasma may not be sufficient to correct severe factor deficiencies or the multiple severe factor deficiency of high dose oral anticoagulant therapy and can lead to false positive results.

Phospholipid dependence

Crucial to the demonstration of an LA is confirmation of phospholipid dependence. This is usually achieved by performing the screening test in an identical fashion, apart from markedly increasing the concentration of the phospholipid. This has the effect of swamping the antibody so that competition for phospholipid binding between the LA antibody and clotting factors is reduced, thereby leading to a reduction in the clotting time compared to that of the screening test. Such reagents are referred to as **confirm reagents**.

Other abnormalities—such as factor deficiencies, therapeutic anticoagulation, and non-phospholipid-dependent inhibitors—will prolong the confirmatory test to a degree similar to the screening test because their effects on clotting times are not related to phospholipid concentration. A typical example of positive testing for LA is given as Case study 15.3.

SELF-CHECK 15.9

What are the laboratory criteria for the detection and confirmation of the presence of a lupus anticoagulant?

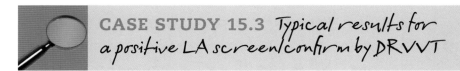

CASE STUDY 15.3 *Typical results for a positive LA screen/confirm by DRVVT*

DRVVT screen ratio	1.45	(RR: 0.85–1.15)
DRVVT confirm ratio	1.00	(RR: 0.86–1.14)

The screen ratio is markedly above the upper value of the reference range and the confirm ratio is significantly lower and within the reference range. This confirms that the abnormality was corrected by the addition of concentrated phospholipid, i.e. a lupus anticoagulant.

The two most common methods employed to increase the phospholipid concentration are:

- Platelet neutralization procedure (PNP)
- High-concentration phospholipid reagents

As its name suggests, reagents for the PNP are prepared from platelets as they contain high concentrations of procoagulant phospholipids. The phospholipids are made available by washing normal platelets and either activating them with a calcium ionophore or repeatedly freezing and thawing them to release the phospholipid by disrupting the platelet membranes. The PNP has been used to confirm phospholipid dependence in APTT, DRVVT, activated seven lupus anticoagulant (ASLA) assay, and Taipan snake venom time (TSVT).

One drawback of using such a reagent prepared from platelets is that it will contain other platelet constituents, in particular **platelet factor 4 (PF4)**. One property of PF4 is that it neutralizes heparin, which can lead to false-positive confirmatory tests in patients receiving therapeutic heparin, as you can see in Case study 15.4.

In practice, investigation for LA in patients whose clinical condition requires anticoagulation by unfractionated heparin is rarely indicated, so PNP confirmatory tests remain in common use.

The most common alternative is to use a confirmatory reagent with a high concentration of the same phospholipid preparation that was diluted in the screening test. Such reagents give comparable results to PNP and are not prone to false-positive interpretations in unfractionated heparin therapy. Such confirmatory reagents have been used in APTT, DRVVT, DPT, and ASLA. The screen and confirm results are interpreted identically to those shown in Case study 15.4.

A variation on this theme is the use of a confirmatory reagent that does not contain concentrated phospholipid but whose constituent phospholipids are nonetheless insensitive to the presence of LA. This is a function of the relative amounts of the individual phospholipids— phosphatidyl choline, phosphatidyl ethanolamine, phosphatidyl serine, and sphingomyelin. This approach is often adopted in APTT testing for LA where an APTT reagent whose phospholipid composition is sensitive to LA is used as the screening test, accompanied by an LA-insensitive APTT reagent for the confirmatory test. Reagents rich in phosphatidyl serine are insensitive to LA, so screening reagents are more sensitive if they have a low phosphatidyl serine content.

platelet factor 4

A small cytokine released from activated platelets that modulates the effects of heparin-like molecules, stimulates protein C activation and is chemotactic for neutrophils and monocytes.

CASE STUDY 15.4 *False-positive LA screen in a patient on unfractionated heparin when using PNP in the DRVVT confirmatory test*

PT (s)	11.1	(RR: 10.0–14.0)
APTT (s)	70.0	(RR: 32.0–42.0)
Thrombin time (s)	101.2	(RR: 9.0–11.0)
Reptilase time (s)	15.1	(RR: 14.2–16.0)
DRVVT screen ratio	1.90	(RR: 0.85–1.15)
DRVVT confirm ratio	1.30	(RR: 0.86–1.14)

The coagulation screening results are indicative of the presence of heparin. The heparin is causing the elevation of the DRVVT screen, but its effect is partly neutralized in the confirmatory test due to the presence of PF4 in the PNP reagent. This can be mistaken for the presence of an LA. It is, of course, possible that a patient on unfractionated heparin does indeed have an LA, but it is impossible to tell in this scenario, so some regent manufacturers add a heparin neutralizer to both the screen and confirm reagents.

How do we assess whether the correction of the screen ratio by the confirm ratio is significant?

In theory, the screen and confirmatory tests should give identical results unless an abnormality is phospholipid-dependent. So in a patient with a factor deficiency, both screen and confirm results should be prolonged by a similar degree. Similarly, if we performed a confirmatory test on a patient with a normal screening test result they should give identical results. In practice, however, we have to allow for a degree of analytical error inherent in any method and partial corrections may be seen. We approach this by applying calculations to assess the degree of correction against a predefined cut-off point. Although much of the research has been done on DRVVT, the calculations can be applied to any assay. The most commonly used calculations in the UK are outlined below.

1. *Percent correction of ratio*
   The degree of correction of the screening test ratio by the confirmatory test ratio is calculated as follows:

   {(Screening test ratio–confirmatory test ratio) × 100}/Screening test ratio

   Provided other causes of elevated clotting times have been excluded, ≥10% correction is considered indicative of the presence of an LA.

2. *The normalized ratio*

The screening test ratio is divided by the confirmatory test ratio to generate a third ratio, which is the normalized ratio.

Screening test ratio/Confirmatory test ratio

A normalized ratio of >1.2 is considered positive for LA, although this cut-off point should be derived locally based on the reagents and analytical equipment in use.

3. *Percent correction of clotting time*

The clotting time of the control for the screening test is subtracted from the clotting time of the test, and the product is then divided by the clotting time for the control. This result is termed the screen ratio. The same is carried out for the confirmatory test and the following equation applied:

{(Screen ratio–confirm ratio) × 100}/Screen ratio

A value of >65% is considered significant.

4. *The test/confirm ratio*

The clotting time of the screening test is divided by the clotting time of the confirmatory test. A ratio above a locally derived reference range is considered positive for LA.

Look at Table 15.4 which demonstrates how to incorporate raw data into each of the calculations above in a patient with a lupus anticoagulant.

There is no consensus on the optimal method. Some laboratories use the calculations recommended by the manufacturers of particular reagents, whilst others adopt a locally preferred calculation for specific assay types. Apart from cases where there is minimal elevation of the screening test above the reference range, correction back into the reference range is strong evidence for the presence of an LA. Some workers have reported that the percent correction of ratio and percent correction of clotting time give the most reliable results, the former being recommended in the initial British guidelines. The test/confirm ratio is not recommended for the same reasons that results are expressed as ratios, as discussed earlier.

Before you read and work through the case studies that follow, look through the flow chart in Figure 15.10 to understand the diagnostic strategies used to detect LA in the clinical haemostasis laboratory.

TABLE 15.4 Worked through examples of calculations for phospholipid dependence on DRVVT testing in a patient with a lupus anticoagulant.

Raw data		
DRVVT screen (test)	60 s	Screen ratio $= \dfrac{60}{32} = $ **1.88** (Reference range: 0.85 – 1.15)
DRVVT screen (normal control)	32 s	
DRVVT confirm (test)	31 s	Confirm ratio $= \dfrac{31}{30} = $ **1.03** (Reference range: 0.86 – 1.14)
DRVVT confirm (normal control)	30 s	

Calculation for percent correction of ratio	Calculation for percent correction of clotting time
$\dfrac{(1.88 - 1.03) \times 100}{1.88} = 45.2\%$	$\dfrac{\left(\dfrac{60-32}{32}\right) - \left(\dfrac{31-30}{30}\right) \times 100}{\left(\dfrac{60-32}{32}\right)} = 96.6\%$

Calculation for normalized ratio	Calculation for test/confirm ratio
$\dfrac{1.88}{1.03} = 1.83$	$\dfrac{60}{31} = 1.94$

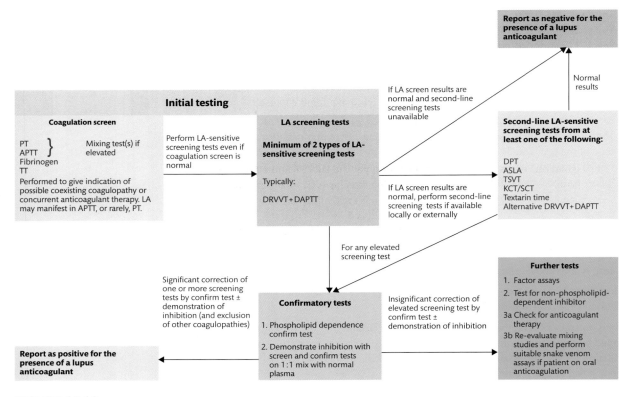

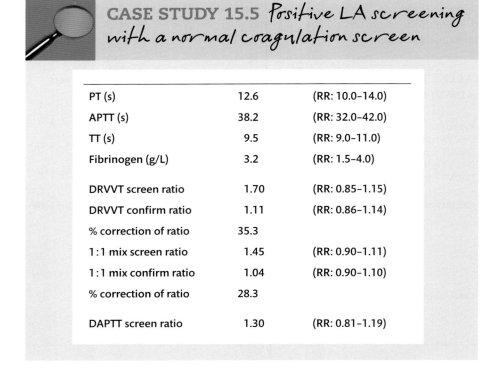

FIGURE 15.10

Flow chart for the laboratory detection of lupus anticoagulants.

DAPTT confirm ratio	0.98	(RR: 0.82–1.17)
% correction of ratio	24.6	
1:1 mix screen ratio	1.24	(RR: 0.84–1.14)
1:1 mix confirm ratio	1.00	(RR: 0.85–1.12)
% correction of ratio	19.4	

The coagulation results shows no abnormalities, yet the DRVVT and DAPTT test are clearly positive. The DRVVT and DAPTT screening tests have 1:1 mixtures with normal plasma are elevated, indicating inhibition; and, with the confirmatory reagent, correct by > 10% and back into the reference range. The LA appears more potent with DRVVT than DAPTT. Some antibodies react better in some systems than others. The routine APTT reagent is insensitive to this particular LA.

Exclusion of other causes of elevated clotting times

Interpretation of the screening and confirmatory procedures we have met so far assumes that no other abnormalities are present, and so the results can be accepted at face value. When another coagulation abnormality coexists, interpreting the result is difficult because you cannot necessarily tell how much each abnormality is contributing to screening test elevation, and, hence, whether the confirmatory test has corrected the effect of an LA.

The starting point for the exclusion of other abnormalities is the coagulation screen as it will give an immediate indication of the presence of abnormalities. The phospholipid in routine thromboplastin reagents is concentrated so it is rare for LA to cause an elevation of the prothrombin time. Routine APTT reagents vary widely in their sensitivity for LA so results will not always be elevated when an LA is present. As you will see in Chapter 16 therapeutic anticoagulants can generate specific result patterns in coagulation screening and they will alter the way in which results are interpreted. Presented below are some case studies to demonstrate interpretation.

The next Case study (15.6) presents with an abnormal coagulation screen, so it is important to find an explanation before taking the LA assays at face value.

CASE STUDY 15.6 A 32-year-old male presented with a deep vein thrombosis

PT (s)	13.0	(RR: 10.0–14.0)
APTT (s)	63.1	(RR: 32.0–42.0)
TT (s)	10.1	(RR: 9.0–11.0)
Fibrinogen (g/L)	2.8	(RR: 1.5–4.0)

1 At first sight these results suggest a factor deficiency in the intrinsic. Before embarking on time-consuming and expensive factor assays, an APTT on a 1:1 mixture with normal plasma was performed and gave the following result:

APTT 1:1 mix (s) 59.1 (RR: 32.0–42.0)

Although slightly shorter than the APTT in neat plasma, this result is nowhere near the reference range and suggests the presence of an inhibitor and not a factor deficiency. In view of the thrombotic presentation, LA screening was performed.

DRVVT screen ratio	1.01	(RR: 0.85–1.15)
DAPTT screen ratio	2.32	(RR: 0.81–1.19)
DAPTT confirm ratio	1.40	(RR: 0.82–1.17)
% correction of ratio	39.7	
1:1 mix screen ratio	1.80	(RR: 0.84–1.14)
1:1 mix confirm ratio	1.11	(RR: 0.85–1.12)
% correction of ratio	38.3	

The DRVVT is normal, yet there is a clear LA in the DAPTT in both neat plasma and the mixing tests. The confirmatory test in neat plasma does not return to the reference range but significantly corrects the screening test result. The screening test in the mixture gives a lower result than in neat plasma due to a dilution effect. The results demonstrate a phospholipid-dependent inhibitor (i.e. LA) that is reacting only in APTT-based asssys.

Key Points

As long as one assay (and its confirmatory tests) demonstrate the presence of an LA, that is sufficient to confirm positivity. Some LA are detectable by only one type of test.

Case study 15.7 demonstrates the importance of performing confirmatory tests for phospholipid-dependence and inhibition in order to distinguish LA from other inhibitors.

 CASE STUDY 15.7 An inhibitor is demonstrated in the coagulation screen but is it an LA?

PT (s)	13.1	(RR: 10.0–14.0)
APTT (s)	110.0	(RR: 32.0–42.0)
APTT 1:1 mix (s)	90.3	(RR: 32.0–42.0)
Fibrinogen (g/L)	3.2	(RR: 1.5–4.0)

DRVVT screen ratio	2.40	(RR: 0.85–1.15)
DRVVT confirm ratio	2.30	(RR: 0.86–1.14)
% correction of ratio	4.2	
1 : 1 mix screen ratio	1.89	(RR: 0.90–1.11)
1 : 1 mix confirm ratio	1.92	(RR: 0.90–1.10)
% correction of ratio	–1.6	
DAPTT screen ratio	3.23	(RR: 0.81–1.19)
DAPTT confirm ratio	3.30	(RR: 0.82–1.17)
% correction of ratio	–2.2	
1 : 1 mix screen ratio	2.87	(RR: 0.84–1.14)
1 : 1 mix confirm ratio	2.86	(RR: 0.85–1.12)
% correction of ratio	0.3	

The LA tests reveal a non-phospholipid-dependent inhibitor as there are no significant differences between screen and confirm assays in neat plasma or mixing tests. Further tests gave the following results:

TT (s)	>120	(RR: 9.0–11.0)
RT (s)	14.5	(RR: 14.2–16.0)

The patient was receiving unfractionated heparin, and the DRVVT and DAPTT confirm reagents were not PNP-based.

Case study 15.8 is an example of antibody heterogeneity and reagent variability.

 CASE STUDY 15.8 *A patient was being investigated for thrombophilia, but was not on medication*

The following results were obtained:

PT (s)	15.0	(RR: 10.0–14.0)
APTT (s)	35.8	(RR: 32.0–42.0)
TT (s)	9.9	(RR: 9.0–11.0)
Fibrinogen (g/L)	3.9	(RR: 1.5–4.0)
DRVVT screen ratio	0.94	(RR: 0.85–1.15)
DAPTT screen ratio	0.99	(RR: 0.81–1.19)

The only abnormality is a slight elevation of the PT, which could indicate a mild FVII deficiency. Measurement of FVII activity gave a normal result and the patient was not on any drugs. Further tests showed the following:

ASLA screen ratio	1.51	(RR: 0.85–1.14)
ASLA confirm ratio	1.10	(RR: 0.88–1.12)
% correction of ratio	27.1	
1:1 mix screen ratio	1.30	(RR: 0.90–1.12)
1:1 mix confirm ratio	1.01	(RR: 0.89–1.11)
% correction of ratio	22.3	

Some LA will not be detected in the most commonly used LA assays, such as DRVVT and DAPTT, and this LA was detected in an extrinsic pathway-based assay.

Oral anticoagulation

As you will read in Chapter 16 oral anticoagulation treatment with vitamin K antagonists (such as warfarin) leads to acquired functional deficiencies of factors II, VII, IX, and X. Since this inevitably results in elevated clotting times in screening tests for LA, we have to rely on mixing studies to correct the deficiencies and thus allow LA to manifest, as shown in Case study 15.9.

There are occasions where the confirmatory tests in the mixing studies do not go back into the reference range but do correct the screening test by >10%, in which case the results are suggestive of the presence of an LA rather than conclusive.

Often the mixing studies are negative, but because dilution of the LA can prevent it from prolonging the screening test, you cannot be certain that the testing is truly negative.

SELF-CHECK 15.10

Why do we have to use more than one screening test and a battery of confirmatory tests to detect lupus anticoagulants?

Testing for LA in orally anticoagulated patients using snake venoms

The venoms from the Coastal Taipan (*Oxyuranus scutellatus*) and Australian Eastern Brown Snake (*Pseudonaja textilis*) contain FII activators, which are capable of activating the abnormal FII produced during warfarin therapy to an altered version of thrombin that will clot *in vitro*. This means that the TSVT and Textarin times (see Table 15.3) will give normal results in orally anticoagulated patients who do not have LA or deficiencies of FII and fibrinogen.

The Textarin time utilizes a novel confirmatory test, the Ecarin time, which uses venom from the Saw-scaled Viper (*Echis carinatus*). Like Taipan and Textarin venoms, the Ecarin

CASE STUDY 15.9 *Results from a patient receiving warfarin therapy*

PT (s)	36.7	(RR: 10.0–14.0)
APTT (s)	51.8	(RR: 32.0–42.0)
TT (s)	9.2	(RR: 9.0–11.0)
Fibrinogen (g/L)	4.5	(RR: 1.5–4.0)
DRVVT screen ratio	2.90	(RR: 0.85–1.15)
DRVVT confirm ratio	2.30	(RR: 0.86–1.14)
% correction of ratio	20.7	
1 : 1 mix screen ratio	1.54	(RR: 0.90–1.11)
1 : 1 mix confirm ratio	1.03	(RR: 0.90–1.10)
% correction of ratio	33.1	
DAPTT screen ratio	1.84	(RR: 0.81–1.19)
DAPTT confirm ratio	1.44	(RR: 0.82–1.17)
% correction of ratio	21.7	
1 : 1 mix screen ratio	1.30	(RR: 0.84–1.14)
1 : 1 mix confirm ratio	0.99	(RR: 0.85–1.12)
% correction of ratio	23.8	

As described above, even though the neat plasma results show > 10% correction of the screen ratio, they are not necessarily reliable. The screening tests in the mixing studies remain elevated, and the confirmatory tests correct by > 10% and back into the reference range, indicating that the normal plasma has corrected the factor deficiencies of warfarin therapy and thus allowed the LA manifest. Similar results would be seen with an isolated hereditary factor deficiency plus lupus anticoagulant.

venom directly activates FII but in a phospholipid- and calcium-*independent* manner, so it is impossible for LA to interfere with the clotting times. Ecarin venom can also activate the FII formed in warfarin therapy. If Textarin and Ecarin venoms are titrated to give similar clotting times with a normal control, dividing the patient's Textarin time by their Ecarin time generates a Textarin/Ecarin ratio, which, if above 1.3, is indicative of the presence of an LA.

The Ecarin time can also be used as a confirmatory test for the TSVT too and is more sensitive to the presence of LA in orally anticoagulated patients than using a PNP confirmatory test. The results are interpreted using the percent correction of ratio.

Pre-analytical variables

Along with the usual considerations for obtaining a high-quality sample, a crucial consideration for LA testing is ensuring that the contamination of the plasma by platelets is minimized, and in any case, the residual platelet count is $<10 \times 10^9/L$. This is because residual platelet material can 'neutralize' LA, particularly the weaker or low-titre antibodies. Most laboratories freeze plasma aliquots in order to batch their LA assays so that the freeze-and-thaw process lyses platelet membranes, thereby releasing procoagulant phospholipid in a similar fashion to the process used to produce PNP reagents. Platelets can be removed from plasma to an appropriate level by filtering or double-centrifugation. The normal control plasma must also be similarly platelet-free.

There is variation in analytical performance between different reagents, even those used for the same test but prepared by different manufacturers. This results in the necessity for locally derived reference ranges specific to the reagents and analytical equipment in use. It is insufficient to use manufacturers' stated reference ranges or those quoted by other laboratories or in research papers.

15.4 Thrombosis

Risk of venous thrombosis

Not all subjects with a hereditary or acquired thrombophilia go on to have a thrombosis. However, the risk of thrombosis for an individual with one of these factors is higher than for someone without the defect. As you saw earlier, the risk of thrombosis in someone with heterozygous protein C, protein S or antithrombin deficiency is approximately five to seven times higher than in an unaffected individual. Since only about 1/1000 people per year suffer a thrombosis, and that figure includes all other causes of thrombosis, this risk is still relatively small. However, subjects with thrombophilia are more likely to suffer a thrombosis at a relatively young age (<40 years old). In addition, certain high-risk situations (such as surgery, using the oral contraceptive pill, or hormone replacement therapy) can increase the risk of thrombosis, and subjects who know they have thrombophilia may need to consider alternative options or receive prophylactic anticoagulation at certain times. Identifying heritable thrombophilia in a subject can also have implications for close relatives, who may also wish to be screened.

Treatment of thrombophilia

Because anticoagulants such as heparin and warfarin are associated with a relatively high risk of bleeding, subjects with thrombophilia are not usually treated until they have had a thrombotic episode, or are placed in a high-risk situation, such as needing surgery. At present, it is also difficult to predict which patients will suffer recurrent thrombosis (up to 30% of individuals who have had a VTE will suffer a further event within 5 years, but individuals with no obvious cause for the first event are at least as likely to suffer a recurrence as those with thrombophilia). At present, therefore, long-term oral anticoagulant therapy is only recommended for subjects with recurrent spontaneous thrombosis, a single thrombosis at an unusual or life-threatening site, a single thrombosis with antithrombin deficiency or lupus anticoagulant, or co-inheritance of two or more genetic defects. These recommendations may change as the findings of ongoing studies are reported.

Other types of thrombosis-related disorders

Although investigation for hereditary and acquired thrombophilias represents a considerable part of the workload in more specialized haemostasis laboratories, other disturbances in haemostasis can result in thrombotic disease.

Arterial thrombosis

You learnt in the introduction to this chapter that thrombophilia, and the causes of thrombophilia, generally refer to venous thromboembolic disease. Thrombosis can also occur in the arterial system but the causes are different. Arterial thrombosis is often preceded by **atherosclerosis**, where the blood vessel is narrowed through deposits of **atheroma**. The composition of the vessel wall and flow characteristics also result in clots forming that are rich in platelets, and treatment of arterial thrombosis will often include antiplatelet therapy. The risk of arterial thrombosis is increased by a number of factors including smoking, **hypertension**, diabetes and obesity. Antiphospholipid syndrome is also associated with an increased risk of arterial thrombosis.

atheroma
An accumulation of lipids, macrophages, and connective tissue causing thickening of the inner wall of the arteries in patches, or plaques.

hypertension
Increased blood pressure.

Heparin-induced thrombocytopenia (HIT)

In approximately 5% of patients receiving unfractionated heparin (UFH) therapy, antibodies against heparin-platelet factor 4 complexes develop, resulting in platelet activation. This typically takes place around 5 days after treatment begins, and may also occur with low molecular weight heparin therapy. A marked drop in the platelet count is seen, and, additionally, both arterial and venous thrombus formation may occur. It is important that heparin therapy is stopped and replaced with an alternative anticoagulant regime.

Cross reference
HIT antibodies and their laboratory detection are covered in detail in Chapter 16.

Thrombotic thrombocytopenic purpura (TTP) and haemolytic uraemic syndrome (HUS)

TTP

von Willebrand factor (VWF) is involved in the normal primary haemostatic mechanisms involving platelet adhesion. VWF subunits combine covalently to form multimers of differing sizes, and larger multimers have a greater facility to promote platelet aggregation. You saw in Chapter 13 how the size of the VWF multimers in plasma is regulated by the metalloprotease ADAMTS13 which breaks down large multimers of VWF into smaller, less reactive multimers. Deficiency of ADAMTS13 leads to a condition called **thrombotic thrombocytopenic purpura** (TTP), which can be either congenital or acquired.

In congenital TTP, also known as the **Upshaw–Schulman syndrome**, mutations cause a deficiency of ADAMTS13, which generally affects the synthesis or secretion of the enzyme rather than causing production of dysfunctional molecules. In acquired TTP, an IgG inhibitory antibody prevents the normal action of ADAMTS13. Each mechanism results in an excess of ultra-large VWF multimers being produced from the Weibel–Palade bodies which become anchored to the endothelium, where they can bind platelets via GpIbα on the platelet membrane. This cancause aggregation of platelets, which results in microvascular thrombosis and haemolytic anaemia. Coagulation screening tests are usually normal or only slightly disturbed, which helps to distinguish TTP from disseminated intravascular coagulation, although thrombocytopenia and a **microangiopathic haemolytic anaemia** will be evident from a full blood count and blood film. Haemoglobin is usually below 105 g/L but the MCV will be normal unless there is marked red cell fragmentation, which will be evident from the blood film. The red cell fragments arise from being sheared as they travel past and through the micro-thrombi, which is the cause of the intravascular haemolysis. Reticulocytes are increased, which can increase the MCV, and nucleated red cells can be seen in the peripheral blood, both indicators of a bone marrow response to the haemolysis. Serum lactate dehydrogenase is also elevated. Neurological signs, such as coma, stroke, seizures and even personality change, are a presenting feature due to formation of thrombi in the cerebral circulation.

Specific assays for ADAMTS13, both functional and immunological, will show plasma levels to be reduced or absent. Antibodies to ADAMTS13 are detected with ELISA techniques.

HUS

A clinically similar disorder, **haemolytic uraemic syndrome** (HUS), occurs primarily in infants and young children and occasionally in the elderly. Typical HUS occurs acutely following gastrointestinal infections with *Escherichia coli* 0157:H7, or less commonly, *Shigella dysenteriae*, both of which produce Shiga-toxins. Most patients will have experienced episodes of bloody diarrhoea during the infection. The Shiga-toxin enters the bloodstream and attaches to glomerular endothelial cells because in infants, young children and the elderly, these cells are rich in the membrane receptor globotriaosyl ceramide (Gb$_3$). The toxin–receptor complex is endocytosed, which leads to the activation of endothelial cells and consequent thrombosis in the renal microvasculature. ADAMTS13 levels are usually normal. The acute renal failure can be so severe that haemodialysis is required. Neurological signs are far less common than in TTP. The microangiopathic haemolytic anaemia can also be severe and the platelet count can fall below 60×10^9/L.

Familial HUS accounts for about 5–10% of all cases and results from the deficiency or dysfunction of **complement factor H**, a regulator of the complement system that ensures the system is directed against pathogens and not self. The deficiency results in excessive activation of complement component 3 (C3), which is deposited on membranes and leads to renal cell injury. Atypical HUS, which is non-diarrhoea related, is distinguished from TTP by the predominance of renal symptoms and absence of neurological signs. It is commonly associated with the post-partum period or exposure to certain drugs, such as quinine, cyclosporin, and ticlopidine.

Cross reference

See definition and further detail of microangiopathic anaemia in Chapter 6.

SELF-CHECK 15.11

What are the main similarities and differences between TTP and HUS?

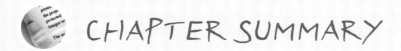

CHAPTER SUMMARY

- Thrombophilia is an increased risk of venous thrombosis caused by the inheritance of certain genetic defects, and it can also be acquired.

- Inherited causes include deficiency of protein C, protein S or antithrombin, and mutations in the factor V gene (FV Leiden) or the prothrombin gene.

- Acquired defects, such as lupus anticoagulants, high homocysteine levels, or increased levels of certain clotting factors, are also associated with thrombophilia.

- Different assays are available to measure levels of protein C, protein S, and antithrombin. Some assays measure the level of protein in plasma (immunological assays), whilst others measure the activity of the protein (functional assays).

- Some individuals have defects which only affect the activity of these proteins, termed type II defects. It is important therefore to use functional assays to investigate thrombophilia.

- Mutations such as FV Leiden and the G20210A prothrombin mutation may be detected through genetic investigations.

- Not all patients with a heritable thrombophilia will go on to develop thrombosis.

- However, detection of thrombophilia may provide an explanation for a thrombotic event, and may indicate the need for prophylaxis (in the form of anticoagulation) in high-risk situations.

- The tests recommended for inclusion in a **thrombophilia screen** are shown in Table 15.5.

- Antiphospholipid syndrome is an autoimmune disorder characterized by thrombotic disease or pregnancy morbidity accompanied by the presence of persistent antiphospholipid antibodies.

- Antiphospholipid antibodies are subclassified depending on whether they are detectable in solid-phase assays such as ELISA, or in coagulation-based tests.

- Anticardiolipin antibodies and anti-β_2GPI antibodies are detected in solid-phase assays and lupus anticoagulants are detected in coagulation tests.

- Antibodies detected in solid-phase assays can be quantified by comparison with affinity-purified standards.

- Lupus anticoagulants are detected by their interference with phospholipid-dependent coagulation assays, and their presence confirmed with tests for inhibition and phospholipid dependence.

- Antibody heterogeneity and reagent variability mean that no single reagent, or reagent type, will detect all lupus anticoagulants. Some antibodies react more strongly in one test than another, and others may only be identifiable by one type of test.

TABLE 15.5 Tests commonly employed in thrombophilia screening.

Thrombophilia screening test	Method	Comments	Further tests if abnormal
Prothrombin Time APTT Thrombin Time	Routine screening reagents (but be aware of the LA sensitivity of your reagents)	May detect LA (prolonged APTT), dysfibrinogenaemia (prolonged TT), high FVIII (shortened APTT). More importantly, will detect effects of heparin or warfarin, or liver disease affecting vitamin K-dependent clotting factors—protein C and S	Mixing tests with normal plasma, LA screening, fibrinogen assay, factor assays
Antithrombin assay	Amidolytic/chromogenic assay using bovine thrombin or factor Xa as substrate	Not all molecular defects are detected equally by all functional assays	Immunological assay Genetic screening
Protein C assay	Amidolytic/chromogenic assay or Clotting assay	Clotting assay affected by FV mutations conferring APC resistance and other variables	If a clotting assay is used, it is important to follow up abnormal results with chromogenic assays and/or immunological assays to exclude a falsely reduced assay. Genetic screening may be performed
Protein S assay	Clotting assay or Free PS antigen	Clotting assay affected by FV mutations conferring APC resistance and other variables	Free PS antigen (if clotting assay used) Total PS antigen Genetic screening
APC resistance/ FV-Leiden screening	APC resistance test without FV-deficient plasma, or APC resistance test with FV-deficient plasma, or DNA screening	Test without FV-deficient plasma may detect APC resistance in the absence of FV mutations conferring APC resistance—not specific for FVL	DNA screening if either APC resistance test is abnormal
Prothrombin G20210A mutation screening	DNA screening	FII levels may be elevated, but overlap with reference range precludes screening with a factor assay	
Antiphospholipid syndrome screening	Solid-phase assays Prolongation of phospholipid-dependent coagulation tests (e.g. DRVVT)	Recommended guidelines exist for LA screening	Evidence of an inhibitor (mixing studies). Confirmation of the phospholipid-dependence (e.g. DRVVT with high-concentration phospholipid). Further tests should be considered if screen is negative
Homocysteine assay	FPIA, ELISA, HPLC, LIA		Some centres also screen for methylene tetrahydrofolate reductase (MTHFR) C677T mutation
Factor VIII assay, other assays	Routine factor assays	May be employed to try and help explain a thrombotic history; however, utility of this test in individual cases is debatable	

DISCUSSION QUESTIONS

15.1 Why could it be that having an inherited thrombophilia doesn't inevitably lead to the development of thrombotic disease?

15.2 What is the difference between type I and type II defects?

15.3 In the contexts of hereditary and acquired thrombophilia, what might be gained by measuring a particular analyte by more than one type of analytical method?

15.4 Why do we need so many screening and confirmatory tests to detect lupus anticoagulants?

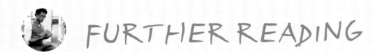 FURTHER READING

- **Greaves M, Cohen H, Machin SJ, Mackie I. Guidelines on the investigation and management of the antiphospholipid syndrome.** *British Journal of Haematology* 2000:**109**;704–15.

  Guidelines written by the Haemostasis Task Force of the British Committee for Standards in Haematology, with recommendations for lupus anticoagulant screening.

- **Hoffbrand AV, Catovsky D, Tuddenham EGD (ed.).** *Postgraduate Haematology*, **5th edn. Blackwell Publishing Ltd, Massachusetts–Oxford–Carlton, 2005.**

  Includes a chapter on arterial and venous thrombosis, thrombophilia testing and treatment options.

- **Lewis SM, Bain BJ, Bates I (ed.).** *Dacie and Lewis Practical Haematology*, **10th edn. Churchill Livingstone, Elsevier, 2006.**

  Includes a chapter on investigation of thrombophilia.

- **Moore GW, Savidge GF. The dilution effect of equal volume mixing studies compromises confirmation of inhibition by lupus anticoagulants even when mixture specific reference ranges are applied.** *Thrombosis Research* 2006:**118**;523–8.

- **Moore GW, Smith MP, Savidge GF. The ecarin time is an improved confirmatory test for the taipan snake venom time in warfarinised patients with lupus anticoagulants.** *Blood Coagulation and Fibrinolysis* 2003:**14**;307–12.

- **Pengo P, Tripodi A, Reber G, Rand JH, Ortel TL, Galli M, de Groot PG. Update of the guidelines for lupus anticoagulant detection.** *J Thromb Haemost* 2009: **7**: 1737–40.

- **Walker ID, Greaves M, Preston FE. Investigation and management of heritable thrombophilia.** *British Journal of Haematology* 2001:**114**;512–28.

  Guidelines written by the Haemostasis Task Force of the British Committee for Standards in Haematology, with recommendations for thrombophilia screening.

Answers to self-check questions, case study questions, and discussion questions are provided in the book's Online Resource Centre, visit www.oxfordtextbooks.co.uk/orc/moore

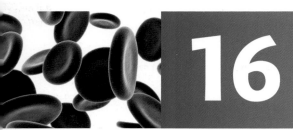

16

Haemostasis and anticoagulation

Gary W. Moore and Jane M. Needham

In this chapter you will encounter an outline for the reasons for anticoagulant therapy, mode of action and use of therapeutic agents, laboratory assays for monitoring treatment, and associated clinical services for patient care.

Learning objectives

After studying this chapter you should confidently be able to:

- Explain the reasons for anticoagulant therapy.
- Understand the mode of action of anticoagulants.
- Understand the importance of anticoagulant management and associated clinical risks.
- Know how to monitor anticoagulant therapy in the laboratory.
- Be aware of hereditary or acquired conditions that can influence treatment outcomes.
- Demonstrate awareness of interacting drugs.
- Demonstrate awareness of models of clinical services.

16.1 Reasons for anticoagulation therapy

In Chapter 15 you learnt about the defects and deficiencies that are associated with thrombophilia and can lead to an imbalance in the haemostatic mechanism regulating the activation or inhibition of the haemostatic process. This has the potential of establishing a **hypercoagulable state** which increases the risk of thrombosis. The formation of a thrombus results in a firm fibrin clot within veins or arteries. It is a serious condition occurring in approximately 1 in 1000 individuals per year in the United Kingdom and can be fatal.

The exact trigger for a venous thrombotic event is still unclear, but it has been established that certain individuals have a higher disposition to thrombosis. This risk is associated with the following:

- Having an inherited or acquired thrombophilia defect
- Medical conditions that can lead to thrombosis secondary to the primary condition
- Events or environment that lead to blood stasis, such as immobility

hypercoagulable state
An increased tendency towards blood clotting.

The aims of prescribing anticoagulant therapy are to:

1. Prevent the growth of an existing **thrombus** or **embolus** through the **vasculature**.
2. Prevent the recurrence of venous thrombotic events.
3. Prevent the occurrence of a thrombosis in 'high risk' medical conditions or during surgical procedures and periods of immobility.

Venous thromboembolism

Venous thromboembolism (VTE) is considered to be one disorder, which includes both deep vein thrombosis (DVT) and pulmonary embolism (PE). It is a common medical condition that can occur in individuals with a hereditary thrombotic defect, an associated high disposition to thrombosis, 'spontaneously' with no identified cause or risk factors, or secondary to other clinical conditions, particularly malignancy. VTE has a high rate of **morbidity** and **mortality** if not correctly diagnosed and treated.

The clinical event normally occurs with the formation of a blood clot in a deep vein within the leg, or very rarely in the arm. The exact sequence of events is still not fully understood. Although local venous **stasis** is necessary, this is not thought to be sufficient on its own to cause thrombosis. Increased turbulence of blood around the valves in veins may initiate DVT. It has been suggested that endothelial damage occurs with the migration of white cells through the vessel wall during stasis, causing platelet activation and subsequent thrombus formation; an alternative hypothesis is clot formation due to localized trapped activated clotting factors which are not exposed to the body's natural inhibitors. As there is no rupture to the vessel wall in the formation of a DVT to involve platelets, the composition of the thrombus is predominantly coagulation factors, particularly fibrin. The lower shear rates in the venous circulation compared to the arterial circulation can also contribute to the formation of venous thrombosis.

DVT below the knee is unlikely to cause acute complications. Presenting symptoms include pain and swelling of the calf due to blocked veins. However a clot formed above the knee has the increased risk of breaking away and forming a life-threatening PE within the lungs, usually resulting in shortness of breath and chest pain, and the need to seek urgent medical attention.

A long-term complication following a DVT, called '**post-thrombotic syndrome**', can occur due to tissue damage following diversion of blood into other veins to avoid the blockage. This presents with a range of symptoms including calf pain and swelling, with ulceration of the skin in severe cases.

SELF-CHECK 16.1

What are the key aims of anticoagulant therapy?

SELF-CHECK 16.2

Where does a blood clot usually initially form in VTE and where can it move to?

Diagnosis of VTE

The diagnosis of DVT or PE is not without difficulties; in the fairly recent past many patients were diagnosed on clinical symptoms alone. Advances in both laboratory assays and radiological investigations have seen the introduction of clinical assessment scores, which you can see in Tables 16.1(a) and (b), and use of D-dimer assays within a flow-chart algorithm as shown

---

thrombus
A blood clot that usually develops in a deep vein of your body, normally in the calf or higher up the leg in the thigh.

embolus
A blood clot or part of a blood clot that migrates through the bloodstream and then lodges in another vessel causing a blockage.

vasculature
The network of blood vessels through your body or organs.

morbidity
High rate of sickness and medical complications compared to the normal population.

mortality
Increased risk of death compared to the normal population.

stasis
A condition in which the normal flow of blood through a vein is slowed or halted.

TABLE 16.1(a) Wells' DVT pre-test probability (PTP) score.

Clinical assessment	Score
Active malignancy (treatment is ongoing, within previous 6 months, or palliative)	1
Paralysis, recent immobility	1
Recently confined to bed >3 days	1
Major surgery within previous 12 weeks	1
Entire leg swollen	1
Swollen calf	1
Pitting oedema (fluid retention) in symptomatic leg	1
Collateral superficial veins (small veins that have grown around a blockage)	1
Previous DVT	1
Alternative diagnosis to DVT as likely or more likely	−2

PTP score <2   **DVT unlikely**; if D-dimers normal, DVT is excluded, if they are elevated, medical imaging is performed.

PTP score ≥ 2   **DVT likely**; perform D-dimers and medical imaging.

TABLE 16.1(b) Wells' PE pre-test probability score.

Clinical assessment	Score
Clinical signs and symptoms of DVT	3.0
Alternative diagnosis of PE is less likely	3.0
Heart rate >100 beats/min	1.5
Immobilization in previous 4 weeks	1.5
Surgery in previous 4 weeks	1.5
Previous DVT/PE	1.5
Active malignancy (treatment is ongoing, within previous 6 months or palliative)	1.0
Haemoptysis (coughing up blood/blood-stained sputum from the lungs)	1.0

PTP score <2.0   low probability of PE
PTP score 2.0–6.0   moderate probability of PE
PTP score >6.0   high probability of PE
Use PTP score to follow the algorithm in Figure 16.1.

Cross reference

You saw in Chapter 13 that D-dimers are cross-linked D fragments that are breakdown products of fibrin. Elevated levels can indicate the presence of a thrombus.

in Figure 16.1. The clinical assessment score, or **Wells' score**, assigns a numerical value to the presence of specific signs and symptoms. The higher the total score, the more likely that a DVT or PE is present, and hence informed decisions can be made about the initiation of diagnostic procedures. If used correctly, this initial assessment reduces the frequency of having to perform invasive procedures (which can have clinical complications), and streamlines and improves diagnosis.

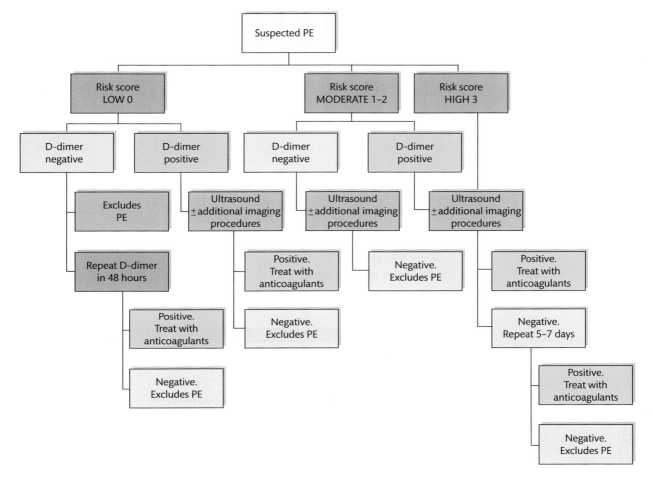

FIGURE 16.1

Example of use of D-dimer within a diagnostic algorithm for suspected PE. The flowchart maps the clinical steps to diagnosis, and treatment with anticoagulant therapy, from initial symptoms, D-dimer result, and medical imaging procedures.

The assays are very sensitive to the presence of D-dimers, but an elevated result is not specific for VTE because D-dimer can be raised in a number of other clinical situations, i.e. post surgery, malignancy, renal failure. Therefore, it is applied as a **negative predictive index** of DVT and clinicians will rarely initiate imaging tests if there is a normal D-dimer level in conjunction with a low clinical probability score. Radiological investigation including **venography** and **compression ultrasonography** is normally performed if D-dimers are elevated and/or there is a raised probability score for suspected DVT. A venograph of a blood clot occluding a leg vein is shown in Figure 16.2.

Patients with a suspected PE normally have a chest X-ray in conjunction with D-dimer and probability scoring, followed by **pulmonary angiography** and **ventilated–perfusion (V/Q)** lung scanning as appropriate.

Normal levels of D-dimers mean it is highly unlikely that a fibrin clot is present. However, fibrinolysis of a small thrombus may not generate sufficient breakdown products to elevate D-dimers above the reference range. A clot that has been *in situ* for more than 10 days may reach a physiological equilibrium, whereby D-dimers that were initially elevated fall back into the reference range.

negative predictive index
The probability that a patient with a normal D-dimer level does not have a DVT or PE.

venography
A radiology procedure where a contrasting agent is injected into the vein to enable a blockage to be visualized on the X-ray.

compression ultrasonography
Used for examining soft tissue; provides real-time images in conjunction with venous compression to diagnose DVT.

pulmonary angiography
Performed to assess blood circulation to the lungs by adding a contrast dye through a catheter into a vein and taking X-rays of the lung.

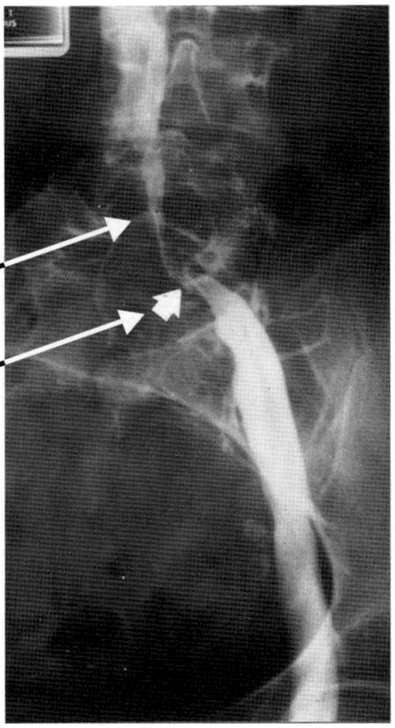

FIGURE 16.2

Example of venograph identifying the presence of a DVT and restricted venous blood flow in the leg. If ultrasound using sound waves to evaluate blood flow in the veins is inconclusive then venography is performed whereby a dye is injected into a vein in the foot; it then travels the length of the suspect vein to make it visible by X-ray, thus allowing any decrease in blood flow or blockage to be visualized. Reproduced by permission from C. Zollikofer & F. Laerum, 2005, *Chapter 20 The Peripheral vessels* in *The NICER Centennial Book 1995—A Global Textbook of Radiology.*

Restricted
blood
flow

DVT

---

ventilated–perfusion (V/Q) scan

A procedure using small amounts of inhaled or injected radioisotopes to measure the flow of blood and air in the lungs. Images taken capture the flow patterns.

stroke

Occurs when the brain's supply of oxygen is cut off by a blockage or interruption to the blood flow, which causes severe neurological damage.

electrocardiography

Procedure for measuring electrical changes in the heart which take place with each beat.

sinus rhythm

A natural heart (cardiac) rhythm generated through the sinus node (normal rate 60–100 beats/min).

cardioversion

Procedure where the heart is stopped, then an electrical current is applied to shock it into restarting with a normal sinus rhythm.

SELF-CHECK 16.3

How is D-dimer testing used to establish a diagnosis of DVT or PE?

Prevention and thromboprophylaxis

Anticoagulant therapy can also be used in certain clinical settings or medical conditions to try and reduce the chance of a thrombotic event occurring and the subsequent risks and complications.

Atrial fibrillation

Atrial fibrillation (AF) is a heart condition where the electrical activity to the atria is disorganized. You can see in Figure 16.3 that AF is characterized by rapid irregular atrial impulses and ineffective atrial contractions. Stasis of blood in the left atrium contributes to the risk of **stroke** and VTE.

A diagnosis of AF is confirmed by **electrocardiography**.

A number of clinical studies have confirmed the benefits of long-term oral anticoagulant therapy (i.e. warfarin) in these patients, unless they are returned to normal **sinus rhythm** with **cardioversion** intervention.

BOX 16.1 *D-dimer assays*

Measuring D-dimer levels for VTE diagnosis is a common request for a routine haemostasis laboratory. The most commonly used assay type is latex-immunoassay (LIA), the principle of which you met in Chapter 2. Other assay types such as ELISA and whole blood agglutination methods are also used.

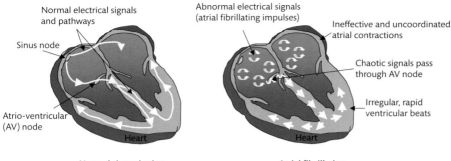

FIGURE 16.3

Atrial fibrillation (AF): identifying area of erratic impulses affecting the normal sinus rhythm within the heart. AF is a heart condition where the electrical activity to the atria is disorganized and is characterized by rapid irregular atrial impulses and ineffective atrial contractions. Stasis of blood (lack of movement) in the left atrium contributes to the risk of stroke and VTE.

Thromboprophylaxis

Thromboprophylaxis in the form of anticoagulant therapy to reduce the risk of VTE is now actively prescribed for short-term use in medical or surgical interventions, conditions where research has demonstrated there is an increased risk of thrombosis, or in patients with a previous history of VTE. A risk assessment is performed to ensure the benefits of **prophylaxis** to select the appropriate therapy in individual patients. There is now a national programme aimed at reducing the incidence of hospital-acquired VTE.

Arterial thrombosis

Whereas in VTE the predominant component of the thrombus is coagulation factors, in arterial thrombosis the predominant component is platelets. The main event leading to arterial thrombosis is the rupture of an **atherosclerotic plaque**, which occurs in conditions such as **hypertension** and **atherosclerosis**. This results in the rapid adherence of circulating platelets to the exposed collagen via von Willebrand factor and specific platelet surface receptors, which you met in Chapter 13. Following activation, subsequent aggregation is triggered by the generation of **thromboxane A₂** by platelets. This process is normally controlled by **prostacyclin** found in the vascular endothelium, which inhibits platelet aggregation. The differences in the composition of arterial and venous clots are illustrated in Figure 16.4.

SELF-CHECK 16.4

How do the composition and formation of a venous and an arterial thrombus differ?

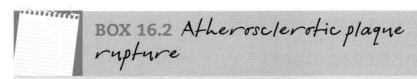

BOX 16.2 *Atherosclerotic plaque rupture*

This leads to thrombus formation, which rapidly slows or arrests blood flow leading to death of the tissues fed by the artery, an event referred to as an **infarction**. When this happens in a coronary artery it is termed a myocardial infarction, otherwise known as a heart attack, and is the most common cause of death in the developed world.

prophylaxis
Procedure to prevent a condition occurring rather than to treat or cure it after it has occurred.

atherosclerotic plaque
Deposit of cholesterol and other fatty material that builds up within the vessel wall, normally an artery.

hypertension
A sustained increase in systolic and/or diastolic blood pressure.

atherosclerosis
Narrowing and hardening of the arteries over time. Associated with age but also other risk factors, e.g. hypertension, high cholesterol.

thromboxane A₂
A potent inducer of platelet aggregation generated through the arachidonic acid pathway within the platelet.

prostacyclin
A potent inhibitor of platelet aggregation generated through the arachidonic acid pathway within the vessel wall.

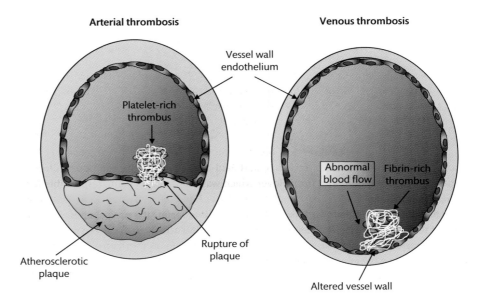

FIGURE 16.4

Differences in clot composition between arterial and venous clots. Arterial thrombosis results from the rupture of an atherosclerotic plaque after a build up of cholesterol under the arterial wall and thrombus formation with a high platelet composition. Venous thrombosis can result from stasis of the blood or imbalance in levels of pro-coagulant clotting factors and their natural inhibitors, which causes damage to the surface of the vessel wall and subsequent thrombus formation with a high fibrin concentration.

16.2 Current therapeutic anticoagulant pharmaceuticals for VTE

Pharmaceutical intervention, in the form of anticoagulant therapy, is the mainstay in the treatment of established venous thromboembolism (VTE) or as prophylactic treatment in conditions with a high risk of thrombosis, such as AF. These agents inhibit or reduce the normal function of coagulation proteins. Heparin and heparin derivatives are delivered by injection, either **intravenously** or **subcutaneously**, whilst coumarins, e.g. warfarin and phenindione, are currently the only available oral preparations for long-term prescribing. Major drug developments to provide improved alternatives are ongoing.

Anticoagulant therapy regimes for VTE have little benefit for the prevention of arterial thrombosis because of its significant platelet component. Until recently, therapy has been limited to aspirin, which inhibits the platelet generation of thromboxane A_2, but recently a new generation of antiplatelet drugs have become available.

Oral anticoagulants

All oral anticoagulants currently prescribed generate their therapeutic effect by antagonizing the action of vitamin K. By doing so they inhibit the production of functional vitamin K-dependent clotting factors II, VII, IX, and X, the naturally occurring inhibitor protein C and its cofactor protein S, and protein Z. Although patients on oral anticoagulation continue to manufacture the vitamin K-dependent factors, they have impaired function and are referred

intravenous

Administration of a drug in liquid form into the body by injection through a vein.

subcutaneous

Administration of a drug in liquid form into the body by injection to just under the skin.

BOX 16.3 *A brief history of warfarin*

The basis of warfarin anticoagulant therapy goes back to the winter of 1921 when an epidemic of haemorrhagic disease devastated herds of cattle in Canada. It was found that this problem only occurred when cattle were fed on sweet clover, a new fodder crop. In 1924 the vet Schofield made the observation that the toxic effect was only associated with spoiled sweet clover. Following a further outbreak in Wisconsin in the 1930s, unclotted cattle blood and spoiled sweet clover were sent to the local university for analysis. After many years of research, Karl Paul Link extracted the compound dicoumarol (4-hydroxycoumarin) from clover which was identified as being responsible for the clotting defect. Damp storage of sweet clover had led to its spoiling by bacterial action which caused the oxidation of **coumarin**, (the compound that gives freshly cut hay its sweet smell), to dicoumarol. Stahmann, a graduate student, went on to develop a large-scale isolation of dicoumarol. Dicoumarol was first used as an anticoagulant in humans by Butt in 1941, although not with widespread use because of toxicity fears. Link continued to investigate coumarin compounds in a search for an anticoagulant with improved pharmacological properties. Amongst over 150 compounds synthesized was 3-(α-acetonyl-benzyl)-4-hydroxycoumarin, which proved to be well suited for clinical use. As the research was funded by the Wisconsin Alumni Research Foundation (WARF) the compound was named warfarin by combining the organization's acronym with the last four letters of coumarin. It was originally marketed as a rodenticide, for which it is still used. Warfarin was approved for human use in 1954 and, since the 1960s, has become the main therapeutic agent for the prevention of thromboembolic disease.

to as 'proteins induced by vitamin K absence/antagonism' (PIVKA). Oral anticoagulants need to be carefully monitored using the INR system to ensure their clinical effectiveness and safety. The most commonly used oral anticoagulant is **warfarin**.

For the majority of conditions, patients receive a warfarin dose that aims to maintain their INR within a therapeutic range of 2.0–3.0, which significantly reduces their thrombotic risk. Those with a higher risk of thrombosis are maintained within a therapeutic range of 3.0–4.0.

There are three widely used oral anticoagulant drugs—warfarin, acenocoumarin, and phenoprocoumarin—which are all derivatives of 4-hydroxy coumarin. Warfarin contains one asymmetrical carbon atom and exists in two **enantiomeric** forms (R and S), with chemical synthesis resulting in a **racemic mixture**. Warfarin is readily absorbed from the gastrointestinal tract, with over 90% bound to serum albumin. R-warfarin has a half-life of about 37–89 hours and S-warfarin 21–43 hours, although S-warfarin has two to five times more anticoagulant activity than R-warfarin. Warfarin is removed from the system by oxidation in the liver and the metabolites excreted in the urine.

Vitamin K is essential for the formation of biologically active vitamin K-dependent clotting factors. These clotting factors are initially non-functional when first synthesized by hepatocytes

Cross references

You will meet INR system in the section below covering laboratory assays.

The clinical management of patients on oral anticoagulant therapy is covered in the final section of this chapter.

enantiomeric

Two stereoisomers that are complete mirror images of each other.

racemic mixture

Equal amounts of two stereoisomers of an optically active substance which does not rotate plane-polarized light.

BOX 16.4 *The first warfarinized VIP*

An early recipient of warfarin was US President Dwight D. Eisenhower who was prescribed the drug after experiencing a heart attack in 1955.

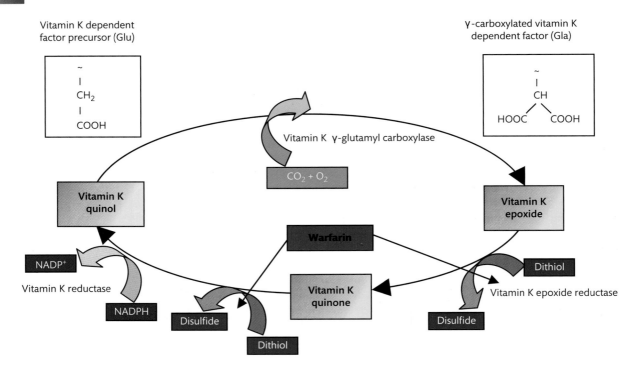

FIGURE 16.5

Coumarin-based drugs and the vitamin K cycle. Coumarins inhibit the action of the vitamin K epoxide reductase enzyme, which results in decreased concentrations of vitamin K and vitamin K hydroquinone. This leads to inefficient carboxylation of vitamin K-dependent factors by the glutamyl carboxylase enzyme.

VKDF, vitamin K-dependent factor.

in the liver. Vitamin K is an essential coenzyme for the post-translational carboxylation of these factors. The glutamyl residues of these proteins are converted by the liver enzyme carboxylase to gamma-carboxyglutamyl residues and comprise the Gla domain, which in the presence of calcium ions are essential for anchoring with the negatively charged phospholipids on cellular membranes.

The concentration of vitamin K-dependent clotting factors is determined by a dynamic equilibrium between synthesis and degradation. Although the rate of synthesis is independent of plasma concentration, the rate of degradation is proportional to the plasma concentration and is influenced by the half-life of the respective clotting factors. The effect of warfarin is to reduce the rate of synthesis of functioning vitamin K-dependent clotting factors, which results in the establishment of a new equilibrium within the plasma. The concentration of coagulation factors will be reduced to the same extent as the rate of synthesis.

The human body has a limited ability to store vitamin K so it is recycled by the liver thousands-fold before it is catabolized into inactive degradation products. This recycling process occurs by the reduction of vitamin K to its hydroquinone form KH_2, followed by oxidation to vitamin K epoxide, KO. This reaction is coupled to the carboxylation of glutamate residues to give gamma-carboxyglutamate and the enzymatic reduction of epoxide with NADH as cofactor, regenerating vitamin K to the KH_2 form. Figure 16.5 shows you that warfarin blocks this reaction by competitively inhibiting the enzyme epoxide reductase and hence preventing the reduction of vitamin K epoxide.

Cross references

You met Gla domains and their function in Chapter 13.

You can find the half-life values of vitamin K-dependent clotting factors in Table 13.3 of Chapter 13.

Drugs

Acenocoumarin

Acenocoumarin has the same anticoagulant properties as warfarin. The difference between the two medications relates to the activity of the R- and S-enantiomer forms of acenocoumarin. Unlike warfarin, it is the R-enantiomer which has the greater anticoagulant activity.

Phenprocoumarin

Phenprocoumarin also has the same anticoagulant properties as warfarin; it is in more wide-spread use in mainland Europe. Phenprocoumarin has a long half-life, 144 hours compared to warfarin's 40 hours. Its clearance from the body is not so dependent on the cytochrome P450 system and there is significant excretion of unchanged drug in urine.

Phenindione

Phenindione, in the form of dindevan, was once the most commonly prescribed oral anticoagulant; its anticoagulant mode of action is identical to coumarin's. It has largely been replaced by warfarin due to its severe side-effects (including pink urine), and now tends to be used as an alternative therapy in the rare cases of patients experiencing adverse reactions to warfarin, such as skin irritation.

Risks of oral anticoagulant therapy

There are two main and potentially life-threatening risks of prescribing oral anticoagulant therapy.

The first is bleeding, which can occur even if treatment is within the therapeutic range. The anticoagulant effect of warfarin or phenindione can be effectively reversed with oral or intravenous vitamin K. The dose needs to reflect the level of the INR and the severity of bleeding. In cases of life-threatening bleeding immediate reversal of the anticoagulant effect may be achieved with a specific clotting factor concentrate containing factors II, VII, and X, or, if unavailable, **fresh-frozen plasma**.

Key Points

It is crucial to remember at all times that anticoagulant therapy is a balance between hyper- and hypocoagulability. An overdose of anticoagulant can precipitate potentially dangerous bleeding symptoms. Underdosing can allow the thrombotic risk factor(s) to precipitate the thrombotic event that the anticoagulation was prescribed to prevent.

---

fresh-frozen plasma
Whole blood contains cells and fluid. The fluid component, plasma, contains all the plasma proteins including coagulation factors. It is prepared at the time of donation when the unit of blood is centrifuged after collection to separate the plasma from the cells. The plasma is removed under sterile conditions and stored frozen to preserve the activity of the coagulation factors. When required it is thawed and transfused through a vein.

The second potential complication is warfarin-induced skin necrosis, which although rare is a very serious complication of therapy. The incidence is higher in patients with a thrombophilia defect, particularly protein C deficiency. It usually presents during the first 3–5 days of initiation of therapy, where levels of functional vitamin K clotting factors are falling, but this also includes the vitamin K-dependent naturally occurring inhibitors, namely proteins C, S, and Z. Because protein C has a short half-life compared to most other vitamin K-dependent factors its level falls sooner, generating a relative protein C deficiency in the early stages of treatment. This can result in the formation of microthrombi in the skin, leading to reduced oxygen supply to surrounding tissue and ultimately cell death.

TABLE 16.2 **Features of new anticoagulants compared to warfarin.**

Key features	Warfarin	Dabigatran	Rivaroxaban
Site of effect	VKOR	Factor IIa	Factor Xa
Oral	Yes	Yes	Yes
Immediate anticoagulant effect	No	Yes	Yes
Monitoring	Yes	No	No
Dosing	Variable	Fixed dose (× 2 daily)	Fixed dose (× 1 daily)
Use in pregnancy	No	No	No
Antidote	Yes	No	No

SELF-CHECK 16.5

Explain the anticoagulant effect of warfarin.

Oral anticoagulants: future developments

Developing an alternative oral anticoagulant to warfarin that requires minimal monitoring and fewer risks is a major area of pharmaceutical research. In recent years some new oral medications have been introduced. Their characteristics compared to warfarin are outlined in Table 16.2. Currently, they are limited to short-term use in patients undergoing elective surgery for knee or hip replacement in order to cover the increased thrombotic risk over the postoperative period. Clinical trials are underway for these and other new anticoagulants, to assess their safety and efficacy for long-term therapeutic use. Their sites of action in coagulation biochemistry are shown in Figure 16.6.

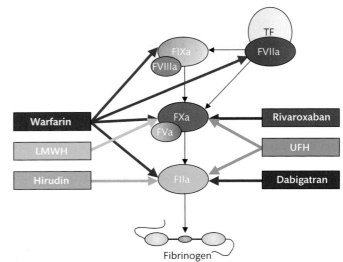

FIGURE 16.6

Summary of areas of coagulation affected by current and newly developed anticoagulant drugs. Warfarin affects the production of vitamin K-dependent factors and thus has an effect at various stages of coagulation biochemistry. UFH predominantly affects factors IIa and Xa, whereas LMWHs predominantly affect factor Xa. Rivaroxaban inhibits FXa, whilst hirudin and dabigatran are direct thrombin inhibitors.

Parenteral anticoagulants

Heparin–mode of action

The anticoagulant properties of heparin were identified in 1916 by a USA medical student, J. McLean, who was investigating coagulation activation by phosphatides. He discovered that a preparation from liver prolonged the clotting time of plasma; it was subsequently found to be heparin. The chemical structure of this naturally occurring **glycosaminoglycan** was determined by a Swedish chemist, J. Erik Jorpes, in 1936. Following purification, the first use in humans was in 1937 when a heparin–saline solution was injected into the brachial artery, resulting in prolongation of clotting time and no detrimental side-effects. Now heparin, one of the oldest drugs, and its derivatives, are some of the most widely used anticoagulants in clinical practice. However, it is only suitable for short-term use as it is associated with **osteoporosis**—it decreases the bone-forming cells, osteoblasts, and increases the activity of osteoclasts which reabsorb bone. Heparin is essential in suspected cases of VTE to prevent thrombus extension through the vasculature, as demonstrated in the first clinical trial during the 1960s.

Unfractionated heparin

Unfractionated heparin (UFH) is a heterogeneous mixture of negatively charged sulphated glycosaminoglycans. It is composed of alternating uronic and glucuronic acid resides with polysaccharide chains, ranging in molecular weight from 3000 to 30 000. Heparin is isolated from porcine intestinal mucosa or bovine lung for manufacture into a therapeutic agent. The structure of a heparin subunit is shown in Figure 16.7.

The anticoagulant activity of heparin is contained in just one-third of the molecule, and consists of a pentasaccharide sequence with high-affinity binding properties to antithrombin, the major serpin found in plasma. Heparin brings about a conformational change in antithrombin which significantly enhances its inhibition of factors IIa (thrombin), IXa, and Xa. Heparin inhibition is most effective against thrombin. You can see in Figure 16.8 that heparin forms a template to which antithrombin and thrombin bind thus generating a **ternary complex**.

Therapeutic use

The clinical advantage of heparin is that the anticoagulant effect is seen immediately because it is administered intravenously and binds straight away to antithrombin. Intravenous administration means that UFH is only suitable for use within a hospital setting. Dosage depends on the level of anticoagulant effect required and is calculated based on the individual's weight. It can be prescribed either as an 8-hourly injection to provide intermittent cover, or as a continuous infusion. The plasma half-life is about 100 minutes, with little anticoagulant effect seen after six hours. Heparin is partly excreted in the urine or destroyed in the liver.

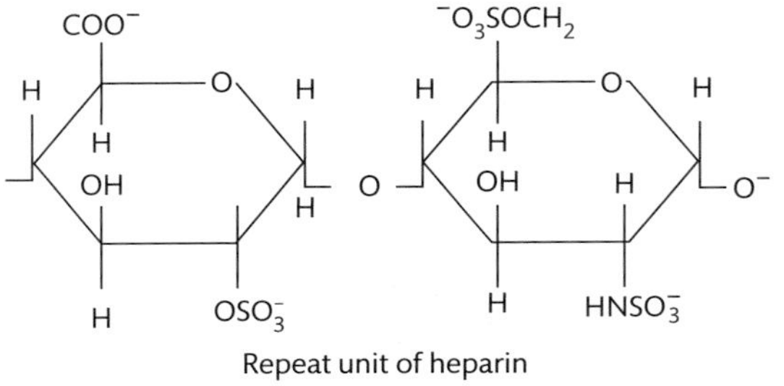

parenteral
Not given orally through the alimentary canal, but administered by injection.

glycosaminoglycan
Group of high molecular weight polysaccharides that includes chondroitin sulfates, dermatan sulfates, heparan sulfate and heparin.

osteoporosis
A skeletal disease that leads to loss of bone mass and structure resulting in an increased risk of fractures.

ternary complex
A complex containing three different molecules.

COO⁻   ⁻O₃SOCH₂

Repeat unit of heparin

FIGURE 16.7

Single unit of unfractionated heparin. Heparin is a mucopolysaccharide structured with alternate units of sulphated glucosamine and glucuronic acid. It is a strongly negatively charged molecule, which facilitates its binding to and inactivation of the positively charged coagulation factors, predominantly IIa and Xa. Reproduced by permission from Quader, Stump & Sumpio, Low molecular weight heparins: current use and indications, *Journal of the American College of Surgeons*, 1998.

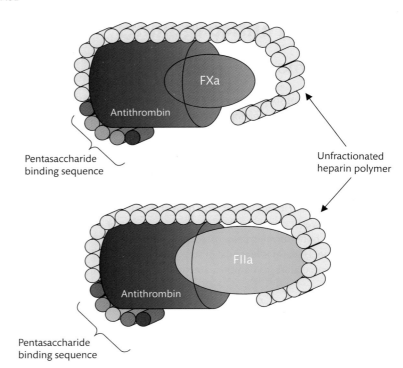

FIGURE 16.8

Illustration of unfractionated heparin (UFH) binding to antithrombin and thrombin or FXa in a template-complex formation. UFH promotes anticoagulant activity by binding to antithrombin and enhancing its major inhibitory effect on factors IIa and Xa. The binding of UFH to antithrombin is through a unique pentasaccharide molecule randomly distributed in the heparin molecule. Binding of the AT–UFH complex to FXa causes a conformational change resulting in the inactivation of FXa. With thrombin binding, however, UFH has to simultaneously bind to AT and thrombin, which requires a longer chain of heparin (saccharide units).

bioavailability

The degree to which a drug or other substance is absorbed or becomes available where it is required physiologically and can act on its target.

therapeutic range

A concentration range within which a drug is clinically effective whilst minimizing risk factors and side-effects.

Monitoring of UFH is essential to ensure clinical effectiveness whilst minimizing the risk of over- or under-anticoagulation, potentially resulting in bleeding or further thrombosis respectively. In the case of UFH this is determined by achieving a defined anticoagulant effect *in vitro*, as assessed by prolonging the normal clotting time of the activated partial thrombo-plastin time (APTT), although there is considerable *in vivo* variation between individuals to the same dosage. This is mainly due to differences in **bioavailability** (about 50%) as heparin also binds to endothelium, macrophages, and plasma proteins including platelet factor 4 (PF4), fibrinogen, factor VIII, and histidine-rich glycoprotein. It is therefore not possible to administer a fixed dose because individual responses to UFH are unpredictable. There is also considerable *in-vitro* variation in APTT reagent sensitivity to heparin; therefore the lower and upper limit of clotting times that identifies effective and safe anticoagulant therapy, termed a **therapeutic range**, needs to be locally established. You can see in Table 16.3 that therapeutic ranges are reagent and analyser combination-specific.

TABLE 16.3 Examples of APTT reagent-dependent therapeutic ranges for UFH monitoring based on *in-vivo* anti-Xa chromogenic heparin assays.

Reagent + analyser	Therapeutic range APTT ratio
General guidelines	1.5–2.5
Heparin level by anti-Xa assay	0.3–0.7 u/mL
Reagent A + analyser 1	2.5–4.0
Reagent B + analyser 2	2.0–3.0
Reagent C + analyser 1	1.5–3.5
Reagent D + analyser 3	1.8–4.1

Risks of heparin therapy

There are two main and potentially life-threatening risks of prescribing heparin anticoagulant therapy.

The first is bleeding, which can occur even if treatment is within the therapeutic range. It is, of course, more likely if the patient becomes over-anticoagulated. The anticoagulant effect of unfractionated heparin can be effectively reversed with protamine sulphate, a protein which is strongly basic and neutralizes acidic heparin.

The second is **heparin-induced thrombocytopenia** (HIT). When platelets are activated they release platelet factor 4 (PF4), some of which binds to the platelet surface. Due to opposite charges, heparin will bind to PF4 on the platelet surface, exposing **neoepitopes** which are immunogenic and lead to antibody production as depicted in Figure 16.9. Thrombocytopenia is due to the removal of antibody-coated platelets via the **reticuloendothelial system**.

neoepitope

An epitope is a localized area of a molecule that is recognized by an antibody; a neoepitope is a structure that is recognizable by an antibody which is only exposed upon formation of a complex.

reticuloendothelial system

The phagocytic system of the body involved in the removal of foreign matter.

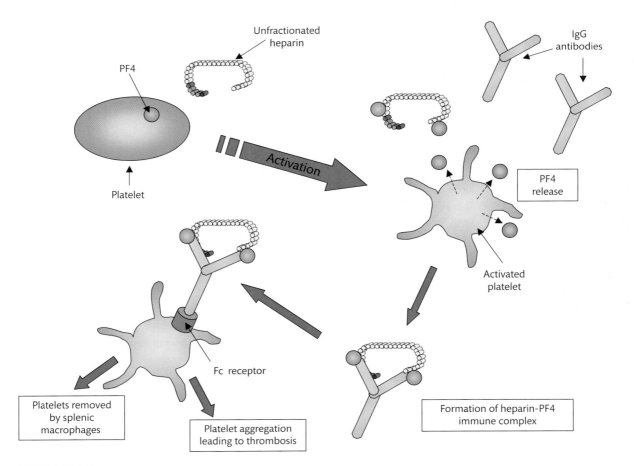

FIGURE 16.9

Pathophysiology of type II heparin-induced thrombocytopenia. Platelets release platelet factor 4 (PF4) and heparin binds to it, resulting in a PF4–heparin complex. IgG antibodies bind to this complex forming a PF4–heparin–IgG immune complex which then binds to Fc receptors on the platelet surface inducing platelet activation. This releases more PF4, thus feeding the cycle and resulting in microthrombi and thrombocytopenia.

HIT can occur in two forms:

- Type I is benign and is associated with an early (within 4 days), usually mild decrease in the platelet count, which rarely falls below 100×10^9/L. The platelet count quickly returns to normal after stopping heparin, and will often do so even if heparin treatment continues. It occurs as a result of the mild direct activation of platelets by heparin and is not immune-mediated. Type I HIT is associated with no major clinical complications and occurs primarily in the setting of high-dose intravenous UFH.

- Type II is caused by an immune response to the heparin and PF4 complex, and is associated with thrombosis. It is reported to occur in 1–5% of patients on UFH, usually between days 5 and 10 of therapy, and treatment needs to be stopped and anticoagulant therapy changed to a **direct thrombin inhibitor** (DTI), e.g. Lepirudin (see p. 582). If the patient has previously been treated with heparin the thrombocytopenia can occur immediately the drug is administered.

Interestingly, bleeding is rarely a problem but thrombosis can be life-threatening. The immune complexes of PF4–heparin bound to antibody bind to Fc receptors on platelets and endothelial cells. This activates the platelets which release more PF4 and form platelet aggregates, further reducing the platelet count. Pro-coagulant platelet microparticles are also formed. Excess PF4 that has not bound to heparin binds to endothelial heparan sulphate which can also generate antibody formation and subsequent endothelial damage by immune complexes. Damaged endothelium can lead to thrombus formation or disseminated intravascular coagulation.

Type II HIT is more common in surgical than medical patients, varies with the dose of heparin, and is more common with bovine- than porcine-derived heparin.

Cross references

You will meet direct thrombin inhibitors later in this section.

Assays for detecting HIT antibodies are covered in Section 16.4 (Laboratory methods).

Low molecular weight heparin

Low molecular weight heparins (LMWHs) are commercially produced from unfractionated heparin by a process of chemical or enzymatic depolymerization, resulting in a heparin with a lower molecular weight than unfractionated heparin. This process produces LMWHs that retain the unique pentasaccharide sequence for specific binding to antithrombin and effective anti-Xa activity, but with reduced ability to inhibit thrombin. You can see in Figure 16.10 that

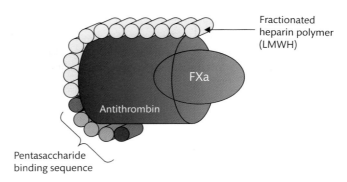

FIGURE 16.10

Illustration of low molecular weight heparin (LMWH) binding to antithrombin and factor Xa in a template-complex formation. LMWHs are fragments of UFH derived from depolymerization processes and are about one-third the size of the original molecule. The LMWH binds to AT through a unique pentasaccharide binding sequence, enhancing the inhibitory activity of AT. However, as LMWH is a much shorter molecule it exerts its anticoagulant effect predominantly on FXa.

FXa inhibition by LMWH does not require a template mechanism, unlike thrombin, IXa, and XIa, which need both enzyme and antithrombin bound to the same heparin chain.

Due to the reduction in their molecular weight, LMWHs have:

- Reduced affinity for other proteins, thereby improving bioavailability
- A longer half-life
- A more predictable anticoagulant response to standard treatment doses
- Reduced side-effects relating to bleeding, osteoporosis, or HIT

LMWH is not readily neutralized by PF4 and has reduced binding to endothelial cells which increases the half-life to about 4 hours and has a bioavailability of 90–100%. Therefore, LMWH can be administered as a single subcutaneous daily injection. LMWH also interacts less with platelets which decreases the risk of HIT. Although a number of manufacturers produce a range of LMWH preparations (albeit with variations in properties), with a few exceptions, they are considered clinically identical.

Due to the predictable bioavailability of LMWH only a few high-risk clinical situations require laboratory monitoring. In most patients, dosage is based on bodyweight and the intensity of anticoagulant effect required. However, due to the targeting of FXa by LMWHs, traditional APTT and thrombin times are relatively insensitive and, therefore, specific anti-Xa assays need to be performed to estimate anticoagulant levels. With the significant benefits outlined, LMWH is now used in the majority of clinical situations requiring immediate short-term anticoagulation. There are, however, some situations where UFH is preferable to LMWH:

- Renal failure where the drug can accumulate
- Patients with replacement heart valves (LMWH is not licensed for use in this group)
- Situations where rapid reversal may be required, such as emergency obstetric or invasive procedures

Cross reference

You will meet the anti-Xa assay for LMWH monitoring in Section 16.4 below, covering laboratory methods.

Risks of LMWH therapy

A number of clinical trials have demonstrated a reduced risk of bleeding with LMWH compared to UFH, particularly when used in conjunction with oral anticoagulants. However, as LMWH is cleared predominantly by the kidneys, it has to be carefully assessed for use in patients with renal failure, in whom it can accumulate in the circulation. If required, LMWH can be reversed with **protamine sulphate**, although not as effectively as UFH, and only about 60% is inactivated.

SELF-CHECK 16.6

What are the therapeutic differences between unfractionated heparin and LMWH?

Direct thrombin inhibitors

The most potent natural thrombin inhibitor is **hirudin**, which is extracted from leeches (*Hirudo medicinalis*) and was the first anticoagulant used in humans, in 1905. Hirudins for therapeutic use are now produced by **recombinant technology** using yeast and administered parenterally, normally by intravenous injection. Although differing slightly in structure from natural hirudin, recombinant (r)-hirudin is still highly specific for thrombin.

recombinant technology
Artificial production of a molecule produced by inserting foreign DNA into a host DNA which will manufacture the product.

Cross reference
You will meet assays for monitoring DTIs in Section 16.4 below covering laboratory assays.

FIGURE 16.11

Illustration of a hirudin-direct thrombin inhibitor (DTI) binding to thrombin. DTIs can directly block the active site of thrombin, or the substrate binding site, i.e. fibrinogen/fibrin or both, without the need for a cofactor, e.g. antithrombin. This enables the inactivation of both soluble and fibrin-bound thrombin, which potentially offers benefits over other anticoagulants.

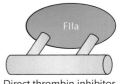

Direct thrombin inhibitor

You can see in Figure 16.11 that, unlike UFH and LMWH, hirudin inhibits thrombin directly in a 1 : 1 irreversible complex independent of any cofactor. Hirudin is also referred to as bivalent as it can bind to thrombin at more than one site. Also, unique to DTIs, they can inhibit thrombin that is free, clot-bound, or bound to fibrin degradation products, but have minimal interaction with plasma proteins. This provides a more predictable anticoagulant response to a given dosage, with a bioavailability of nearly 100% via subcutaneous administration. Therefore it is not considered clinically necessary to regularly monitor therapy, although laboratory assays exist that will detect the effects of DTIs if required.

Currently, three hirudin-based DTIs are available:

- **Lepirudin**, which binds to thrombin irreversibly and is cleared by the kidneys.
- **Bivalirudin**, which binds reversibly to thrombin and is eliminated predominantly by proteolysis, not involving the liver or kidneys.
- **Argatroban**, which binds reversibly to thrombin and is cleared by the liver.

Following clinical trials, hirudins are currently clinically approved for two indications: anticoagulation in patients diagnosed with HIT complicated by thrombosis, and thromboprophylaxis after major orthopaedic surgery.

Risk factors

Pharmacokinetics of most hirudin-based anticoagulants are very dependent on renal function, which makes predicting dosage in the elderly and critically ill patients difficult. Renal impairment is also associated with an increased risk of bleeding. Unlike other anticoagulants there is no specific antidote to DTIs. In patients with minor bleeding, merely stopping therapy is usually effective because DTIs have a short half-life (approximately 2 hours). In cases of major bleeding, haemodialysis or haemofiltration are the only viable methods of reducing the concentration of the circulating anticoagulant.

16.3 Current therapeutic anticoagulant pharmaceuticals for arterial thrombosis

cardiac
Relating to the function of the heart and associated medical conditions.

vascular
Relating to the network of blood vessels in the body, namely arteries, veins, and capillaries and associated medical conditions.

Pharmaceutical intervention for the prevention of arterial thrombosis is currently focused on inhibiting platelet aggregation. These drugs are now increasingly being prescribed in clinical practice for a wide range of **cardiac** and **vascular** conditions.

- Aspirin binds to cyclooxygenase and inhibits the arachidonic acid pathway, thereby preventing the generation of the platelet agonist thromboxane A_2, which you can see illustrated in Figure 16.12. Risks associated with aspirin include intestinal bleeding and the recently identified phenomenon of aspirin resistance (see below).
- Dipyridamole enhances activity of the platelet function inhibitor prostacyclin and inhibits phosphodiesterase enzymes which regulate platelet signalling.

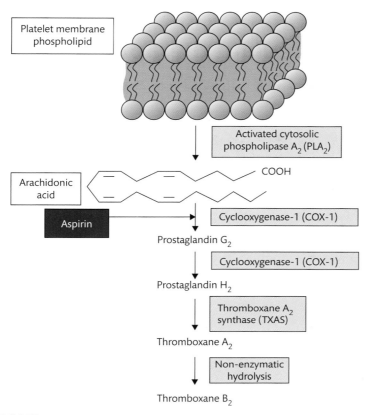

FIGURE 16.12

Anticoagulant effect of aspirin on the arachidonic acid (AA) pathway. Upon platelet activation, cytosolic phospholipase A_2 liberates AA from membrane phospholipids. Once released, AA is oxygenized by cyclooxygenase-1 (COX-1) to prostaglandin G_2 (PGG_2) and then reduced to prostaglandin H_2 (PGH_2), also by COX-1. PGH_2 is then isomerized to thromboxane A_2 (TXA_2) by thromboxane A_2 synthase (TXAS) and TXA_2 is released to function as a platelet activator. TXA_2 is unstable and is rapidly hydrolysed non-enzymatically to its metabolite thromboxane B_2. Aspirin, and other NSAIDs, exert their anticoagulant effect by inhibiting COX-1 activity, thereby preventing the generation of TXA_2 to facilitate platelet activation. The action of aspirin is immediate and irreversible and platelets are affected for the remainder of their lifespan.

- Abciximab is a monoclonal antibody that selectively binds with glycoprotein IIbIIIa on the platelet surface reducing platelet-to-platelet aggregation through fibrinogen.
- Clopidogrel is a potent non-competitive inhibitor of ADP-induced platelet aggregation; it acts by preventing the binding of ADP to its platelet membrane receptor.

Monitoring the clinical effectiveness of these medications is not routinely required. However, the impairment of platelet function means that assessment is occasionally necessary, e.g. prior to surgery to clarify bleeding risk, or to establish the presence of ineffectual therapy (aspirin resistance).

Cross reference

Some of the platelet function assays that you met in Chapter 14 for diagnosing bleeding disorders are described below in their role as tools for monitoring antiplatelet therapy.

SELF-CHECK 16.7

What is the anticoagulant effect of aspirin?

16.4 **Laboratory monitoring of anticoagulant therapy**

The nature of different anticoagulants and test design means that no single test can be used to monitor each drug.

Laboratory monitoring of warfarin

The prothrombin time (PT) is the most commonly used laboratory test for monitoring warfarin therapy. It was first described by Quick in 1935, before the discovery of oral anticoagulants, and was initially introduced as a screening test for coagulation defects. As you saw in Chapter 14, it remains in everyday use for that purpose.

The PT measures the time a patient's plasma takes to clot in the presence of optimal concentrations of tissue factor, phospholipids, and calcium ions. Since there is no contact activator in the assay system, it means that factor XII remains dormant and subsequent components of the intrinsic pathway take no part in the generation of factor Xa to begin the common pathway. Therefore, the PT reflects the combined activities of three vitamin K-dependent factors (factors II, VII, and X) and two non-vitamin K-dependent factors (factor V and fibrinogen). Reduced fibrinogen levels will only prolong a PT if they are marked (<1.0g/L) and factor V deficiency is extremely rare. Therefore, the major determinants of the clotting times are vitamin K-dependent factors, making PT an ideal tool for warfarin monitoring. Whilst the activated partial thromboplastin time (APTT) is also affected by reductions in vitamin K-dependent factors (II, IX, and X), there are more stages involving non-vitamin K-dependent factors that contribute to the clotting time, so it is less sensitive as a warfarin monitoring tool.

Standardization

Most laboratory reagents for common analyses are available from a variety of manufacturers. Whilst each type will be broadly similar, the differences in reagent composition can lead to variation in analytical performance. For instance, in the diagnostic setting when investigating for a factor deficiency, the PT of a patient's plasma with thromboplastin A may give a clotting time of 10s but 16s with thromboplastin B. This could result in the patient being considered normal if analysed with the first reagent but abnormal with the second, leading to the initiation of further investigations to characterize the apparent deficiency. An alternative explanation is that, although the clotting times are different, the reagents are still measuring the same factors but have different performance characteristics and sensitivities. Thus, the reference range for thromboplastin A is 10–13 s and for thromboplastin B is 15–17 s. As long as reagent (and analyser) -specific reference ranges are used then these differences can be accounted for and the patient above would be considered normal by both reagents.

The situation is different when using the PT to monitor warfarin therapy because the results are not compared to a reference range but a therapeutic range, which needs to be the same wherever and however the PT is done. Since it would be impossible to supply every laboratory worldwide with the same thromboplastin reagent to monitor warfarinized patients, alternative measures are used to achieve an acceptable degree of inter-laboratory standardization based on the known properties of thromboplastin reagents.

BOX 16.5 *Recombinant thromboplastins*

In 1986, native human brain preparations were withdrawn from general use due to potential infection risks during manufacture, particularly in relation to Creutzfeldt–Jakob disease and the human immunodeficiency virus. Rabbit brain thromboplastins were the initial replacement. Thromboplastin reagents containing highly purified recombinant human tissue factor produced in *E. coli* and reconstituted into synthetic phospholipid vesicles became available in the early 1990s. The vesicles must contain phospholipids with a net negative charge to function effectively during *in-vitro* coagulation, the most effective being phosphatidyl serine. Consequently, recombinant thromboplastins are composed entirely of defined ingredients making them potentially superior to the relatively crude tissue extract reagents of human or animal tissues.

Thromboplastin reagents

Quick's original thromboplastin reagent was prepared from rabbit brain, the brain being an organ rich in both tissue factor and lipid. When PT monitoring of warfarin therapy was first introduced, most thromboplastin reagents were prepared locally from cadaver brains as they were easily obtained from the hospital mortuary. Other tissues have since been used as a source of thromboplastin such as bovine brain, rabbit lung, and human placenta.

As there was no standardization for the local preparation of thromboplastin reagents, variations in analytical performance existed between batches within a given laboratory and from one laboratory to another. The problems were exacerbated by reporting PTs in seconds because a stably anticoagulated patient could have a very different clotting time when tested with different batches of thromboplastin, whether at the same hospital over time or a different hospital using its own reagent. This resulted in unwarranted dose alterations, and thereby increased the risks of bleeding and thrombosis. Commercial supplies of thromboplastin were introduced in the 1950s that relieved hospital staff of the burden of local reagent preparation. Standardization was assumed—but not necessarily delivered—between preparations from alternative manufacturers, and poor inter-laboratory agreement remained evident.

The late 1960s saw the availability in the UK of a standardized thromboplastin, the Manchester Comparative Reagent (MCR), a phenolized extract of human brain. PT results were expressed as a **PT ratio**, where the patient's PT with the MCR was divided by that of the PT of a normal pooled control plasma analysed with the same MCR. Whilst this greatly improved inter-laboratory agreement it was impossible to manufacture enough reagent to supply other countries. An alternative model was needed to standardize PT analysis for warfarin monitoring on a worldwide scale and this came in the form of the **International Normalized Ratio** (INR).

The International Normalized Ratio

The INR was adopted as the World Health Organization (WHO) international PT standardization scheme in 1983. Theoretically, the INR obtained with a given thromboplastin gives the PT ratio that would have been generated if the patient's plasma was analysed with a WHO standard thromboplastin.

The INR is derived by first calculating the PT ratio from a previously determined **geometric mean normal prothrombin time** (GMNPT) for that thromboplastin. The sensitivity of the thromboplastin to the oral anticoagulant effect relative to the WHO standard is defined by a numerical value, the **International Sensitivity Index** (ISI). The INR is calculated from the PT ratio and ISI as follows:

$$INR = \{Patient\ PT\ (s)/GMNPT\ (s)\}^{ISI}$$

Cross reference

More details are given on GMNPT later in this section.

Therefore, accurate ISI assignment is crucial to the generation of accurate INRs. ISIs are assigned to thromboplastins after calibration against the WHO standard or a secondary standard that has been calibrated against it.

SELF-CHECK 16.8

How is an INR calculated?

Thromboplastin calibration and ISI assignment

The original WHO International Reference Preparation (IRP), designated 67/40, was a human brain thromboplastin, but it is no longer available. Replacement IRPs were calibrated against 67/40 before supplies were exhausted, and subsequent IRPs have been/will be calibrated against them. Thus, all IRPs will have had their ISIs defined in terms of 67/40. The inevitable degree of uncertainty in the accuracy of ISI assignment to new IRPs is limited by assigning ISIs using large, multicentre calibration exercises. These involve collaboration between 20 laboratories or more from at least 10 different countries. Currently, there are WHO standard preparations for thromboplastins of recombinant human, native rabbit, and native bovine origin.

Any new IRP is calibrated against all existing IRPs. The ISI assigned to the new IRP is taken as the mean ISI obtained from the calibration with each current IRP. Each collaborating laboratory identifies a minimum of 20 healthy individuals and 60 stably orally anticoagulated patients with INRs spread throughout the range of 1.5–4.5. Each day, fresh plasma samples from two of the healthy individuals and six of the orally anticoagulated patients are tested by PT with each of the current IRPs and the new IRP being calibrated. PTs on each sample are typically

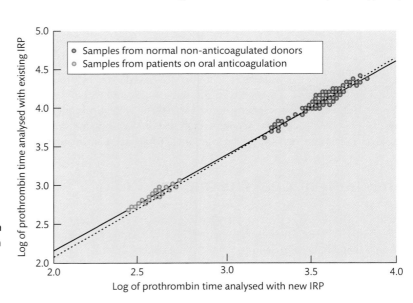

FIGURE 16.13

Orthogonal regression line for ISI calibration prepared by plotting the log of prothrombin times (PT) with the new thromboplastin against the log of PTs with the International Reference Preparation (IRP).

performed in quadruplicate. An **orthogonal regression line** is prepared from the natural logarithms of the PTs, which you can see in Figure 16.13.

The orthogonal regression model assumes that a single line can be drawn through both populations yet you can see in Figure 16.13 that the line may deviate between them. This lack of coincidence can be corrected using Tomenson's correction calculation. The slope of the orthogonal regression line through both populations is used to calculate the ISI of the new IRP.

> **SELF-CHECK 16.9**
>
> How is the ISI of a new IRP generated?

National reference preparations and manufacturer's working standards are considered to be secondary standards and should be calibrated against the IRP for the corresponding species. Large, multicentre calibration exercises are impractical for generating secondary standards, but the exercises should be performed in at least two laboratories to minimize the effects of inter-laboratory variation. Secondary standards are used to calibrate manufacturers' commercial reagents. Each reagent batch should be calibrated against a secondary standard from the same tissue of the same species that has been prepared using a similar manufacturing process. These calibrations can be performed using pooled normal plasmas and pooled plasmas from orally anticoagulated patients. Plasmas artificially depleted of vitamin K-dependent factors are also available. The advantage of using pooled plasmas means that far fewer PT estimations need to be performed to generate the regression line than if fresh individual samples were used. Similarities between the secondary standard and the reagent being calibrated, coupled with the reduction of biological variation between individual samples due to pooling, result in minimal data point scatter about the regression line.

> **SELF-CHECK 16.10**
>
> How is the ISI of a new secondary standard thromboplastin generated?

Local calibration

Commercial thromboplastins are supplied with assigned ISI values in order to contribute to a reduction in the inter-laboratory variation of INR results. However, this is not the full story because there are other variables that impact on raw clotting times apart from thromboplastin variability, principal amongst them being the different analytical platforms used to deliver reagents and detect fibrin clot endpoints. Each platform has innate characteristics and limitations that impact on the clotting time, even if the same plasma sample and thromboplastin are analysed by each method.

Consequently, the ISI assigned by the manufacturer is only valid for their equipment and method(s) of analysis. Hospital laboratories should calibrate each batch of thromboplastin they use to assign a local ISI based on the specific reagent/technique/endpoint detection method(s) in local use. Some manufacturers do provide instrument-specific ISIs, but a local-system ISI should still be undertaken to account for local variations in technique, analyser programming, and maintenance procedures.

A reliable local system ISI can be derived from a minimum of 7 normal and 20 abnormal (warfarinized) plasmas, although 3 normals and 10 abnormals can be used for low ISI reagents. Sets of normal and abnormal artificially depleted lyophilized plasmas can be purchased for local system ISI calibration that are described as 'substantially equivalent to a full fresh plasma ISI calibration'. However, the preparation process for lyophilized plasmas can prolong PTs if analysed with a low ISI thromboplastin, and some practitioners prefer to use frozen plasmas. Frozen plasmas tend

orthogonal regression line
Generating a best-fit line through a series of points commonly involves ordinary regression, which minimizes the sum of the squares of the vertical distances from each point to the line. Ordinary regression assumes the measurements were made without error. Orthogonal regression allows for random error by minimizing the sum of squares of the perpendicular distances between each point and the line.

Cross reference
You met the analytical platforms of tilt-tube techniques, mechanical clot detection, and photo-optical clot detection in Chapter 2.

CASE STUDY 16.1 Impact of analytical platform variation on INR generation

As part of a local quality check, plasma from a patient on warfarin had a PT performed by the manual tilt-tube technique and automated photo-optical clot detection using the same thromboplastin. The patient's target INR range was 3.0–4.0. The manufacturer's assigned ISI was 1.05. The results were as follows:

	Patient PT (s)	INR
Tilt-tube (GMNPT: 15 s)	59.0	4.2
Automated analyser (GMNPT: 12 s)	43.2	3.8

Note that the GMNPT and patient PT by each method are quite different. Analysis by the tilt-tube technique would lead to dose alteration, but the patient would have remained on the same dose if clinical decision-making was based on the automated INR.

The thromboplastin was then calibrated for each method and gave an ISI of 1.00 for the tilt-tube technique and 1.04 for the automated method. Recalculation of the INRs gave the following results:

	Patient PT (s)	INR
Tilt-tube (GMNPT: 15 s)	59.0	3.9
Automated analyser (GMNPT: 12 s)	43.2	3.8

There was virtually no difference between the manufacturer's ISI and that generated locally for the automated analysis, probably because the manufacturer calibrated using a similar instrument. The ISI for the manual technique was sufficiently different to make a clinically significant difference to the INR when adopting the manufacturer's ISI, which reverted to a clinically equivalent result when the local ISI was applied.

to show a lower degree of INR variability between thromboplastins, but there can be difficulties in preserving sample integrity during shipment and storage which increases their cost.

The plasmas are each assigned a PT value by the manufacturer using an IRP thromboplastin and analysed by a manual technique. IRPs are calibrated using manual techniques. The local laboratory performs PTs on each plasma, ideally in quadruplicate and in the same working session, using the local analytical platform(s) and determines the ISI as described above.

An alternative method is to use plasmas that are assigned INR values rather than PT values by the manufacturer. The PTs are analysed using the local analytical platform(s) and the logs of the PTs are plotted against the logs of the reference INR, which you can see in Figure 16.14. Patient INRs are generated from local PT analysis by direct interpolation from the orthogonal regression line, thereby negating the need to determinate the ISI or GMNPT. Look again at Figure 16.14 and you will note that the regression line is generated from only four PT results because each plasma sample is a pool.

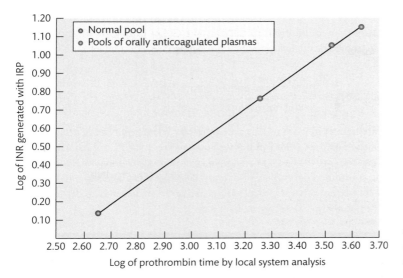

FIGURE 16.14

Local ISI calibration prepared by plotting the log of prothrombin times with the new thromboplastin against the logs of INRs with the reference thromboplastin.

Manufacturers of certified plasmas should specify the reagent/analyser combinations for which their products have been shown to operate reliably. Local ISI calibration should ideally be derived using certified PT or INR values derived from the same species thromboplastin.

SELF-CHECK 16.11

How is a local system ISI generated?

Geometric mean normal prothrombin time (GMNPT)

For the reasons mentioned earlier, the local system for analysing PT will affect the GMNPT as well as the ISI, and so the GMNPT must also be derived locally in order to generate accurate INR results. GMNPT is used in preference to an arithmetic mean because there is a log–normal distribution of PTs in a healthy adult population. Calculating the GMNPT effectively performs a log transformation of the data to normalize the distribution before calculating the mean itself. Although mathematically correct, there is rarely a significant enough difference between the arithmetic and GMNPT to adversely affect INR values, yet most laboratories apply the GMNPT to account for the rare occasions where its benefit might be realized.

A GMNPT is generated from the PTs of a minimum of 20 fresh plasmas from normal adult donors from both sexes and analysed over a period of several days for each analyser and technique in local use. Sophisticated automated analysers will deteriorate over time, even with regular and effective maintenance, so GMNPT may also alter over time. In reality, any drift will be minimal but re-assessment of GMNPT warrants consideration if the internal or external quality control schemes suggest a deterioration in PT/INR performance. A major equipment service may necessitate re-assigning the GMNPT and/or ISI.

Commercially prepared plasmas specifically for GMNPT evaluation are not available, even though in theory GMNPT should be locally assessed for every new thromboplastin batch. PTs for GMNPT assessment should be performed on fresh plasma, not frozen or lyophilized, because routine warfarin monitoring is performed on fresh plasma. Few laboratories have the donor availability to do this and tend to rely on the fact that GMNPT drift, if it occurs at all, is usually minimal. One way round this is to calculate the GMNPT from the PT and INR of a lyophilized or frozen pooled normal plasma obtained for the ISI calibration exercise, as shown below:

$$\text{Theoretical GMNPT} = \frac{\text{PT of normal pooled plasma (s)}}{\text{INR of normal pooled plasma}}$$

Commercial normal plasma pools are usually prepared from a large number of donors, often in excess of 100. Calculating the GMNPT in this way assumes that the PT of such a large pool does indeed equate to the GMNPT had it been derived from a group of separate donors. Fresh plasmas can only be substituted by lyophilized or frozen plasmas if the laboratory has demonstrated that the mean result of replicate PTs of lyophilized or frozen plasmas analysed by local procedures is identical to that of fresh plasma samples.

SELF-CHECK 16.12

How is a GMNPT generated?

Point-of-care testing

Efficient delivery of an outpatient anticoagulant clinic often requires fast turnaround times of INR results, which are not necessarily achievable via a remote centralized laboratory. A common response to this problem is for biomedical scientists to use **point-of-care test** (POCT) instruments in the environs of the clinic itself. POCT devices are portable, semi-automated analysers that perform only a single type of test or a very limited repertoire. The reagents and blood samples are loaded manually and endpoint detection is automatic.

Most POCT devices for PT/INR testing are designed to analyse whole blood samples from capillary punctures, although many can also analyse plasma. The biomedical scientist performs the capillary puncture, often referred to as a finger-prick, and the non-anticoagulated whole blood is immediately applied to a disposable test strip or cartridge containing thromboplastin in a dry state. The blood reconstitutes the thromboplastin and the strip/cartridge is immediately inserted into the analyser for clot detection. Interestingly, fresh capillary blood contains sufficient calcium ions to facilitate *in-vitro* coagulation and some strips/cartridges do not contain calcium within the reagent.

A number of POCT instruments for INR generation are available that use a variety of clot detection principles, as summarized below:

- As the whole blood starts to clot, the reduction and eventual cessation of red cell motion is detected using optical pattern recognition by changes in laser interference.
- Integral to the reagent once it has been reconstituted are paramagnetic iron oxide particles. Alternating magnetic fields cause pulsation of the particles which slows and stops as the blood clots. The changes in particle motion are detected optically.
- A reaction tube containing a magnet rotates slowly. Clot formation changes the position of the magnet and is detected because it removes the magnet from a magnetic field.
- Whole blood enters small-bore channels in a cartridge and is pumped back and forth. Clot formation reduces the oscillation and is detected photo-optically.
- Clot formation generates thrombin, which is reacted with a fluorescent substrate.
- Clot formation is detected by a change in the electrical impedance of blood that occurs when fibrinogen is converted to fibrin.

Performance issues with POCT instruments

Many research studies have been published comparing the analytical performance of POCT analysers between each other and standard laboratory equipment in the context of warfarin monitoring. Some studies have concluded that there is strong agreement between POCT devices and standard analytical techniques, whilst others have reported systematic bias or agreement only up to a certain point within the therapeutic range, typically when the INR is between 3.0 and 4.0. Although the two methods may give statistically different results, the degree of difference may be small enough that decisions on dosing are not markedly affected, in which case the methods can be considered clinically equivalent. If a haematology department uses standard analyses in the centralized laboratory and POCT devices in the anticoagulant clinic it is important to be aware of the degree of correlation. Analytical parity within the therapeutic range is important because patients may be tested by both methods during a given period of anticoagulation. It is common for POCT results to be checked by standard analysis when INRs are beyond the point where the methods have been shown to agree.

One additional factor that contributes to differences between POCT and standard analysis is the fact that most thromboplastins for POCT are dry reagents. Upon reconstitution of dry reagents, FVII is exposed to thromboplastin in intermediate states which can affect the clotting time. Liquid reagents used in standard testing contain a stable and fully hydrated thromboplastin immediately available for interaction with FVII. Consequently, recombinant reagents are better suited to POCT analysis because their uniform composition results in a sharp phase transition from the dry state to the liquid state.

Effective ISI calibration of a POCT device requires a calibration exercise comparable to that of a secondary standard. This would need relatively large numbers of normal donors and orally anticoagulated patients to provide fresh capillary blood, and is thus a prohibitive exercise for routine hospital laboratories. Consequently, manufacturers assign the ISIs to batches of test strips/cartridges using an IRP, and the ISI is adopted by all users of the instrument and its specific reagent strip/cartridge. To a large extent, this practice in effect generates a local system ISI, although operator and individual device variability are not accounted for.

POCT instruments are necessarily portable and relatively easy to operate. This has led to their operation by non-laboratory personnel such as nurses and pharmacists in clinics and primary-care settings. As long as appropriate training is provided and quality control is monitored by biomedical scientists, this appears to be a safe and effective addition to the armoury of anticoagulant monitoring. Some patients are suited to self-testing and even self-management but they must be carefully selected, and not all patients are willing to do so or can be successfully trained.

SELF-CHECK 16.13

What are the main differences between performance of INR by routine automated analysis and POCT?

Inter-laboratory INR variability

Although we know that a local system ISI corrects for major differences in PT/INR results between systems, a surprising number of laboratories adopt the manufacturer's assigned ISI, irrespective of the analytical platforms in local use. This is often a resource issue but it may reflect a lack of awareness of the clinical gains to local calibration. Reports from the UK National External Quality Assurance Scheme (UK NEQAS) reveal that inter-laboratory agreement remains a problem. Even for those laboratories who do undertake local calibration, there are important variables to take into account and they are detailed in Table 16.4.

TABLE 16.4 Variables affecting ISI calibration.

Variable	Potential effect on calibration
Calibration against an inappropriate IRP	Using a thromboplastin derived from a different species will impact on raw clotting times and alter the slope of the calibration curve.
Insufficient sample numbers	Calibration has to be based on a sufficiently representative set of donors, otherwise the calibration curve will not equate to the patient population.
Distribution of INRs in the orally anticoagulated donors	These samples must have INRs distributed within the range of 2.0–4.5 and have representative numbers of low, medium, and high values in order to equate to the patient population. If calibrating with pooled plasmas, it is the responsibility of the manufacturer to ensure an appropriate spread of INRs amongst the donors.
Calculation errors	Mathematical errors will generate an incorrect ISI.
Analyser malfunction	If the calibration is performed on an analyser that is malfunctioning, which isn't always immediately obvious to the operator, the calibration will be irrelevant to INRs generated once the fault is repaired.
Operator variability	This is particularly relevant to manual and semi-manual techniques where relative experience and quality of training will impact on competence.

Key Points

Patients whose INR is beyond the therapeutic range or who are unstable (variable INR) are less likely to give good agreement between methods, and these are the patients most likely to be investigated for analytical anomalies.

Even if an effective calibration is undertaken, performance of PTs in the diagnostic/monitoring setting is subject to the effects of pre-analytical variables, which themselves will impact on ISI generation if the samples used for calibration are thus affected.

Use of the arithmetic mean normal PT in place of GMNPT can potentially affect the accuracy of INR results, even if the calibration was well performed. Errors in the generation of GMNPT will affect INR accuracy, such as an unrepresentative donor population, analyser/technical faults or complications in pre-analytical variables.

Cross references

The types and effects of pre-analytical variables on coagulation testing are detailed in Chapters 2 and 14.

Causes of warfarin resistance are detailed later in the chapter.

Other factors interfering with the INR for oral anticoagulant monitoring

Some patients require immediate anticoagulation and may be given UFH or LMWH therapy until the oral anticoagulant effect has reached a therapeutic INR value. It is possible for

UFH to further prolong a PT and give a false impression of the degree of anticoagulation achieved by the warfarin. In practice, it is rare for therapeutic levels of UFH to interfere with PT analysis because of the powerful stimulus of a significant excess of tissue factor in thromboplastin reagents. Some manufacturers add heparin neutralizers to thromboplastin reagents to further reduce the potential for UFH interference, although they are only effective up to certain UFH concentrations. The main problems are encountered when blood samples are taken from central lines that have not been flushed sufficiently to prevent UFH entering the sample. Use of LMWH, which does not interfere with PT analysis, is becoming more common.

It is rare for lupus anticoagulants (LA) to cause an elevated PT, because the high concentration of phospholipid in thromboplastin reagents swamps most LA and prevents them from manifesting in this test. Warfarin is used in the treatment of antiphospholipid syndrome, so patients with clinically significant PT-reacting LA can be difficult to monitor because there is an ever-present risk of overestimation of anticoagulation. Such patients can usually be monitored with an alternative thromboplastin if it is shown to be unresponsive to that patient's LA. However, it should be borne in mind that LA-reactivity characteristics can alter over time in the same patient. Where this is unachievable, one-stage clotting assays for FII or FX can be used, because the additional dilutions integral to the assay design abolish the inhibitory effect of all but the most potent LA. Chromogenic factor X assays are available for patients whose LA overcomes even the dilution effect. A factor X level around 40% of normal equates to an INR of 2, and a level around 15% equates to an INR of 3.

Despite its limitations the INR system has significantly decreased inter-laboratory variability and facilitated the adoption of standard therapeutic ranges worldwide.

Investigating warfarin resistance

Individual patients vary in their response to a given warfarin dose, hence the need for monitoring therapy by INR. Some may require 0.5 mg daily to achieve a therapeutic INR, whilst others may need 15 mg daily to reach a similar INR. Some patients respond poorly to warfarin, even at increasing doses, which can be due to a phenomenon called **warfarin resistance**.

The patient is given an oral dose of warfarin under supervision and serial blood samples are taken over the course of three days for INR determination and direct assay of warfarin. Measurement of warfarin concentration over time allows determination of the bioavailability of warfarin and its **half-life** in that patient. Measuring the INR over time in response to a single dose of warfarin reveals information about the **pharmacodynamic** response.

half-life
The time taken for the amount of drug in the body to reduce its initial concentration by one-half.

pharmacodynamics
The action, effect, and breakdown of drugs in the body.

Key Points

Apparent warfarin resistance may be due to non-compliance; the dose of warfarin has to be supervised to ensure that the patient has correctly taken the drug.

Sampling is more frequent on the first day to ascertain the peak warfarin concentration and assess the degree of absorption. Daily measurements are sufficient after that at 48 and 72 hours post-dose in order to calculate the half-life. In the rare cases where the results suggest warfarin malabsorption, a further study using intravenously administered warfarin is necessary to assess warfarin resistance due to causes post-absorption. These regimes tend to be undertaken only in specialist laboratories.

Laboratory monitoring of heparins

Assays

The activated partial thromboplastin time (APTT) is the most widely used test for monitoring UFH therapy. The APTT is considered to be a sensitive test to the presence of UFH, with some reagents demonstrating prolongation of the APTT when the plasma heparin concentration is as low as 0.1 IU/mL. However, numerous APTT reagents are commercially available, but the variation in their phospholipid composition and concentration results in marked variability in heparin sensitivity.

Similar to warfarin monitoring, patients are assessed for adequate levels of anticoagulation by reference to a therapeutic range. This is often taken as 1.5–2.5 times the APTT of the normal plasma pool if reported in seconds, or an APTT ratio between 1.5 and 2.5. In view of the reagent variability, which is compounded by the type of analytical platform in local use, arbitrary use of these ranges is inappropriate. Instead, individual laboratories should calibrate their APTT therapeutic range to equate to plasma heparin concentrations between 0.3 and 0.7 IU/mL as measured by a chromogenic factor Xa inhibition assay, or 0.2 and 0.4 IU/mL if measured by protamine sulphate titration. The plasmas used for the calibration should be obtained from patients receiving UFH rather than spiking normal plasma, in order to reflect the effects of patient physiology on circulating UFH.

Another limitation to the use of APTT in UFH monitoring is that the APTT response is affected by other aspects of the patient's haemostasis. In particular, elevated FVIII levels—which can occur postoperatively or associated with acute illness, malignancy, or pregnancy—can reduce the APTT and give the impression that the patient is less anticoagulated than is actually the case. Markedly elevated fibrinogen can have a similar, although less marked, effect. Conversely, patients on concomitant oral anticoagulation, with factor deficiencies (e.g. DIC), or lupus anticoagulants may further prolong an APTT and give the impression of a greater degree of anticoagulation than has actually been achieved.

The short plasma half-life of UFH and the possibility of a degree of neutralization by platelet factor 4 means that blood samples for monitoring purposes should be centrifuged and analysed within 2 hours of collection. This is not always logistically possible and can lead to misleading results because the sample may contain significantly less available UFH by the time it is analysed. Taking the sample into a cooled collection tube and keeping it on ice until it reaches the laboratory can reduce these effects.

BOX 16.6 APTT and PT ratios

The APTT ratio is derived from dividing the patient's APTT by that of the normal plasma pool or a mean APTT value from a panel of normal donors. Some laboratories report their diagnostic screening APTT results in ratio format in place of the raw clotting time in seconds. This makes no difference to diagnostic efficacy as long as reference ranges are determined locally.

Similarly, some laboratories report diagnostic PTs as a PT ratio or even an INR. Use of INR in diagnostic screening is contentious, as it was designed to improve analytical parity in the context of the oral anticoagulant effect rather than disease states.

In recognition of the variables that affect UFH monitoring by APTT, use of factor Xa inhibition assays, so-called **anti-Xa assays**, is becoming more common. They are predominantly chromogenic assays and thus unaffected by many of the variables that affect clotting based tests. The requirement to analyse within a short time-frame remains; although as long as the sample is cooled and the plasma is separated from the cells in time, it can be stored frozen until analysis.

Some patients who require large doses of UFH to prolong their APTT are said to exhibit **heparin resistance**. This can be due to AT deficiency, short heparin survival *in vivo* associated with large thrombi, elevated FVIII or fibrinogen, circulating activated coagulation factors, or HIT (as a result of platelet factor 4 release from aggregating platelets which neutralizes heparin).

SELF-CHECK 16.14

What are the problems associated with monitoring UFH by APTT?

Anti-Xa assays

Anti-Xa assays use the same principle as the assay you met in Chapter 15 for measuring AT levels, except that the patient's plasma 'supplies' a different variable. In the antithrombin assay, the variable supplied by the patient's plasma is AT itself, which is reacted with fixed amounts of excess exogenous heparin and factor Xa to form AT–heparin–factor Xa complexes. The residual factor Xa is measured via its reaction with a chromogenic substrate, the intensity of the resultant coloured product being inversely proportional to the patient's AT concentration; i.e. the more AT that was present in the plasma the more factor Xa will complex with AT–heparin, thereby leaving less residual factor Xa to react with the chromogenic substrate.

In the anti-Xa assay for heparin monitoring, the variable 'supplied' by the patient's plasma is the circulating UFH which is reacted with fixed amounts of excess exogenous antithrombin and factor Xa, as shown below. In this case, the residual factor Xa that reacts with the chromogenic substrate is inversely proportional to the UFH concentration. So if the UFH concentration is high, there will be less residual FXa and the colour intensity of the final reaction will be low. Results are read from a standard curve.

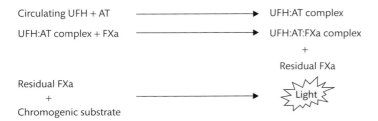

Most patients will have normal levels of circulating AT, but some may be deficient. The anti-Xa assay principle is based on there being an excess of AT, which is provided in the reagent, so the results are unaffected by the patient's own antithrombin levels. Additionally, this ensures that all heparin becomes complexed with AT, which would not necessarily happen if the assay relied on the patient's AT alone, and therefore measures 'free' heparin and provides a truer estimate of the concentration. Some commercially available assays do not employ the AT excess principle, relying instead on the patient's AT alone to complex with the exogenous factor Xa. This is not necessarily inferior because, although methods using excess AT may be more accurate in terms of estimating the actual concentration of circulating heparin, they may not provide a true reflection of the actual degree of anticoagulation. For instance, a patient with reduced antithrombin will generate a heparin concentration value that appears to be within the therapeutic range when measured by an AT-excess assay. However, the heparin will not be providing sufficient anticoagulant effect because the patient has insufficient circulating AT for the heparin to exert its full effect *in vivo*. The APTT of course gives a direct indication of the anticoagulant effect.

Clot-based assays exist for measuring anti-Xa activity in heparinized patients which rely on the patient's AT to complex with an excess of factor Xa. The residual factor Xa is then reacted with bovine plasma containing prothrombin, factor V and fibrinogen, which also contains optimal concentrations of calcium chloride and phospholipid to allow clot formation. The clotting time is directly proportional to the heparin concentration; i.e. a high heparin concentration results in less residual factor Xa and hence longer clotting times. Results are read from a standard curve.

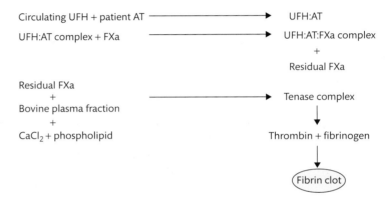

The superior bioavailability and longer half-life of LMWHs means they are administered in lower doses than UFH, and subcutaneously rather than intravenously. Therefore, LMWHs rarely interfere with routine coagulation screening tests and have to be monitored with anti-Xa assays. Routine laboratory monitoring of LMWHs is however unnecessary for most patients because there is a predictable dose–response. Situations requiring monitoring include morbid obesity, pregnancy, renal failure, low body weight, young children, and patients on long-term therapy to detect drug accumulation.

SELF-CHECK 16.15

What are the principles of anti-Xa assays for monitoring heparin therapies?

Anti-Xa performance considerations

Standard curves for anti-Xa assays are prepared by spiking normal plasma with heparin at different concentrations and assaying each concentration for anti-Xa activity. A crucial consideration when undertaking anti-Xa assays for heparin monitoring is that UFH preparations from different manufacturers can vary in their biochemical composition. Consequently, different preparations will yield different values for standard curves. Ideal practice dictates that the standard curve should be prepared from the same preparation that the patient is receiving. The variation is greater between LMWHs because the manufacturers use alternative methods of chemical or enzymatic depolymerization of UFH.

Anti-Xa assays are more complex than APTT to perform by manual techniques. Most hospital laboratories have automated equipment capable of performing anti-Xa assays, yet they are

BOX 16.7 Do APTT and anti-Xa assays mirror the full clinical picture in heparin monitoring?

Although LMWHs are considered to have predominantly anti-Xa activity, the variation in manufacture results in some preparations having appreciable anti-IIa activity. These are usually the preparations that may interfere with coagulation screening tests. Measuring only anti-Xa activity may not provide a complete picture of the degree of anticoagulation of UFH or LMWH when anti-IIa activity is also present. Additionally, heparins induce the release of tissue factor pathway inhibitor, which will also contribute to anticoagulation by downregulating the initiation stage of coagulation.

considerably more expensive than APTT and may not be a financially viable proposition for laboratories with a low demand.

Thrombin time

The concentration of thrombin used when the thrombin time (TT) is employed diagnostically makes the TT oversensitive to UFH. The TT will often be unmeasurable when the APTT indicates a therapeutic anticoagulant response. The TT can be modified to employ a higher concentration of thrombin for UFH monitoring. However, this requires having two types of TT in the repertoire, one of which has limited applications and results in resource wastage. Use of TT for UFH monitoring is largely historical and APTT is now used by the vast majority of laboratories that opt to monitor with a coagulation screening test.

Some LMWHs have sufficient anti-IIa activity to elevate a TT, and occasionally APTT, but not to such an extent that therapeutic ranges can be applied.

Protamine sulphate neutralization test

Protamine sulphate, which is strongly basic, binds to heparin, which is strongly acidic, and forms a stable salt lacking anticoagulant effect. This test is based on the TT and uses a range of protamine sulphate concentrations that are added to the patient's plasma before the addition of thrombin. The TT normalizes when all the UFH is neutralized, and the concentration of UFH is calculated from the amount of protamine sulphate required to produce this effect. The test can also be used to calculate the amount of protamine sulphate required to reverse the anticoagulant effect of UFH *in vivo*, for instance after cardiopulmonary surgery or haemodialysis.

BOX 16.8 The link between heparin neutralization and fish

Protamine sulphate was first isolated from salmon sperm, and subsequently from other fish. Patients with fish allergies can react violently to the drug so it is administered slowly. Protamine sulphate is now primarily produced using recombinant biotechnology.

Laboratory detection of heparin-induced thrombocytopenia antibodies

Type II HIT occurs in about 3% of patients treated with UFH, and the haemostasis laboratory plays an important role in confirming the clinical diagnosis. The clinical probability of the presence of HIT II is assessed using the 4Ts scoring system, which you can see in Table 16.5. HIT antibodies are detected in the laboratory by immunological assays and platelet activation assays.

Immunological HIT assays

Cross references

You met the principle of indirect ELISA in the Method box on p. 543 in Chapter 15, which described its use in the detection of anticardiolipin antibodies.

In Chapter 15 you met a similar principle of swamping an antibody with an antigen excess to reduce its *in-vitro* effect in the high phospholipid confirmatory tests used in lupus anticoagulant detection.

The most commonly used immunological assays for HIT antibodies are the indirect enzyme-linked immunosorbent assays (ELISA). Antibodies in patient plasma are captured by surface-bound PF4–heparin or PF4–polyvinylsulphate complexes. Binding of PF4 to polyvinylsulphate generates a cryptic autoepitope in the PF4 that is recognizable to HIT antibodies.

The ELISAs do not quantify HIT antibodies against a standard curve. Rather, reagents are provided with batch-specific cut-off points for optical density values. Patient samples whose optical density exceeds the cut-off value are reported as positive for the presence of HIT antibodies. If a patient is positive then the ELISA can be repeated in the presence of a high concentration of heparin. If this inhibits the reaction and causes a >50% reduction in the optical density value, it is considered characteristic of HIT antibodies.

The ELISA assays have a high sensitivity for the presence of HIT antibodies (~90%), but a lower specificity for HIT II. This is because patients on heparin without clinical HIT II, and even healthy subjects, can generate positive results in the ELISA assays. Clearly, heparin-treated patients can make the antibodies without developing clinical symptoms of HIT II. In healthy patients, the apparent positivity may be due to a conformational change in PF4 upon binding to the microtitre wells that allows antibodies non-specific for PF4–heparin complexes to bind. Alternative immunological assays are available that circumvent the latter scenario because their design does not involve binding of PF4–heparin complexes to a solid surface, and these have been shown to have improved specificity. A fluorescence-linked immunofiltration assay (FLIFA) immobilizes antibodies in the patient's serum on a nitrocellulose membrane, which

TABLE 16.5 The 4Ts scoring for probability of the presence of HIT II.

Category	2 points	1 point	0 points
Thrombocytopenia	> 50% reduction or nadir $\geq 20 \times 10^9$/L	30–50% reduction or nadir $10-19 \times 10^9$/L	<30% reduction or nadir $<10 \times 10^9$/L
Timing of reduction in platelet count	Days 5–10 or ≤ day 1 with heparin exposure in past 30 days	> Days 10 or ≤ day 1 if heparin exposure in past 30–100 days	< Day 4 (no recent heparin exposure)
Thrombosis or other sequelae	Proven thrombosis, skin necrosis, or acute systemic reaction after bolus of heparin	Progressive, recurrent, or silent thrombosis; erythematous skin lesions	None
Other potential causes of thrombocytopenia	Not apparent	Possible reasons	Definite reasons

Score 6–8—High probability of HIT (leads to replacement of heparin with DTI)
Score 4–5—Moderate risk for HIT (clinical judgement whether to alter treatment)
Score 0–3—Low risk for HIT

are then detected fluorimetrically with PF4–heparin complexes conjugated with fluorescein isothiocyanate (FITC). An enzyme-linked immunofiltration assay (ELIFA) immobilizes the antibodies in the same way, but detects them using an enzymatic chromogenic reaction using peroxidise-linked, PF4–heparin complexes.

A strongly positive result indicates a greater likelihood of HIT II than a weak positive that minimally or moderately exceeds the cut-off optical density (OD) value. Cut-off values tend to be in the region of 0.4 OD units and results of >1.0 have been associated with an increased risk of thrombosis. Only IgG antibodies require detection.

The above assays are quite time-consuming and can take up to four hours to complete. A rapid gel particle-agglutination technique is available that employs polystyrene beads coated with PF4–heparin complexes that act as the solid phase. The beads are mixed with patient serum in a well containing a gel. Any HIT antibodies present in the patient serum bind to the immobilized PF4–heparin complexes. A secondary anti-human immunoglobulin antibody is used which acts as a bridge between beads that are coated with HIT antibodies, leading to agglutination. The well is centrifuged for 10 minutes and the results are interpreted visually. You can see in Figure 16.15 that if HIT antibodies are present, the red polystyrene particles agglutinate and

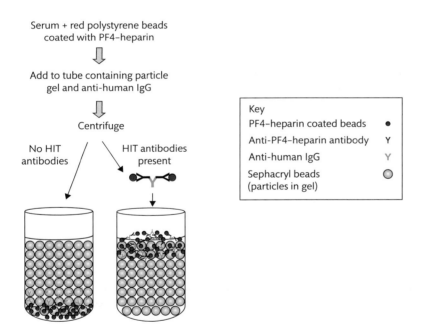

FIGURE 16.15

Gel particle-agglutination technique for the detection of HIT antibodies. Patient serum is incubated with PF4–heparin-coated polystyrene beads at 37 °C for 5 minutes. The serum + bead mixture is then added to a well containing sephacryl beads and anti-human immunoglobulin antibody. The well is then centrifuged for 10 minutes. HIT antibodies in the patient serum bind to the PF4–heparin complexes on the polystyrene beads, whereupon the anti-human immunoglobulin antibody binds to the HIT antibodies on different beads leading to agglutination. When centrifuged, the agglutinated beads are too large to pass through the particles in the gel and remain at the top. If no HIT antibodies are present, no agglutination occurs and the beads are centrifuged to the bottom of the well. The results are read by eye, a red band at the top of the gel being positive and one at the bottom being negative. Weak antibodies can generate a diffuse red colour throughout the gel.

remain on top of the gel after centrifugation. If HIT antibodies are absent the polystyrene particles are centrifuged to the bottom of the gel.

Platelet activation assays

This group of assays is based on the platelet-activating capacity of PF4–heparin–antibody complexes. HIT antibodies bound to PF4–heparin complexes activate platelets via interaction of the antibody's tail with the FcγIIa receptor on the platelet surface. Patient serum is incubated in the presence of fresh donor platelets and heparin to activate the platelets and cause them to aggregate. The most commonly used method to detect that the platelets have been activated is a standard platelet aggregometer. If a patient demonstrates aggregation with heparin at a concentration of 0.1–0.5 IU/mL that is abolished in a separate test using heparin at a concentration of 100 IU/mL, the presence of HIT antibodies is confirmed. Figure 16.16 shows the aggregation plots from a patient with HIT antibodies.

Other endpoints can be used to detect the platelet activation, such as the measurement of the release of radioactive serotonin from the platelets or ADP release in lumiaggregometry. The serotonin-release assay is considered to be the 'gold standard', but it is technically demanding and is rarely routinely available. A flow cytometric method has been described where patient serum and donor platelets are incubated together with high and low concentrations of heparin. The low concentration of heparin should activate the platelets in the presence of HIT antibodies, but the activation is abolished with the high concentration. The platelets are then incubated with fluoresceinated annexin V which interacts with the anionic phospholipids exposed on the platelet surface after activation. The degree of binding of annexin V is assessed by flow cytometry. Platelets activated by PF4–heparin–antibody complexes can exhibit a 300-fold increase in binding compared to resting platelets. This method has been shown to have comparable diagnostic performance to that of the serotonin-release assay.

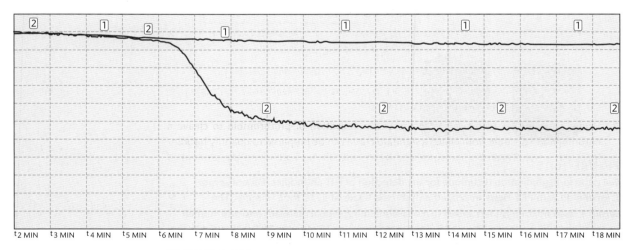

t_2 MIN t_3 MIN t_4 MIN t_5 MIN t_6 MIN t_7 MIN t_8 MIN t_9 MIN t_{10} MIN t_{11} MIN t_{12} MIN t_{13} MIN t_{14} MIN t_{15} MIN t_{16} MIN t_{17} MIN t_{18} MIN

FIGURE 16.16

Platelet aggregation plots for the detection of HIT antibodies. Tracing 2 exhibits a full aggregation pattern because the therapeutic concentration of heparin leads to the formation of PF4–heparin complexes to which the HIT antibodies attach and then activate the platelets. Tracing 1 exhibits no aggregation because the antibodies are swamped by an excess of antigen.

The functional assays have a lower sensitivity for HIT antibodies, but a higher probability of identifying cases that have the clinical hallmarks of HIT II. The sensitivity can be improved if the donor platelets are washed to remove potential interfering or masking factors in the donor's plasma, such as IgG, acute-phase proteins (i.e. fibrinogen) or variation in calcium concentration. A major influence on test sensitivity is the significant variation between donors of the activation response of their platelets to HIT antibodies.

Some patients may be positive by immunoassay but not platelet activation assay, and vice versa; so both types of assay are necessary for HIT diagnosis.

SELF-CHECK 16.16

What are the two main types of assay used to detect HIT antibodies, and what are their basic principles?

Laboratory monitoring of direct thrombin inhibitors

Theoretically, the thrombin time should lend itself to monitoring direct thrombin inhibitor (DTI) therapy. However, as you saw with UFH, the concentration of thrombin used in standard tests makes the thrombin time oversensitive to DTIs.

DTIs can be monitored similarly to UFH by using a therapeutic range of APTT ratios between 1.5 and 2.5. There are also similar reagent considerations because APTT reagents also have variable responses to DTIs. As you saw for UFH, the sensitivity of APTT reagents to other aspects of the patient's haemostasis compromises their effectiveness in monitoring DTIs. APTT reagents do not exhibit a linear response to DTIs and give a poor indication of anticoagulant response at high and low doses. This can be resolved by using the Ecarin fraction from the venom of the Saw-scaled Viper to activate *in-vitro* coagulation via prothrombin.

Cross reference

In Chapter 15 you met the Ecarin time in its role as a confirmatory test for lupus anticoagulants.

Ecarin has been shown to give a linear response to hirudin and lepirudin over a wide range of concentrations and can be used in three ways for monitoring purposes:

1. Comparing the raw Ecarin clotting time to a therapeutic range.

2. Using Ecarin clotting times of spiked normal plasma to generate a standard curve which can be used to quantify hirudin/lepirudin levels.

3. Using the thrombin generated from the Ecarin activation of prothrombin to cleave a chromogenic substrate from which a standard curve can be prepared to quantify hirudin/lepirudin levels. Thrombin is neutralized by the hirudin/lepirudin, and the amount of residual thrombin is inversely proportional to the hirudin/lepirudin concentration.

An alternative snake venom-based assay for monitoring DTIs is the **prothrombinase-induced clotting time** (PiCT). The factor V activator from Russell's Viper venom activates the patient's factor V, which is then reacted with reagents containing factor Xa, phospholipid and calcium ions to form the prothrombinase complex and promote clot formation. The time taken to clot is directly proportional to the DTI concentration. A standard curve is generated by spiking normal plasma with different concentrations of the DTI that the patient has received. The PiCT is a stable and reliable assay for levels of DTIs throughout and above therapeutic concentrations, but it can be affected by patient levels of factors II, V, and X below 25% of normal and by lupus anticoagulants. Patients on concomitant oral anticoagulant therapy will have reduced levels of factors II and X and cannot be monitored by PiCT.

Monitoring antiplatelet therapy

The effects of antiplatelet therapy can be monitored by the platelet aggregometry techniques used for detecting platelet function disorders. Although effective at demonstrating an overt physiological response, they may not detect more subtle changes of altered platelet function. Biochemical assays can be used as surrogate markers by measuring receptor changes/occupancy upon drug binding, enzyme function, or changes in surface proteins after activation. The biochemical assays may detect more subtle changes but may not reflect the degree of anticoagulation. Flow cytometry can be used to detect some of these changes. These techniques are time-consuming and technically demanding, and often require fresh platelets from the patient which cannot be routinely available. Consequently, monitoring of antiplatelet therapy is not routinely undertaken.

The PFA-100, which you met in Chapter 14 as a screening tool for primary haemostatic disorders, has been used to monitor antiplatelet therapy, particularly aspirin in terms of identifying non-compliance and **aspirin resistance**. Some patients appear under-responsive to standard doses of aspirin according to their PFA-100 results with the collagen–epinephrine cartridge. However, it is unclear whether this *in-vitro* phenomenon of apparent resistance to the effects of aspirin equates to a genuine clinical failure of aspirin to protect the patient from thrombotic events. Many patients who appear aspirin-resistant from their PFA-100 results demonstrate a reduced response to arachidonic acid by light-transmission platelet aggregometry (i.e. aspirin sensitive). The PFA-100 also lacks sensitivity to the platelet aggregation inhibitory effect of clopidogrel. The low sensitivity of PFA-100 to the effects of antiplatelet drugs is due to the many variables that impact on results, such as platelet count, anaemia, and inherent platelet reactivity to collagen. High levels of von Willebrand factor have been shown to affect PFA-100 results and may be the reason why some patients appear to be aspirin-resistant by this method.

True aspirin resistance occurs when the drug fails to completely inhibit thromboxane formation. Thromboxane A_2 is unstable under physiological conditions so measurement of its metabolite, **thromboxane B_2**, as an indicator of cyclooxygenase activity is the best way to detect clinical aspirin resistance. Thromboxane B_2 can be assayed by ELISA techniques.

A POCT analyser called VerifyNow™ has been designed specifically for the rapid monitoring of antiplatelet agents. Similar to the PFA-100, it is a cartridge-based, semi-automated device that tests whole blood samples. The VerifyNow™ was originally developed to assess the effects of GpIIbIIIa inhibitors by measuring the agglutination of fibrinogen-coated beads by platelets that have been stimulated by the thrombin receptor agonist peptide (TRAP). The TRAP-activated platelets bind to the beads and fall out of solution, and the rate of change in light transmittance is reported as Platelet-Aggregation Units (PAU). Cartridges using arachidonic acid as the agonist are available for aspirin monitoring, the reactivity reported as Aspirin Reaction Units (ARU). The effect of clopidogrel on the $P2Y_{12}$ ADP receptor is monitored using a cartridge containing ADP as the agonist and reported in $P2Y_{12}$ Reaction Units (PRU). The principle of the VerifyNow™ system is shown in Figure 16.17.

Direct measurement of drug levels is rarely helpful because of their pharmacological behaviour. For instance, the effects of aspirin are immediate and irreversible and remain long after the drug has been cleared from the plasma. Abciximab binds to platelets very quickly and is released very slowly, so most remains platelet-bound and measurement of plasma levels does not reflect the anticoagulant effect.

Although there are tests that demonstrate inhibition of platelet function by antiplatelet drugs, an important question is whether they are effective or even necessary. More data from clinical trials is needed to ascertain whether specific limits of laboratory values can be used to alter dosing decisions such has been achieved with the INR in warfarin monitoring. Less than 5% of

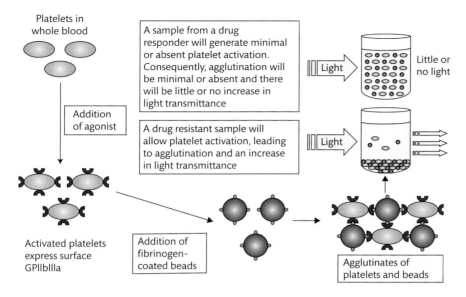

FIGURE 16.17

Principle of the VerifyNow™ system for monitoring antiplatelet agents. The appropriate agonist is added to a whole blood sample to maximally activate the platelets and promote surface expression of the fibrinogen receptor GpIIbIIIa. The blood is mixed with fibrinogen-coated beads and leads to the formation of platelet–bead agglutinates which fall out of solution. Light transmittance through the sample increases in proportion to the degree of agglutination.

patients are poor aspirin responders, some of which are due to non-compliance, so laboratory monitoring is difficult to justify. Since platelet function testing does not predict clinical events, regular testing does not guarantee effective monitoring. Existing tests can, however, indicate in most patients that the drugs are reaching their targets and exerting the desired pharmacological effect.

16.5 Management of oral anticoagulant therapy

Oral anticoagulants, normally in the form of warfarin in the UK, have been in use since the 1940s. Their clinical use declined in the 1960s due to concerns over their effectiveness in the management of myocardial infarction. However, improvements in safety due to analytical standardization and the demonstration of improved patient outcomes from better designed clinical trials, has resulted in increased prescribing for medical conditions where anticoagulant therapy is known to be clinically beneficial.

Anticoagulant therapy is considered effective if it prevents stroke and thromboembolism in patients with AF or the recurrence of thrombosis in patients with a confirmed venous thromboembolic event. To achieve this, oral anticoagulant therapy is routinely monitored by the INR, which you met earlier in this chapter. Adoption of this method by the WHO has resulted in a global improvement in the safety and effectiveness of oral anticoagulant therapy. Depending on the clinical condition, a patient is assigned an INR target range and the warfarin dosage is adjusted to maintain the INR within that range, as detailed in the British Committee

TABLE 16.6 Examples of INR therapeutic ranges for specific conditions.

Clinical condition	Therapeutic range INR
Atrial fibrillation	2.0–3.0
VTE (first event)	2.0–3.0
VTE (recurrent on warfarin)	3.0–4.0
Mechanical mitral valve replacement	3.0–4.0
Antiphospholipid syndrome (with VTE)	3.0–4.0

Within each therapeutic range a patient will have a target INR; for instance a patient with a therapeutic range of 2.0–3.0 will have a target INR of 2.5. If the dosing practitioner aims to keep the patient at the target INR then they are less likely to fall outside the therapeutic range.

for Standards in Haematology (BCSH) guidelines. Therapeutic ranges for the main conditions requiring oral anticoagulant therapy are given in Table 16.6.

Crucial to safe and effective therapy is patient counselling to ensure they understand the reason for therapy, associated risks and the 'do's' and 'don'ts' whilst on anticoagulation therapy. Good communication links between patients and those managing anticoagulant therapy are essential.

Need for management

Unlike the majority of prescription medication that does not need regular monitoring for effectiveness or side-effects, it is essential for safety in those patients prescribed the current oral anticoagulants. Monitoring is necessary to ensure that therapeutic reduction of functioning vitamin K coagulation factors has been achieved, and to reduce the risk of life-threatening haemorrhage or stroke by timely intervention with dosage adjustment.

There is no mathematical relationship between the amount of warfarin prescribed and the reduction of functional vitamin K-dependent coagulation factors. Warfarin dosage has to be tailored to the individual, which will be influenced by various factors, including age, lifestyle, diet, alcohol intake, genetic factors, ethnicity, other medical conditions, and importantly, interaction of other medication in association with liver function.

cytochrome P450

A large superfamily of haem-containing proteins that take part in electron transfer reactions.

Warfarin clearance from the body occurs in the liver via **cytochrome P450** catalysed oxidation of warfarin. Many other drugs influence the liver and activity of the various cytochromes, which can increase warfarin clearance and reduce the anticoagulant effect, or inhibit clearance and enhance the anticoagulant effect. Other influences of therapy involve drugs that inhibit the intestinal flora that produce vitamin K, notably antibiotics.

All these factors contribute to the requirement to regularly monitor a patient's INR and adjust the warfarin dosage accordingly. National targets exist to maintain patients in the therapeutic range and reduce adverse events.

Treatment risks

The specific risks of haemorrhage and thrombosis associated with anticoagulant medication were detailed earlier. However, the experience of most anticoagulant clinics is that these risks are exacerbated by other underlying causes. Most common is the cessation or introduction of medication for other clinical conditions without reference to the interaction with warfarin.

Patients with additional medical conditions that affect diet and the gastrointestinal tract can have adverse effects on vitamin K levels and warfarin absorbance. Patient non-compliance, either in taking medication or attending for monitoring, can result in very high INRs and an increased risk of life-threatening **cerebral haemorrhage**.

Although rare there are also some genetic factors that can influence the effectiveness and management of warfarin therapy. The term warfarin resistance has been attributed to patients requiring significantly higher than average dosage to achieve a therapeutic INR. This has now been identified as a genetic mutation in the vitamin K epoxide reductase enzyme at the warfarin binding site (vitamin K epoxide reductase complex subunit 1–VKORC1), which reduces its inhibitory effect on vitamin K metabolism. In contrast the term **warfarin sensitivity** has been attributed to patients requiring significantly less than the average dosage to achieve a therapeutic INR. This has been now been identified as being due to polymorphism variants in cytochrome P450 CYP2C9, which results in slower breakdown and clearance of the more potent enantiomer S-warfarin.

cerebral haemorrhage
A rupture of a blood vessel in the brain or leakage of blood from a vessel resulting in impaired oxygen supply to the area and subsequent brain damage of variable severity.

Drug interactions

Drug interactions have been discussed in other sections of this chapter in relation to the safety and effectiveness of anticoagulant therapy. If clinically indicated, most medication can be prescribed alongside warfarin, but close INR monitoring is required to ensure warfarin dosage adjustment occurs at the beginning of any interacting effect.

Interactions fall into three groups:

- Enhanced warfarin effect with a risk of bleeding
- Reduced warfarin effect with a risk of thrombosis
- Variable effect can enhance or reduce response

Also requiring consideration is other anticoagulant medication, predominantly antiplatelet drugs. Unless prescribed by a clinician these should not be taken concurrently with warfarin as they increase the risk of bleeding due to the combined effects of impaired platelet function and reduced functional coagulation factors.

Contraindications (liver disease)

Other medical conditions should be carefully considered prior to commencing anticoagulant therapy to assess clinical benefit versus clinical risk. It is particularly important to perform a coagulation screen prior to starting therapy in case there is an underlying coagulation defect or abnormal liver function which would make achieving a safe stable dosage difficult because coagulation factors are mainly produced in the liver.

Dosing regimes

There are national guidelines both from professional bodies and the National Patient Safety Agency on initial dosage (loading doses) regimes as well as algorithms to assist with subsequent prescribing. A typical dosing algorithm for a patient with AF is shown in Table 16.7.

Warfarin is manufactured as 0.5, 1.0, 3.0, and 5.0 mg colour-coded tablets. It is recommended that patients are provided with a range of tablets to enable 'fine tuning' of dosage, prevent the need to break tablets in half and to provide a consistent dosage throughout the week.

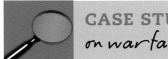

CASE STUDY 16.2 *Effect of antibiotics on warfarin therapy*

Target INR range   3.0–4.0

Stable INR (mean = 3.5) for the last 14 months–average daily warfarin dose 2.14 mg

Day 1   Patient presents in the Emergency Department feeling 'unwell'

INR = 2.0

C-reactive protein (marker of infection/inflammation) = 129 mg/L (ref. range: 0–5 mg/L)

Diagnosed as having bacterial endocarditis, which is an infection of the heart's inner lining or the heart valves that can damage or destroy the heart valves.

Patient started on antibiotics and admitted.

Day 3   INR = 12.0 (no evidence of bleeding)

Given 2.0 mg vitamin K (antidote)

Day 4   INR = 1.8

Restarted on a reduced dose of warfarin.

What caused the increased INR and why?

What implications for management does this have?

Patients fall into two categories:

Cross reference

The commonly used guideline documents are cited in the Further reading list at the end of this chapter.

- Patients with VTE or prophylaxis for VTE where is it is critical to obtain a therapeutic INR as soon as possible. LMWH will need to be continued until two INRs are within the therapeutic range.

- Patients with AF who can be started on a low dose and then increased gradually until their INR is in the therapeutic range.

TABLE 16.7 Example of warfarin dosing initiation algorithm for a patient with AF.

INR	Day	Dose (mg)
1.1	1	6
	2	6
	3	3
If, e.g., 2.0–2.5	4	3 mg daily, test INR in 3 days

Why must warfarin be regularly monitored?

Duration of oral anticoagulation

The reason a patient is receiving oral anticoagulation dictates not just the therapeutic range and target INR, but also the duration of anticoagulant therapy. The British Committee for Standards in Haematology recommend the following:

- Anticoagulation for one month is inadequate treatment after an episode of VTE.
- At least 6 weeks' anticoagulation is recommended after calf vein thrombosis.
- At least 3 months' anticoagulation is recommended after proximal DVT or PE.
- Anticoagulation for 3 months should be sufficient for patients with temporary risk factors and a low risk of recurrence.
- At least 6 months' anticoagulation is recommended for idiopathic VTE or permanent risk factors.

Service models

Service models by healthcare professionals

Over the last 15 years, service models of care for the provision of anticoagulant therapy have undergone major changes, and continue to do so due to the increasing numbers of patients requiring therapy and today's prolonged life expectancy. There are a number of approaches to service delivery that are very dependent on local needs and geographical area.

Traditionally, patients were seen in a hospital-based, medical consultant-led, face-to-face clinic service. This model of service is still provided in some hospitals, but in most this service has undergone significant change. Although still under consultant clinical direction, service is delivered by a range of healthcare professionals—i.e. nurses, biomedical scientists, or pharmacists—often working as multidisciplinary teams.

Many hospital-based clinics now offer face-to-face clinics for a patient's initial visit to explain the therapy and provide advice for any problems or queries. Subsequently, patients are either bled in the community (usually provided by their GP's surgery), or attend hospital-based phlebotomy; the samples are then sent to the local haematology laboratory that provides the INR and anticoagulant management service. Information about changes in dose, or maintenance of current dose, is returned to the patient by post, telephone or text. Many patients are given a yellow booklet where the INR and any dosage changes are recorded at every visit. Patients are advised to keep it with them at all times. Most hospital-based anticoagulant services use a computerized anticoagulant management system as a tool to manage all aspects of the service, including dosage decisions, appointments, length of treatment, and information about interacting drugs. This provides a comprehensive record and audit tool on all aspects of service.

In some areas, GPs provide an anticoagulant management service either in conjunction with the local laboratory to provide INR testing or using one of the POCT devices available for INR testing.

It is important that the same level of quality assurance is applied to all aspects of the service, whether delivered as a hospital- or GP-based service. A flow chart for dosing by healthcare staff is given in Figure 16.18, showing the different models that can be adopted.

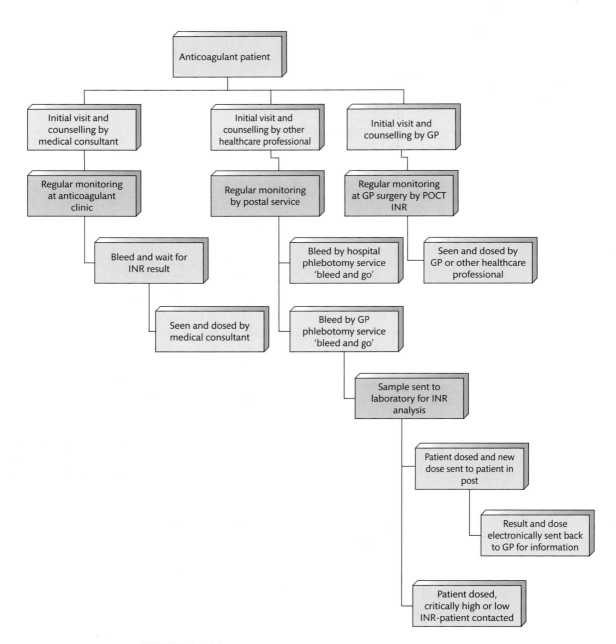

FIGURE 16.18

Service models of anticoagulant management by healthcare professionals. The flowchart illustrates options for the delivery of anticoagulant services provided either by a medical consultant, other healthcare professionals, or GP. They range from traditional 'face-to-face' clinics to community-based sample collection, with postal and phone dosing service. It also identifies the integral role of the diagnostic laboratory service within each model.

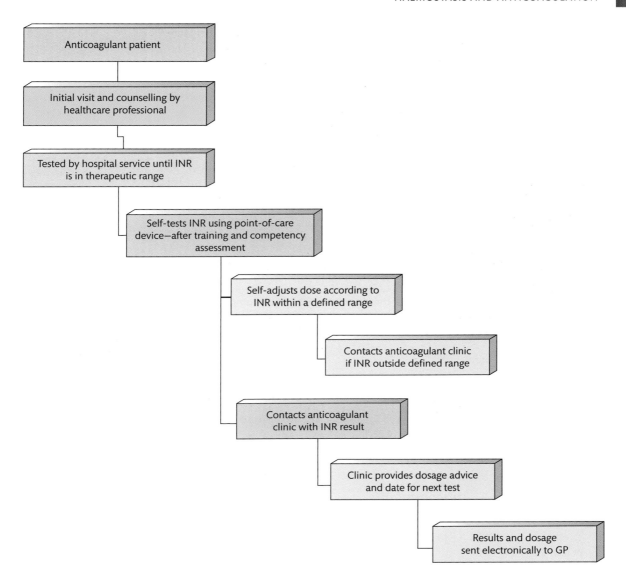

FIGURE 16.19

Service models of anticoagulant monitoring via patient self-testing. The flowchart illustrates procedures for patients and healthcare professionals to provide the option of patient self-testing and self-dosing, if appropriate. This enables patients to perform INR at home using a point-of-care device and adjusting their own dose within defined limits, and interacting with the anticoagulant clinic for management support and advice.

Service models by patients

With the increased availability and reliability of point-of-care devices there is evidence that self-testing may be a viable alternative for patients suitably trained in testing procedures, quality assurance, and procedures for clinical supervision. Relatively small numbers of patients currently elect to self-test and contact their local anticoagulant management service with their

INR result, which then provides warfarin dosage instructions. Figure 16.19 presents a flow chart for patient self-testing using POCT devices.

There have been some trials on patients self-testing and self-dosing as more patients seek autonomy and control over their medical condition and treatment. Safety and quality assurance aspects are paramount, and there are now national guidelines on patient self-testing and monitoring to address these issues.

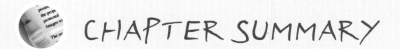 CHAPTER SUMMARY

General

■ Anticoagulant therapy is provided to prevent the genesis or growth of a thrombus and to reduce the risk of re-thrombosis.

■ Aetiology of thrombosis formation and composition is dependent on its occurrence in a vein or an artery.

■ Anticoagulants work indirectly or directly against coagulation proteins to reduce the risk of thrombosis.

Diagnosis of VTE

■ D-dimer levels can be used as a negative predictive indicator of VTE, and so rapidly exclude a diagnosis of DVT.

■ Confirmation of VTE requires radiological investigation.

Anticoagulants

■ UFH or LMWH provide an immediate anticoagulant effect, and are primarily used to provide cover until warfarin therapy is established.

■ Coumarins, notably warfarin and phenindione, are currently the only oral anticoagulants licensed for long-term use in the UK.

■ Monitoring of warfarin is essential to reduce the risk of catastrophic haemorrhage or further thrombosis. Overdosing can lead to the former and underdosing to the latter.

Laboratory monitoring

■ Oral anticoagulant therapy is monitored using the INR system.

■ Effective ISI calibration at international, manufacturer, and local levels is crucial to generating accurate INR results.

■ UFH is usually monitored by APTT but this test can be markedly affected by concomitant haemostatic abnormalities or anticoagulant therapies. APTT reagents from different manufacturers vary in their sensitivity to UFH, and therapeutic ranges should be locally assigned with respect to UFH levels measured by anti-Xa or protamine sulphate titration assays.

- LMWH rarely needs monitoring and is performed using anti-Xa assays utilizing the same preparation administered to the patient to generate the standard curve. Anti-Xa assays can be used to monitor UFH.

- Type II HIT is a clinically significant complication of heparin therapy. It is detected in the laboratory using immunological assays and platelet activation assays.

- DTIs can be monitored using APTT, assays based on Ecarin venom or PiCT.

- Antiplatelet therapy is not routinely monitored. Platelet aggregometry, functional markers, PFA-100, thromboxane B_2 levels, and VerifyNow™ can be used when necessary.

Management of anticoagulation

- Genetic mutations in the form of vitamin K epoxide reductase enzyme at the warfarin-binding site (VKORC1) and polymorphism variants in cytochrome P450 CYP2C9 have been identified as causes of anticoagulant management difficulties in some patients.

- A number of service models are available for the delivery of anticoagulant management; currently, most common is a postal service. Use of confidential electronic media is under development.

- New therapeutics may change monitoring and service requirements for the management of VTE in the future.

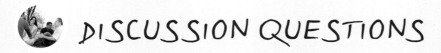

DISCUSSION QUESTIONS

16.1 Why do some anticoagulants need to be monitored and not others?

16.2 Why does the site of thrombus formation influence selection of anticoagulant therapy?

16.3 How do laboratory assay principles and limitations affect their effectiveness in monitoring anticoagulant therapy and what measures are taken to overcome or limit these effects?

16.4 What developments could lead to changes in how anticoagulant management services are provided?

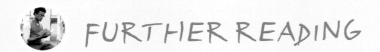

FURTHER READING

- **Baglin TP, Keeling DM, Watson HG (for the BCSH).** Guidelines on oral anticoagulation (warfarin): 3rd edition—2005 update. *British Journal of Haematology* 2005:**132**;277–85.

- **Baglin T, Barrowcliffe TW, Cohen A, Greaves M (for the BCSH).** Guidelines on the use and monitoring of heparin. *British Journal of Haematology* 2006:**133**;19–34.

- **Blann AD.** Deep vein thrombosis and pulmonary embolism: A guide for practitioners. MeK Update, Keswick UK, 2009.

- Fitzmaurice DA, Gardiner C, Kitchen S, Mackie I, Murray ET, Machin SJ. An evidence-based review and guidelines for patient self-testing and management of oral anticoagulation. *British Journal of Haematology* 2005:**131**;156–65.

- Keeling DM, Mackie IJ, Moody A, Watson HG (for the BCSH). Diagnosis of deep vein thrombosis in symptomatic outpatients and the potential for clinical assessment and D-dimer assays to reduce the need for diagnostic imaging. *British Journal of Haematology* 2004:**124**(1);15–25.

- Keeling D, Davidson S, Watson H (for the BCSH). The management of heparin-induced thrombocytopenia. *British Journal of Haematology* 2006:**133**;259–69.

- Moore GW, Henley A, Cotton SS, Tugnait S, Rangarajan S. Clinically significant differences between point-of-care analysers and a standard analyser for monitoring the international normalised ratio: a multi-instrument evaluation in a hospital outpatient setting. *Blood Coagulation and Fibrinolysis* 2007:**18**;287–92.

- National Patient Safety Agency. Actions that can make anticoagulant therapy safer: Alert and other information (http://nrls.npsq.nhs.uk/resources/?entryid45=59814)
  Crucial reading regarding required competencies of healthcare professionals involved in anticoagulant therapy.

Answers to self-check questions, case study questions, and discussion questions are provided in the book's Online Resource Centre, visit www.oxfordtextbooks.co.uk/orc/moore

Glossary

Acenocoumarin An oral anticoagulant.

Acetylation The addition of acetyl groups to histone lysine residues to induce an open chromatin configuration.

Acquired von Willebrand's disease VWF deficiency is secondary to other disease states (i.e. non-hereditary).

Actin-binding protein Proteins that bind actin.

Activated partial thromboplastin time A coagulation screening test for global assessment of intrinsic and common pathways.

Activated protein C The activated form of the naturally occurring inhibitor of the activated forms of factor V and factor VIII.

Activated protein C resistance A hereditary or acquired abnormality where the anticoagulant action of normal activated protein C is reduced by other factors, e.g. factor V Leiden.

Activin receptor-like kinase 1 An endothelium bound growth factor receptor involved in angiogenesis.

ADAMTS-13 An enzyme that degrades ultra-large VWF multimers.

Aetiology The cause(s) of a disorder/disease.

Afibrinogenaemia The absence of plasma fibrinogen.

Agonists Molecules that activate cell functions via surface receptors.

Alkylation The transfer of an alkyl group (C_nH_{2n+1}) from one molecule to another.

ALL Acute lymphoblastic leukaemia or acute lymphocytic leukaemia.

All-*trans* retinoic acid (ATRA) A vitamin A derivative which interacts with the PML–RARα fusion protein in acute promyelocytic leukaemia and, at pharmacological concentrations, can induce differentiation of cell cycle arrested promyelocytes, allow their maturation and induction of apoptosis.

Alleles Different forms of a specific gene.

Alloantibodies Antibodies directed against substances from a member of one's own species that are recognized as foreign to self.

Alpha antiplasmin Prime inhibitor of plasmin.

Alpha granules Platelet storage granules containing numerous large molecules necessary for haemostasis and wound repair.

Alpha macroglobulin 'Back-up' inhibitor for antithrombin and α_2-antiplasmin.

Alpha and beta spectrin The major structural components of the matrix that provide 'skeletal' support for the structure of the red blood cell.

Amastigote Asexual replication phase of *T. cruzi*, *L. donovani*, and *L. infantum*.

AML Acute myeloid leukaemia.

Amplification The activation of various haemostatic components by the trace thrombin formed at initiation of coagulation.

Anaemia The principal disease of red blood cell, characterized by reduced haemoglobin and oxygen-carrying capacity, and symptoms such as tiredness and lethargy.

Aneuploidy The numerically abnormal chromosomal complement of a cell.

Angiogenesis Blood vessel formation.

Angiogenic The promotion of blood vessel formation.

Anisocytosis The variation in the size of the red blood cells when viewed by light microscopy.

Annexin V A phospholipid-binding protein with inhibitory activity towards blood coagulation.

Anti beta 2 GPI antibody A type of antiphospholipid antibody detected in solid-phase assays.

Anticardiolipin antibody A type of antiphospholipid antibody detected in solid-phase assays.

Anticoagulant A physiological or pharmacological mechanism that retards clotting processes.

Anticoagulation The clinical practice of minimizing the risk of thrombosis with anticoagulants.

Antigen presenting cell A cell that expresses MHC class II molecules in conjunction with antigenic material to elicit a T-cell response.

Antiphospholipid antibodies A heterogeneous group of autoantibodies that bind to phospholipid, complexes of phospholipid and protein, or phospholipid-binding proteins. Persistent presence of such antibodies is associated with thrombotic disease.

Antiphospholipid syndrome A disorder of haemostasis that predisposes patients to arterial or venous thrombosis and pregnancy morbidity, which occur in the presence of autoimmune antiphospholipid antibodies.

Antithrombin A naturally occurring inhibitor which predominantly acts on thrombin and activated factor X.

Antithrombin Cambridge II An antithrombin variant associated with mild increase in thrombotic risk.

Antithrombotic A molecule, process or therapy that prevents or interferes with the processes that form a blood clot.

Anti-Xa assay Assays based on inhibition of FXa that are used for measuring the effects of unfractionated heparin, low molecular weight heparin and antithrombin.

Aplastic anaemia An anaemia associated with pancytopenia and generally caused by suppression and/or damage to the bone marrow that results in low numbers of red blood cells and haemoglobin.

Apoptosis The process of programmed cell death involving the ordered removal of organelles and cells. One of the functions of apoptosis is to prevent acquired genetic mutations being passed on to daughter cells.

Apotransferrin The carrier protein transferrin when free of iron is called apotransferrin.

Argatroban A direct thrombin inhibitor derived from hirudin.

Aspirin resistance A condition where the platelets of some patients appear under-responsive to standard doses of aspirin, although evaluation of the phenomenon is method dependent.

Atherogenesis The process of the development of atherosclerosis, often involving blood vessel damage, thrombosis and hypercholesterolaemia.

Atheroma The accumulation of lipids, macrophages and connective tissue causing thickening of the inner wall of the arteries in patches, or plaques.

Atherosclerosis The narrowing and hardening of the arteries over time leading to impaired blood flow. Associated with age but also other risk factors, e.g. hypertension, high cholesterol.

Atherosclerotic plaque A deposit of cholesterol and other fatty material that builds up within the arterial wall.

Atrophy Wasting of a structure with subsequent loss of function.

Auer rods Eosinophilic primary granules abnormally assembled into rod-like structures and used as a marker of myeloid malignancies.

Autoantibodies Antibodies that are directed against an organism's own tissues or native proteins.

Autoimmune haemolytic anaemia (AIHA) Anaemia that follows the destruction of red cells by an inappropriate antibody produced by the patient themselves.

Babesiosis Parasitic protozoan infection by *Babesia* organisms.

Background staining Uptake of Romanowsky stain by plasma-derived paraprotein fixed on the microscope slide.

Band 3 Component of the membrane of the red cell that provides recognition, transport, and anchorage sites.

Band form An immature granulocyte with a horse-shoe shaped nucleus.

Banding pattern A method of identifying chromosomes based upon their appearance following staining.

Basophil A granulocyte characterized morphologically by large violet or black granules that may partially or completely obscure the bilobed nucleus.

Basophilia An increase in the number of basophils, beyond the upper limit of the reference range.

Bence-Jones protein Paraproteins found in the urine.

Bernard-Soulier syndrome A bleeding disorder characterized by defects of the GPIb–IX–V platelet surface receptor complex.

Beta 2 glycoprotein-I Plasma protein with procoagulant and anticoagulation properties.

Bethesda assay The method used to quantify an inhibitor that requires prolonged incubation to detect progressively acting FVIII inhibitors.

Bilirubin The major breakdown product of haem: high plasma levels cause the clinical sign jaundice.

Biliverdin A primary breakdown product of haem that is converted into bilirubin.

Bioavailability The degree to which a drug or other substance is absorbed or becomes available where it is required physiologically and can act on its target.

Bivalirudin A direct thrombin inhibitor derived from hirudin.

Blackwater fever A sudden intravascular haemolysis followed by fever and haemoglobinuria in patients infected with *P. falciparum*.

Blast An early stage of differentiation of a blood cell as it passes from the stem cell stage to the mature cell stage that should only be found within the bone marrow in low numbers. Blasts may be further characterized by their lineage; e.g. myeloblasts are of the myeloid lineage, lymphoblasts are of the lymphoid lineage.

Blast threshold The minimum number of blasts required to diagnose a leukaemia as acute. WHO currently specifies 20% blasts to make this diagnosis.

Blood coagulation The process where specialized proteins interact to form a clot.

Blood film A stained smear of drop of blood that, when viewed through a microscope, provides additional information on red blood cells, white blood cells and platelets.

Blood transfusion The science of ensuring the safe transfer of blood and other substances from one person to another.

Bone marrow Soft tissue located inside hollow bones responsible for production and maturation of blood cells.

Bone marrow aspiration The process of obtaining a sample of liquid bone marrow.

Breakpoint Describes an area of a chromosome, usually within a gene, where a region of chromosomal material is lost or exchanged with another chromosome.

Breakpoint cluster region (BCR) An area of a gene where DNA breakages tend to occur.

Bromodomains Originally identified in the Drosophila protein brahma. A bromodomain comprises a sequence of 110 amino acids derived from a four-helix bundle. When the helices interact, they produce a hydrophobic binding pocket with a conserved amino acid sequence that recognizes acetyl lysine.

C/EBP CCAAT enhancer binding protein, a factor important for the transcription of certain genes.

C4b-binding protein A component of the complement system that forms a high-affinity complex with protein S.

Calabar swellings Characteristic subcutaneous swellings of *Loa loa* filariasis.

Carbaminohaemoglobin A sub-type of haemoglobin characterized by binding to carbon dioxide.

Cardiac Relating to the function of the heart and associated medical conditions.

Cardiolipin A phospholipid found in high concentrations in metabolically active cells used as a capture antigen for the detection of anticardiolipin antibodies in the diagnosis of antiphospholipid syndrome.

Cardioversion Procedure of atrial fibrillation where heart is stopped, then an electrical current is applied to shock it into restarting with a normal sinus rhythm.

Cascade theory of coagulation Compartmentalized *in vitro* model of coagulation comprising three converging pathways that involve a series of enzyme and cofactor reactions to ultimately generate fibrin.

CD34 A molecule of the surface of stem cells that is a marker of these cells and so allows their identification and collection, (see also Cluster of differentiation).

Cell cycle arrest Occurs when the G1–S–G2–M transitions become disrupted. Arrest usually occurs in late GI or S phases as a consequence of the activation of tumour suppressor proteins in an attempt to initiate DNA repair. Alternatively, it can be seen during S phase where synthesis of DNA is disrupted.

Cellularity The proportion of cells within the bone marrow.

Centrifuge A commonplace but essential item of laboratory equipment for separating solid material (e.g. blood cells) from liquids (e.g. serum or plasma).

Centroblasts Highly proliferative cells found within the early germinal centre following antigenic stimulation.

Centrocyte A small non-dividing cell found within the germinal centre. The nucleus contains a cleft.

Centromere A prominent structure that joins two identical sister chromatids.

Cerebral haemorrhage A rupture of a blood vessel in the brain or leakage of blood from a vessel resulting in impaired oxygen supply to the area and subsequent brain damage of variable severity.

Cerebral malaria Invasion of the central nervous system by cytoadherance of *P. falciparum* infected red cells to the vascular endothelium and rosetting of non-infected cells around the adhered infected cells.

Charcot-Leyden (crystal protein) A type of enzyme found within eosinophils and basophils that has the propensity to form crystals. Evidence of crystals in body fluids indicates allergy.

Chemotaxins Any group of small molecules that can induce chemotaxis.

Chemotaxis The process whereby chemical signals, for example, complement components C3a and C5a, and bacterial products, such as lipopolysaccharide, disseminate forming a concentration gradient for granulocytes to follow.

Chemotherapy (treatment using drugs) Generally held to be treatment of a cancer with cytotoxic drugs, although the use of any drug, such as an antibiotic, is also chemotherapy.

Chimeric protein Following translocation, the protein product obtained containing elements of both fused genes.

Chitin The principal component of arthropod exoskeletons.

Chromatids Subunits of chromosomes separated by a centromere. Chromatids become chromosomes following division of the centromere during mitosis.

Chromatin The DNA histone composite found within chromosomes.

Chromogenic substrate A substrate that mimics the natural substrate of an enzyme, to which a dye, such as paranitroalinine is added. The enzyme will cleave the substrate to release the dye, causing a measurable colour change.

Class switching recombination The process of generating different types of immunoglobulin.

Clauss fibrinogen assay Assay based on the thrombin time that quantifies fibrinogen activity.

Clinical Pathology Accreditation (UK) Ltd Accreditation body for pathology laboratories in the UK.

Clone A cell, group of cells, or organism descended from and genetically identical to a single common ancestor.

Cluster of differentiation (CD) antigen The standardized notation used to describe a range of molecules associated with the differentiation and maturation of cells. CD markers can be measured using epitope-specific monoclonal antibodies.

Coagulation The process where specialized proteins interact to form a clot.

Coagulation factors Circulating inert enzymes and cofactors that become activated to operate in concert to ultimately generate fibrin in a blood clot.

Coagulation screen A group of tests that assess global functionality of plasma clotting factors.

Coagulopathy Hereditary or acquired abnormality of blood coagulation.

Cobalamin The chemical basis of vitamin B_{12} and related molecules.

Collagen A long protein fibre that connects and strengthens numerous tissues.

Collagen-binding activity assay An ELISA assay to quantify the collagen binding capacity of VWF.

Colony-forming unit A lineage specific stem cell, responsible for the production of only one type of blood cell.

Colony-stimulating factor A cytokine that participates in the regulation of haemopoiesis by acting on precursor cells to induce their differentiation into colonies of themselves or into the next stage of differentiation.

Common pathway Compartment within the cascade theory of coagulation involving a sequence of enzyme activation reactions starting with activation of FII (prothrombin) by FXa and cofactors of FVa, phospholipid and calcium ions. The activated FII (thrombin) converts fibrinogen to fibrin.

Co-morbidities Two or more co-existing diseases.

Complement A series of inflammatory and defensive proteins that normally assemble on the surface of pathogens such as bacteria, helping to cause their destruction. However, inappropriate complement activation can occur on the cells of the body (such as red blood cells) also contributing to their destruction.

Complement factor H A regulator of the complement system that ensures the system is directed against pathogens and not against self.

Complement system An enzyme cascade triggered by antigen-antibody complex formation and resulting in the activation of a series of defence mechanisms, including inflammation and cell lysis.

Complementarity determining region The region of an antibody that complements the structure of its associated antigen.

Complex karyotype Describes the situation where more than three acquired cytogenetic abnormalities are found within a population of tumour cells.

Compression ultrasongraphy Used for examining soft tissue; provides real-time images in conjunction with venous compression to diagnose DVT.

Confirm reagent A reagent used to demonstrate phospholipid dependence when the presence of a lupus anticoagulant is suspected.

Conformational change Alteration in the structure and shape of a protein that can alter biochemical properties.

Constitutionally Pertaining to an entity's composition.

Continuing professional development Practical and educational activities that maintain up to date and informed professional practice.

Coumarin A plant toxin that is the precursor for a number of anticoagulants, notably warfarin.

CpG islands Regions of the genome that are composed of dinucleotides of cytosine and guanine.

Cross-links Covalent bonds between adjacent fibrin molecules introduced by activated FXIII.

Cryoglobulins Proteins that precipitate and aggregate at low temperatures.

Cryptic translocation This occurs when the original morphology and banding pattern of a chromosome is maintained following translocation. This means the translocation may go undetected.

Cutaneous Pertaining to the skin.

Cyclin-dependent kinases A group of enzymes, requiring cyclins, that are involved in the transfer of phosphate groups to enable the progression of the cell cycle.

Cytochemistry A technique that uses chemical stains that react with cytoplasmic components and so define different cells in the blood and bone marrow.

Cytochrome P450 A large superfamily of haem-containing proteins that take part in electron transfer reactions.

Cytokines Small hormone-like intercellular mediators with a diverse range of functions including the stimulation of the immune system in response to an encounter with a pathogen.

Cytopenia A reduction in one or more cell lineages within the peripheral blood. If all lineages (red cells, white cells and platelets) are reduced, this is termed pancytopenia.

Cytoreductive therapy A form of therapy effective at reducing high blood cell counts. An example of cytoreductive therapy is the use of hydroxycarbamide.

2,3-diphosphoglycerate (2,3-DPG) A red blood cell metabolite product of anaerobic respiration but which may also partially regulate in oxygen carriage by haemoglobin.

D-dimer Terminal degradation product of cross-linked fibrin.

De-novo leukaemia A primary leukaemia; of unknown cause.

Deep vein thrombosis A condition where a blood clot forms in one or more of the deep veins, commonly in the inner thigh or lower leg.

Deletion loss of chromosomal material.

Dense bodies Platelet storage granules containing numerous small molecules necessary for haemostasis.

Dense tubular system Platelet internal membrane system facilitating internal platelet biochemistry.

Deoxyhaemoglobin Haemoglobin that is not carrying oxygen.

Desmopressin Synthetic antidiuretic drug that stimulates release of FVIII and VWF.

Diamond–Blackfan anaemia The principal congenital cause of pure red cell aplasia.

Diapedesis The movement of neutrophils, between the vascular endothelial cells, from the blood into the tissues.

Dimer A molecule composed of two linked subunits.

Dimorphic A population of two distinct populations of red cells in the same FBC sample.

Diploid Chromosomal complement of a normal somatic cell, containing 22 pairs of autosomes and two sex chromosomes.

Direct antiglobulin test (DAT) A laboratory test to search for an antibody on the surface of red blood cells. Commonly used in the diagnosis of AIHA.

Direct thrombin inhibitor Anticoagulant drug that interacts directly with thrombin without the need for cofactors.

Disseminated intravascular coagulation A potentially life threatening condition resulting from excessive activation of coagulation plus loss of control and localization mechanisms.

Divalent metal transporter-1 The molecule at the surface of the enterocyte through which iron passes into the body.

DNA methyltransferases A family of enzymes responsible for the transfer of methyl groups to DNA leading to gene silencing.

Döhle bodies Cytoplasmic remnants of endoplasmic reticular material. Blue-grey in colour.

Domain A discrete section that is part of the structure of a protein.

Drumstick Small nuclear protrusion often expressed by neutrophils on a blood film and found in females (and some males) comprising a condensed X chromosome.

Dry tap An unsuccessful bone marrow aspirate which yields either no bone marrow material, or insufficient amounts for analysis. A dry tap could be caused by poor technique, but is more likely to be due to bone marrow fibrosis or hypercellularity.

Dyserythropoiesis Abnormal red cell development.

Dysfibrinogenaemia Functional deficiency of fibrinogen.

Dyskaryorrhexis Abnormal bursting of a cell's nucleus.

Dysplasia The abnormal development or maturation of cells, tissues or organs.

Dysregulation Describes the abnormal function of one or more regulated processes within a cell.

Ecchymoses Bruises caused by the leakage of blood from blood vessels.

Eclampsia One or more convulsions occurring during or immediately after pregnancy.

Ectoparasite A parasite that lives on the external surface of the host.

EDTA An anticoagulant chemical that, when added to whole blood, allows a full blood count to be undertaken.

Effector Describes a fully functional, mature cell.

Electrocardiography A procedure for measuring electrical changes in the heart which take place with each beat.

Electrophoresis The migration of dispersed particles (perhaps molecules) relative to a fluid under the influence of an electric field.

Embden–Myerhof glycolytic pathway A complex series of metabolic reactions whereby energy (in the form of ATP, NADH, and NADPH) is generated from glucose.

Embolus A blood clot or part of a blood clot that migrates through the bloodstream and then lodges in another vessel causing a blockage.

Enantiomeric Two stereoisomers that are complete mirror images of each other.

Endoglin A membrane glycoprotein involved in angiogenesis.

Endoparasite A parasite that lives within the body of the host.

Endothelial cell A specialized cell that forms the internal lining of the blood vessels and sinuses: damage/dysfunction promotes thrombosis and hypertension.

Endothelial protein C receptor Transmembrane receptor that binds protein C to enhance its activation.

Enzyme-linked immunosorbent assay (ELISA) An immunoassay that employs an enzyme linked to an antibody or antigen as a marker for the detection and quantification of proteins/antibodies.

Eosinophil A granulocyte characterized morphologically by large red-brown granules that may partially or completely obscure the bilobed nucleus.

Eosinophil cationic protein A bactericidal and helminthotoxic protein that can also induce degranulation of mast cells.

Eosinophil-derived neurotoxin/eosinophil protein X Is not restricted to eosinophils, but can also be found in basophils and monocytes.

Eosinophil peroxidase An enzyme forming reactive singlet oxygen and hypobromous acid in the presence of H_2O_2 and bromide ion.

Epidermotropic A preference to existing within the epidermis.

Epimastigote Replication phase of *T. cruzi* in the vector gut.

Epistaxis Nosebleeds.

Erythroblast/normoblast Blast of the erythrocyte (red blood cell) pathway.

Erythroblastic island A highly specialized microenvironment in the bone marrow where erythropoiesis takes place.

Erythrocyte A red blood cell, carrier of haemoglobin.

Erythrocyte sedimentation rate A physical property of blood defined by the rate of settling of the blood by gravity.

Erythrocytosis Increased numbers of circulating red blood cells, generally the consequence of the bone marrow's response to loss of mature red cells.

Erythroderma Red and scaling skin caused by inflammation.

Erythropoiesis The process of the development of red blood cells.

Erythropoietin A growth factor, generally derived from the kidney, that promotes the development of red blood cells.

Essential thrombocythaemia A clonal proliferation of megakaryocytes leading to an increased platelet count.

Euchromatin Describes regions of DNA with an open chromatin structure possessing active genes.

Euploid Containing 46 chromosomes.

Exflagellation Extension of flagella from a malarial microgametocyte.

Exocytosis Binding of cytoplasmic vesicles to the cell membrane leading to the release of the vesicle's contents into the extracellular environment.

External Quality Assessment Where a central agency supplies all registered laboratories with blood samples for analysis with locally employed techniques to enable performance comparisons.

Extramedullary haemopoiesis Haemopoiesis occurring outside the bone marrow, such as in the liver, spleen and lymph nodes.

Extravascular haemolysis Haemolysis outside the blood vessels, generally in the liver and spleen.

Extrinsic pathway A compartment within the cascade theory of coagulation involving activation of FX by FVIIa and cofactors of tissue factor, phospholipid and calcium ions.

Extrinsic tenase complex Enzyme/cofactor/substrate complex (FVIIa/TF/FX + phospholipid and calcium ions) that generates the initial activated factor X.

Exudative tonsillitis Enlarged red tonsils covered in white patches.

Factor deficiency Reduced concentration and/or function of a coagulation factor that may predispose to a bleeding tendency.

Factor V Cambridge Arg306Thr mutation in the factor V gene, rendering the FV molecule resistant to inactivation by activated protein C.

Factor V Hong Kong Arg306Gly mutation in the factor V gene. It does not cause activated protein C resistance.

Factor V Leiden A mutation in the factor V gene, rendering the FV molecule resistant to inactivation by activated protein C.

Factor V Liverpool Ile359Thr mutation in the factor V gene, rendering the FV molecule resistant to inactivation by activated protein C.

Factor VIII binding capacity A chromogenic/ELISA assay to quantify the FVIII binding capacity of VWF.

Faggot cells Immature granulocytes that contain bundles of Auer rods. These are commonly seen in acute promyelocytic leukaemia.

Fanconi's anaemia The principal congenital cause of pancytopenia, also linked with skeletal and other abnormalities.

FcγR A receptor that recognizes a particular region (called the Fc region) on an IgG antibody.

Ferritin The main storage protein for iron: can be present in cells or in the serum.

Ferroportin A component of the cell membrane enterocytes, macrophages and hepatocytes controlling the export of iron into the circulation.

Fibrin Insoluble polymer strands derived from fibrinogen that form part of a blood clot and strengthen it.

Fibrinogen Fibrin precursor and ligand that facilitates platelet–platelet aggregation and forms a mesh that is the basis of the thrombus.

Fibrinolysis Regulated mechanism of fibrin clot destruction.

Fibrinopeptide A Peptide that shields polymerization site on fibrinogen Aα chain.

Fibrinopeptide B Peptide that shields polymerization site on fibrinogen Bβ chain.

Fibroblast A cell found in the bone marrow and numerous other sites in the body that synthesizes many products such as collagen, but also maintains structural integrity and contributes to wound healing, and tissue repair.

Fibronectin A multifunctional glycoprotein involved in cell adhesion, differentiation, growth and wound healing.

Fibrosarcoma A tumour developing in the fibrous connective tissue.

Field's stain A rapid Romanowsky stain used on unfixed thick films of peripheral blood for malarial parasite detection.

Filariasis Parasitic nematode infections by *W. bancrofti*, *B. malayi*, *B. timori* (lymphatic filariasis), and *L. loa* (Loa loa filariasis).

Flow cytometer Machine that analyse cells treated with fluorescent dyes and moving in a liquid stream past a laser beam. Analysis is based on the size, granularity and fluorescence of the individual cell.

Flow cytometry A technique that identifies blood and bone marrow cells according to size and granularity. Also used in conjunction with fluoresceinating antibodies to determine the presence of different molecules on the cell surface or in the cytoplasm.

Fluorochrome A chemical which, when excited by light of a particular wavelength, will emit light of a different but predictable wavelength, measurable using a photodetector.

Folate Essential micronutrient requirement in the development of the red blood cell.

Follicular dendritic cell (FDC) Cells with long branching processes found within lymphoid follicles. FDCs are important for enabling B-cell maturation.

Forssman antibody An antibody directed against the Forssman antigen.

Forssman antigen A glycosphingolipid found on cell membranes in many different species. Antibodies directed against the Forssman antigens are caused by a number of infectious agents, although are not associated with infectious mononucleosis.

Forward scatter A flow cytometric measurement to determine the size of a cell.

Frameshift mutation An alteration in the codon structure, changing the reading frame.

Fresh frozen plasma A therapeutic that contains plasma proteins including coagulation factors and used clinically to restore haemostasis.

Full blood count The most common and important laboratory test in haematology; it provides information on red blood cells, white blood cells and platelets.

Fusion protein Following translocation, the protein product containing elements of both fused genes. Also called chimeric protein.

Gain-of-function mutations Mutations that result in increased concentrations or interactions with target molecules.

Gastric parietal cells Cells of the luminal wall of the stomach which synthesize and secrete the vitamin B_{12} carrier molecule intrinsic factor, essential for the absorption of the vitamin.

Gating The process of selecting a particular population of cells being analysed by flow cytometry on which to base further immunophenotyping analysis.

Geometric mean normal prothrombin time Locally derived mean value from a minimum of 20 healthy donors used in calculation of PT ratios and INRs.

Gla domain Calcium binding portion of vitamin K dependent factors comprising γ-carboxyglutamic acid residues.

Glanzmann's thrombasthenia Bleeding disorder characterized by defects of the GPIIbIIIa platelet surface receptor.

Globin That part of the haemoglobin molecule that is protein.

Glucose-6-phosphate dehydrogenase (G6PD) A metabolic enzyme involved in the generation of NADPH.

Glutathione A metabolite that provides protection against toxic reactive oxygen species.

Glycophorin A and glycophorin C Component of the membrane of the red cell that provides recognition, transport, and anchorage sites.

Glycoproteins Proteins with carbohydrate chains.

Glycosaminoglycan Group of high molecular weight polysaccharides, commonly adopting structural functions, that includes chondroitin sulfates, dermatan sulfates, heparan sulfate and heparin.

Go The part of the cell cycle when it is not actively proliferating but is resting.

Granules Small bodies within the cytoplasm of granulocytes that contain bioactive molecules such as enzymes.

Granulocyte A white blood cell with granules in the cytoplasm. Neutrophils, eosinophils and basophils all have prominent granules (and an irregular nucleus); monocytes may have granules but this is rare.

Granulopoiesis The growth, differentiation and maturation of granulocytes.

Gray The unit of measurement for the absorbed dose of radiation (i.e the amount deposited in the mass of a particular material). One Gray = one joule per kilogram.

Growth factors Cytokines produced by one type of cell that initiate or promote the growth or differentiation of another cell.

Haem The non-protein part of the haemoglobin molecule that contains iron.

Haemarthrosis Bleeding into joint spaces that can lead to joint damage and disability.

Haematinic Nutrients required for effective red cell and haemoglobin production.

Haematocrit The proportion of blood that is made up of red blood cells.

Haemato-oncology The study of cancers of the haemopoietic system.

Haematuria Presence of blood in urine.

Haemodilute When aspirated contents of the bone marrow are excessively diluted with peripheral blood.

Haemoglobin A specialized iron-containing protein within the red blood cell that transports oxygen.

Haemoglobinopathy Disease (such as thalassaemia and sickle cell disease) resulting from mutations in the globin genes and so abnormal haemoglobin synthesis.

Haemolysis The inappropriate destruction of red blood cells that commonly leads to anaemia.

Haemolytic anaemia The consequence of inappropriate destruction of red blood cells in the circulation and/or liver and spleen, perhaps due to a defect in the red cells themselves, or due to a pathological condition acting on otherwise healthy cells.

Haemolytic uraemic syndrome Thrombotic microangiopathy occurring mainly in young children following gastrointestinal illness accompanied with diarrhoea.

Haem-oncology Cancers of the blood.

Haemopexin A plasma protein that complexes with, and thus removes.

Haemophilia Hereditary bleeding disorder caused by a deficiency in a clotting factor.

Haemophilia A FVIII deficiency.

Haemophilia B FIX deficiency.

Haemophilia C FXI deficiency.

Haemopoiesis The process of producing the cellular constituents of the blood: red blood cells, white blood cells, and platelets.

Haemoproliferative disorder A condition characterized by inappropriately increased numbers of circulating blood cells and their precursors.

Haemorrhage Excessive bleeding caused by a breakdown in haemostasis.

Haemorrhagic disease Disorders that lead to excessive bleeding.

Haemosiderin A granular and storage form of iron normally present in cells such as those of the liver, spleen and bone marrow.

Haemostasis The interplay of cellular and molecular processes that maintain blood fluidity and also generate blood clots at sites of injury, regulate clot formation, and degrade clots.

Haemoxygenase A key enzyme in the recycling pathway of the haem molecule that generates iron, carbon monoxide, and biliverdin.

Haemozoin Product of haemoglobin digestion by malarial parasites comprised of polymerized insoluble haem residues.

Half-life The period of time for the amount of drug in the body to reduce its initial concentration by one-half.

Haploinsufficiency Occurs when one of a pair of genes on homologous chromosomes is silenced through deletion or mutation. The intracellular concentration of the 'normal' gene product is insufficient to complete its intended biological role.

Haptoglobin A plasma protein that complexes with, and thus removes, haemoglobin and free haem from the circulation.

Helix–loop–helix domain Contained by a family of transcription factors, called helix–loop–helix proteins, these domains facilitate the activation of dimers from inactive monomers.

Helminth A parasitic worm commonly found within the intestines.

Heparin A natural anticoagulant often added to blood to allow additional analyses of white blood cells.

Heparin resistance Some patients require large doses of UFH to prolong the APTT due to AT deficiency, short heparin survival *in vivo* associated with large thrombi, elevated FVIII or fibrinogen, circulating activated coagulation factors or HIT.

Heparin-induced thrombocytopenia Reduction in platelet count associated with heparin and LMWH therapy. Type I disease is benign and results from the activation of platelets by high-dose UFH. Type II disease is caused by an immune response and associated with thrombosis.

Hepatocytes Liver cells involved in protein synthesis and storage.

Hepatomegaly Increase in the size of the liver.

Hepatosplenomegaly Increase in the size of the spleen and liver.

Hepcidin A liver-derived molecule that regulates the movement of iron into the blood.

Hereditary haemochromatosis The principal congenital cause of iron overload, most often due to a mutation (termed C282Y) in the gene for the iron regulator HFE.

Hereditary haemorrhagic telangiectasia Fragile blood vessel disorder.

Heterochromatin Contains hypoacetylated histones and a closed chromatin configuration. Genes within these areas are switched off.

Heterophile antibody An antibody that reacts with antigens expressed on the surface of cells derived from an unrelated species.

Heterozygous Inheritance of two different copies of an allele at a particular locus (compare Homozygous).

High molecular weight multimers The largest VWF subunits; the main contributors to GpIb and collagen binding capacity.

High-pressure [/performance] liquid chromatography Column chromatography technique used to separate, identify, and quantify compounds.

Hirudin Direct thrombin inhibitor extracted from leech saliva.

Histidine-rich glycoprotein A regulator of fibrinolysis.

Histiocyte A type of macrophage found within connective tissue.

Histone deacetylase A class of enzyme that removes acetyl groups from histones, thereby inhibiting DNA transcription.

Hodgkin and Reed-Sternberg cell Characteristic mutated B-cell associated with Hodgkin lymphoma.

Homeobox Genes encode transcriptional regulators which are expressed at particular times and in particular places within an organism – for example during embryonic development, or in cell differentiation.

Homeostasis The maintenance of stable physiological systems.

Homozygous Inheritance of two identical copies of an allele at a particular locus.

Human leukocyte antigen (HLA) Specialized cell membrane proteins that help defend us from infection with viruses but severely restrict the success of transplants.

Hypercalcaemia Raised plasma calcium concentration.

Hypercellular Denotes an increase in the size of the haemopoietic compartment of the bone marrow, or an increase in the number of cells within the marrow.

Hypercellularity Increase in the number of cells within the bone marrow.

Hypercoagulable state An increased tendency towards blood clotting.

Hyperdiploidy Human cells containing in excess of 46 chromosomes.

Hypermethylation The process of switching off genes through the addition of methyl groups.

Hypersegmented Greater than 3% of the neutrophil population showing in excess of 5 nuclear lobes.

Hypersegmented neutrophil A principal blood film sign of vitamin B_{12} deficiency. The nucleus of the normal neutrophil may have perhaps three or four lobes; in vitamin B_{12} deficiency the number of lobes may rise to seven or eight.

Hypertension A sustained increase in systolic and/or diastolic blood pressure.

Hyperviscosity Increased blood viscosity.

Hypnozoite A dormant stage in the life cycles of *P. vivax* and *P. ovale*.

Hypocellular A reduction in the size of the haemopoietic component of the marrow and an increase in the size of the yellow marrow (fatty marrow) compartment.

Hypochromic On a blood film, a red blood cell lacking in colour and therefore very likely to be lacking in haemoglobin.

Hypofibrinogenaemia Low concentration of functionally normal fibrinogen.

Hypomethylation The process of removing methyl groups from DNA, leading to gene activation.

Hyposegmented A neutrophil with two nuclear lobes or fewer.

Iatrogenic Describes a disease or condition caused by medical intervention.

Imatinib mesylate A signal transduction inhibitor which can be used to target the ATP binding pocket conserved on the Abl transcript of BCR–ABL but which can also inhibit c-Kit and the platelet derived growth factor receptor (PDGFR).

Immature B-cell An early B-cell, more mature than the pre-B cell, that expresses intact IgM.

Immune complex The combination of an antibody bound to its target antigen.

Immune paresis Reduction of all immunoglobulins in a patient's serum, except for the paraprotein.

Immunocompetent Fully functioning immune system.

Immunodeficiency Any inherited or acquired inability to mount a fully effective immunological response to a microbial pathogen.

Immunophenotyping A technique that labels cells with antibodies to identify the presence or absence of cell surface or cytoplasmic markers to characterize lineage.

Inclusion body An abnormal body within the red blood cell generally associated with a particular pathology.

Indirect antiglobulin test (IAT) A laboratory test to search for an antibody on the surface of red blood cells. Commonly used in the diagnosis of AIHA.

Ineffective haemopoiesis A state in which the bone marrow produces a large number of precursor cells, which perish (usually via apoptosis) before entering the peripheral blood.

Infarction The process that results in the generation of an area of necrotic (dead) tissue caused by the loss of an adequate blood supply.

Infection The presence of sufficiently high numbers of a microorganism that invoke clinical symptoms and provoke a defensive response.

Inhibitor In haemostasis, inhibitors are pathological antibodies that interfere with function of haemostatic molecules or initiate their immune-mediated removal from the circulation.

Initiation Events that start coagulation biochemistry via tissue factor and activated factor VII.

Interleukin A cytokine that passes instruction messages from one leucocyte to another.

Internal quality control Samples of known values that are analysed simultaneously with patient samples to monitor performance of an assay.

Internal tandem duplications Arise from the duplication of sequences from within a gene. In relation to FLT3, ITD of the juxtamembrane region of the gene result in constitutive activation of FLT3.

International Normalized Ratio A system established by the WHO to standardize prothrombin time (PT) reporting for patients receiving oral anticoagulants.

International sensitivity index Calibrated numerical value defining the sensitivity of a thromboplastin to the oral anticoagulant effect relative to the WHO standard.

Interstitial deletion Loss of chromosomal material from within a chromosome.

Intravascular haemolysis Haemolysis occurring in the circulation.

Intravenous Administration of a drug in liquid form into the body by injection into a vein.

Intrinsic pathway Compartment within the cascade theory of coagulation involving a sequence of enzyme activation reactions starting with contact activation of FXII leading to activation of FX via PK, HMWK, FXI, FIX, FVIII and cofactors of phospholipid and calcium ions.

Intrinsic tenase complex Enzyme/cofactor/substrate complex (FIXa/FVIIIa/FX + phospholipid and calcium ions) that generates activated factor X on the platelet surface.

Ionizing radiation Radiation in the form of either high-energy waves or particles which, when interacting with atoms, can remove electrons, thus producing a charge (ion).

Iron-deficiency anaemia An anemia that results from insufficient iron being delivered to the bone marrow.

Jak2 An enzyme activated by the binding of erythropoietin to its receptor that ultimately results in cell proliferation and differentiation.

James's dots Multiple small brick-red dots inside red cells infected with *P. ovale* that are darker than the Schüffner's dots seen inside red cells infected with *P. vivax*.

Jaundice A yellow coloration of the skin caused by high levels of bilirubin that may in turn be a sign of excessive haemolysis and/or liver damage.

Kala-azar Alternative name for visceral leishmaniasis.

Karyotype Description of the chromosomal complement of a cell.

Kinetoplast Mitochondrial DNA.

Kinins A family of proteins that play an important role in inflammation, haemostasis and pain.

Köhler illumination The mechanism to set up a microscope ready for use.

Lamellipodia Extensions of the cell cytoskeleton; they comprise actin projections which aid cell locomotion.

Large granular lymphocytes A population of large lymphocytes containing cytoplasmic granules.

Lectin Mannose Binding Protein 1 Intracellular transport protein for FV and FVIII.

Left-shift Describes an increase in the number of immature neutrophils within the peripheral blood.

Lepirudin A direct thrombin inhibitor developed from hirudin.

Lethargy Tiredness or fatigue.

Leucocyte An alternative name for the white blood cell.

Leucocytosis An increase in the white blood cell count.

Leucoerythroblastic blood picture A blood film showing nucleated red cells and immature white cells.

Leukaemia A haemoproliferative disorder usually characterized by inappropriately increased numbers of white blood cells and their precursors in the circulation. There may also be abnormalities in red blood cells and platelets.

Leukaemic phase Describes the presence of malignant leukaemic cells that have entered the peripheral blood from their associated lymphoid organ(s).

Leukaemogenesis The development of leukaemia.

Leukaemoid reaction A white cell count greater than $50 \times 10^9/L$ with all stages of maturation present within the peripheral blood.

Leukotrienes A type of lipid related to prostacyclins involved in inflammation and allergic reactions.

Ligands Molecules that bind other structures, such as cell surface receptors.

Light chain restriction An overexpression of either kappa or lambda light chains. This overexpression of a single type of light chain would be the product of a monoclonal population of B cells.

Lineage-specific growth factors Growth factors that act on only one set of cells and not on any other, e.g. on cells of the red cell series and not on cells of the granulocyte series.

Lineage-specific stem cell A stem cell that will give rise to only one type of blood cell, e.g. red blood cells alone, not red blood cells and/or granulocytes.

Lineage-restricted A particular immunophenotypic marker that is only expressed on one particular cell lineage.

Lipoprotein (a) Competitive inhibitor of plasmin.

Low molecular weight heparin A depolymerized form of unfractionated heparin that retains anticoagulant activity, mainly towards FXa, but with more predictable and favourable pharmacokinetics.

Lupus anticoagulant A type of antiphospholipid antibody specifically detected in coagulation assays.

Lymphadenopathy Swollen or enlarged lymph nodes, possibly the consequence of infection or a malignancy such as lymphoma.

Lymphoblast A blast of the lymphocyte pathway that ultimately develops into the mature lymphocyte.

Lymphocyte A small white blood cell with a round and regular nucleus that occupies approximately 95% of the cell. It has immunological properties, such as antibody production or destruction of cells infected with viruses.

Lymphocytosis A raised lymphocyte count above the upper end of the reference range.

Lymphomagenesis The development of lymphoma.

Lymphomas Malignancies of lymphoid cells largely restricted to the lymphoid organs (spleen or lymph nodes), although are sometimes encountered in patients with extranodal lymphomas (those originating outside the lymphoid organs).

Lymphopenia A reduction in the number of lymphocytes, below the lower end of the reference range.

Lymphopoiesis The growth, differentiation and maturation of lymphocytes within primary lymphoid organs.

Lymphoproliferative Inducing cells of lymphoid origin to proliferate at a rate greater than that usually observed in healthy individuals.

Lyonization Switching off an X chromosome in females through chromatin condensation. This chromatin condensation prevents the transcription and translation of genes contained within the additional X chromosome.

Lysosomes Organelles that contain digestive enzymes.

Macrocyte A large red blood cell.

Macrocytic Describes an anaemia where the MCV is above the top of the reference range.

Macrogametocyte Female malarial gametocyte.

Macroglobulinaemia Large amounts of big proteins circulating in the blood, for example IgM antibodies.

Macrophage A specialized white blood cell that is found in the tissues and derived from circulating monocytes.

Major basic protein Disrupts the lipid bilayer of parasites and target cells through interactions with anionic regions on targets.

Malaria An infectious disease found in tropical and subtropical regions. It is caused by parasites of *Plasmodium* species that are carried by mosquitoes.

Maltese Cross formations Tetrad of *Babesia* ring form trophozoites.

Margination Adherence to the vascular endothelium.

Maturational arrest Occurs in malignant cells when they are unable to develop beyond a particular stage of maturation. This failure in development prevents the production of a population of mature and functional effector cells.

Mature B-cell Surface expression of both IgM and IgG, these cells are yet to encounter antigen. Also called naive B-cells.

Maurer's clefts Irregular red/mauve dots inside red cells infected with *P. falciparum* that are larger and fewer in number than Schüffner's dots.

Mean cell haemoglobin (MCH) The amount of haemoglobin inside the 'average' red blood cell.

Mean cell haemoglobin concentration (MCHC) The concentration of haemoglobin inside the 'average' red blood cell.

Mean cell volume (MCV) The size of the 'average' red blood cell.

Mediastinum This defines the area within the thorax between the lungs containing the heart, trachea, oesophagus, and thymus.

Megakaryoblast The precursor cell to the megakaryocyte.

Megakaryocyte The bone marrow cell that gives rise to platelets.

Megaloblastic anaemia A type of anaemia defined by the presence of large erythroblasts (megaloblasts) in the bone marrow and generally caused by lack of vitamin B_{12}.

Melanosome Pigment-containing organelle.

Menorrhagia Heavy menstrual bleeding.

Merosome Structure within which malarial merozoites exit hepatocytes.

Merozoite The stage of the malarial parasite life cycle resulting from schizont multiplication.

Metacyclic A biochemical term for the extension of a cyclic group by another cyclic group.

Metacyclic trypomastigotes Infectious stage of trypanosome life cycle that expresses variant surface antigens.

Metamyelocyte The final stage of the development of a granulocyte before it becomes a mature polymorphonuclear leucocyte.

Methaemoglobin A subtype of haemoglobin characterized by the presence of iron in its oxidised state.

Microangiopathic haemolytic anaemia Loss of, or damage to, red blood cells through destruction caused by factors in the small blood vessels leading to haemolysis and anaemia.

Microcyte A small red blood cell.

Microcytic Describes an anaemia where the MCV is below the bottom of the reference range.

Microdeletion A submicroscopic deletion within a chromosome.

Microgametocyte Male malarial gametocyte.

Micronutrients Essential minerals and vitamins absorbed from the diet and required in trace amounts for the correct function of a cell or biochemical process.

MicroRNAs Small fragments of RNA, 20–23 nucleotides in length, which bind in a complementary fashion to mRNA to inhibit translation.

Mimetic A compound that mimics properties of another.

Missense mutation Encodes a different amino acid following a single nucleotide exchange.

Mitogen Any chemical or substance capable of inducing mitosis.

Mixing tests Mixing patient plasma with normal plasma and performing coagulation tests can indicate the presence of a factor deficiency or inhibitor.

Monoblasts and promonocytes Immature cells that are bone marrow precursors of mature monocytes.

Monoclonal antibodies (mAbs) Are manufactured to recognize a particular epitope on a specific antigen. Although mAbs produced by different manufacturers may have the same name, they may recognize a different epitope on the specified antigen.

Monocyte A large white blood cell whose nucleus is regular and generally round, and which occupies 60% to 80% of the cell. It has immunological and secretory properties and, in the tissues, develops into a macrophage.

Monomer A molecule that can combine with others to form a polymer; the smallest repeating unit of a polymer.

Mononuclear leukocyte A white blood cell with a round and regular nucleus. Generally, these cells do not have granules in their cytoplasm.

Monosomy Loss of a particular chromosome.

Morbidity High rate of sickness and medical complications compared to the normal population.

Morphological Pertaining to external appearances of cells.

Morphology The shape or appearance of a cell.

Mortality Increased risk of death compared to the normal population.

M-protein A monoclonal protein or paraprotein.

Multimer A protein composed of more than one peptide chain.

Multimerization Formation of multimers.

Multiple coagulation factor deficiency 2 Cofactor for lectin mannose binding protein 1.

Musculoaponeurotic A fibrous or membranous sheath that connects muscle to bone.

Mutagen A chemical substance known to induce DNA mutations.

Myeloablative therapy The process whereby the bone marrow is destroyed by high doses of chemotherapeutic agents in preparation for stem cell transplantation. Stem cell transplantation provides a potential cure for patients receiving this therapy.

Myeloblast A blast of the myeloid pathway.

Myelodysplasia Abnormal development of myeloid cells.

Myelofibrosis A bone marrow condition characterized by overgrowth of normal haemopoietic tissue by fibroblasts.

Myeloma A malignancy of white blood cells within the bone marrow, characterized by anaemia and, generally, a high ESR and increased plasma viscosity.

Myelosuppression The failure of the myeloid component of the bone marrow to produce red cells, white cells and platelets as a consequence of either a therapeutic agent or a malignant clone.

Myocardium Heart muscle.

Naive B-cell Surface expression of both IgM and IgD, these cells are yet to encounter antigen. Also called mature B-cells.

Naturally occurring inhibitors (non-pathological) Molecules that regulate secondary haemostasis by inhibiting activated clotting factors.

Negative predictive index The probability that a patient with a normal D-dimer level does not have a DVT or PE.

Neoepitope An epitope is a localized area of a molecule that is recognized by an antibody; a neoepitope is a structure, recognizable by an antibody, that is only exposed upon formation of a complex.

Neoplasia An abnormal proliferation of cells that can be benign or progress to malignancy.

Nephelometry Measurement of the intensity of light scatter when transmitted through a reaction mixture containing particulate matter by detecting light at an angle (usually at right angles or about 75°).

Neutropenia A neutrophil count below the lower limit of the reference range.

Neutrophil A granulocyte characterized morphologically by small granules that generally do not obscure the multilobed nucleus.

Neutrophilia A neutrophil count above the upper limit of the reference range.

NFκB Is a transcription factor that is involved in cell development, growth, and apoptosis. Overexpression of NFκB is associated with a number of diseases including cancer.

Nijmegen modification Altered version of Bethesda inhibitor assay that reduces pH drift.

Nonsense mutation A mutation in a DNA sequence that generates a codon not encoding an amino acid.

Normoblast, or Erythroblast Blast of the erythrocyte (red blood cell) pathway.

Normocellular The percentage of haemopoietic cells to bone marrow falls within the expected range based on a patient's age.

Normocyte A normal sized red blood cell.

Normocytic Describes an anaemia where the MCV is within the reference range.

Normocytic normochromic anaemia A particular form of anaemia associated with red cells of a normal size and coloration. Although there can be a number of causes, in the context of a malignancy, the most likely causes are anaemia of chronic disease or myelosuppression.

Nucleated red blood cell A stage in the development of the red blood cell when it still retains a nucleus and before it becomes a reticulocyte.

Nucleocytoplasmic ratio The ratio between the size of a cell's nucleus and its cytoplasmic volume.

Nucleolus (plural nucleoli) An area of the nucleus composed of genes that encode ribosomal RNA essential in the translation of transcribed proteins.

Ocular adnexa Accessory structures of the eye including the eyelids, lacrimal glands, orbit and paraorbital areas.

Oligomer A molecule containing a small number of repeating units; oligo means 'few' in Greek.

Oncogenic The process of producing cancer.

Oncology The area of medicine that deals with the development, diagnosis, treatment, and prevention of tumours.

One-stage coagulation assay Assay based (mainly) on prothrombin time or activated partial thromboplastin time that quantifies activity levels of individual coagulation factors.

Oocyst Spore phase.

Ookinete Motile malarial zygote.

Opportunistic infection An infection caused by organisms that do not normally cause disease in the presence of a competent immune system.

Opsonins Molecules coating the surface of cells which enhance the recognition and destruction of these coated cells by phagocytes.

Orthogonal regression line Generating a best-fit line through a series of points commonly involves ordinary regression, which minimizes the sum of the squares of the vertical distances from each point to the line. Ordinary regression assumes the measurements were made without error.

Osteolytic lesions Regions of bone degradation due to the overactivity of osteoclasts.

Osteoporosis A skeletal disease that leads to loss of bone mass and structure resulting in an increased risk of fractures.

Oximetry A non-invasive method for determining the amount of oxygen within arterial blood.

Oxyhaemoglobin Haemoglobin that is carrying oxygen.

Palatal petechiae Small blood spots within the oral cavity (see also Petechiae).

Pallor A pale coloration to the skin.

Pancytopenia Low levels of all blood cells due to bone marrow invasion, suppression, or another pathology.

Pappenheimer bodies Iron-containing granules within siderocytes.

Paracaspase A caspase-related protein.

Paracentric inversion A region of a particular chromosomal arm rotated through 180°.

Parasitaemia Quantitation of the number of parasitized red blood cells (normally expressed as a percentage).

Parasitism A form of symbiosis where the parasitic organism benefits from the association to the detriment of the host organism.

Parasitophorous vacuole Vacuole that forms around a malarial parasite upon entering a red cell.

Parasitophorous vacuole membrane Invagination of the red cell membrane that forms the membrane of the vacuole that surrounds a malarial parasite when invading a red cell.

Parenterally Not given orally through the alimentary canal, but administered by injection.

p-arm Located above the centromere; this is the shorter chromosomal arm.

Pelger–Hüet anomaly Hyposegmented neutrophils with a single or bilobed nucleus.

Peptidases Enzymes that cleave peptide bonds in proteins.

Peptide Short amino acid chain.

Pericentric inversion Rotation of chromosomal material through 180° and involving the centromere.

Peripheral blood The blood that is contained within the circulatory system.

Perls' stain The principal stain of blood, bone marrow, or tissues such as the liver for deposits of iron.

Pernicious anaemia The anaemia defined by autoimmune destruction of gastric parietal cells and/or intrinic factor, which causes vitamin B_{12} deficiency.

Petechiae Red pinpoint-sized haemorrhages of small capillaries in the skin or mucous membranes that form as a consequence of blood leaking from vessels.

Peyer's patches A group of lymph nodes in the wall of the ileum.

Phagocytosis The process of the ingestion and destruction of foreign and unwanted material, such as bacteria and effete red blood cells. Phagocytosis is performed by phagocytes: principally neutrophils and monocytes/macrophages.

Phagolysosome Membrane-enclosed vesicle formed from fusion of a lysosome (organelle containing digestive enzymes) and a phagosome (vacuole formed around foreign body inside a phagocytic cell).

Phagosome Neutrophil membrane forming a vacuole around the membrane of an ingested bacterium.

Pharmacodynamics The action, effect and breakdown of drugs in the body.

Pharyngitis Inflammation of the pharynx caused by an infection.

Phenindione An oral anticoagulant and inhibitor of vitamin K metabolism.

Phenprocoumarin An oral anticoagulant and inhibitor of vitamin K metabolism.

Philadelphia chromosome This denotes the derived chromosome 22der (22q−) not to be confused with t(9;22). The translocation process is abbreviated to t(9;22).

Phosphorylation The process of adding a phosphate group (PO_4) to an organic molecule.

Placental insufficiency Placental failure to supply nutrients to the foetus and remove toxic waste.

Plasma The clear, straw-coloured fluid which remains when all blood cells have removed from blood.

Plasma cell Antibody secreting terminal stage in B-cell maturation following exposure to antigen.

Plasma viscosity A global property of the 'thickness' or 'thinness' of the plasma.

Plasmin An enzyme that degrades fibrin.

Plasminogen The circulating zymogen of plasmin.

Plasminogen activator inhibitor type 1 The prime inhibitor of tissue plasminogen activator.

Plasminogen activator inhibitor type 2 An intracellular molecule involved in cell proliferation that is also produced by the placenta and exerts some activity against t-PA and u-PA.

Plasminogen activator inhibitor type 3 An inhibitor of activated protein C.

Platelets A blood cell that helps prevent blood loss by combining with other platelets and certain proteins to form a clot, or thrombus.

Platelet activating factor A phospholipid released from platelets that contributes to maintenance of vessel endothelial cell junctions.

Platelet adhesion Process of adhering platelets to exposed subendothelium via ligands and receptors.

Platelet clumps Aggregates of platelets within a FBC, demonstrable on a blood film. Often artefactual, it can be facilitated by the presence of EDTA in blood tubes.

Platelet factor 4 A small cytokine released from activated platelets that modulates the effects of heparin-like molecules, stimulates protein C activation and is chemotactic for neutrophils and monocytes.

Platelet shape change Platelet shape alteration from discoid to a spiny sphere.

Pleomorphic Variations in the appearance of a particular type of cell.

Ploidy Describes the number of homologous chromosomes within a cell.

Pluripotent stem cell A stem cell that has the potential to give rise to many other different types of stem cells.

Poikilocytosis A variation in the shapes of the red cell population. Causes include abnormal erythropoiesis and myelofibrosis.

Point mutation The alteration of a single nucleotide in a gene sequence.

Point-of-care test Tests analysed on portable analytical devices that can be used on wards, in clinics, GP surgeries and even by patients themselves.

Polychromasia A finding on blood film that translates as 'many colours'. In practice there will be red blood cells of a normal colour, but others (reticulocytes) with a blue tinge.

Polycythaemia A haemoproliferative disorder characterized by inappropriately increased numbers of red blood cells.

Polycythaemia vera Characterized by an increase in an individual's red cell mass >25% above the patient's mean predicted value.

Polymorphism Variations in the sequence of a particular gene between individuals.

Polymorphonuclear leukocyte (polymorph) A white blood cell with an irregular nucleus. Neutrophils, eosinophils and basophils are all polymorphs.

Polyploidy The presence of more than one complete set of chromosomes.

Porphyria A disease caused by abnormalities in the production of haem characterized in the laboratory by anaemia and increased iron.

Post-thrombotic syndrome A late complication of DVT where tissue damage occurs from diversion of blood into other veins to avoid blockage.

Pre-B cell An early B cell containing cytoplasmic IgM.

Pre-eclampsia Pregnancy-induced high blood pressure associated with protein in the urine. The only cure is delivery or abortion of the fetus.

Primary care Often the initial stages of healthcare where people seek help from their general practitioner.

Primary haemostasis The initial haemostatic response that results from interplay between vessel endothelium, von Willebrand factor and platelets.

Primary lymphoid organs Includes the bone marrow and thymus as main sites of lymphopoiesis.

Procoagulant Physiological or pharmacological mechanism that promotes coagulation processes.

Professional body A learned organization that represents a particular profession.

Pro-inflammatory cytokines Regulatory cellular-communication signalling molecules that favour and promote inflammation.

Prolymphocyte A stage in lymphoid development between lymphoblast and lymphocyte.

Promastigote The infective stage of *L. donovani* and *L. infantum*.

Propagation The activation of various haemostatic components by the trace thrombin formed at initiation of coagulation.

Prophylaxis A procedure to prevent a condition occurring rather than treat or cure it after it has occurred.

Prostacyclin A potent inhibitor of platelet aggregation generated through the arachidonic acid pathway within the vessel wall.

Prostacyclins A member of the eicosanoid family of lipids related to arachidonic acid: it is found in vascular endothelial cell, causes vasodilation, and plays an inhibitory role in platelet aggregation.

Prostaglandin A lipid derived potent physiological mediator.

Protamine sulphate A strongly basic heparin neutralizer used therapeutically and analytically.

Protease nexin-2 A naturally occurring inhibitor of FXIa, FIXa, and FXa.

Protein C The zymogen of activated protein C, the naturally occurring inhibitor of the activated forms of factor V and factor VIII.

Protein S The non-enzymatic cofactor for activated protein C.

Proteolytic Enzymes that digest or lyse proteins into smaller sections or amino acids are said to be proteolytic.

Prothrombin time A coagulation screening test for global assessment of extrinsic and common pathways.

Prothrombin time (PT) ratio Derived from dividing the patient prothrombin time(s) by that of a normal pooled control preparation or previously determined mean normal value.

Prothrombinase complex The enzyme/cofactor/substrate complex (FXa/FVa/FII + phospholipid and calcium ions) that generates activated factor II on the platelet surface.

Prothrombinase-induced clotting time A snake venom-based assay for monitoring direct thrombin inhibitors.

Prothrombotic The promotion of processes that form a blood clot.

Proto-oncogene The normal counterpart of a gene that, when mutated, can produce an abnormal protein which will lead to increased proliferation or cell survival.

Prozone A concentration of antibody or antigen is so high that the optimal concentration for maximal reaction with antigen is exceeded and binding is reduced or does not occur.

Pulmonary angiography A technique performed to assess blood circulation to the lungs by adding a contrast dye through a catheter into a vein and taking X-rays of the lung.

Pulmonary embolism A fragment of a clot (the embolus) that travels through the circulation and lodges in the pulmonary artery or one of its branches causing partial or total blockage. It is potentially fatal.

Punched-out lesions Caused by the catabolic effects of osteoclast activating factors on bony structures.

Pure red cell aplasia A condition of suppression of the production of red blood cells which does not influence white blood cells or platelets.

Purpura fulminans A life-threatening disorder characterized by cutaneous haemorrhage and necrosis (tissue death), and disseminated intravascular coagulation.

Pyrexia A rise in the body's core temperature.

Pyruvate kinase A metabolic enzyme of the glycolytic pathway involved in the generation of ATP.

q-arm Located below the centromere, this is the longer of the chromosomal arms.

Qualitative Non-numerical data; for example, the ability of a platelet to function correctly.

Quantitative Types of data that deal with numerical values; for example, the number of platelets in one litre of blood.

Quantitative buffy coat Laboratory technique for concentrating blood parasites and staining their DNA for microscopical detection.

Racemic mixture Equal amounts of two stereoisomers of an optically active substance which does not rotate plane-polarized light.

Receptor A molecule on the surface of (or in) a cell that acts as a recognition site for other molecules that bind in order to promote specific functions.

Recombinant technology The artificial production of a molecule produced by inserting foreign DNA into a host DNA which will produce the product.

Red blood cell count The number of red blood cells in a sample of blood.

Red blood cells Blood cells that carry oxygen.

Red cell distribution width A quantitative method for describing anisocytosis. The greater the variation in red cell size, the greater the RDW. If the RBCs are of a uniform size, the RDW is low.

Refractory anaemia An anaemia that does not respond to B12, folate or iron therapy.

Release reaction Secretion of platelet granule contents via surface connected open canalicular system.

Reptilase time Coagulation screening test employing a snake venom enzyme that mainly assesses fibrinogen activity but is not affected by the action of heparin.

Respiratory burst An increase in a phagocyte's oxygen consumption followed by the release of reactive oxygen species.

Restriction enzymes Enzymes that recognize specific nucleotide sequences and can cut DNA wherever the sequence occurs. This selective cutting allows fragments to be formed which can be indicative of mutations within a specified sequence through the loss or gain of these restriction sites.

Reticulocyte The final stage of the development of the red blood cell before it reaches maturity.

Reticuloendothelial system A collection of white blood cells (such as macrophages) present in organs such as the liver, spleen and lymph nodes, with roles in immunology, phagocytosis and in scavenging debris and dead cells.

Reversed ratio A lymphocyte count that is higher than the neutrophil count.

Rheology/rheological The study of the physical nature of blood or plasma principal measurement are ESR and viscosity.

Rhesus-associated glycoprotein Component of the membrane of the red cell that provides recognition, transport, and anchorage sites.

Rheumatoid arthritis An inflammatory disease that mainly affects the joints.

Rhoptry Organelle found in malarial parasite merozoites.

Right-shifted Greater than 3% of the neutrophil population showing in excess of five nuclear lobes.

Ring sideroblasts Abnormal erythroblasts with iron granules arranged in a ring around the nucleus.

Risk assessment The determination and documentation of the quantitative or qualitative value of risk related to a specific situation/procedure and a recognized hazard.

Ristocetin cofactor assay A platelet aggregation assay to quantify the GPIb binding capacity of VWF.

Ristocetin-induced platelet aggregation test A platelet aggregation assay that subjects VWF to decreasing concentrations of ristocetin in order to identify Type 2B VWD and pseudo-VWD.

Romanowsky A type of stain specially developed to enable the examination of different blood cells.

Schistocytes Distortions and fragments of red cells that are very common in different types of haemolytic anaemia. Consequently, they are not diagnostic of a particular condition, but may be useful in confirmation.

Schizogony Asexual reproductive process of multiple fission in malarial parasites.

Schizont The stage of the malarial parasite life cycle resulting from asexual reproduction in the liver of the human.

Schüffner's dots Multiple small brick-red dots inside red cells infected with *P. vivax* or *P. ovale*.

Scissile Easily split or cleaved.

Secondary care The stage in health care subsequent to primary care, where people are referred to the hospital.

Secondary haemostasis Regulated and localized formation of fibrin polymers via interplay of clotting factor enzymes and cofactors.

Secondary leukaemia Leukaemia attributable to prior treatment for another disease.

Self-peptides Short protein sequences presented to developing lymphocytes in order to inactivate self-reactive lymphocytes.

Self-renewal A normal property of stem cells enabling the stem cell population to be regenerated without necessarily undergoing differentiation of daughter cells into specific cell lines.

Sequester To remove or separate.

Seropositive Identification of specific antibodies within a patient's serum.

Serotonin Also known as 5-hydroxytryptamine (5-HT), a hormone that acts as a neurotransmitter in the brain and contributes to haemostasis by initiating vasoconstriction.

Serum The fluid that remains after the blood has been allowed to clot.

Shear forces Forces produced when surfaces are pressed together or move over each other.

Sickle cell disease A qualitative haemoglobin disorder generally characterized in the laboratory by a chronic haemolytic microcytic anaemia, and in the clinic by infection and microvascular occlusion.

Side scatter In terms of a flow cytometric measurement, represents the internal complexity of a cell as may be due to granules.

Sideroblastic anaemia An anaemia that results from impaired inclusion of iron into haem, and thus into haemoglobin.

Sideroblasts An erythroblast—therefore generally found in the bone marrow—containing granules of non-haem iron complexed to other molecules.

Siderocytes Red blood cells characterized by the presence of iron granules as a consequence of sideroblastic anaemia.

Sinus rhythm A natural heart (cardiac) rhythm generated through the sinus node (normal rate 60–100 beats/min).

Smear cells Lymphocytes that have broken apart due to mechanical damage when making a blood film—commonly seen in leukaemia.

Sodium citrate An anticoagulant chemical added to blood to allow the measurement of coagulation proteins, pro-thrombin time and the activated partial thromboplastin time.

Somatic hypermutation Occurs within the germinal centre and incorporates point mutations within the variable region of immunoglobulin in order to improve antigenic binding.

Spherocyte An abnormal and small red blood cell characterized by the lack of central pallor.

Splenectomy The procedure of removing the spleen that generally increases the lifespan of cells and as such is a ther-apeutic option for individuals with certain diseases of the haemopoietic system.

Splenomegaly Enlarged spleen.

Sporozoite The stage of the malarial parasite life cycle result-ing from sexual reproduction in the midgut of the mosquito.

Standard operating procedure Document that explicitly states how every aspect of a given procedure must be per-formed.

Stasis A condition in which the normal flow of blood through a vein is slowed or halted.

Stem cell The cell in the bone marrow that gives rise to all the mature peripheral blood cells.

Stoichiometric The quantitative relationship between reac-tants and products in a balanced chemical reaction.

Streptokinase Exogenous plasminogen activator produced by some strains of *Streptococcal* bacteria.

Stroke A clinical condition where the brain's supply of oxygen is cut off by a blockage or interruption to the blood flow, which causes severe neurological damage.

Subcutaneous Administration of a drug in liquid form into the body by injection just under the skin.

Sulphaemoglobin A sub-type of haemoglobin characterized by binding to sulphur-rich compounds.

Superoxide A toxic form of oxygen and powerful oxidizing agent than can attack and destroy many components of the red cell.

Superoxide dismutase, catalase Antioxidant enzymes that neutralize toxic reactive species such as superoxide and hydrogen peroxide.

Surface-connected open canalicular system Intracellular network of channels/canals inside platelets that facilitate release of platelet granule constituents.

Symbiosis Close interaction between different species.

Systemic lupus erythematosus A chronic autoimmune disease with multiple organ/system involvement that is often associ-ated with antibodies directed against cell nuclei.

Talin Ubiquitous cytoskeletal protein linking integrins to the actin cytoskeleton.

Terminal deletion The loss of the end of a chromosomal arm.

Ternary complex A complex containing three different molecules.

Tertiary care When a patient is passed from one hospital to a specialist referral centre, often part of a university teaching hospital.

Tetramer Complex comprised of 4 subunits.

Thalassaemia A quantitative haemoglobinopathy caused by a mutation in alpha, beta, or both genes that leads to a reduction, or even abolition, in the expression of alpha or beta globin.

Therapeutic anticoagulation The use of anticoagulants as a treatment for the increased risk of thrombosis.

Therapeutic range The range of concentrations at which a therapeutic agent is effective. For anticoagulants that are monitored with screening tests such as INR and APTT, the therapeutic range is referred to in units of the test not con-centration of the drug.

Thrombin The activated form of factor II (i.e. factor IIa) whose prime functions are coagulation factor activation, such as converting fibrinogen to fibrin, and activating protein C.

Thrombin-activable fibrinolysis inhibitor Inhibitor of fibri-nolysis activated by thrombin bound to thrombomodulin.

Thrombin time Coagulation screening test that mainly assesses fibrinogen activity.

Thrombocytopenia Low numbers of platelets in the blood, often cited as less than 100×10^9/L.

Thrombocytosis When the platelet count exceeds the top end of the reference range.

Thrombogenic Causing blood to clot; causing thrombosis.

Thrombomodulin A transmembrane receptor that binds and modifies thrombin to facilitate activation of protein C and thrombin activable fibrinolysis inhibitor.

Thrombophilia A defect in the haemostatic system predisposing an individual to increased risk of venous thromboembolism.

Thromboplastin A reagent used in the prothrombin time containing tissue factor and phospholipid in order to assess the extrinsic and common pathways. Calcium ions may be integral to the reagent or added separately.

Thrombopoiesis The development of platelets (also known as thrombocytes).

Thrombopoietin A growth factor that stimulates megakaryo-cyte maturation and platelet production.

Thrombosis Inappropriate or pathological formation of a blood clot in an artery or vein.

Thrombospondin Adhesive glycoprotein with roles in platelet aggregation, angiogenesis and plasmin inhibition.

Thrombotic disease Disorders that lead to thrombosis, which is a partial or complete obstruction of a blood vessel by a blood clot.

Thrombotic thrombocytopenic purpura A thrombotic microangiopathy characterized by spontaneous formation of platelet thrombi in the microvessels leading to mechanical haemolysis and thrombocytopenia.

Thromboxane A$_2$ A platelet agonist produced from membrane arachidonic acid as part of the cyclooxygenase pathway within platelets.

Thromboxane B$_2$ Metabolite of thromboxane A$_2$ which can be measured as a marker of cyclooxygenase activity and thus of the effect of aspirin.

Thrombus A blood clot that usually develops in a deep vein of the body, normally in the calf or higher up the leg in the thigh (the saphenous vein).

Thymocytes Immature T-cells entering the thymus.

Tissue factor The initiator of coagulation by acting as a cofactor to activated factor VII; often found at the surface of cells such as the monocyte but also in plasma.

Tissue factor pathway inhibitor The inhibitory regulator of the initiation phase of coagulation.

Tissue plasminogen activator The prime activator of plasminogen.

Toxic granulation Occurs when neutrophils have been mobilized to fight an infection. The primary granules are more abundant in preparation for fighting infection and have a higher concentration of acid mucosubstances, which have prominent azurophilic-staining characteristics.

Trabeculae Bony processes which extend from the outer bony tables into the marrow cavity.

Transcobalamin The molecule that carries vitamin B$_{12}$ in the blood and present in two forms: transcobalamin I and transcobalamin II.

Transcription factor A protein which plays a regulatory role in the transcription of particular genes.

Transferrin Iron is actively carried through the blood as transferrin.

Transient abnormal myelopoiesis In children with trisomy 21, a brief period in which myeloid production within the bone marrow becomes grossly abnormal.

Trephine The process of obtaining a sample of bone that includes both bone tissue and bone marrow.

Trisomy The gain of a particular chromosome.

Trophoblasts Cells of the outer layer of the blastocyst ('pre-embryo') that attach a fertilized ovum to the uterine wall and develop into the placenta.

Trophozoite The feeding stage in the life cycle of malarial parasites.

Tropical pulmonary eosinophilia Nocturnal cough, wheezing, fever, and eosinophilia arising from marked sensitivity to microfilariae in the lungs.

Trypanosome Flagellated *Trypanosoma* trypomastigotes.

Trypanosomiasis Parasitic protozoan infection by *Trypanosoma* organisms.

Trypomastigotes *Trypanosoma* life cycle stages.

Tumour burden The size of an individual's tumour or the number of tumour cells involved in a particular malignant case.

Tumour lysis syndrome The release of a number of intracellular components following lysis of tumour cells.

Tumour suppressor genes Encode proteins that can protect the genome from DNA damage by, for example, inducing DNA repair or apoptosis.

Turbidimetry Measurement of the loss of intensity of light transmitted through a reaction mixture containing particulate matter; unscattered light is measured.

Two-stage factor assay Assays to measure activity of coagulation factors (usually FVIII) where the first stage involves generation of FXa which then reacts with either a chromogenic substrate or exogenous clotting factors in the second stage.

Type I defect Reduced concentration of a normally functioning protein.

Type II defect dysfunctional proteins which are often produced in normal amounts.

Ubiquitination The addition of ubiquitin monomers to a peptide which allows for degradation of the peptide via the proteosome.

Unfractionated heparin Highly sulphated glycosaminoglycan with high negative charge used as an immediate acting therapeutic anticoagulant due to its potentiating effect on circulating antithrombin. Its use must be monitored by the APTT.

Upshaw–Schulman syndrome Hereditary thrombotic thrombocytopenic purpura due to ADAMTS-13 deficiency.

Uraemia The accumulation of urea within the blood.

Urinary plasminogen activator Plasminogen activator with minor role in blood clot lysis (sometimes called urokinase).

Vacutainer A glass tube with an inbuilt vacuum that draws blood directly from the vein without the use of syringe. Vacutainer is a brand name; there are other types of evacuated tubes.

Variable region Generates antigen binding diversity within a specific class of antibodies.

Vascular Relating to the network of blood vessels in the body, namely arteries, veins, and capillaries and associated medical conditions.

Vasculature The network of blood vessels through the body or organs.

Vasoconstriction A narrowing of the diameter of a blood vessel.

Venepuncture The process of obtaining intravenous access to obtain a sample of blood via a needle.

Venography A radiology procedure where a contrasting agent is injected into the vein to enable a blockage or obstruction to be visualized by X-ray examination.

Venous thromboembolism A disorder that encompasses both deep vein thrombosis (DVT) and pulmonary embolism (PE).

Ventilated–perfusion (V/Q) scan A procedure using small amounts of inhaled or injected radioisotopes to measure flow of blood and air in the lungs. Images taken capture the flow patterns.

Vitamin B$_{12}$, and B$_6$, and folate Micronutrients essential for erythropoiesis: their absence results in anaemia.

Vitamin K Cofactor in the γ-carboxylation of glutamic acid side chains in factors II, VII, IX, and X and the inhibitor molecules protein C, protein S, and protein Z.

Vitronectin A multifunctional protein that stabilizes PAI-1, contributes to binding of platelets to vascular cell walls and promotes adherence, migration, proliferation, and differentiation of many different cell types.

von Willebrand factor A large protein that enables platelets to bind to exposed sub-endothelium and also stabilizes FVIII.

von Willebrand's disease Deficiency of von Willebrand factor.

Warfarin Most commonly used oral anticoagulant that works by antagonizing the action of vitamin K in the production of functional factors II, VII, IX, and X and the inhibitory proteins C, S, and Z.

Warfarin resistance Present in patients who require higher than average warfarin dosage to achieve a therapeutic INR and due to a genetic mutation in the vitamin K epoxide reductase enzyme which reduces its inhibitory effect on vitamin K metabolism.

Warfarin sensitivity Present in patients who require less than average warfarin dosage to achieve a therapeutic INR; it is due to polymorphism variants in cytochrome P450 CYP2C9, which result in slower breakdown and clearance of the more potent enantiomer S-warfarin.

Weibel–Palade bodies Intracellular storage bodies for von Willebrand factor in endothelial cells.

Wells' score A clinical assessment method based on scoring the presence of specific symptoms in order to ascertain a probability of the presence of VTE.

White blood cell differential A breakdown of the numbers of the different white blood cells in a sample of blood.

White blood cells Blood cells that function primarily as defence against infection.

Wild-type DNA Denotes germline DNA. Mutations found within tumour cells when compared to wild-type DNA are considered to be acquired.

Zygote Derived from the Greek for 'joined', it is the unicellular product of joining male and female genetic material— the product of fertilization.

Zymogen Inactive precursor of an enzyme, also called proenzyme.

References

British Committee for Standards in Haematology (BCSH). *Guidelines for the Diagnosis, Investigation and Management of Polycythaemia/Erythrocytosis*. Blackwell Publishing, 2005 (diagnostic algorithm updated 2007). Available at http://www.bcshguidelines.com

Burkitt D. A sarcoma involving the jaws in African children. *British Journal of Surgery* 1958:**46**(197);218–23.

Delsol G, Lamant L, Mariamé B, Pulford K, Dastugue N, Brousset P, Rigal-Huguet F, al Saati T, Cerretti DP, Morris SW, Mason DY. A new subtype of large B-cell lymphoma expressing the ALK kinase and lacking the 2;5 translocation. *Blood* 1997:**89**(5);1483–90.

Draper G, Vincent T, Kroll ME, Swanson J. Childhood cancer in relation to distance from high voltage power lines in England and Wales : a case-control study. *BMJ* 2005:**330**(7503);1290.

Köhler G, Milstein C. Continuous cultures of fused cells secreting antibody of predefined specificity. *Nature* 1975:**256**;495–7.

Nowell P, Hungerford D. A minute chromosome in chronic granulocytic leukemia. *Science* 1960:**132**;1497.

Pratt G, Harding S, Holder R, Fegan C, Pepper C, Oscier D, Gardiner A, Bradwell AR, Mead G. Abnormal serum free light chain ratios are associated with poor survival and may reflect biological subgroups in patients with chronic lymphocytic leukaemia. *British Journal of Haematology* 2009:**144**(2);217–22.

Index

A

abciximab 583
acenocoumarin 575
acetylation 291
acid phosphatase 321, 323
activated partial thromboplastin time
(APTT) 40, 41, 486-7, 547, 578
  inhibitor screening 499
  reference range 41
acute leukaemias of ambiguous
lineage 360-1
  bilineal leukaemia 361
  biphenotypic leukaemia 360-1
acute lymphoblastic leukaemias
(ALL) 265, 335, 391-5
  cytogenetic analysis 335
  FAB classification 393
  WHO classifications 391-3
acute megakaryoblastic leukaemia
(M7) 344, 346
acute monoblastic/monocytic
leukaemia (M5) 344-5
acute myeloid leukaemia (AML)
  cytogenetic analysis 335
  FAB classification 344-5
  IPSS scoring 363-4
  maturation states (MO, M1, M2)
344-5
  related precursor neoplasms 348-55
    AML with myelodysplasia-related
changes 355-6
    AML not otherwise
specified 358-9
    AML with recurrent genetic
abnormalities 349-55
  WHO classification 348-55
  WHO scoring 364
acute myelomonocytic leukaemia
(M4) 344-6
acute promyelocytic leukaemia
(and variant) (M3) 344-5
acute-phase response 136
ADAMTS-13 439, 560
ADP, platelet agonist 520
African trypanosomiasis (sleeping
sickness) 214-15
  clinical features 215
  life cycle of parasites 214-15

alcohol abuse 136
alkylating agents, therapy-related
myeloid neoplasms 356
alleles 279
alloantibodies 145
alloimmune haemolysis 145-8
alloimmune haemolytic anaemia 148
alpha-granules 58, 439, 442, 443
  disorders of 512
alpha-methyldopa 152
alpha-naphthyl acetate esterase
(ANAE) 322
alpha$_2$-antiplasmin 462, 471
alpha$_2$-macroglobulin 465, 471
Alport syndrome 521
American trypanosomiasis
(Chagas disease) 215-16
  clinical features 216
  life cycle of *T. cruzi* 216
amnionless 127
anaemias 105-7
  aplastic 5, 108-10
  causes 4, 109, 110
  classification 106
  congenital dyserythropoietic
(CDAs) 108-9
  definitions 105, 107
  iron-deficiency anaemia 114-16
  of malaria 198-9
  megaloblastic anaemia 232
  pernicious anaemia 128
  signs and symptoms 106
anaemias (bone marrow) 108-13
  chemotherapy 111-12
  haemopoietic cancer 110-11
  laboratory investigations 112-13
  pancytopenia 109-10
  pure red cell aplasia 108-9
  treatment 112
anaemias of chronic disease
(ACD) 136-41
  cancer 110-11, 138-9
  endocrine disease 137-8
  gastrointestinal disease 137
  kidney 137
  laboratory studies 139-40
  liver 136
  reproductive organs 137
  rheumatoid arthritis 136

  systemic inflammatory disease 138
anaemias (haemolytic anaemias)
144-52
anaemias (vitamin deficiency) 126-35
  consequences 135
  folate 129
  laboratory investigations 130-5
  treatment 129-30
  vitamin B$_6$ 129
  vitamin B$_{12}$ 126-9
anaplastic large cell lymphoma,
ALK-positive 427
aneuploidy 282
angioimmunoblastic T-cell lymphoma
(AITL) 427
anisocytosis 98
ankyrin 80-1
Anopheles mosquitoes 191
anti-Xa assays 596-7
antibodies
  Forsmann 251
  heterophile 250
  Paul–Bunnell 250
antibody-directed cellular cytotoxicity
(ADCC) 249
anticoagulation 18-20, 566-612
  antiplatelet therapy 602-3
  arterial thrombosis 582-3
  direct thrombin inhibitors 601-3
  heparins 594-601
  laboratory monitoring 584-603
  new 576
  oral therapy management 558,
603-10
  screening tests for haemostasis 42-3
  service models 607-10
  venous thromboembolism
(VTE) 567-82
  warfarin 584-93
  see also lupus anticoagulants (LA)
antigen-presenting cells (APCs) 247
antihuman globulin (AHG) 146-8
antiphospholipid antibodies 541-58
  detection in solid-phase
assays 543-4
  lupus anticoagulants (LA) 544-58
antiphospholipid syndrome 539, 541-4
antiplatelet therapy 602-3
antithrombin 42, 463-4

Haematology

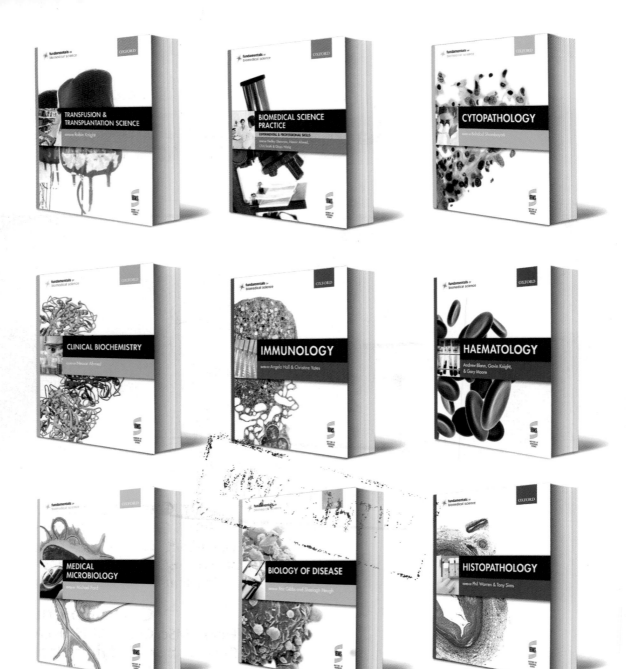

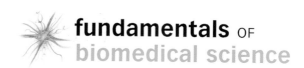

fundamentals OF
biomedical science